Gastrointestinal Pathology

Gastrointestinal Pathology

Correlative Endoscopic and Histologic Assessment

Edited by

Gregory Y. Lauwers, MD, FAGPS
Senior Member and Director, Gastrointestinal Pathology Service
Department of Pathology, Moffitt Cancer Center
Professor, Departments of Pathology and Cell Biology and Oncologic Sciences
University of South Florida
Tampa, FL, USA

Michael B. Wallace, MD, MPH
Consultant – Gastroenterology and Hepatology
Fred C. Andersen Professor of Medicine, Mayo Clinic School of Medicine
Jacksonville, FL, USA

Associate Editor:

Till S. Clauditz, MD
Associate Professor, Head of Gastrointestinal Pathology Service
Department of Pathology with Section Molecular Pathology and Cytology
University Medical Center Hamburg-Eppendorf,
Hamburg, Germany

WILEY Blackwell

This edition first published 2021

Registered Offices
John Wiley & Sons, Inc., 111 River Street, Hoboken, NJ 07030, USA
John Wiley & Sons Ltd, The Atrium, Southern Gate, Chichester, West Sussex, PO19 8SQ, UK

Editorial Office
9600 Garsington Road, Oxford, OX4 2DQ, UK

For details of our global editorial offices, customer services, and more information about Wiley products visit us at www.wiley.com.

Wiley also publishes its books in a variety of electronic formats and by print-on-demand. Some content that appears in standard print versions of this book may not be available in other formats.

Library of Congress Cataloging-in-Publication Data applied for

HB ISBN: 9780470658369

Cover Design: Wiley
Cover Images: © Gregory Y. Lauwers and Michael B. Wallace

Set in 9.5/12.5pt STIXTwoText by SPi Global, Pondicherry, India

Printed in Singapore
M043281_250321

Contents

List of Contributors

Thomas Arnason
Queen Elizabeth II Health Sciences Centre and Dalhousie University
Halifax
Nova Scotia
Canada

Ian Brown
Envoi Specialist Pathologists
Brisbane
Australia

Till S. Clauditz
Department of Pathology
University-Medical-Center
Hamburg
Germany

Tze Sheng Khor
PathWest Laboratory Medicine
Queen Elizabeth II Medical Centre
Nedlands
Western Australia
Australia

K. Kim
Samsung Medical Center
Sungkyunkwan University School of Medicine
Seoul
South Korea

Bence Kővári
Department of Pathology
University of Szeged
Szeged
Hungary

Priyanthi Kumarasinghe
Department of Anatomical Pathology
PathWest, QE II Medical Centre
Univ. of Western Australia
Perth
Australia

Gregory Y. Lauwers
Moffitt Cancer Center
Tampa
Florida
USA

Jun Haeng Lee
Samsung Medical Center
Sungkyunkwan University School of Medicine
Seoul
South Korea

Laurence de Leval
Institute of Pathology
University of Lausanne
Lausanne
Switzerland

Anthony R. Mattia
Newton-Wellesley Hospital
Newton, MA
USA

Christophe Rosty
Envoi Specialist Pathologists
Brisbane
Queensland
Australia

Yutaka Saito
National Cancer Center
Tokyo Japan

Mounir Trimeche
Institute of Pathology
University of Lausanne
Lausanne
Switzerland

Michael B. Wallace
Mayo Clinic
Jacksonville
Florida
USA

Herbert C. Wolfen
Mayo Clinic
Jacksonville
Florida
USA

Naohisa Yahaghi
Keio University Cancer Center
Tokyo
Japan

1

General Principles of Biopsy Diagnosis of GI Disorders

Herbert C. Wolfen[1], Michael B. Wallace[1], Naohisa Yahaghi[2] and Yutaka Saito[3]

[1] *Mayo Clinic, Jacksonville, Florida, USA*
[2] *Keio University Cancer Center, Tokyo, Japan*
[3] *National Cancer Center, Tokyo Japan*

Tissue sampling of the gastrointestinal tract at the time of endoscopy is the cornerstone of many gastrointestinal diagnoses. The development of a flexible endoscope and the subsequent ability to directly acquire tissue under optical guidance has been one of the most important advancements in the field of gastroenterology throughout its history. Although tissue sampling can be performed through nonendoscopic devices, the ability to directly correlate precise locations and target biopsies to specific areas of disease is critical to our ability to diagnose and further understand gastrointestinal pathology. Many of the advancements in our understanding of the basic pathology and molecular biology of gastrointestinal disease can be directly attributed to our ability to acquire tissue for histological, molecular, and genetic analyses. An excellent example is our deep understanding of the molecular pathology of colorectal cancer development from normal colonic epithelium to adenoma to colorectal cancer, a discovery made possible because of colonoscopic access to precursor lesions such as adenomatous polyps and early cancers.

In this chapter, we will review general principles of tissue acquisition at the time of endoscopy including the following topics:

- Endoscopic equipment for obtaining tissue including endoscopic accessory channels, biopsy forceps, snare devices, needle aspiration and cytology brush.
- General principles of optimal sampling technique.
- Methods of tissue preparation in the endoscopy laboratory to optimize diagnostic accuracy.
- The role of endoscopic ultrasound (EUS)-guided fine-needle aspiration cytology.

Endoscopic Equipment for Tissue Sampling

Modern endoscopic equipment can be divided in two general categories: the endoscope that allows access to the gastrointestinal tract and accessory devices that are typically passed through the working channel of the endoscope to directly acquire tissue, including biopsy forceps, snares, fine-needle aspiration devices, and cytology brushes. Recent developments in tissue sampling include devices that are capable of wide-field, often definitive, endoscopic resection of early neoplasia and invasive carcinoma.

A modern endoscope is a remarkably robust and versatile instrument including a light source, optical lenses with a video capture device, image processing, and display equipment, and importantly for the purposes of tissue acquisition, an accessory channel ranging from 1 to 6 mm (typically 3–4 mm), which allows passage of devices for mechanical collection of tissue (Figures 1.1 and 1.2).

There is a general trade-off between the diameter of the instrument and the ease and comfort with which it can be passed through the natural orifices of the body such as the mouth and anus. In general the larger the outer diameter, the larger the accessory channel is to accommodate larger instruments for tissue acquisition. A fundamental limitation of most flexible endoscopes, as opposed to surgical instruments, is that all accessories pass through a single access point of the endoscope. As compared to surgical instruments with multiple access points, the endoscopic devices do not typically allow triangulation to acquire a large bulk tissue or resect entire organs. For this reason, most tissue is sampled through pinch forceps, needle

Gastrointestinal Pathology: Correlative Endoscopic and Histologic Assessment, First Edition. Edited by Gregory Y. Lauwers and Michael B. Wallace.

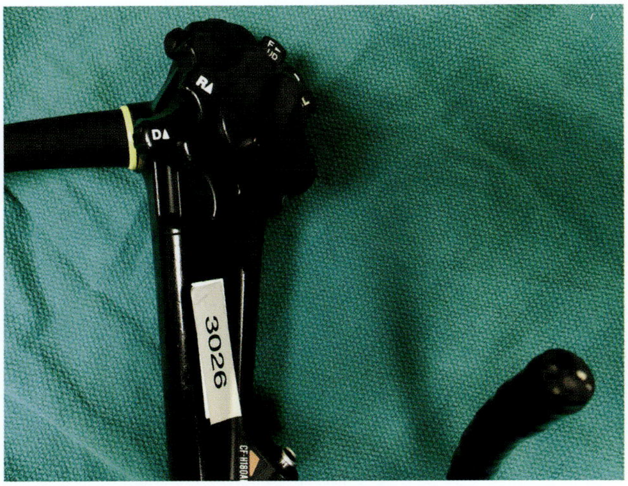

Figure 1.1 Endoscope with control handle and tip. The tip contains a light source, imaging window, and accessory channel through which various tissue acquisition devices can be passed.

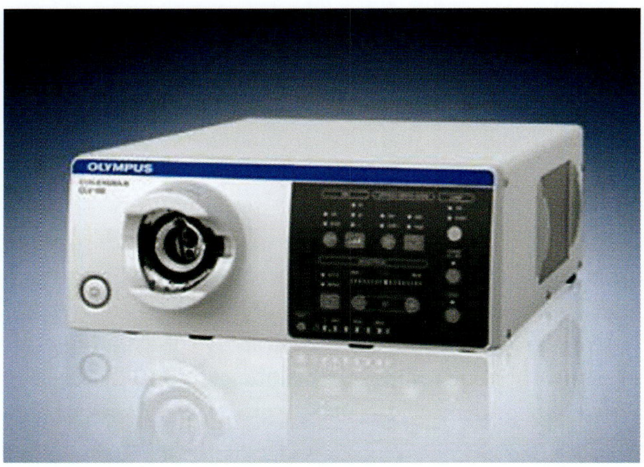

Figure 1.2 Endoscopic processor, which converts the light captured from the endoscope tip into a visible image for display. *Source:* Olympus America, Inc. With permission.

aspiration, or wire loop snare devices. More recently, electrosurgical needles and other cutting tools have been developed, which have allowed wide-field resection of tissues of virtually any diameter (Figure 1.3).

Pinch Biopsy Forceps

The flexible pinch biopsy forceps have been one of the most versatile of all instruments for tissue acquisition. These typically involve a flexible steel cable and lever device with two sharp-edged cups, which can be opened and closed to acquire tissue (Figure 1.4).

Standard endoscopic sampling typically acquires tissue from the mucosa and occasionally a submucosal depth of the intestinal wall; however, large-capacity forceps as well as multiple sampling including "bite on bite" allow sampling of the deeper layers. Pinch biopsy forceps come in multiple sizes from very small instruments such as a pediatric forceps, which can be passed through very small working channels. Recent development of very tiny forceps makes it possible to pass them through special endoscopes into the bile or pancreas duct and to pinch biopsy outside of the traditional gastrointestinal lumen (Figure 1.5).

Studies comparing jumbo forceps to standard forceps have generally not shown significant advantages of larger capacity forceps. A limitation of most forceps is the inability to sample tissue in the submucosa routinely. This is highlighted in studies looking for Barrett's esophagus after the surface epithelium has been ablated. Biopsy forceps can remove tissue with mechanical closure alone or with electrocautery ("hot biopsy") although the use of hot biopsy has diminished significantly due to increased risks of complication and tissue damage in the biopsy specimen.

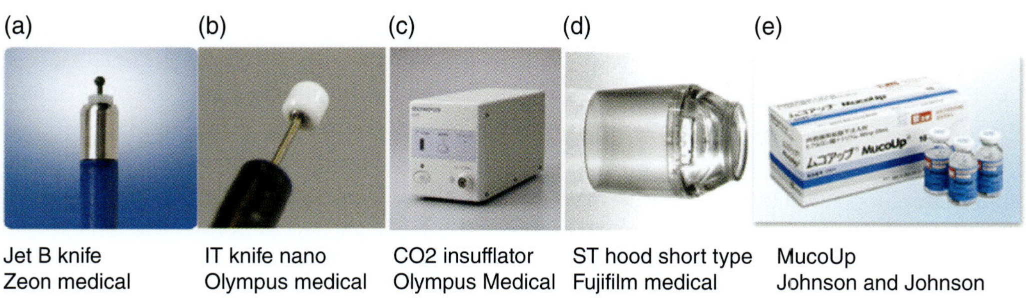

Figure 1.3 (a) Tools for performing endoscopic resection including endoscopic submucosal dissection (ESD). *Source:* Zeon Medical. (b) Standard and insulated tip electrocautery knives for incision and dissection. *Source:* © 2017 Korean Society of Gastrointestinal Endoscopy. (c) CO_2 insufflator for luminal distension, which is preferred to air given rapid reabsorption. *Source:* Olympus. (d) Distal attachment hood to facilitate maintaining view within the submucosal space. *Source:* Fujifilm medical. (e) Injection fluid (hyaluronic acid; Mucoup [Johnson and Johnson]) for submucosal lifting. *Source:* Gut and Liver.

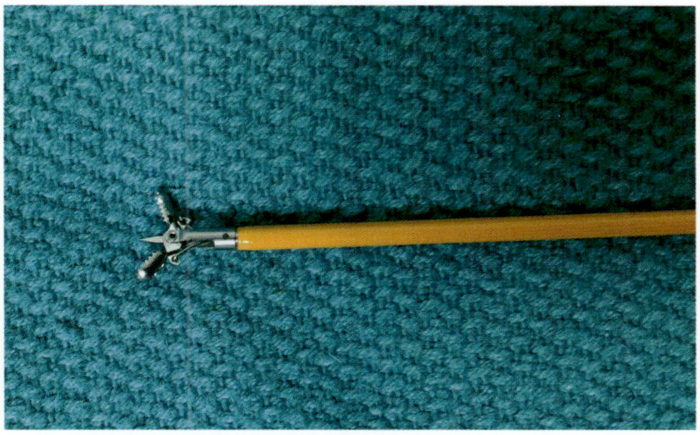

Figure 1.4 Endoscopic biopsy forceps in the open position. The needle-like pin in the center holds the tissue in place so one to two samples can be obtained per pass.

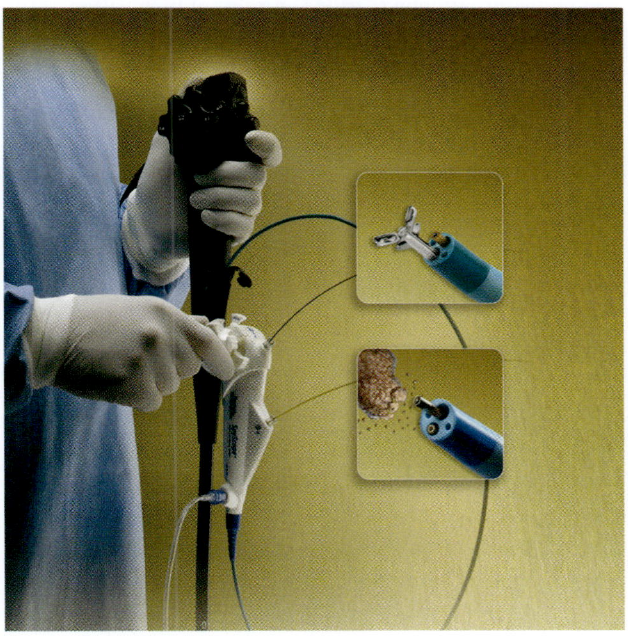

Figure 1.5 Micro biopsy forceps <1 mm in diameter, which can be passed through specialized endoscopes into the bile duct, pancreas duct, or via 19-gauge needles for extraluminal tissue sampling. *Source:* Boston Scientific Corporation with permission.

Endoscopic Snare Devices

Endoscopic snare devices have also been widely used for resection of polypoid as well as flat lesions throughout the gastrointestinal tract. They have been remarkably versatile and effective over the past four decades. Endoscopic snares typically involve a metallic wire, which may braided or monofilament (Figure 1.6).

A wire loop is generally constrained within a small caliber plastic catheter. At the distal end of the catheter, the wire loop can be opened to various sizes to grasp and resect polyps of different sizes. Typical sizes include loops 5–30 mm in diameter. There are numerous different shapes including

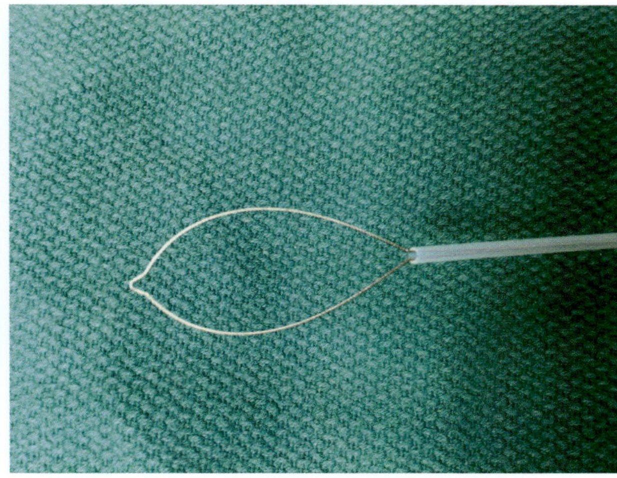

Figure 1.6 Endoscopic snare for polypectomy. The wire loop is extended in the open position outside the plastic sheath. When closed, the wire loop is strangulated and resects the polyp tissue.

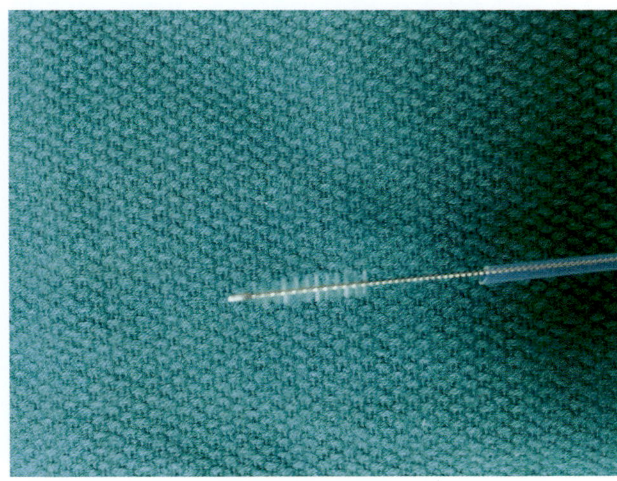

Figure 1.7 Endoscopic cytology brush. Note the abrasive brush extended beyond the protective plastic sheath.

oval, hexagonal, and asymmetric "duck bill." Snares also come in various degrees of stiffness, which allow resection of lesions of many shapes and sizes. Tissue can be resected with mechanical closure alone (so-called "cold snare") or with mechanical plus electrosurgical cutting ("hot snare"). Recent studies suggest that cold snare is associated with lower risk of bleeding and bowel wall injury.

Endoscopic Brush Cytology

Abrasive brush cytology has been used in many different fields of tissue sampling. Typical endoscopic brush is constrained within a plastic catheter similar to endoscopic snares (Figure 1.7).

After passing through the accessory channel of the endoscope, the abrasive brush is exposed and rubbed against the area of tissue sampling. This is most commonly applied to obtain specimens for microbiology, particularly fungal specimens. These have also been widely applied in the biliary tract for sampling of suspicious biliary strictures. More recent advances include a highly abrasive wide-area tissue sampling system that has been recently studied and Barrett's esophagus as an alternative to pinch forceps, as well as nonendoscopic abrasive sponge sampling, which has the potential to offer inexpensive population-based screening for esophageal neoplasia (Figure 1.8).

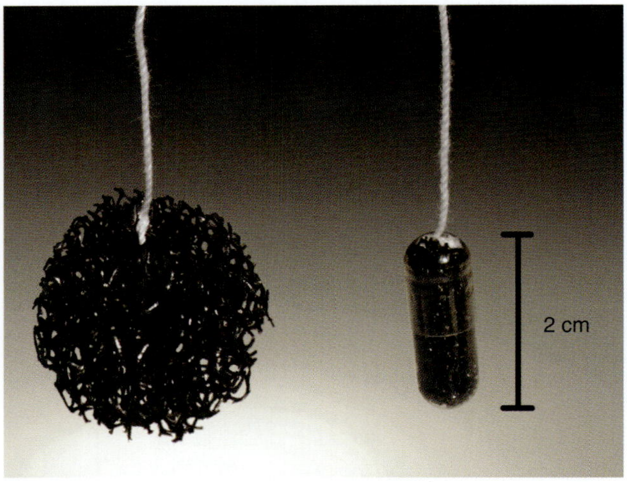

Figure 1.8 Nonendoscopic abrasive cytology brush. *Source:* From Kadri, S.R., Lao-Sirieix, P., O'Donovan, M. et al. (2010). Acceptability and accuracy of a non-endoscopic screening test for Barrett's oesophagus in primary care: cohort study. *BMJ* 341: c4372. doi: https://doi.org/10.1136/bmj.c4372. Open access article.

Endoscopic Fine-Needle Aspiration (FNA) Devices

The most common application of FNA devices in endoscopy is endoscopic ultrasound-guided tissue sampling (EUS-FNA). The development of endoscopic ultrasound in the 1970s and 1980s significantly expanded the reach of endoscopic tissue sampling into the pancreas and other extraluminal organs such as lymph nodes and now virtually any organ within reach of the proximal or distal GI tract lumen (Figure 1.9).

Other needle aspiration devices include biliary sampling needles often used in conjunction with forceps and brush sampling, or so-called "triple sampling." EUS-FNA devices come in various sizes from 19- to 25-gauge. These devices are typically attached to a handle, which allows the endoscopist to puncture and make to-and-fro movements within the target lesion and also apply negative pressure. With various methods, both cytologic and histologic material can be obtained through these needle devices. Recent efforts to develop Tru-Cut devices have been met with variable success.

Tissue Processing in the Endoscopy Laboratory

An excellent recent review on the topic of tissue acquisition has been published by the American Society for gastrointestinal endoscopy. For most routine tissue sampling the biopsy material is placed in formalin and subsequently embedded in paraffin for histological analysis. Other specific preparations include sampling for microbiological evaluation, molecular or genetic testing, and electromicroscopy. These

(a) (b)

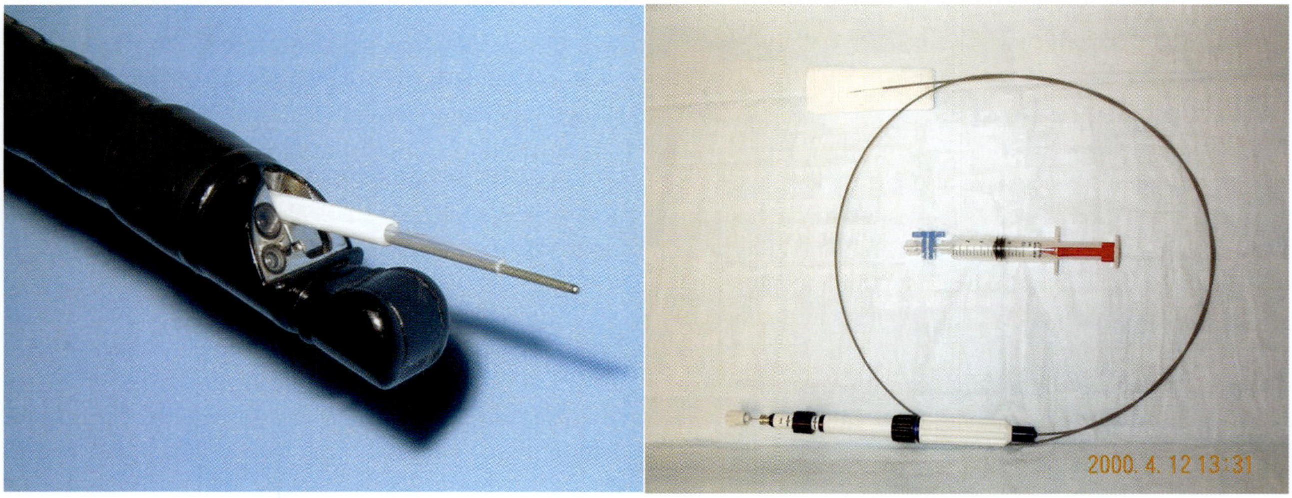

Figure 1.9 (a) and (b) Endoscopic ultrasound endoscope and guided fine-needle aspiration (EUS-FNA) device.

special samples should be handled according to local institutional guidelines. In general, samples that are obtained for culture should be obtained prior to placing forceps into formalin as formalin residue can destroy or inactivate live microbial tissue.

Non-oriented Samples

Most pinch biopsy samples are placed directly in formalin without orientation. This is also true for small polyps where the likelihood of invasive cancer is very low. The sample is placed directly into a small formalin jar. The needle or forceps should be rinsed if it comes in direct contact with formalin as subsequent contact with living tissue can cause chemical injury.

Oriented Samples

Increasingly, endoscopic resection is being used for definitive oncologic removal of precancerous and invasive lesions. In these cases it is advantageous to orient the specimen so that precise staging as well as margin assessment can be performed. A typical situation is in endoscopic resection of early neoplasia in the esophagus such as Barrett's esophagus. In this case a sample is frequently obtained through endoscopic mucosal resection. Large pieces of tissue, typically 1–2 cm in diameter, can be obtained to a depth of the submucosa. In this case the sample should be removed from the patient in a way that does not damage or distort the tissue. This is typically performed by suctioning the tissue into a distal attachment cap/hood and then removing the endoscope. Alternative retrieval devices include a modified snare with a protective net. These tissues should then be immediately oriented at the bedside typically by placing them on a paraffin or similar firm block. The tissue should be flattened typically with the mucosal side up and the edges carefully pinned so that the tissue remains flat (Figure 1.10).

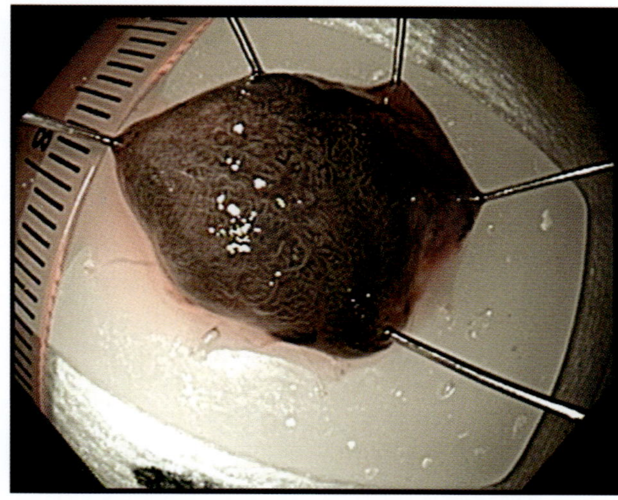

Figure 1.10 Pinned and oriented resection tissue from Barrett's esophagus-associated neoplasia. Note the mucosal side facing up and the lateral margins pinned to prevent curling of the edges.

Cytology Samples

Cytology samples obtained from either brush or fine-needle aspiration can be processed in a variety of ways. Most commonly these are prepared as thin smear on glass slides, which can be evaluated either immediately as an air-dried sample stained with a modified Romanowsky stain, or as an alcohol-fixed slide evaluated with Papanicolaou staining. It is often helpful to place additional excess material in a cytological preservative or formalin. Special handling is required for samples where lymphoproliferative disease is considered. Typically these include cytological preservatives such as Roswell Park Memorial Institute (RPMI) medium that allow subsequent flow cytometry. As a practical matter, placement in such a preservative should be considered even when likelihood is low since cells preserved in such solution can always be examined with routine cytological methods; however, cells that are placed in formalin or alcohol cannot be evaluated for flow cytometry. The use of rapid on-site evaluation (ROSE) cytology has been shown in many studies to increase diagnostic yield and reduce the need for repeated procedures.

Culture Samples

Samples obtained for culture should be placed in a sterile specimen container. Sterile saline maybe needed to prevent drying of the specimen. Attention should be paid to minimize contamination although it is recognized that the endoscope and the organs throughout which it is passed are not sterile and is not possible to obtain a purely sterile access into the gastrointestinal lumen. Contamination with oropharyngeal organisms or colonic organisms is not uncommon.

Specific Organ Sampling Methods

Esophagus

Diagnostic Sampling

Indications for diagnostic sampling of the esophagus include Barrett's esophagus and other suspected neoplastic disorders, inflammatory disorder such as eosinophilic esophagitis, gastroesophageal reflux disease, and infectious esophagitis.

The most common indication in Western countries for tissue sampling from the esophagus is likely Barrett's esophagus. There are established guidelines for sampling of the esophagus. These have traditionally been based on the notion that early neoplasia is not visible endoscopically and thus random sampling of the mucosa should be performed to ensure adequate detection of early neoplasia. The most widely used standard is the so-called Seattle protocol. The American Society for Gastrointestinal Endoscopy (ASGE) guideline for tissue sampling calls for surveillance of nondysplastic Barrett's esophagus in four quadrants every 2 cm with a large-capacity forceps for the entire Barrett's mucosa. Patients with established low-grade dysplasia sampling should be more intensive with four-quadrant biopsies every 1–2 cm. For patients who choose to undergo surveillance for high-grade dysplasia, sampling every 1 cm should be performed; however, more recent evidence suggests that patients with established low-grade and high-grade dysplasia should likely undergo therapy to eradicate the Barrett's esophagus. Advances in endoscopic imaging, such as high-definition narrow-band imaging, confocal laser endomicroscopy, and chromoendoscopy, have significantly increased the yield of biopsy and allow much more targeted sampling although these have not yet replaced the need for random biopsy. These advances are likely to reduce the need for random biopsies and focus more on targeted sampling.

For eosinophilic esophagitis the ASGE recommends two to four biopsies from the proximal esophagus and two to four biopsies from the distal esophagus. Biopsy should also be obtained from the gastric antrum and duodenum when diffuse eosinophilic gastroenteritis is suspected.

For suspected infectious esophagitis, multiple biopsies from the margin and base of a visualized ulcer should be obtained and the sample should be sent for standard histology as well as immunohistochemical and possibly viral cultures and PCR. For candidal esophagitis, multiple biopsies of the affected area as well as cytology brushings may be complementary to biopsy.

Therapeutic Sampling

Increasingly, endoscopic resection methods are being applied to early neoplasia the esophagus, particularly Barrett's esophagus and early squamous cell carcinoma. These are largely confined to tumors suspected to be T1 or nodular high-grade dysplasia. Endoscopic mucosal resection (EMR) methods generally involve an EMR device such as a modified band ligator followed by snare resection of the pseudopolyp (Figure 1.11–1.13).

Other methods include endoscopic submucosal dissection (ESD) in which the lateral margins of the suspected area are incised with electrocautery knife followed by dissection along the submucosal plane to obtain an en bloc specimen. EMR devices can typically obtain samples 1–2 cm in diameter into

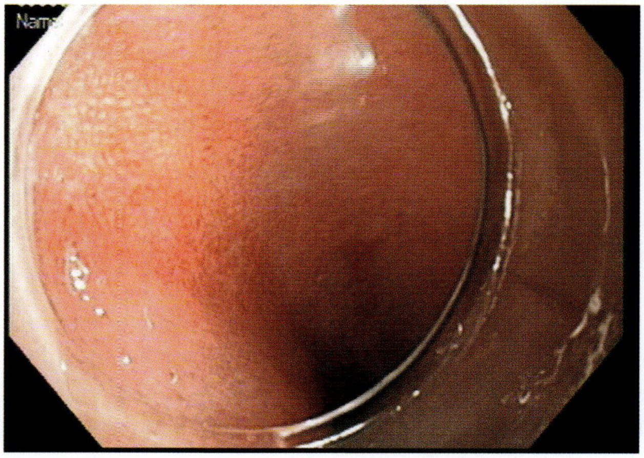

Figure 1.11 Barrett's esophagus with flat neoplasia (9 o'clock) for targeted endoscopic resection.

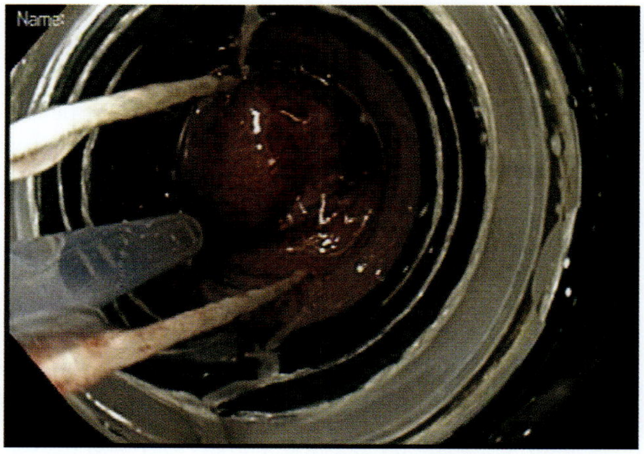

Figure 1.12 Multiband mucosectomy device. The black rubber bands are mounted on the outside of a plastic cap. The tissue is suctioned into the cap and a band deployed to create a pseudopolyp, which is then removed by snare.

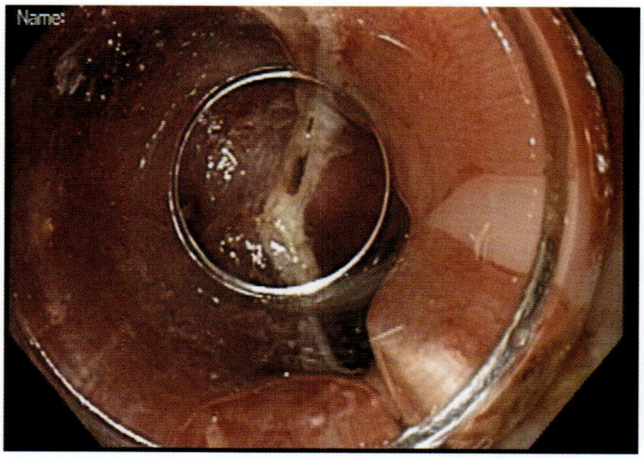

Figure 1.13 Area of resection at 6–12 o'clock includes the entire region of suspected neoplasia at 9 o'clock. The remaining tissue at the 9 o'clock area represents intact deep submucosa and muscularis propria.

the depth of the mid-submucosa. Endoscopic submucosal dissection can obtain samples of any lateral diameter and generally to the base of the submucosa.

One major advantage of these techniques is the ability to perform wide-field or en bloc resection and orient the sample. Samples should be retrieved without causing trauma to the tissue, preferably by removal through the endoscopic cap or through a snare-net as opposed to suctioning via the accessory channel, which can traumatize or fragment the tissue. Once retrieved the tissue should be handled as with other endoscopic resection specimens by orienting the specimen and pinning it on a fixed material such as a paraffin block. En bloc specimens can be oriented in terms of the oral and anal side of the lesion and assessed for lateral and deep margins. For resections that are performed piecemeal such as with multiband mucosectomy, the lateral margins cannot be accurately assessed and so complete resection relies on the endoscopic inspection intraluminally. The specimens should still be oriented and assessed for the deep margin.

Stomach

Diagnostic Sampling

Major indications for diagnostic sampling of the stomach include assessment for *Helicobacter pylori* infection, diagnosis of gastritis, metaplastic atrophic change, gastric polyps, and suspected neoplasia, particularly in the setting of gastric ulceration or early gastric cancer.

H. pylori Sampling Biopsy is one of several recommended methods for *H. pylori* sampling that also includes urease breath testing and stool testing for *H. pylori* antigen. When using endoscopic tissue sampling, there are two general methods including non-histological testing of the tissue for the presence of urease using the traditional Campylobacter-like organism test (CLO-test). In this case, the tissue should be placed in the standard agar well and visually inspected for a pH change following the instructions for use in this product. Histological sampling can also be performed with one of two methods. One method is to take three biopsies including one from the angularis corpus antrum junction, one from the greater curvature of the corpus, and one from the greater curvature of the antrum. Alternatively, the updated Sydney protocol may be followed, which includes five biopsies including one from the antrum lesser curve, antrum greater curve, gastric corpus lesser curve, and greater curve, and one from the angularis of the stomach.

Environmental Metaplastic Atrophic Gastritis (EMAG) Current guidelines recommend 7–12 biopsies including 4-quadrant biopsies including an antrum, 2 from the angularis, 4 from the corpus, and 2 from the cardia.

Gastric Polyps Gastric polyps are very frequently encountered, particularly in patients who are on chronic proton pump inhibitor therapy. Current ASGE guidelines for management of gastric polyps suggest that polyp should be sampled by biopsy. Fundic gland polyps larger than 1 cm should be removed by polypectomy. Hyperplastic polyps larger than 5 mm should be removed by polypectomy, and all adenomatous polyps should be removed by polypectomy. In patients who have numerous polyps, particularly where endoscopic inspection is highly consistent with fundic gland polyps, the largest of the polyps should be removed by polypectomy and representative sampling performed of smaller polyps.

Ulcer Disease Because of the potential for neoplasia in the setting of ulcers, numerous biopsies should be obtained from the base as well as the margins of the ulcer to exclude malignancy. Cytology may also be helpful. Sampling for concurrent *H. pylori* infection should be performed as suggested above.

Therapeutic Sampling

Endoscopic resection in early gastric cancer is now widely performed throughout the world. The endoscopic resection methods include endoscopic mucosal resection typically with a cap-assisted device as in the esophagus, or injection of a submucosal agent such as saline followed by snare resection of the lifted tissue. Lesions larger than 1–2 cm should generally be removed en bloc by endoscopic submucosal dissection when early gastric cancer is suspected. Tissue should be handled in the same manner as discussed above in esophagus.

Small Intestine

Major indications for tissue sampling of the small intestine include celiac disease as well as resection of early neoplasia.

Diagnostic Sampling

Currently established protocols for sampling for celiac disease recommend four to six biopsies from the duodenum including the duodenal bulb and distal duodenum.

All other suspicious areas should be sampled using routine biopsy technique. Sampling of the papilla should be performed with caution as biopsy in this area can cause pancreatitis. When a suspected neoplastic lesion is seen in the region of the papilla, it is preferred to take a biopsy that does not immediately injure the orifice of the bile duct or the pancreas duct.

Therapeutic Sampling

Adenomatous polyps of the duodenum are handled in a similar manner to adenomatous lesions anywhere in the gastrointestinal tract. Endoscopic mucosa resection can be performed with injection followed by snare. There appears to be higher risks of bleeding and perforation associated with endoscopic resection of duodenal lesions. This is particularly true were using cap-assisted devices where the thin wall of the duodenum is suctioned into the cap leading to inadvertent full-thickness resection.

Special attention is required for resection of lesions involving the ampulla of Vater. In these cases, typically the lesion is resected followed by placement of a stent in the pancreatic and bile duct orifice to prevent stricturing of these and acute pancreatitis.

Another special situation is polypoid lesions in the distal small intestine, which can now be accessed with deep enteroscopy methods. Polyps are generally removed in the same manner as polypoid lesions elsewhere in the gastrointestinal tract by snare polypectomy. Special circumstances include numerous polyps such as those developed in patients with Peutz–Jeghers syndrome. These can be particularly large and numerous. It may not be possible to resect and retrieve all tissues. Because of the laborious process of deep enteroscopy, it is often not feasible to extract the endoscope with each large polypoid tissue. Thus diagnostic sampling can be performed by biopsy of the lesion or fragmentation of the lesion with a snare followed by complete therapeutic excision of the lesion.

Colon

Major indications for diagnostic sampling of the colon include detection of both overt and microscopic colitis and surveillance for dysplasia in inflammatory bowel disease.

Perhaps the most commonly performed tissue sampling in the field of gastroenterology involves removal of colorectal polyps and tissue sampling of more advanced colorectal neoplasia.

Diagnostic Sampling

In patients with chronic diarrhea and suspected microscopic colitis, random biopsies should be taken throughout the colon including at least two biopsies from the right, transverse, descending, and sigmoid colon. For limited sampling the flexible sigmoidoscopy is also a reasonable approach. In this case at least two biopsies should be obtained from the sigmoid and descending colon as well as transverse colon if this can be reached with the sigmoidoscope.

In the setting of inflammatory bowel disease, biopsy sampling should be performed to establish the diagnosis and to assess the extent. For the initial diagnosis, the American Society for gastrointestinal endoscopy recommends two biopsies from each of five sites including the ileum and rectum.

Surveillance of inflammatory bowel disease is a special circumstance and is evolving. Traditionally, random biopsies were obtained throughout the colon. Current guidelines recommend biopsy of each colonic segment with four-quadrant biopsies every 10 cm from the cecum to the rectum for a minimum total of 33 biopsy samples. In cases where the entire colon is not affected, four samples should be obtained every 10 cm of the affected areas. More recently, it has been shown that using dye spray such as indigo carmine or methylene blue can identify areas of dysplasia with high accuracy and thus guide directed sampling without the need for random biopsy. Biopsies should however also be assessed from each colonic segment to assess for inflammation.

Therapeutic Sampling

Endoscopic resection methods of flat and lateral spreading colorectal polyps has expanded rapidly over last 10 years. Most noninvasive neoplastic lesions of the colon can now be removed through advanced endoscopic methods such as EMR or ESD avoiding the need for surgery. Lesions less than 2 cm can typically be removed en bloc with endoscopic mucosal resection involving injection of a fluid cushion under the lesion followed by snare resection. Where there is suspected early (mucosal or superficial submucosal) invasive carcinoma, en bloc resection should be performed using either EMR or ESD depending on the size of the lesion. The tissue processing should be the same as for other neoplastic lesions with orientation of the specimen and pinning of the specimen to assess the lateral and deep margins (Figure 1.14).

The final histological analysis allows for detailed staging, as well as matching the corresponding histological and endoscopic findings; note the lavender line overlays indicating sites of advanced neoplasia. The close collaboration between pathologists and endoscopists further improves the accuracy of each procedure (Figure 1.15).

Summary

The role of pathology in gastrointestinal endoscopy remains critical. Gastroenterologists should have a thorough knowledge of optimal methods of tissue removal and initial processing to allow optimal diagnosis and therapeutic results. Advances in endoscopic resection have allowed complete resection of many early cancers but require closer cooperation between the endoscopist and pathologist to ensure the tissue is properly handled and staged. With EUS-FNA, the direct interaction of pathologist with rapid on-site cytological evaluation has led to higher accuracy, and reduced the need for repeat procedures. Finally, advances in imaging will continue to improve the targeting of tissue sampling and reduce the need for low-yield random sampling methods.

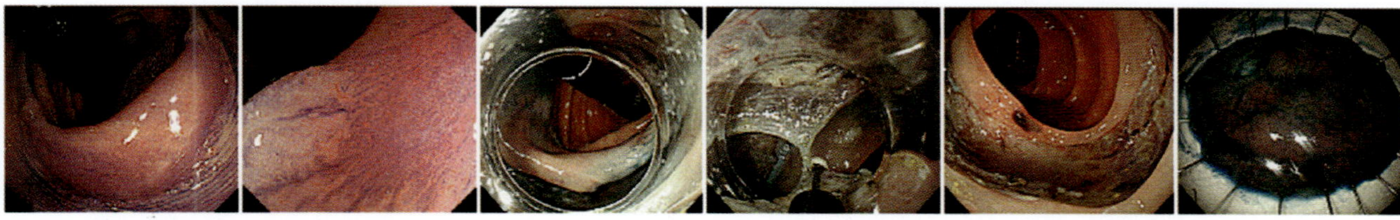

Figure 1.14 Endoscopic submucosal dissection (ESD) procedure. A flat neoplastic lesion is seen in panel 1–2 after staining with cresyl violet. The margins are incised (panel 3) with the endoscope retroflexed (black tube). The submucosal plane is dissected with a needle knife (panel 4). The final resection site (panel 5) and corresponding resection specimen prepared for pathology processing (panel 6).

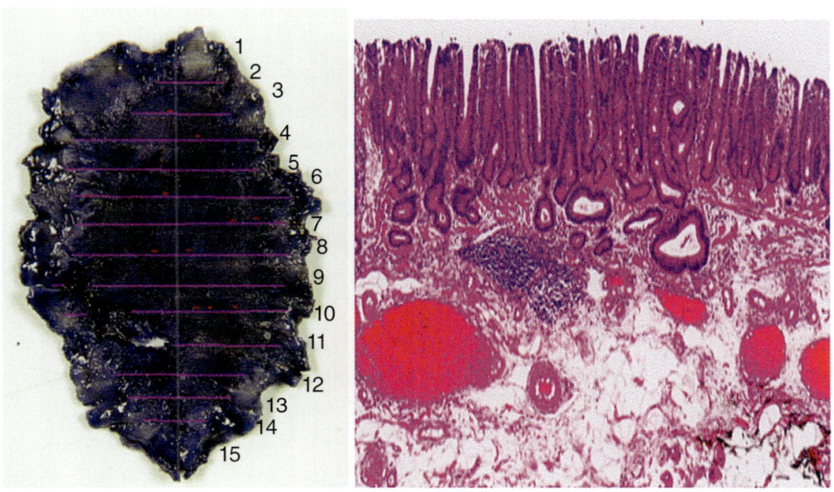

Figure 1.15 Endoscopically resected en bloc well-differentiated adenocarcinoma 28 × 17 mm with superficial submucosal invasion and no lymphovascular invasion and negative horizontal and vertical margins. This sample meets criteria for endoscopic curative resection.

Figure 1.16 Large mediastinal lymph node sampled with EUS-FNA. The needle is seen entering from the upper right of the screen into the tumor in the center of the image.

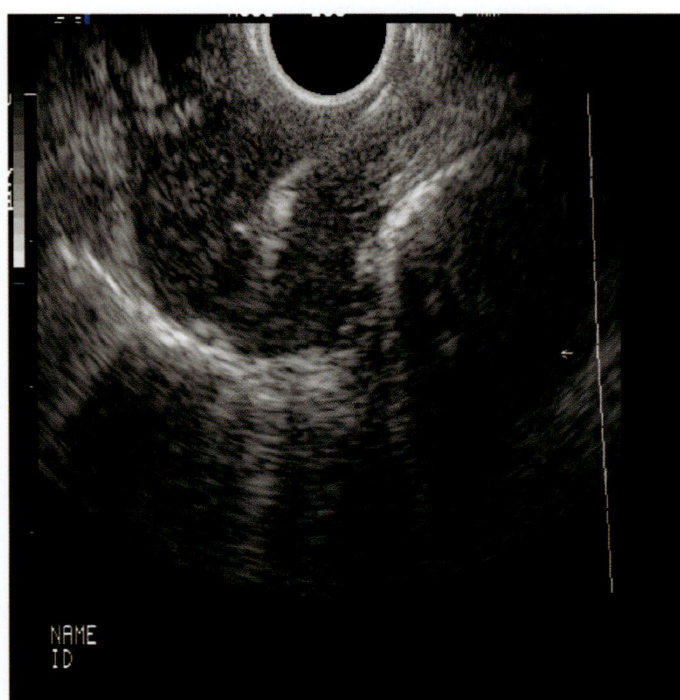

Further Reading

Al-Haddad, M. and Eloubeidi, M.A. (2008). Diagnostic and therapeutic applications of endoscopic ultrasound-guided punctures. *Dig. Dis.* 26 (4): 390–397.

Basford, P., George, R., Nixon, E. et al. (2014). Endoscopic resection of sporadic duodenal adenomas: comparison of endoscopic mucosal resection (EMR) with hybrid endoscopic submucosal dissection (ESD) techniques and the risks of late delayed bleeding. *Surg. Endosc.* 28 (5): 1594–1600.

da Cunha Santos, G., Boerner, S.L., and Geddie, W.R. (2011). Maximizing the yield of lymph node cytology: lessons learned from rapid onsite evaluation of image- and endoscopic-guided biopsies of hilar and mediastinal lymph nodes. *Cancer Cytopathol.* 119 (6): 361–366.

Eloubeidi, M.A., Tamhane, A., Jhala, N. et al. (2006). Agreement between rapid onsite and final cytologic interpretations of EUS-guided FNA specimens: implications for the endosonographer and patient management. *Am. J. Gastroenterol.* 101 (12): 2841–2847.

Falk, G.W., Rice, T.W., Goldblum, J.R., and Richter, J.E. (1999). Jumbo biopsy forceps protocol still misses unsuspected cancer in Barrett's esophagus with high-grade dysplasia. *Gastrointest. Endosc.* 49 (2): 170–176.

Gupta, N., Mathur, S.C., Dumot, J.A. et al. (2012). Adequacy of esophageal squamous mucosa specimens obtained during endoscopy: are standard biopsies sufficient for postablation surveillance in Barrett's esophagus? *Gastrointest. Endosc.* 75 (1): 11–18.

Hikichi, T., Irisawa, A., Bhutani, M.S. et al. (2009). Endoscopic ultrasound-guided fine-needle aspiration of solid pancreatic masses with rapid on-site cytological evaluation by endosonographers without attendance of cytopathologists. *J. Gastroenterol.* 44 (4): 322–328.

Humphris, J.T.J., Kwok, A., and Katelaris, P.H. (2007). Cold snare polypectomy for diminutive polyps: an assessment of the risk of incomplete removal of small adenomas. *Gastrointest. Endosc.* 69: AB207.

Ichise, Y., Horiuchi, A., Nakayama, Y., and Tanaka, N. (2011). Prospective randomized comparison of cold snare polypectomy and conventional polypectomy for small colorectal polyps. *Digestion* 84 (1): 78–81.

Ikematsu, H., Yoda, Y., Matsuda, T. et al. (2013). Long-term outcomes after resection for submucosal invasive colorectal cancers. *Gastroenterology* 144 (3): 551–559. quiz e514.

Johanson, J.F., Frakes, J., and Eisen, D. (2011). Computer-assisted analysis of abrasive transepithelial brush biopsies increases the effectiveness of esophageal screening: a multicenter prospective clinical trial by the EndoCDx Collaborative Group. *Dig. Dis. Sci.* 56 (3): 767–772.

Kadri, S.R., Lao-Sirieix, P., O'Donovan, M. et al. (2010). Acceptability and accuracy of a non-endoscopic screening test for Barrett's oesophagus in primary care: cohort study. *BMJ* 341: c4372. https://doi.org/10.1136/bmj.c4372.

LeBlanc, J.K., Emerson, R.E., Dewitt, J. et al. (2010). A prospective study comparing rapid assessment of smears and ThinPrep for endoscopic ultrasound-guided fine-needle aspirates. *Endoscopy* 42 (5): 389–394.

Levy, M.J., Reddy, R.P., Wiersema, M.J. et al. (2005). EUS-guided trucut biopsy in establishing autoimmune pancreatitis as the cause of obstructive jaundice. *Gastrointest. Endosc.* 61 (3): 467–472.

Mann, N.S., Mann, S.K., and Alam, I. (1999). The safety of hot biopsy forceps in the removal of small colonic polyps. *Digestion* 60 (1): 74–76.

Monkemuller, K.E., Fry, L.C., Jones, B.H. et al. (2004). Histological quality of polyps resected using the cold versus hot biopsy technique. *Endoscopy* 36 (5): 432–436.

Phoa, K.N., van Vilsteren, F.G., Weusten, B.L. et al. (2014). Radiofrequency ablation vs endoscopic surveillance for patients with Barrett esophagus and low-grade dysplasia: a randomized clinical trial. *JAMA* 311 (12): 1209–1217.

Qumseya, B.J., Wang, H., Badie, N. et al. (2013). Advanced imaging technologies increase detection of dysplasia and neoplasia in patients with Barrett's esophagus: a meta-analysis and systematic review. *Clin. Gastroenterol. Hepatol.* 11 (12): 1562–1570. e1561–e1562.

Sakamoto, T., Matsuda, T., Nakajima, T., and Saito, Y. (2012). Efficacy of endoscopic mucosal resection with circumferential incision for patients with large colorectal tumors. *Clin. Gastroenterol. Hepatol.* 10 (1): 22–26.

Sharaf, R.N., Shergill, A.K., Odze, R.D. et al. (2013). Endoscopic mucosal tissue sampling. *Gastrointest. Endosc.* 78 (2): 216–224.

Trier, J.S. (1971). Diagnostic value of peroral biopsy of the proximal small intestine. *N. Engl. J. Med.* 285 (26): 1470–1473.

Vogelstein, B., Fearon, E.R., Hamilton, S.R. et al. (1988). Genetic alterations during colorectal-tumor development. *N. Engl. J. Med.* 319 (9): 525–532.

Wang, K.K. and Sampliner, R.E. (2008). Updated guidelines 2008 for the diagnosis, surveillance and therapy of Barrett's esophagus. *Am. J. Gastroenterol.* 103 (3): 788–797.

Watanabe, T., Itabashi, M., Shimada, Y. et al. (2012). Japanese Society for Cancer of the Colon and Rectum (JSCCR) guidelines 2010 for the treatment of colorectal cancer. *Int. J. Clin. Oncol.* 17 (1): 1–29.

Wu, L., Li, P., Wu, J. et al. (2012). The diagnostic accuracy of chromoendoscopy for dysplasia in ulcerative colitis: meta-analysis of six randomized controlled trials. *Color. Dis.* 14 (4): 416–420.

2

Esophagus Inflammatory Conditions

Anthony R. Mattia[1], *Gregory Y. Lauwers*[2], *Michael B. Wallace*[3] *and Till S. Clauditz*[4]

[1] *Newton-Wellesley Hospital, Newton, MA, USA*
[2] *Moffitt Cancer Center, Tampa, Florida, USA*
[3] *Mayo Clinic, Jacksonville, Florida, USA*
[4] *Department of Pathology, University-Medical Center, Hamburg, Germany*

Normal Histology, Variations

The esophagus has a pearly white and smooth surface under which a network of small vessels is seen (Figure 2.1) except for the distal esophageal sphincter where prominent longitudinal and palisading vessels (exceeding 100 mm in diameter) are observed and used to define the esophagogastric junction.

Microscopic Features

The esophageal mucosa is composed of a non-keratinizing flat stratified squamous epithelium, lamina propria, and muscularis mucosae (Figure 2.2; Table 2.1). The squamous epithelium is 10–20 cell layers thick measuring 300–500 μm in thickness. The prickle cells contain a large quantity of cytoplasmic glycogen, which stains positively with periodic acid–Schiff (PAS). The basal proliferative zone, the cuboidal or polyhedral basal and parabasal cells account for 15% or less of the epithelial thickness. A small number of specialized cell types, including T lymphocytes, Langerhans cells, endocrine cells, and melanocytes are also present in the deep/parabasal epithelium. The lamina propria consists of loose connective tissue with scattered inflammatory cells, vessels, nerves, and small mucous glands. The lamina propria papillae normally extend into the epithelium for 1/3–1/2 of its thickness. The muscularis mucosae is a thick layer of smooth muscle bundles oriented longitudinally. In the distal 1–2 cm of the esophagus, the basal zone, papillae, and intraepithelial cells may be more prominent, and include rare eosinophils. Esophageal mucosal biopsies typically include the squamous epithelium and scant lamina propria. The muscularis mucosae is seldom present, and better identified in esophageal mucosal resection specimens.

Infectious Esophagitis

Definition, General Features, Predisposing Factors

Infection is a common cause of esophagitis, particularly in immunocompromised patients but can also occur in apparently immunocompetent hosts with certain predisposing conditions. Fungi (*Candida* species) and viruses are responsible for most cases of infectious esophagitis, and dual infections may be encountered. Bacterial, mycobacterial, and parasitic esophagitis (e.g. Chagas disease due to *Trypanosoma cruzi*) are rarely encountered in esophageal biopsy material.

Fungal Esophagitis

Fungal infection due to *Candida albicans* is the most common cause of infectious esophagitis.

Predisposing conditions are broad and include HIV infection/AIDS, other immunosuppressed conditions such as organ transplant, prolonged corticosteroid therapy as well as other conditions such as diabetes, malignancy, antibiotic therapy, acid-suppressive therapy, and pregnancy. Infection due to *Candida tropicalis* and *Candida (Torulopsis) glabrata has* also been described, as well as infection due to other fungi such as *Histoplasma capsulatum* and *Aspergillus* species.

Viral Esophagitis

Herpes simplex (HSV) is the most common etiology of viral esophagitis, and also occurs primarily in the setting of immunosuppression, such as solid organ and bone marrow transplantation, underlying malignancy, chemotherapy, and HIV infection (AIDS). These patients may also have disseminated infection at the time of diagnosis. It can also develop in healthy adults including pregnant women and

Gastrointestinal Pathology: Correlative Endoscopic and Histologic Assessment, First Edition. Edited by Gregory Y. Lauwers and Michael B. Wallace.

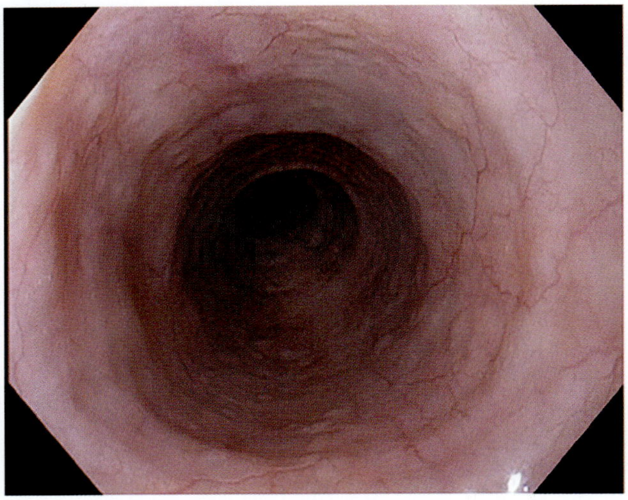

Figure 2.1 Endoscopic appearance of distal esophagus with normal squamous mucosa.

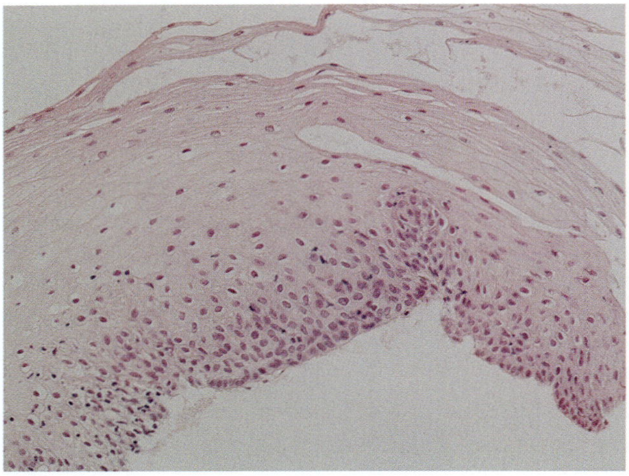

Figure 2.2 Normal esophagus squamous mucosa with normal stratified non-keratinizing epithelium.

Table 2.1 Normal esophageal mucosa.

Epithelium:
Non-keratinizing squamous epithelium
Glycogen rich
10–20 cells thick (300–500 μm)
Basal proliferative zone up to 15%
Few scattered parabasal T lymphocytes and other specialized cells
Lamina propria:
Papillary length 1/3 to 1/2 of epithelial thickness
Muscularis mucosae

children. Both HSV types 1 and 2 can infect the esophagus with type 1 being most common. Infection by varicella-zoster virus (VZV) may also rarely occur in immunocompromised hosts.

Cytomegalovirus (CMV)-induced esophagitis also typically occurs in the immunosuppressed population, particularly in the setting of HIV infection/AIDS, organ transplantation, chemotherapy, corticosteroid therapy, and other forms of long-term immunosuppression. CMV may rarely cause esophagitis in immunocompetent patients, especially in the elderly.

Bacterial Esophagitis

Clinically significant bacterial esophagitis occurs almost exclusively in immunocompromised patients. Secondary bacterial colonization of areas of prior esophageal injury and ulceration is more common. Bacterial invasion of squamous mucosa or the deeper layers is required to establish a diagnosis of primary bacterial esophagitis. Gram-positive bacteria are the most common causative organisms (including *Staphylococcus aureus, Staphylococcus epidermidis, Streptococcus viridans*, and beta-hemolytic streptococci).

Mycobacterial Esophagitis

The rare mycobacterial esophagitis typically occurs in the setting of advanced immunosuppression. Both *Mycobacterium tuberculosis* complex and *Mycobacterium avium* complex can be encountered.

Parasitic Esophagitis

Chagas disease involving the esophagus is an important cause of esophageal dysfunction (dysphagia) in endemic regions, such as Latin America. However, the organism and its pathologic effects are typically not identified on biopsy specimens.

Clinical Features and Endoscopic Characteristics

Clinical and endoscopic features are specific to each condition. For candidal esophagitis, symptoms vary from none (especially in patients with mild disease from chronic inhaled steroids) to severe dysphagia and odynophagia in immunosuppressed patients. *Candida* appears as a white, cottage cheese-like exudate, which is partially adherent to the epithelium (Figure 2.3). HSV and CMV both cause ulcerations. HSV ulcers are typically small, 1–3 mm, whereas CMV ulcers may be both deep and wide. Biopsy yield for the virus is highest from the edge of HSV ulcers and from the center of CMV ulcers. In practice, both are usually obtained. Other infections' etiologies may have nonspecific findings. The inflammatory

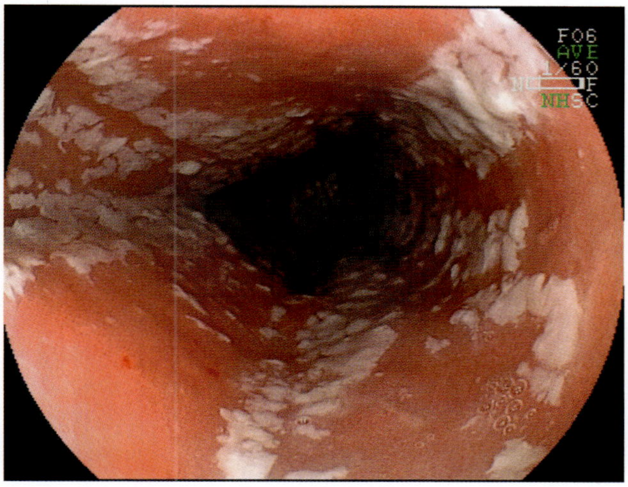

Figure 2.3 Endoscopic appearance of white exudate typical of *Candida albicans* in a patient on chronic inhaled corticosteroid.

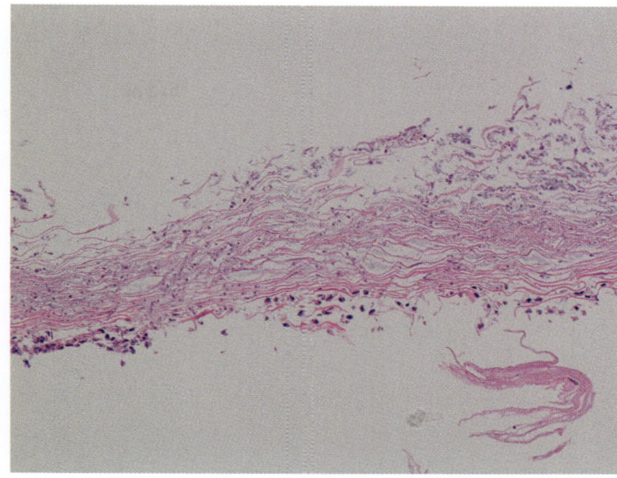

Figure 2.4 Debris of slough off superficial squamous epithelium with fungal hyphae and acute inflammation.

reaction of tuberculous esophagitis often imparts a radiologically detectable mass-like lesion, whereas mucosal changes include linear ulcers and induration that preferentially affects the mid-portion of the esophagus. Fistula formation and perforation may occur. Chagas disease presentation is similar to that of achalasia with manometric findings of a poorly relaxing lower esophageal sphincter and an aperistaltic esophagus body.

Microscopic Features

Candida

The biopsies typically show an active esophagitis with a mixed inflammatory infiltrate of neutrophils, lymphocytes, and eosinophils. Neutrophils are often present in small, superficial clusters associated with parakeratosis or squamous debris, which may be a diagnostic clue. Prominent intraepithelial neutrophils may be associated with abscesses, erosions, or ulcerations. The inflammatory response may be minimal in severely immunocompromised patients.

Yeast forms of *C. albicans* and pseudohyphae (with refractile cell walls) are usually present in superficial desquamated keratin debris (Figure 2.4). The yeast are 3–5 μm in diameter basophilic oval forms while the, nonseptate sausage-like pseudohyphae are 3–5 μm in diameter and are arranged perpendicular to the epithelial surface. Occasional septate hyphae can be present. The presence of psuedohyphal and hyphal forms correlates with active infection. Most infections are superficial with isolated, intraepithelial fungal forms, and organisms in detached squamous cells. However, in immunocompromised hosts, deeper tissue invasion within ulcers and erosions may be seen. *Candida* are often conspicuous in routinely stained sections, although their appearance is enhanced with periodic acid–Schiff (PAS, Figure 2.5) or Grocott methenamine silver (GMS) stains. In *Candida (Torulopsis) glabrata* infections, only small budding yeast forms are seen, which may mimic histoplasmosis.

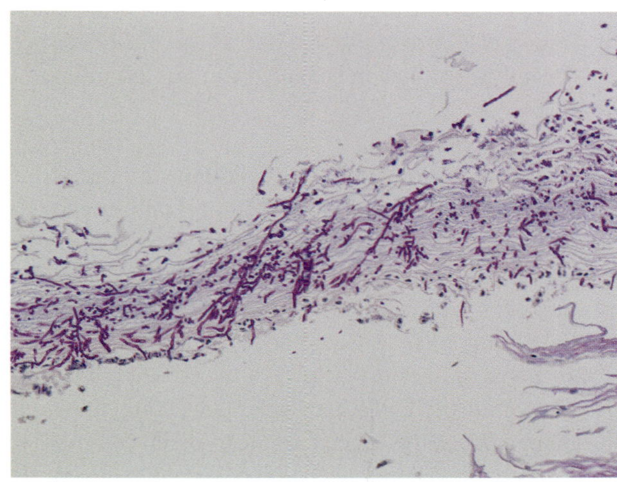

Figure 2.5 PAS stain of Figure 2.4 illustrating the fungal elements of *Candida albicans*.

Candida can colonize preexisting ulcers or damaged mucosa of any etiology, and in such cases the possibility of dual infection or pathology should be considered. Also, when *Candida* yeast forms are present only in desquamated keratin debris unassociated with inflammation or endoscopic findings, carry over from an oral infection should be suspected.

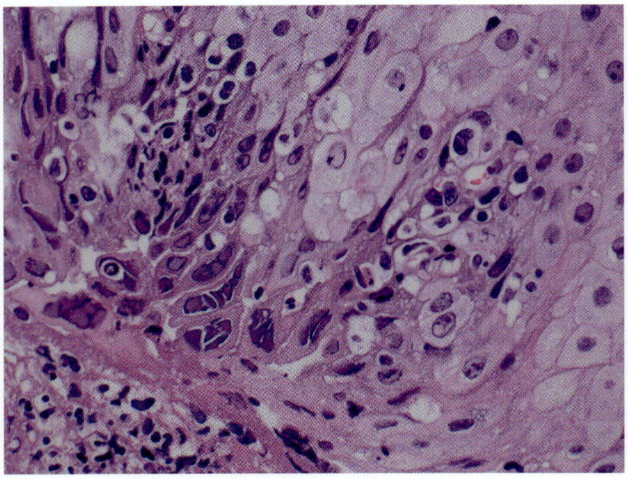

Figure 2.6 Multinucleated basal keratinocytes typical of HSV esophagitis.

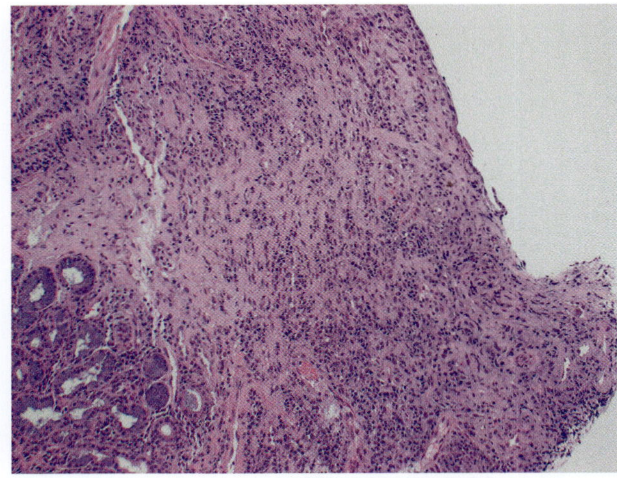

Figure 2.7 Erosive esophagitis with prominent granulation and atypical cellular elements.

Cytologic brushings are also very useful in the diagnosis of *Candida* esophagitis, as the organisms are readily identified on Papanicolaou stained smears.

Herpes Simplex (HSV)

If HSV infection is suspected, in addition to biopsies for histology, fresh tissue can be sent for viral culture to confirm the diagnosis and identify strains that may be resistant to acyclovir. HSV infection is associated with ulceration and a mixed inflammatory infiltrate of intraepithelial neutrophils, eosinophils, and lymphocytes, as well as aggregates of macrophages that can be a diagnostic clue. HSV infects squamous cells of intact or denuded epithelium and is best identified at the edge of an ulcer and in cells within the ulcer slough. Therefore, optimal histologic diagnosis requires sampling of the ulcer edge rather than the ulcer bed. The typical viral cytopathic effects include multinucleation, ground glass nuclei, and dense intranuclear eosinophilic inclusions with a thickened nuclear membrane and a clear halo (Cowdry type A inclusion bodies) (Figure 2.6). Viral inclusions and multinucleated cells are not always identifiable in biopsies, and ancillary immunohistochemistry (IHC) staining for HSV may be required. Concomitant infection of *Candida*, cytomegalovirus, or bacteria can exist, particularly in immunocompromised patients. Varicella Zoster Virus has been associated with esophagobronchial fistula formation.

Cytomegalovirus (CMV)

Culture is not used routinely, and does not distinguish the simple presence of CMV from active infection; however, culture may be useful for identifying drug resistance.

Ulceration and granulation tissue formation with associated acute inflammation is common. In contrast to HSV esophagitis, CMV rarely infects the squamous epithelium, and preferentially involves endothelial cells, stromal cells, and glandular epithelium. Therefore, biopsies of the ulcer bed should preferentially be performed when CMV esophagitis is suspected (Figure 2.7). CMV cytopathic effect is characterized by nuclear enlargement with classic "owl eye" large intranuclear inclusions, and granular, eosinophilic cytoplasmic inclusions (Figure 2.8a). Smaller, atypical intranuclear inclusions may be present and are more subtle, simulating activated fibroblasts. These infected cells are best identified by immunohistochemical staining (Figure 2.8b). CMV may coexist with HSV and *Candida* infection in some cases.

Bacterial Esophagitis

Sheets of bacteria are typically present with associated necrosis and mucosal erosion, highlighted by a tissue Gram stain. Inflammation may be scant or absent in neutropenic patients.

Mycobacterial Esophagitis

Histologic features include subepithelial and mural necrotic and non-necrotic granulomas with fibrosis and chronic inflammation. Acid fast bacilli can be recognized on Ziehl–Neelsen stain in approximately 2/3 of cases.

Immunohistochemical Studies and Molecular Features

IHC staining for HSV (HSV 1 and 2 cocktail stain) may be useful for suspected infections if diagnostic inclusions are not readily identified on H&E sections. Similarly, IHC for CMV is useful to highlight infected cells without typical CMV morphology, and may be more sensitive than light microscopy.

PCR for *M. tuberculosis* may be useful in selected cases.

(a) (b)

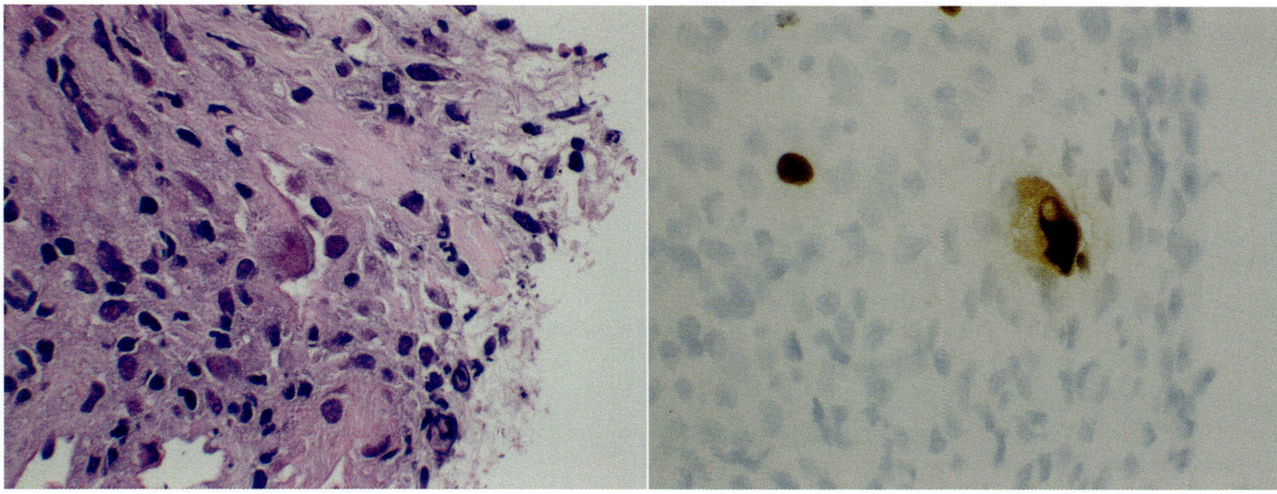

Figure 2.8 High-magnification evaluation of Figure 2.7 demonstrated (a) endothelial CMV infection (b) confirmed by immunohistochemistry.

Differential Diagnosis

Clinical

Inflammatory changes of the esophagus can be seen in many conditions, most commonly acid reflux disease. Behcet's disease may present with focal ulcers, as can pill-induced (associated with an impacted pill, which may or may not be present during exam) ulcers.

Microscopic

The differential diagnosis of *Candida* esophagitis includes reflux esophagitis, drug injury, glycogenic acanthosis, ectopic sebaceous glands, and other infections.

The differential diagnosis of HSV esophagitis includes other etiologies of mucosal ulceration, including other infections, Crohn's disease, HIV-associated ulceration, and drug injury. In some cases, the cytologic atypia induced in the squamous epithelium by the viral cytopathic effects of HSV may be difficult to distinguish from squamous dysplasia/carcinoma, as well as radiation esophagitis.

Prognosis, Evolution, and Clinical Management

Most patients present with dysphagia or odynophagia and undergo upper endoscopy with biopsy. Infectious etiologies are treated with appropriate antimicrobials (e.g. fluconazole for candida), typically with high response rates. In immunosuppressed patients, including those on chronic inhaled steroids, frequent retreatment, or chronic suppressive treatment, may be necessary after full efforts to restore immune function.

Gastroesophageal Reflux Disease

Definition, General Features, Predisposing Factors

The chronic regurgitation of gastroduodenal juice into the esophagus causes gastroesophageal reflux disease (GERD). The mucosal injury results from the effects of refluxed gastric acid, bile, pepsin, and duodenal contents that overwhelm the normal protective antireflux barriers, such as esophageal acid clearance and mucosal resistance. Risk factors and predisposing conditions include obesity, diet, sedentary lifestyle, tobacco and alcohol use, hiatus hernia, reduced lower esophageal sphincter tone, loss of esophageal peristaltic function, gastric hypersecretory states, and delayed gastric emptying. Symptomatic GERD is prevalent worldwide, with considerable geographic variation. Prevalence estimates are approximately 20% in North America and Europe, with only East Asia showing estimates <10%.

Clinical Features and Endoscopic Characteristics

There are several endoscopic classifications of gastroesophageal reflux disease (Figure 2.9). The Los Angeles Classification divides esophagitis into four grades:

Grade A: one or more mucosal breaks, each no longer than 5 mm.

Grade B: at least one mucosal break more than 5 mm long, but not continuous between the tops of 2 mucosal folds.

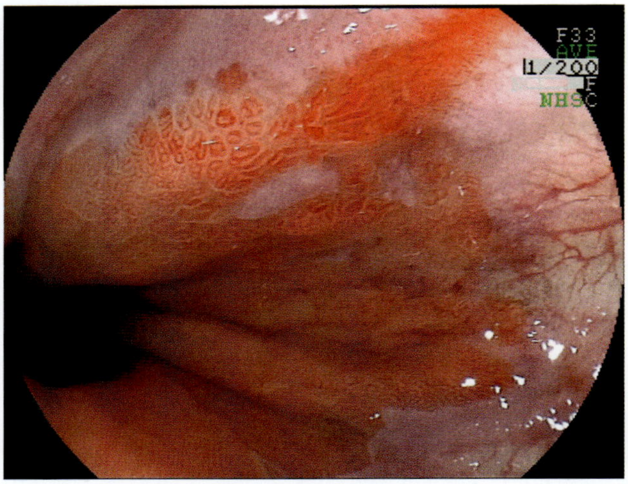

Figure 2.9 Endoscopic appearance of erosive esophagitis in a patient with gastroesophageal reflux disease.

Grade C: at least one mucosal break that is continuous between the tops of 2 or more mucosal folds, but which is not circumferential.

Grade D: a circumferential mucosal break, erosions and ulceration, often resulting in scarring and stenosis if the reflux is recurrent.

Mucosal bridges and esophagogastric fistulae may be encountered.

The endoscopic findings in reflux esophagitis have been classified into three main stages: active, healing, and scarring. Relapse and healing occur repeatedly in patients with gastroesophageal reflux disease (GERD), and a mixture of the stages is often seen in biopsy specimens.

Table 2.2 Histologic features of GERD.

Basal cell hyperplasia (>15%)
Papillary elongation (>50%)
Dilated intercellular spaces (spongiosis)
Intraepithelial inflammation
Neutrophils
Eosinophils
Mononuclear cells

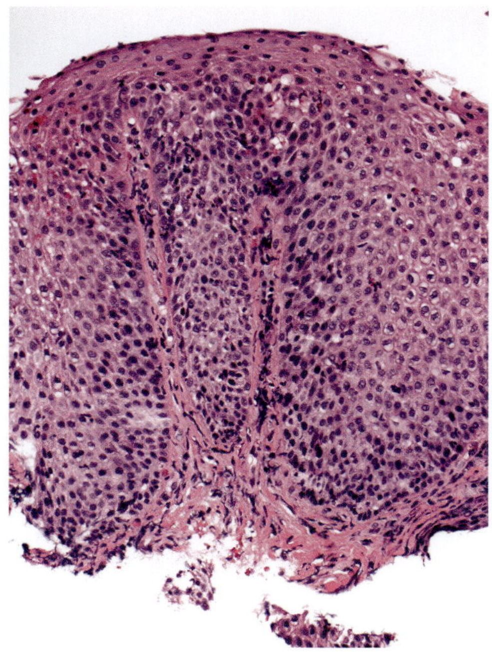

Figure 2.10 Characteristic appearance of low-power view of reflux esophagitis with basal cell hyperplasia, elongation of papillae, lymphocytic and eosinophilic infiltrate.

Microscopic Features

The typical features of GERD are basal cell layer hyperplasia, papillary elongation, dilated intercellular spaces (intercellular edema/spongiosis), and intraepithelial inflammation, including neutrophils, eosinophils, and mononuclear cells (Table 2.2; Figures 2.10, 2.11). However, none of these features is specific for this diagnosis.

The proliferative epithelial changes are more common than inflammatory infiltration. Basal cell hyperplasia is diagnosed when the thickness of the basal layer exceeds 15% in a well-oriented section. Papillary elongation, defined as extending >50% of the epithelial thickness, should also be only assessed in well-oriented sections. Finally, in minimal GERD, dilated intercellular spaces in the basal and parabasal areas may be the only finding.

Esophageal squamous mucosa normally contains few or no inflammatory cells and the inflammatory infiltrate in GERD is highly variable. The presence of occasional eosinophils is typical of GERD, although large numbers of intraepithelial eosinophils mimicking eosinophilic esophagitis may be identified. Notably, eosinophils are not found in all GERD biopsies and can be seen in asymptomatic patients. Neutrophils may be present, and are more numerous in areas of erosion and ulceration. Lymphocytes, often with irregular nuclear contours (squiggle cells), are usually scattered through the epithelium. Finally, severe inflammation with ulceration may be associated with inflammatory pseudotumor formation, with marked atypia of the reactive stromal cells.

In practice, the report should provide a descriptive summary of the histologic features and injury patterns present, as well as their severity. A note can be added to state that the findings are compatible with reflux injury pattern in the appropriate clinical setting.

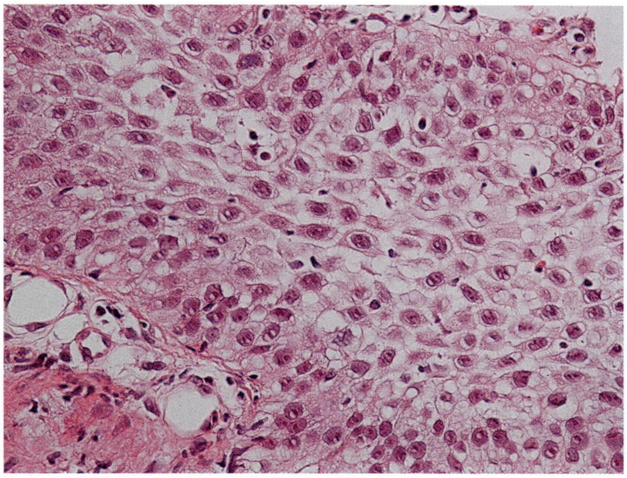

Figure 2.11 High-power magnification of reflux esophagitis with basal cell hyperplasia, spongiosis, and eosinophilic infiltrate.

Differential Diagnosis

Clinical

Clinically, erosive esophagitis from GERD is typically in the lower third of the esophagus and contiguous with the gastroesophageal junction as opposed to other inflammatory or infectious etiologies that may occur more proximally. The presence of a normal distal esophagus with more proximal inflammation virtually excludes GERD-associated inflammation. Typical symptoms are heartburn and regurgitation. Ph- metry (monitoring the acid reflux events by a wired or wireless sensor in the distal esophagus) can be used in challenging cases but is rarely necessary with obvious symptoms and when esophagitis is seen.

Microscopic

As none of the histologic features are specific for GERD, other etiologies such as infection, eosinophilic esophagitis, iatrogenic injuries, Crohn's disease, and inflammatory skin disorders involving the esophagus may enter into the differential diagnosis.

The presence of large numbers of neutrophils in the superficial epithelium should suggest the possibility of fungal infection or superinfection, and special stains (PAS-diastase, GMS) should be performed to exclude *Candida* organisms. Large numbers of intraepithelial eosinophils raising the possibility of eosinophilic esophagitis and correlation with clinical findings and PPI treatment status are required (see Section "Eosinophilic Esophagitis"). Numerous intraepithelial lymphocytes, if predominant, may suggest an alternative diagnosis such as lymphocytic esophagitis or lichen planus-associated esophagitis (see Sections "Lymphocytic Esophagitis" and "Dermatological Diseases Involving the Esophagus").

Ulceration with regenerative squamous epithelial atypia may be difficult to distinguish from in situ-squamous cell carcinoma and dysplasia. The regenerating epithelial cells have round nuclei with minimally thickened nuclear membranes; fine chromatin; and large, irregular nucleoli, and generally have abundant cytoplasm. Further, maturation toward the epithelial surface can usually be found. In difficult cases, additional biopsies should be requested after medical treatment of the esophagitis. However, in some cases, inflammatory pseudotumors with marked atypia of the reactive stromal cells will need to be differentiated from poorly differentiated carcinoma or sarcoma. Cytokeratin immunohistochemistry (IHC) may be helpful when trying to distinguish between reparative reactions and malignancy.

Less commonly, activated lymphocytes in areas of ulceration may appear atypical and raise the suspicion for lymphoma. In some cases, immunohistochemistry and/or flow cytometry may be necessary to assess for clonality.

Prognosis, Evolution, and Clinical Management

GERD management is based on the severity and potential for complications and largely consists of lifestyle modification, anti-acid medications or surgery. Most nonerosive or minimally erosive (Los Angeles Grade A) responds to a combination of lifestyle modifications and low-dose (single daily proton pump inhibitor [PPI] such as omeprazole) anti-acid therapy. Lifestyle modifications include weight loss, avoiding large meals with two to three hours of bedtime (where gravity no long prevents "upward" reflux), and minimizing specific refluxogenic foods (alcohol, mint, fatty food, chocolate, caffeine). PPI therapy is highly effective, even for severe erosive GERD but may require twice-daily therapy. More than 95% of patients will heal erosive disease on PPI therapy.

Surgical therapy is aimed at restoring the lower esophageal sphinter pressure zone and angle of His, and reducing hiatal hernias. Surgery is also highly effective with more than 80% of individuals having sustained elimination or reduction in GERD symptoms and use of PPI. The major side effect of surgery is retention of gas in the stomach ("gas-bloat syndrome") due to the inability to naturally belch swallowed air.

Eosinophilic Esophagitis

Definition, General Features, Predisposing Factors

Eosinophilic esophagitis (EOE) is a chronic, immune-mediated or antigen-mediated inflammatory condition characterized by symptomatic esophageal dysfunction and eosinophil predominant mucosal inflammation. EOE represents a type 2 (Th2) helper T cell and cytokine-mediated disorder involving genetic predisposition, environmental exposures, and allergic background. Food-based antigens appear to be the dominant mediators of EOE, although aeroallergens may also act as triggers in susceptible patients.

Since it was first established as a distinct clinicopathologic entity in 1993, EOE has become an increasingly recognized cause of dysphagia and esophageal dysfunction, particularly among patients refractory to medical treatment of gastroesophageal reflux disease.

EOE is reported worldwide, with highest prevalence in the United States and Western Europe. It occurs more frequently in children and young adults, although it is increasingly recognized in older adults, and is more common in males (male-to-female ratio of 3–4 : 1). A history of other allergic conditions may be present, such as asthma and atopic dermatitis, as well as peripheral eosinophilia, which are more common in children.

Current diagnostic criteria for EOE include a combination of clinical and pathologic features (Table 2.3).

Table 2.3 Definition of eosinophilic esophagitis and diagnostic criteria.

Symptoms related to esophageal dysfunction
Eosinophil-predominant inflammation on esophageal biopsy, characteristically consisting of a peak value of ≥15 eosinophils per high-power field (EOS/HPF)
Mucosal eosinophilia is isolated to the esophagus and persists after a PPI trial
Secondary causes of esophageal eosinophilia excluded (Table 2.5)
A response to treatment (dietary elimination; topical corticosteroids) supports the diagnosis of EOE, but is not required.

Clinical Features and Endoscopic Characteristics

Eosinophilic esophagitis (EOE) is increasing in prevalence and often seasonal with spikes during typically airborne allergy season. It presents with dysphagia to solids, classically with pills sticking. Other atopic symptoms are common. At endoscopy, the esophagus has white punctate spots (eosinophilic microabscess), rings, longitudinal furrows (Figure 2.12), and desquamates easily with insufflation or dilation. In late stages, the esophagus may be very narrowed and poorly distensible.

Microscopic Features

Esophageal biopsies are required to diagnose EOE. Eosinophils are generally absent from the esophageal squamous epithelium in normal individuals. The histologic hallmark is the presence of an increased number of eosinophils within the squamous epithelium (Figure 2.13). Although there is no exact threshold number that establishes a diagnosis, 15 eos/HPF (peak count) in at least one biopsy is considered a "minimum" threshold.

Eosinophilia may be patchy, and it is recommended that two to four biopsies from at least two locations in the esophagus should be taken to maximize diagnostic yield. The distribution of eosinophilia is important, as they may be identified in both proximal and distal biopsies or be more prominent in proximal biopsies. Practically, only intact eosinophils with visible nuclei should be counted and eosinophilic granules should not be included, although degranulated eosinophils may be a useful clue.

Other histologic findings may be present although none of these should be considered pathognomonic. These features include moderate-marked reactive basal hyperplasia,

(a) (b)

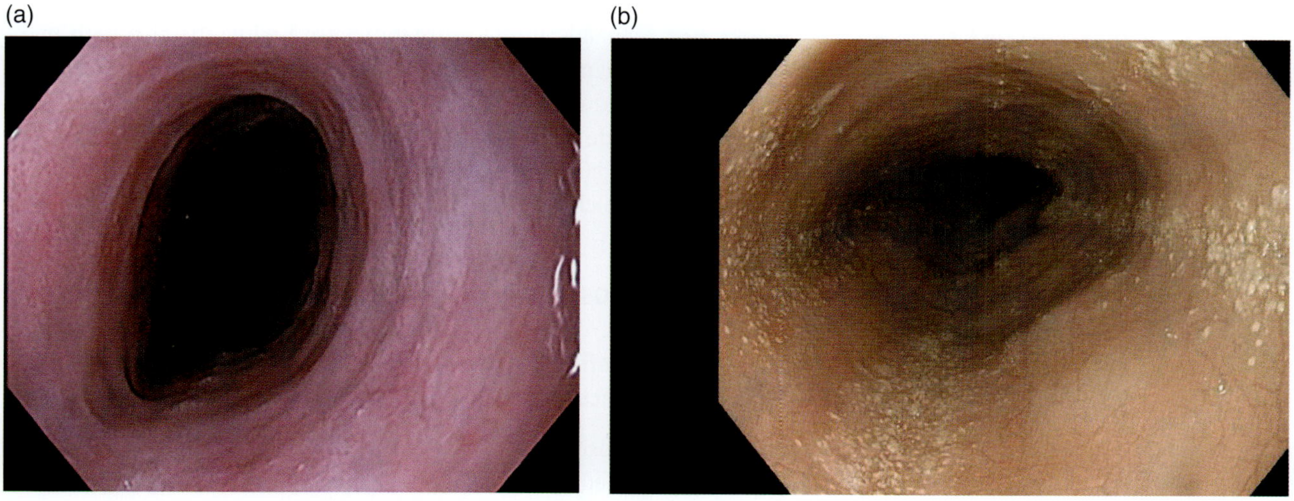

Figure 2.12 Endoscopic appearance of eosinophilic esophagitis (a) with so-called feline esophagus appearance and (b) with extensive white microabcesses. Subtle circular rings and longitudinal furrows also present.

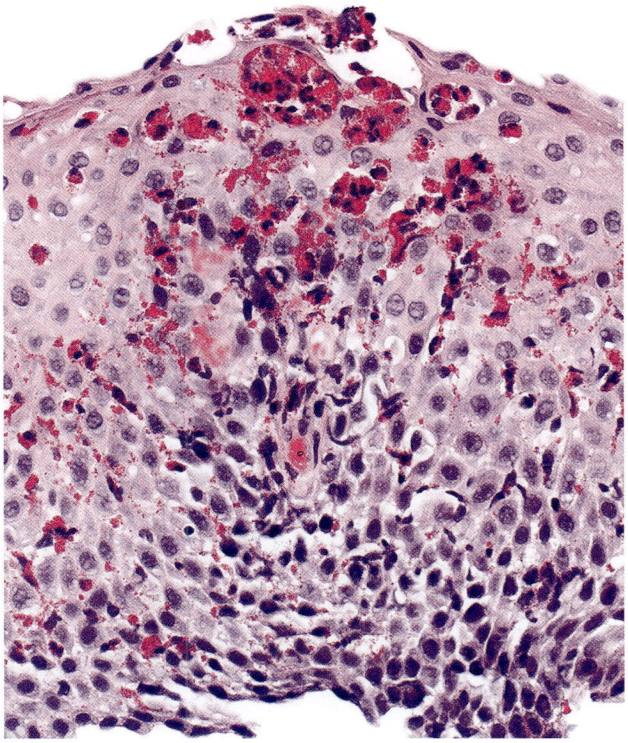

Figure 2.13 Characteristic histology of eosinophilic esophagitis with basal cell hyperplasia, marked eosinophilic infiltrate with eosinophilic microabscesses.

eosinophilic microabscesses (superficial aggregates of ≥4 eosinophils), superficial layering of eosinophils, and subepithelial fibrosis. The presence of subepithelial fibrosis is also associated with eosinophils in the lamina propria and correlates with fibro-stenotic complications of EOE, but may not be identifiable depending on biopsy depth. Other inflammatory cells, such as lymphocytes and mast cells, can also be increased. When reporting the cases, a note is useful to summarize additional relevant histologic features and to provide an overall assessment of the case based on all available biopsies (including prior biopsies, if applicable). For example, active esophagitis with intraepithelial eosinophils (peak count of # per HPF) followed by a note. When large numbers of eosinophils are present (e.g. >40 per HPF), an exact count may be difficult and it is appropriate to report the peak count as such (e.g. "peak count of >40 per HPF").

Immunohistochemical Studies and Molecular Features

Currently, the examination of esophageal mucosal biopsies by hematoxylin and eosin (H&E) stained sections, with clinical correlation, remains the most reliable diagnostic test for EOE. The diagnostic value of ancillary studies in distinguishing eosinophilic esophagitis from gastroesophageal reflux disease and other conditions remains unproven.

Immunohistochemical stains targeting eosinophil peroxidase, major basic protein, and eosinophil-derived neurotoxin, have been reported to enhance detection of eosinophils compared to evaluation of H&E sections, but these stains are not widely used in routine clinical practice. A recent study suggested that the presence of intra-squamous IgG4 deposits by immunohistochemistry may be a useful adjunctive marker for EOE.

Molecular analyses of esophageal tissues, such as gene expression analysis of chemokines such as eotaxin-3 (CCL26), and transcriptome analysis show promise to improve diagnosis and clinical monitoring, and to guide patient-specific therapy.

Differential Diagnosis

Clinical

Dysphagia and rings in the esophagus can occur from any inflammatory condition. Even eosinophils may be present in GERD alone. EOE typically requires a confirmatory biopsy from the upper and lower esophagus showing eosinophilic infiltrates. Desquamative conditions that should be excluded include bullous pemphigoid and lichen planus. These typically require deep biopsies and special immunofluorescence staining; thus, communication between endoscopist and pathologist is critical.

Microscopic

The histologic appearance of EOE is not specific, and mucosal infiltration by eosinophils is a component of a variety of other esophageal inflammatory conditions (Table 2.4).

GERD and PPI-responsive esophageal eosinophilia exhibit considerable histologic overlap with EOE. In an untreated patient, fewer numbers of eosinophils with distal predominance may be suggestive of GERD. Correlation with response to PPI therapy is paramount.

In eosinophilic gastroenteritis, obtaining biopsy specimens from the stomach and duodenum and other clinical symptoms such as nausea, vomiting, and diarrhea may be helpful in establishing a diagnosis.

The presence of granulomas is helpful in diagnosing esophageal involvement by Crohn's disease, but they are uncommon. Eosinophils may also be admixed with neutrophils and lymphocytes, and involvement of other parts of the GI tract is typically present.

Infections are recognized by the identification of viral inclusions (such as HSV), and fungal or parasitic organisms. Mixed inflammation with neutrophils may also be present. Rare cases of HSV esophagitis occurring in a background of EOE have been described.

Table 2.4 Endoscopic and histologic features of the major causes of infectious esophagitis.

Organism	Endoscopic features	Morphological features	Ancillary studies
Candida	Focal or confluent white plaques	Parakeratosis with neutrophils Colonization of ulcers Budding yeast, pseudohyphae, occasional septate hyphae Superficial invasion typical	PAS-diastase, GMS stains
Herpes simplex	Superficial ulcers, multiple	Edge of ulcer—inclusions in squamous cells and/or squamous debris of ulcer slough Multinucleation, ground glass nuclei, dense eosinophilic nuclear inclusions (Cowdry type A)	IHC
CMV	Single deep ulcer, linear ulcers	Base of ulcer—inclusions in endothelial and stromal cells Intranuclear ("owl's eye") and granular cytoplasmic inclusions Atypical inclusions common	IHC

Table 2.5 Conditions associated with esophageal eosinophilia in the differential diagnosis of EOE.

GERD
PPI-responsive esophageal eosinophilia
Eosinophilic gastrointestinal diseases
Crohn's disease
Infection (*Candida*, HSV, parasites)
Hypereosinophilic syndrome
Achalasia
Drug hypersensitivity injury
Vasculitis
Pemphigus
Connective tissue diseases
Graft versus host disease (GVHD)

In drug-induced esophageal eosinophilia, there is a temporal relationship and resolution when the offending agent is withdrawn.

Ancillary Studies (if Applicable)

IHC for virus (HSV) and/or special stains for fungi (GMS, PAS-diastase) are indicated if infection is suspected.

Prognosis, Evolution, and Clinical Management

EOE is initially treated with proton pump inhibitors. There is emerging evidence that PPIs affect specific inhibition of the chemokine, eotaxin, which blunts eosinophil infiltration. It may be difficult to distinguish GERD-associated eosinophilia from EOE in this subgroup. For those that do not respond to PPI, options include identification and avoidance of food antigens (typically through a Six Food Elimination Diet; SFED) or suppression with topical corticosteroids, which can be from a swallowed metered dose inhaler, or from peroral viscous budesonide. For late-stage, fibrotic disease, repeated, carefully monitored esophageal dilation is effective.

Lymphocytic Esophagitis

Definition, General Features, Predisposing Factors

This uncommon and poorly characterized condition is histologically defined as the presence of dense lymphocytic infiltrates involving the esophageal mucosa without concomitant evidence of significant active inflammation. It is described in approximately 1/1000 esophageal biopsies, predominantly affecting older females (median age 63 years). This controversial entity lacks clearly defined clinical associations in adults, and likely represents a nonspecific reaction pattern to a wide variety of mucosal insults (Table 2.6), including GERD, medications, infection, motility disorders, and other immune-mediated disorders. In the pediatric population, lymphocytic esophagitis has been described in association with Crohn's disease and celiac disease.

Clinical and Endoscopic Characteristics

About 75% of patients present with esophageal symptoms, most commonly dysphagia or odynophagia, which may raise the suspicion of eosinophilic esophagitis. Similarly, the endoscopic impression may suggest eosinophilic esophagitis, with the presence of rings, furrows, plaques, and strictures.

Table 2.6 Conditions associated with esophageal lymphocytosis (lymphocytic esophagitis).

GERD
Medications
Infection
Motility disorders
Immune-mediated disorders (e.g. CVID)
Lichen planus/lichenoid esophagitis
Crohn's disease (pediatric)
Celiac disease (pediatric)

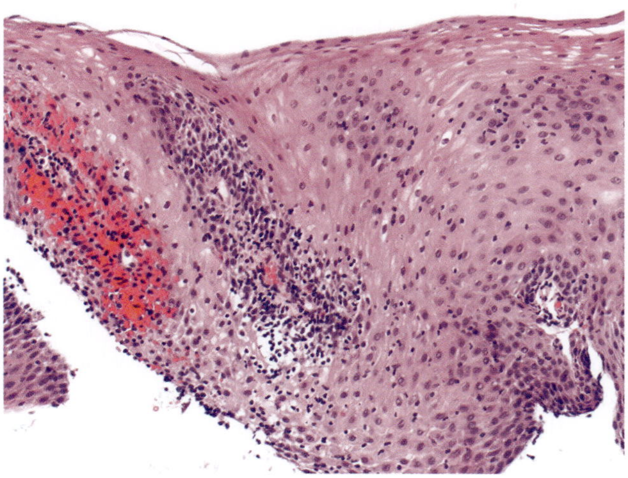

Figure 2.14 Characteristic histology of lymphocytic esophagitis.

Microscopic Features

Recently proposed histologic criteria include the presence of dense lymphocytic infiltrates involving esophageal squamous mucosa with marked spongiosis in the absence of significant numbers of neutrophils or eosinophils (Figure 2.14). The findings are most pronounced in the peripapillary epithelium. There is no required or established "minimum" count or density of intraepithelial lymphocytes, and the pattern and distribution of the lymphocytic epithelial injury is most important.

Immunohistochemical Studies and Molecular Features

Ancillary testing, including the subtyping of the intraepithelial CD3, CD4, and CD8 T cells is generally noncontributory and not required for the diagnosis. A subset of cases with CD4 predominant T cells and dysmotility has been reported.

Differential Diagnosis

The clinical and endoscopic differential diagnosis includes EOE, although by definition eosinophils are rare or absent. If neutrophils are present, special stains for candida may be warranted. Intraepithelial lymphocytes may be prominent in lichen planus esophagitis/lichenoid esophagitis, although the additional presence of a band-like lymphocytic infiltrate in the lamina propria and necrotic keratinocytes is a distinguishing feature. Characteristic direct immunofluorescence findings of lichen planus DIF may or may not be demonstrated. Lymphocytosis may also be associated with esophageal involvement by Crohn's disease in children, although other histologic and clinical features of Crohn's disease are typically present, particularly elsewhere in the gut.

Prognosis

Follow-up clinical and biopsy data are limited, although in some patients sequential biopsies have demonstrated persistent lymphocytosis, suggesting a chronic process.

Drug-Induced Esophagitis

Definition, General Features, Predisposing Factors

Medication-related injury to the esophageal mucosa ("pill esophagitis") is an increasingly recognized complication of orally administered drugs. Mucosal injury is typically caused by prolonged direct contact and local caustic effects of the offending agent, although mechanisms of toxicity may be complex and multifactorial. Numerous drugs have been implicated (Table 2.7). Most cause a nonspecific injury pattern, and the diagnosis is suggested by the clinical history.

Elderly patients and women are most commonly affected. The elderly often have multiple underlying risk factors, and the female predominance is attributed to the more common use of certain medications in this group, such as iron supplements and bisphosphonates. Risk factors include pills taken with little or no water or while recumbent, underlying disorders of esophageal motility (e.g. diabetes, strictures, achalasia) and disorders of local anatomy causing external compression (enlarged left atrium, aortic aneurism). However, many patients do not exhibit abnormal esophageal function or other risk factors.

Clinical and Endoscopic Characteristics

Typically, there is a temporal relationship between the onset of symptoms and ingestion of a potentially injurious drug. Common symptoms include sudden-onset chest

Table 2.7 Medications implicated in causing esophagitis and histologic features.

Medication	Histologic features
NSAIDs	Nonspecific, ± crystalline debris
Antibiotics (e.g. tetracyclines/doxycycline, clindamycin)	Doxycycline—vascular injury
Potassium chloride	Nonspecific
Iron	Bluish-brown crystalline debris, Fe stain +
Bisphosphonates (e.g. alendronate)	Nonspecific, ± crystalline debris and multinucleated squamous cells
Quinidine	Nonspecific
Resins (e.g. kayexalate, bile acid sequestrants)	Kayexalate: Basophilic crystals with "fish scales," AFB (black), PAD, Diff-quick bile acid sequestrants: Orange-black crystals, lack "fish scales," AFB (yellow)
Mycophenolate	Increased apoptosis (GVHD-like)
Taxanes	Mitotic arrest, ring mitoses

pain, odynophagia and/or dysphagia that occur within a few hours or days after taking the medication. Severe reflux injury is often an initial diagnostic concern. The chest pain may be pleuritic in nature, mimicking a pulmonary embolism, or may suggest an acute cardiac syndrome. Hematemesis and perforation are rare complications.

Endoscopically, most lesions occur in the middle third of the esophagus, at the level of the aortic arch, although any level may be involved. Findings include erythema, erosions, ulcers (including "kissing" ulcers), and strictures. Discrete erosions in this region, away from the Z-line, are an important clue suggesting a drug-related etiology (Figure 2.15). Occasionally, a diffuse mucosal sloughing pattern has been described.

Microscopic Features (Table 2.7)

Biopsies most commonly show nonspecific esophagitis characterized by erosions, ulcers, active inflammation with neutrophils and occasionally eosinophils, surface epithelial damage, and granulation tissue. Adjacent mucosa is relatively normal. A careful search of the exudate and ulcer bed for refractile or polarizable foreign material is warranted, which may be an important diagnostic clue. However, in most cases the clinical history is necessary to make the diagnosis.

Some medications are associated with additional characteristic histologic features. Erosions and ulcers associated

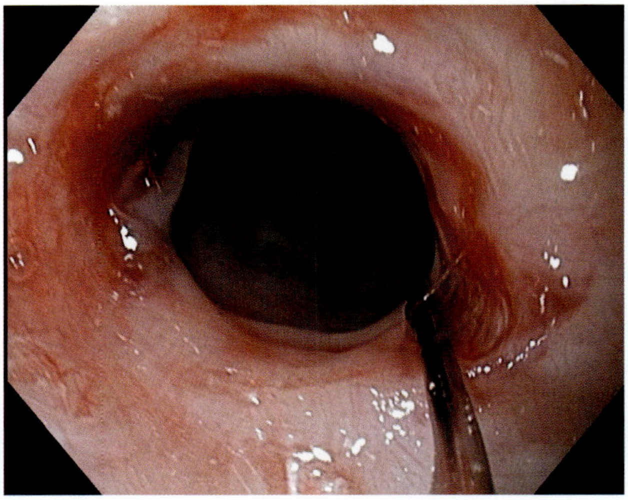

Figure 2.15 Endoscopic appearance of inflammatory stricture of the esophagus with sloughing mucosa.

with doxycycline injury often exhibit a distinct capillary/vascular injury with degenerative changes and possible fibrin thrombi. In iron pill-associated mucosal injury, bluish-brown crystalline iron debris is found adjacent to the surface epithelium, admixed with the inflammatory exudate, or within granulation tissue (Figure 2.16). The iron can be highlighted by a Prussian Blue stain, which may also demonstrate crystalline debris in the lamina propria or underlying vessels. Although iron is well recognized as a caustic agent in the esophagus and elsewhere in the GI tract, some cases may represent secondary deposition in preexisting lesions. Alendronate has been associated with multinucleated squamous cells, in addition to the presence of polarizable crystalline material.

Kayexalate (sodium polystyrene sulfonate) in sorbitol can be recognized by the presence of characteristic lightly basophilic, refractile, nonpolarizable crystals that display a mosaic pattern that resembles fish scales. The crystals can be highlighted by acid fast (black), PAS/Alcian blue and Diff-Quik stains. Bile acid sequestrants (e.g. colestipol, colesevelam, cholestyramine) may be recognized by their orange-black crystals, which lack a striated, fish-scale appearance and may appear pale yellow on acid fast stain.

Mycophenolate, used in solid organ transplantation, is associated with increased apoptosis of esophageal squamous epithelial cells, resembling GVHD. Taxane-based chemotherapy leads to striking mitotic arrest with ring mitoses, along with epithelial necrosis or ulceration.

Differential Diagnosis

The major histologic differential diagnostic consideration is infection, particularly fungal (*Candida*) or viral (HSV, CMV), which may need to be excluded with appropriate histochemical and immunohistochemical stains or

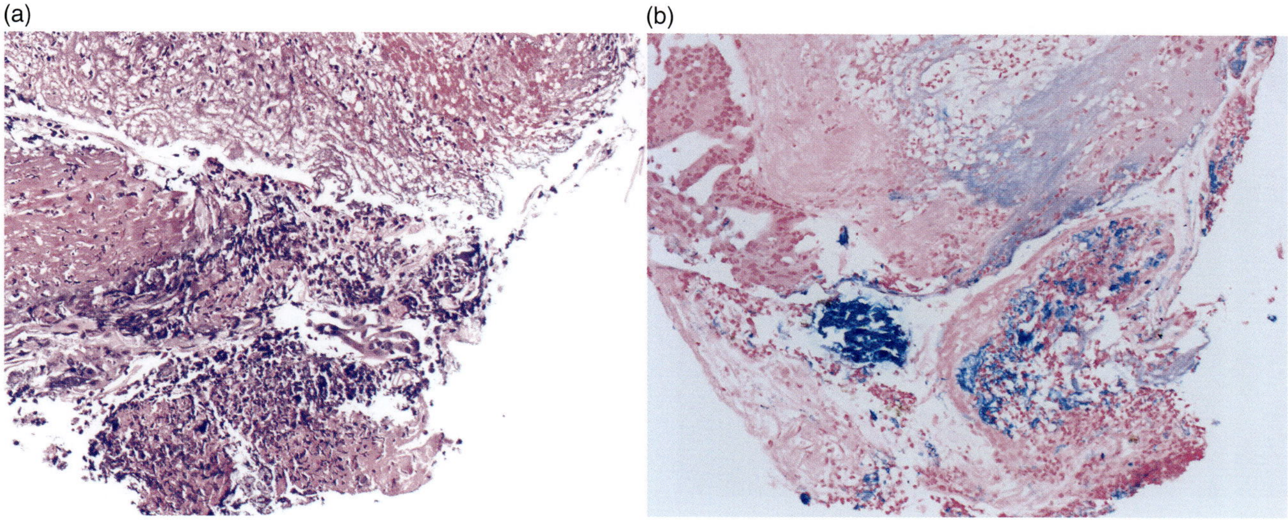

Figure 2.16 (a) Iron tablet erosive esophagitis with fibrinopurulent debris. (b) The Prussian Blue iron stain is diagnostic.

recognized by characteristic viral cytopathic effect. In rare cases, exuberant granulation tissue and excessive exudates mimic the gross appearance of a neoplasm. If eosinophils are prominent, reflux or eosinophilic esophagitis may enter into the differential diagnosis. GVHD should be excluded if prominent apoptosis is present, such as with mycophenolate injury. Finally, lichen planus involvement of the proximal esophagus with stricture formation can also mimic drug injury. In all of these considerations, the clinical context is critical to the evaluation of the histopathologic findings.

Prognosis, Evolution and Clinical Management

Most cases are self-limited and resolve without complications. Discontinuing the suspected caustic agent and supportive management, such as PPI therapy, hydration, sucralfate, or topical anesthetics, typically results in an uneventful recovery. Local epinephrine may be needed for active bleeding. Dilatation may be required if strictures develop, and surgical management is rarely needed for severe complications such as perforation. Most patients can resume their medications with recommendations for proper administration, which will assist in avoiding recurrent injury.

Sloughing Esophagitis

Definition, General Features, Predisposing Factors

Sloughing esophagitis is characterized by extensive superficial squamous mucosal necrosis or desquamation, associated with endoscopic plaques imparting a sloughing appearance to the mucosa. Sloughing esophagitis has also been included under the terms esophagitis dissecans superficialis and acute necrotizing esophagitis, which includes broader inclusion criteria and more diverse causes of esophageal injury. It occurs in middle-aged to older adults (median age 56 years), frequently with debilitating comorbidities and who are commonly on multiple medications, especially central nervous system depressants and drugs known to cause esophageal mucosal injury. It most likely represents a form of direct contact injury, rather than an ischemic injury, and may represent a unique pattern of drug-induced esophagitis. Acute necrotizing esophagitis ("black esophagus") is a rare condition that arises in debilitated patients with severe comorbidities such as hypoperfusion, sepsis, diabetic ketoacidosis, and malignancy, and results from the combining effect of ischemia and corrosive injury of gastric contents. A rare case occurring in a child who was associated with a history of vomiting has also been reported.

Clinical and Endoscopic Characteristics

Dysphagia, odynophagia, chest pain, heartburn, vomiting or cough are reported in 45% of patients, include. The mid-distal esophagus is most commonly involved. Endoscopy reveals white plaques or membranes, and there may be sloughing of the epithelium as well as other nonspecific findings such as erythema, erosions, rings, or webs. In black esophagus, the sloughing necrotic membrane may appear blackened (Figure 2.17). The clinical presentation is distinctive with bleeding and a characteristic diffuse circumferential black mucosal discoloration of the distal esophagus with an abrupt transition at the gastroesophageal junction.

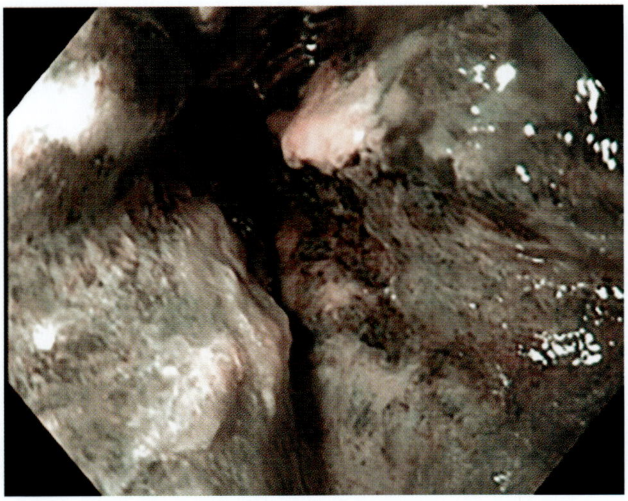

Figure 2.17 Endoscopic appearance of necrotizing esophagitis with appearance of "black esophagus."

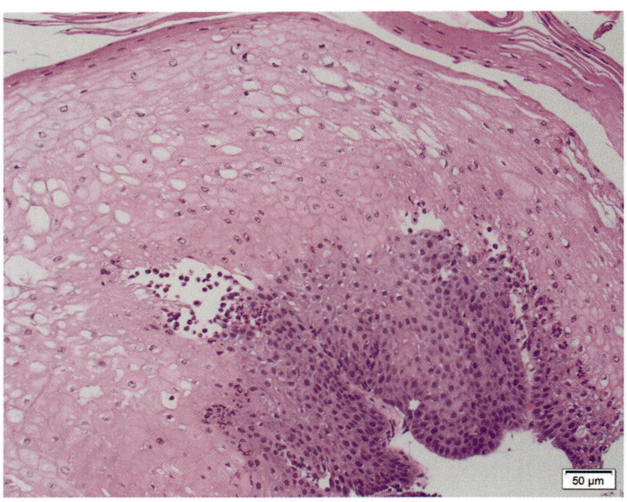

Figure 2.18 Characteristic appearance of sloughing esophagitis with two-tone appearance of the esophageal mucosa.

Microscopic Features

Biopsies show a two-toned appearance, with a superficial zone of necrotic, eosinophilic squamous epithelium and underlying intact squamous mucosa that appears normal or reactive. The necrotic epithelial layer may be partially or completely detached and exhibits pyknotic, parakeratosis-like or faded, ghost-like nuclei. In some cases a neutrophilic infiltrate is seen between the epithelial layers, ranging from mild to severe (Figure 2.18). In black esophagus, biopsies show necrotic squamous epithelium and mucosa, with possible involvement of submucosa. Pill fragments and surface colonization by bacteria or fungal yeasts have also been described.

Immunohistochemical Studies and Molecular Features

Ancillary studies may be necessary to exclude differential diagnostic considerations including special stains for fungal organisms, viruses or direct immunofluorescence for skin disease-associated esophagitis (see below).

Differential Diagnosis

The differential diagnosis includes disorders that may exhibit histologic epithelial necrosis and/or endoscopic plaques. *Candida* esophagitis may exhibit similar white plaques endoscopically. Histologically, the plaques appear flaky and less compact, and special stains (GMS, PAS) are diagnostic. Pill-induced esophagitis is more often associated with nonspecific mucosal ulcers. Corrosive or caustic injury, such as alkali (lye) or acid ingestion, typically shows extensive edema, erythema, and hemorrhage in addition to necrotic exudates. Clinical history is key and the mucosa is seldom biopsied. Esophageal involvement by cutaneous bullous disorders may need to be excluded by immunofluorescence studies for IgG and C3. Severe eosinophilic esophagitis may also exhibit sloughing membranes, but is recognized by the marked intraepithelial eosinophilic infiltration. Black esophagus (i.e. acute esophageal necrosis) is a rare condition that arises in debilitated patients with multiple comorbidities such as hypoperfusion, sepsis, diabetic ketoacidosis, and malignancy. It results from the combining effect of ischemia and corrosive injury of gastric contents. The clinical presentation is distinctive with bleeding and a characteristic diffuse circumferential black mucosal discoloration of the distal esophagus with an abrupt transition at the gastroesophageal junction.

Prognosis, Evolution and Management

The clinical course and outcome in patients with sloughing esophagitis is primarily related to the presence of significant underlying diseases. In the few patients with follow-up biopsies documented, most have shown endoscopic and histologic resolution.

Graft Versus Host Disease of the Esophagus

Definition, General Features, Predisposing Factors

Graft versus host disease (GVHD) is an important complication of allogeneic stem cell transplantation, leading to considerable morbidity and mortality. Gastrointestinal tract involvement is frequent, and endoscopy with biopsy plays a central role in the diagnosis and management of patients with suspected GVHD. Although the pathologic features of GVHD are well described in glandular mucosa, they are less so for the esophagus. Manifestations of esophageal injury may occur in the acute or chronic phases of GVHD. Diagnosis requires correlation of the clinical and pathologic features.

Clinical and Endoscopic Characteristics

Symptoms of esophageal GVHD include dysphagia and odynophagia. Endoscopically, acute presentations of GVHD have been described as showing bullous disease or a desquamative process with mucosal cast formation (Figure 2.19). In the chronic phase, the presence of webs, strictures, or concentric rings involving the mid-upper esophagus on EGD or barium contrast imaging are considered diagnostic features (Figure 2.20).

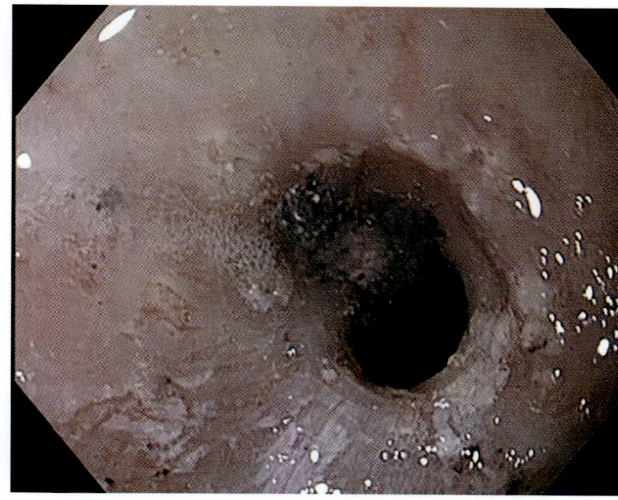

Figure 2.20 Endoscopic appearance of inflammatory stricture with persistent desquamation in chronic esophageal GVHD.

Microscopic Features

The histologic features of esophageal GVHD are similar to those of other sites in the GI tract. The squamous epithelium exhibits apoptosis, intraepithelial lymphocytosis, basal vacuolization, and necrosis in severe cases (Figure 2.21). Apoptotic keratinocytes are prominent in the basal and suprabasal region and the associated lymphocytosis can have a lichenoid interface appearance. The extent of the findings can be graded as mild, moderate, or severe. Severe GVHD is characterized by erosion and/or ulceration. Involvement of deeper layers with submucosal fibrosis has been described in chronic GVHD, but this layer is seldom represented in biopsy samples. Due to potential discordance among the observed clinical severity, endoscopic abnormalities, and histologic findings, it is recommended that a minimum of 8–10 serial H&E stained sections be cut to detect minimal histologic changes of GVHD. Finally, comparison to prior biopsies should be noted in order to assess treatment effects.

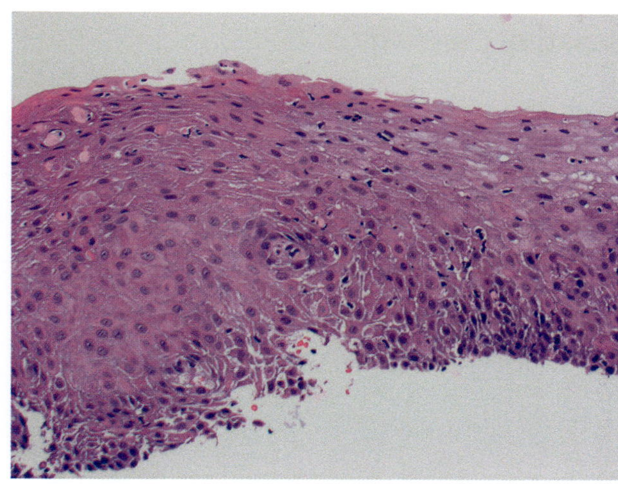

Figure 2.21 Microscopic appearance of acute GVHD of esophagus with basal apoptosis, lymphocytic infiltration, and dyskeratotic epithelial elements.

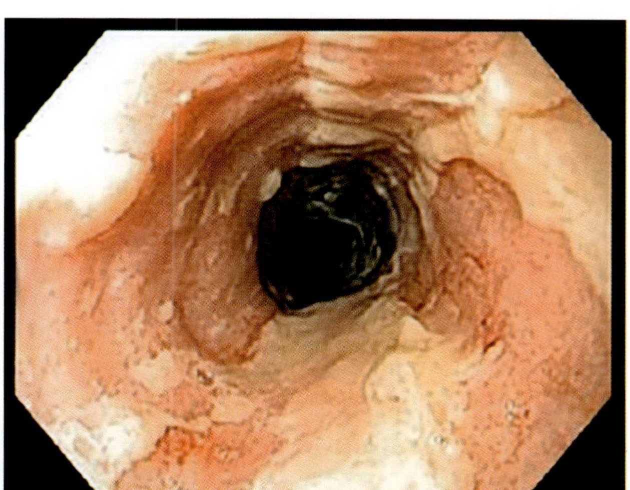

Figure 2.19 Endoscopic appearance of acute GVHD of esophagus with diffuse mucosal desquamation.

Differential Diagnosis

The major differential diagnostic considerations include other types of esophageal mucosal injury that may lead to increased apoptosis, such as drug or infection. Knowledge of the clinical context is important, as epithelial apoptosis in the setting of stem cell transplantation likely represents GVHD, whereas mycophenolate-associated injury occurs in solid organ transplant recipients. Cytomegalovirus infection also causes apoptosis, and may coexist with GVHD, necessitating immunohistochemical staining for exclusion. In cases where bullae or desquamation is observed endoscopically, the differential diagnosis may also include other vesiculobullous dermatologic disorders involving the esophagus.

Prognosis, Evolution, and Clinical Management

Systemic immunomodulatory therapy is indicated for patients with moderate to severe GHVD. Corticosteroids are used as first-line therapy, and other agents considered as options in an algorithmic approach.

Radiation Esophagitis

Definition, General Features, Predisposing Factors

Radiation injury to the esophagus is a dose-limiting toxicity occurring as either an acute or late complication of radiation therapy of thoracic neoplasms. The risk of radiation esophagitis is increased by concurrent chemotherapy and radiation dose–volumetric parameters, which may be related to underlying vascular changes and ischemic injury. Overall, symptomatic radiation esophagitis is rare, affecting <1% of treated patients.

Clinical and Endoscopic Characteristics

Patients with acute esophageal radiation toxicity (which develops within two to three weeks of exposure) complain of dysphagia, odynophagia, and/or substernal chest pain. Late manifestations (≥3 months) include stricture formation, chronic ulcerations, and fistula formation. Endoscopic abnormalities, depending on the time course, include mucositis, ulceration, strictures, or fistulas.

Microscopic Features

Macrocytic changes and cytologic atypia of squamous epithelial cells and stromal cells are common, often associated with multinucleation and bizarre hyperchromatic nuclei. Notably, the cells maintain an abundant cytoplasm and mitosis is rare. Submucosal fibrosis and obliterative vasculitis may also be evident in deeper biopsy specimens.

Immunohistochemical Studies and Molecular Features

Immunohistochemical stains may be useful in the differential diagnosis of viral esophagitis.

Differential Diagnosis

The squamous epithelial cytologic atypia may mimic carcinoma, which can be of particular concern for recurrent or persistent tumor in patients being treated for primary esophageal carcinomas, as radiation changes and neoplasia can coexist. Review of the prior tumor histology, if available, and assessment for evidence of invasion can be helpful.

The nuclear changes may also resemble viral infection, particularly *Herpes simplex*, which can be excluded by appropriate immunohistochemical stains for HSV.

Prognosis, Evolution and Clinical Management

The outcome is dependent on the radiation dose and the overall severity of injury. The lesion may heal completely, although severe injury may lead to chronic ulcers, strictures, and fistulas. Oral glutamine therapy may have a protective effect during therapy. Radiation-induced esophageal carcinoma may also be a late complication of therapy for extraesophageal thoracic tumors. Endoscopic dilation and stenting may be required to maintain luminal patency.

Dermatological Diseases Involving the Esophagus

Definition, General Features, Predisposing Factors

The esophagus may be involved in multiple primary dermatologic conditions (Table 2.8). Esophageal manifestation may develop in the presence or absence of skin lesions. As these disorders are generally not well recognized by

Table 2.8 Dermatologic diseases involving the esophagus.

Lichen planus
Bullous diseases
Pemphigus vulgaris
Bullous pemphigoid
Epidermolysis bullosa acquisita
Behcet's syndrome
Toxic epidermal necrolysis/Stevens–Johnson syndrome
Scleroderma

both gastroenterologists and pathologists, they may be overlooked for some time and the diagnosis delayed with potentially important consequences.

Lichen planus involving the esophagus is rare and can occur in conjunction with other mucosal (or cutaneous) lesions or as the sole manifestation. It is predominantly seen in middle-aged women. Oral involvement coexists with skin lesions in approximately 30–50% of patients. Lichenoid esophagitis refers to a subset of patients with an identical lichen planus pattern of histologic injury without oral or cutaneous lesions, negative immunofluorescence studies and some distinct demographics, such as polypharmacy and an association with viral hepatitis or HIV.

The bullous diseases are also difficult to diagnose in the esophagus and correlation of the findings with the clinical manifestations, separate biopsies of the skin lesions, and ancillary immunofluorescence studies can help secure the diagnosis. Pemphigus vulgaris is the most common of the autoimmune mucocutaneous diseases with bulla formation. Men and women are affected equally, with a predominance of middle-aged to elderly individuals, although often asymptomatic, esophageal involvement can be demonstrated in the majority of patients if sought by endoscopy and biopsy. Pemphigus vulgaris is caused by loss of integrity of the normal intercellular attachments within the mucosal epithelium resulting in intramucosal bullae of various sizes. Although esophageal involvement may be a frequent occurrence in active mucocutaneous disease, it may also rarely occur as the sole or initial manifestation.

Bullous pemphigoid is a chronic, immune-mediated, subepidermal blistering skin disease that rarely involves mucosal surfaces and affects the esophagus less commonly than pemphigus vulgaris. It primarily affects patients in the fifth through seventh decades.

Epidermolysis bullosa is a diverse group of inherited skin disorders caused by mutations of genes that encode for structural proteins located at the dermal-epidermal junction. The patients characteristically develop blisters after minor trauma, with a range of clinical phenotypes and severity. Minor trauma from a food bolus may elicit similar esophageal mucosal injury.

There are also rare reports of Behcet's disease involving the esophagus, ranging from asymptomatic to severe stricturing disease. In scleroderma, dysmotility-associated esophageal inflammatory injury is due primarily to reflux and/or candidiasis.

Clinical and Endoscopic Characteristics

Endoscopic evaluation often plays a central role in the evaluation of patients with suspected esophageal manifestations of these dermatologic diseases, although in some cases the procedure must be approached with caution, particularly in the bullous or blistering disorders.

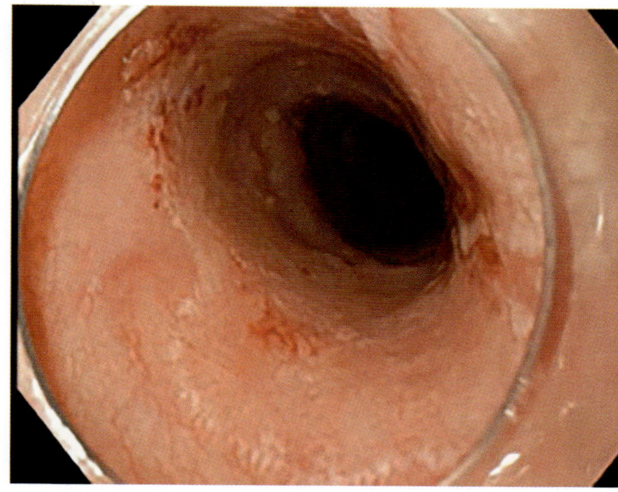

Figure 2.22 Endoscopic appearance of esophageal lichen planus with diffuse mucosal plaques.

In lichen planus, dysphagia and esophageal strictures may clinically suggest GERD. Magnification chromoendoscopy was used in one study showing a high prevalence of esophageal disease. Mucosal stripping, hyperemia, and submucosal plaques (Figure 2.22) are typically limited to the upper and mid-esophagus.

Odynophagia and dysphagia are the usual symptoms of esophageal pemphigus vulgaris, as well as the other mucosal blistering diseases. Endoscopic diagnosis involves both evaluation of the appearance of the lesions and tissue sampling. The mucosa may initially appear normal, with the subsequent appearance of erosions, diffuse longitudinal erythematous lines, or mucosal sloughing. Induction of bullae in normal mucosa by the endoscope (Nikolsky's sign) may be observed.

The esophagus is among the most common sites of GI involvement in epidermolysis bullosa, manifested by symptoms of dysphagia and odynophagia. Clinical phenotypes range from mild to severe with bullae and blister formation, ulceration, scarring, webs, and strictures, most commonly involving the proximal esophagus. The trauma of a food bolus, or the endoscope itself, may precipitate of exacerbate bullae and ulcer formation.

Microscopic and Immunofluorescence Features

In addition to hematoxylin and eosin stained sections, immunofluorescence (IF) studies can be of diagnostic value for the diagnosis of lichen planus and vesiculobullous disorders (Table 2.9). If suspected, additional biopsy samples should be submitted fresh or in an appropriate IF transport medium (e.g. Michel's or Zeus)

Table 2.9 Histologic features of bullous diseases involving the esophagus.

	Cleft	Inflammation	Ancillary IF
Pemphigus vulgaris	Suprabasal with acantholysis	Mixed, with eosinophils	Intracellular IgG and C3
Bullous pemphigoid	Subepithelial	Neutrophils, eosinophils, fibrin, red blood cells	Linear basement membrane IgG and C3
Epidermolysis bullosa	Subepithelial	Minimal or absent	N/A

In lichen planus of the esophagus, the histologic features more closely resemble those seen in oral, rather than cutaneous disease. The characteristic histologic features include a prominent band-like lymphocytic infiltrate involving the epithelium and lamina propria, acanthotic or atrophic mucosal changes, and scattered degenerated or apoptotic keratinocytes (Civatte bodies). The latter are an important diagnostic feature of lichen planus and a distinguishing characteristic from lymphocytic esophagitis. Immunofluorescence studies showing globular IgM deposits at the epithelial-subepithelial junction along with complement staining in apoptotic squamous cells, similar to cutaneous findings, may be useful in establishing the diagnosis.

Histologically, pemphigus vulgaris is characterized by the presence of suprabasal clefting and intraepithelial blisters due to prominent acantholysis. The intact basal epithelial cells may appear similar to a row of tombstones at the base of the cleft. The blister may be accompanied by a mild superficial mixed inflammatory infiltrate, which includes eosinophils. Immunofluorescence shows characteristic intercellular deposition of IgG and C3, although the results can be negative in early stages or in disease remission.

Bullous pemphigoid shows subepithelial clefting, often containing a mixture of fibrin, red cells, neutrophils, and eosinophils. Immunofluorescence studies may demonstrate the deposition of complement components (typically C3), and linear deposits of IgG at the level of the basement membrane, although these studies may be of limited value if the mucosa has been extensively eroded.

In epidermolysis bullosa, the lesions are thought to be similar to those found in the skin, with the esophageal mucosa exhibiting a subepithelial cleavage plane, with little or no associated inflammatory infiltrate.

Differential Diagnosis

The differential diagnosis of lichen planus includes other disorders that may show intraepithelial lymphocytic infiltration, such as drug injury, reflux, infections, Crohn's disease and lymphocytic esophagitis. Clinical correlation is necessary, with particular attention to other mucocutaneous findings, medication or IBD history, location of injury, and response to therapy.

Differentiating bullous diseases from sloughing esophagitis requires clinical and/or IF correlation.

Prognosis, Evolution, and Clinical Management

Esophageal lichen planus has a tendency to cause persistent dysphagia and stricture formation. Systemic treatment is usually required to prevent stricturing disease. Injection of corticosteroids and a response to oral fluticasone have been reported. Squamous cell dysplasia and carcinoma can develop and long-term follow-up is advised.

Mucosal pemphigus vulgaris may remain localized to the mucous membranes or progress to skin involvement. Corticosteroids and immunosuppressive agents are considered first-line treatments.

In epidermolysis bullosa, stricturing disease is common and treatment is symptomatic. Although these patients are at increased risk of skin cancer, esophageal carcinoma is rarely reported.

Scleroderma-associated chronic GERD can lead to Barrett's esophagus with an increased risk of esophageal adenocarcinoma.

Esophagitis and Inflammatory Bowel Disease

Definition, General Features, Predisposing Factors

Isolated esophageal Crohn's disease is rare, and usually associated with established extraesophageal disease. Endoscopic studies report a prevalence of esophageal involvement between 0.2 and 11% in adults with Crohn's disease. However, in children up to 43% may show histological esophageal involvement on mucosal biopsy.

Esophageal inflammation has been documented in patients with ulcerative colitis, although there have been no documented patterns that occur more commonly in ulcerative colitis than in controls.

Clinical and Endoscopic Characteristics

The most common clinical presentation in Crohn's disease is dysphagia. However, esophageal symptoms may be absent or not correlate well with the endoscopic or biopsy findings. In fact, upper gastrointestinal symptoms related to involvement of other organs may predominate.

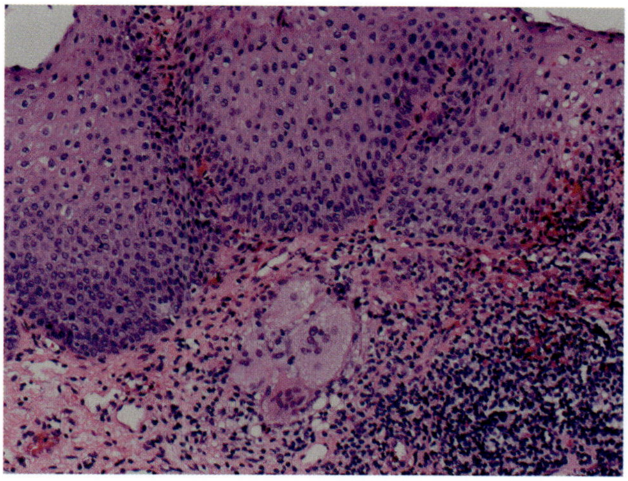

Figure 2.23 Esophageal granuloma in a previously diagnosed patient with Crohn's disease.

Endoscopically, the mid- to distal esophagus is most commonly involved. Findings may include erythema, erythematous nodules, single or multiple erosions, and aphthous or deep punched-out ulcers, which may mimic pill-induced esophagitis, but are usually differentiated by the extensive mucosal involvement. Strictures and fistulas may occur.

Microscopic Features

Histologic features can be found in asymptomatic patients (particularly children) and those with endoscopically normal appearing mucosa. Therefore biopsies are an important diagnostic tool. The findings include focal active mucosal infiltration with neutrophils and eosinophils, erosions, and ulceration. Erosions and ulcers are associated with an inflammatory infiltrate of the lamina propria and submucosa, which may contain histiocytes or small, poorly formed granulomas (Figure 2.23). Epithelioid granulomas are documented in up to 39% of esophageal biopsies, and in the proper clinical setting the presence of granulomas is considered diagnostic of Crohn's esophagitis. Transmural inflammation has been documented in surgical specimens.

Crohn's disease has also been associated with lymphocytic and eosinophilic esophagitis patterns of mucosal inflammation. The lymphocytic pattern is entirely nonspecific. Crohn's disease-related eosinophilic inflammation may be similar to allergic eosinophilic esophagitis, although the underlying immunologic mechanisms appear to differ.

Differential Diagnosis

The histological differential diagnosis includes lymphocytic esophagitis, eosinophilic esophagitis, certain infections (fungal, mycobacterial), and pill esophagitis. The clinical context as well as corroborating histological abnormalities in other mucosal biopsies is a key consideration. Special stains may be indicated to exclude infectious agents.

Prognosis, Evolution, and Clinical Management

Esophageal Crohn's disease is unlikely to progress or lead to recurrent esophageal lesions or symptoms during subsequent disease exacerbations. Esophageal symptoms, when present, typically improve with therapy. Some patients may require dilatation for strictures, or surgery for complications such as fistulae or abscesses.

Further Reading

Abid, S., Mumtaz, K., Jafri, W. et al. (2005). Pill-induced esophageal injury: endoscopic features and clinical outcomes. *Endoscopy* 37: 740–744.

Abraham, S.C., Yardley, J.H., and Wu, T. (1999). Erosive injury to the upper gastrointestinal tract in patients receiving iron medication: an underrecognized entitiy. *Am. J. Surg. Pathol.* 23: 1241–1247.

Abraham, S.C., Cruz-Correa, M., Lee, L. et al. (1999). Alendronate-associated esophageal injury: pathologic and endoscopic features. *Mod. Pathol.* 12: 1152–1157.

Abraham, S.C., Ravish, W.J., Anhalt, G.J. et al. (2000). Esophageal lichen planus: case report and review of the literature. *Am. J. Surg. Pathol.* 24: 1678–1682.

Abraham, S.C., Bhagavan, B., Lee, L. et al. (2001). Upper gastrointestinal tract injury in patients receiving Kayexalate (sodium polystyrene sulfonate) in sorbitol. *Am. J. Surg. Pathol.* 25: 637–644.

Aceves, S.S., Newbury, R.O., Dohil, R. et al. (2007). Distinguishing eosinophilic esophagitis in pediatric patients: clinical, endoscopic, and histologic features of an emerging disorder. *J. Clin. Gastroenterol.* 41: 252–256.

Adler, D.G., Farraye, F.A., and Crawford, J.M. (2015). Gastrointestinal tract endoscopic and tissue processing techniques and normal histology. In: *Surgical Pathology of the GI Tract, Liver Biliary Tract, and Pancreas*, 3e (eds. R.D. Odze and J.R. Goldblum), 4–33. Philadelphia: Saunders.

Almashat, S.J., Duan, L., and Goldsmith, J.D. (2014). Non-reflux esophagitis: a review of inflammatory diseases of the esophagus exclusive of reflux esophagitis. *Semin. Diagn. Pathol.* 31: 89–99.

Armstrong, D., Bennett, J.R., Blum, A.L. et al. (1996). The endoscopic assessment of esophagitis: a progress report on observer agreement. *Gastroenterology* 111: 85–92.

Arnold, M.A., Swanson, B.J., Crowder, C.D. et al. (2014). Colesevelam and colestipol: novel medication resins in the gastrointestinal tract. *Am. J. Surg. Pathol.* 38: 1530–1537.

Attwood, S.E., Smyrk, T.C., Demeester, T.R., and Jones, J.B. (1993). Esophageal eosinophilia with dysphagia. A distinct clinicopathologic syndrome. *Dig. Dis. Sci.* 38: 109–116.

Basseri, B., Levy, M., Wang, H.L. et al. (2010). Redefining the role of lymphocytes in gastroesophageal reflux disease and eosinophilic esophagitis. *Dis. Esophagus* 23: 368–376.

Bennett, A.E., Goldblum, J.R., and Odze, R.D. (2009). Inflammatory disorders of the esophagus. In: *Surgical Pathology of the GI Tract, Liver, Biliary Tract and Pancreas*, 2e (eds. R.D. Odze and J.R. Goldblum), 231–267. Saunders Elsevier: Phildelphia.

Bennett, A.E., Goldblum, J.R., and Odze, R.D. (2015). Inflammatory disorders of the esophagus. In: *Surgical Pathology of the GI Tract, Liver Biliary Tract, and Pancreas*, 3e (eds. R.D. Odze and J.R. Goldblum), 311–314. Philadelphia, PA: Saunders/Elsevier.

Bradley, J. and Movsas, B. (2004). Radiation esophagitis: predictive factors and preventive strategies. *Semin. Radiat. Oncol.* 14: 280–286.

Brown, L.F., Goldman, H., and Antonioli, D.A. (1984). Intraepithelial eosinophils in endoscopic biopsies of adults with reflux esophagitis. *Am. J. Surg. Pathol.* 8: 899–905.

Brownschidle, S.S., Ganguly, E.K., and Wilcox, R.L. (2014). Identification of esophagitis dissecans superficialis by endoscopy. *Clin. Gastroenterol. Hepatol.* 12: e79–e80.

Buckner, F.S. and Pomeroy, C. (1993). Cytomegalovirus disease of the gastrointestinal tract in patients without AIDS. *Clin. Infect. Dis.* 17: 644–656.

Calabrese, C., Fabbri, A., Bortolotti, M. et al. (2003). Dilated intercellular spaces as a marker of oesophageal damage: comparative results in gastrooesophageal reflux disease with and without bile reflux. *Aliment. Pharmacol. Ther.* 8: 525–532.

Calabrese, C., Fabbri, A., Benni, M. et al. (2003). Squamous cell carcinoma arising in esophageal lichen planus. *Gastrointest. Endosc.* 57: 596–599.

Canalejo Castrillero, E., Garcia Duran, F., Cabello, N., and Garcia, M.J. (2010). Herpes esophagitis in healthy adults and adolescents: report of 3 cases and review of the literature. *Medicine* 89: 204–210.

Carmack, S.W., Vemalupalli, R., Spechler et al. (2009). Esophagitis dissecans superficialis ("sloughing esophagitis"): a clinicopathologic study of 12 cases. *Am. J. Surg. Pathol.* 33: 1789–1794.

Caviglia, R., Ribolsi, M., Maggiano, N. et al. (2005). Dilated intercellular spaces of esophageal epithelium in nonerosive reflux disease patients with physiological esophageal acid exposure. *Am. J. Gastroenterol.* 100: 543–548.

Chandran, V.S., Murray, J.A., and Abraham, S.C. (2008). Esophageal lichen planus. *Arch. Pathol. Lab. Med.* 132: 1026–1029.

Chehade, M. and Sampson, H.A. (2008). Epidemiology and etiology of eosinophilic esophagitis. *Gastroenterol. Clin. N. Am.* 18: 33–44.

Chehade, M., Sampson, H.A., Morotti, R.A., and Magid, M.S. (2007). Esophageal subepithelial fibrosis in children with eosinophilic esophagitis. *J. Pediatr. Gastroenterol. Nutr.* 45: 319–328.

Chen, Z., Scudiere, J.R., and Montgomery, E. (2009). Medication-induced upper gastrointestinal tract injury. *J. Clin. Pathol.* 62: 113–119.

Chryssostalis, A., Gaudric, M., Terris, B. et al. (2008). Esophageal lichen planus: a series of eight cases including a patient with esophageal verrucous carcinoma. A case series. *Endoscopy* 40: 764–768.

Cohen, S., Saxena, A., Waljee, A.K. et al. (2012). Lymphocytic esophagitis: a diagnosis of increasing frequency. *J. Clin. Gastroenterol.* 46: 828–832. 51.

Damaschin, O., Dahmani, O., Faibis, F. et al. (2009). Esophageal tuberculosis in a patient on maintenance dialysis: advantages of interferon-gamma release assay. *Ren. Fail.* 31: 248–250.

Daniels, J.A., Loirat, C., and Jacqz-Aigren, E. (2008). Gastointestinal tract changes associated with taxanes: marker of drug toxicity versus effect. *Am. J. Surg. Pathol.* 32: 473–477.

De Petris, G., Caldero, S.G., Chen, L. et al. (2014a). Histopathological changes in the gastrointestinal tract due to drugs: an update for the surgical pathologist (part I of II). *Int. J. Surg. Pathol.* 22: 120–128.

De Petris, G., Caldero, S.G., Chen, L. et al. (2014b). Histopathological changes in the gastrointestinal tract due to drugs: an update for the surgical pathologist (part II of II). *Int. J. Surg. Pathol.* 22: 202–211.

Decker, G.A., Loftus, E.V. Jr., Pasha, T.M. et al. (2001). Crohn's disease of the esophagus: clinical features and outcomes. *Inflamm. Bowel Dis.* 7: 113–119.

Dellon, E.S. (2013). Eosinophilic esophagitis. *Gastroenterol. Clin. N. Am.* 42: 133–153.

Dellon, E.S., Chen, X., Miller, C.R. et al. (2012). Diagnostic utility of major basic protein, eotaxin-3, and leukotriene enzyme staining in eosinophilic esophagitis. *Am. J. Gastroenterol.* 107: 1503–1511.

Dellon, E.S., Gonsalves, N., Hirano, I. et al. (2013). ACG clinical guideline: evidenced based approach to the diagnosis and management of esophageal eosinophilia and eosinophilic esophagitis (EoE). *Am. J. Gastroenterol.* 108: 679–692.

Dellon, E.S., Speck, O., Woodward, K. et al. (2013). Clinical and endoscopic characteristics do not reliably differentiate PPI-responsive esophageal eosinophilia and eosinophilic esophagitis in patients undergoing upper endoscopy: a prospective cohort study. *Am. J. Gastroenterol.* 108: 1854–1860.

DeNardi, F.G. and Riddell, R.H. (2007). Esophagus. In: *Histology for Pathologists*, 3e (eds. S.E. Millse et al.), 565–588. Philadelphia: Lippincott Williams and Wilkins.

Dent, J. (2007). Microscopic esophageal mucosal injury in nonerosive reflux disease. *Clin. Gastroenterol. Hepatol.* 5: 4–16.

Dern, C.B. (2015). Chagas' disease. *N. Engl. J. Med.* 373: 456–466.

Dickens, C.M., Heseltine, D., Walton, S. et al. (1990). The oesophagus in lichen planus: an endo-scopic study. *BMJ* 300: 84.

Diehl, J.T., Thomas, L., Bloom, M.B. et al. (1988). Tracheoesophageal fistula associated with Barrett's ulcer. The importance of reflux control. *Ann. Thorac. Surg.* 45: 449–450.

Dignan, F.L., Amrolia, P., Clark, A. et al. (2012). Diagnosis and management of chronic graft-versus-host disease. *Br. J. Haematol.* 158: 46–61.

Ebach, D.R., Vanderheyden, A.D., Ellison, J.M. et al. (2011). Lymphocytic esophagitis: a possible manifestation of pediatric upper gastrointestinal Crohn's disease. *Inflamm. Bowel Dis.* 17: 45–49.

El-Serag, H.B., Sweet, S., Winchester, C.C. et al. (2014). Update on the epidemiology of gastro-oesophageal reflux disease: a systematic review. *Gut* 63: 871–880.

Eng, J. and Sabanathan, S. (1991). Tuberculosis of the esophagus. *Dig. Dis. Sci.* 36: 536–540.

Ergun, G.A., Lin, A.N., Dannenberg, A.J. et al. (1992). Gastrointestinal manifestations of epider-molysis bullosa. A study of 101 patients. *Medicine (Baltimore)* 71: 121–127.

Faias, S., Lage, P., Sachse, F. et al. (2004). Pemphigus vulgaris with exclusive involvement of the esophagus: case report and review. *Gastrointest. Endosc.* 60: 312–315.

Filipovich, A.H. (2008). Diagnosis and management of chronic graft-versus-host disease. *Best Pract. Res. Clin. Haematol.* 24: 1678–1682.

Fine, J.D., Johnson, L.B., Weiner, M. et al. (2008). Gastrointestinal complications of inherited epidermolysis bullosa: cumulative experience of the National Epidermolysis Bullosa Registry. *J. Pediatr. Gastroenterol. Nutr.* 46: 147–158.

Fiocca, R., Mastracci, L., Riddell, R. et al. (2010). Development of consensus guidelines for the histologic recognition of microscopic esophagitis in patients with gastroesophageal reflux disease: the Esohisto project. *Hum. Pathol.* 41: 223–231.

Fu, B. and Rueda-Pedraza, M.E. (2012). Non-neoplastic disorders of the esophagus. In: *Gastrointestinal and Liver Pathology*, 2e (eds. C.A. Iacobuzio-Donahue and E.A. Montgomery), 26–32. Philadelphia: Elsevier Saunders.

Fukuchi, M., Otake, S., Naitoh, H. et al. (2011). A case of exfoliative esophagitis with pemphigus vulgaris. *Dis. Esophagus* 24: E23–E25.

Furuta, G.T. (2011). Eosinophilic esophagitis: update on clinicopathologic manifestations and pathophysiology. *Curr. Opin. Gastroenterol.* 27: 383–388.

Furuta, G.T. and Katzka, D.A. (2015). Eosinophilic esophagitis. *N. Engl. J. Med.* 373: 1640–1648.

Geboes, K., Ectors, N., and Vantrappen, G. (1991). Inflammatory disorders of the esophagus. *Hepato-Gastroenterology* 38 (Suppl 1): 26–32.

Gill, P., Piris, J., and Warren, B.F. (2003). Bizarre stromal cells in the oesophagus. *Histopathology* 42: 88–90.

Goldstein, N.S. and Amin, M. (2010). Upper gastrointestinal tract in inflammatory bowel disease. *Surg. Pathol.* 3: 349–359.

Greenwald, D.A. and Brandt, L.J. (2002). Esophageal disorders due to systemic diseases. In: *Gastrointestinal Diseases: An Endoscopic Approach* (eds. A.J. DiMarino and S.B. Benjamin), 2231–2243. Thorofare, NJ: Slack Inc.

Grin, A. and Streutker, C.J. (2015). Esophagitis: old histologic concepts and new thoughts. *Arch. Pathol. Lab. Med.* 139: 723–729.

Gupta, K.B., Manchanda, M., and Vermas, M. (2011). Tuberculous oesophago-pleural fistula. *J. Indian Med. Assoc.* 109: 504–505.

Gurvits, G.E. (2010). Black esophagus: acute esophageal necrosis syndrome. *World J. Gastroenterol.* 16 (26): 3219–3225.

Haque, S. and Genta, R.M. (2012). Lymphocytic oesophagitis: clinicopathological aspects of an emerging condition. *Gut* 61: 1108–1114.

Hokama, A., Yamamoto, Y.Y., Taira, K. et al. (2010). Esophagitis dissecans superficialis and autoimmune bullous dermatoses: a review. *World J. Gastrointest. Endosc.* 2: 252–256.

Houman, M.H., Ben Ghorbel, I., Lamloum, M. et al. (2002). Esophageal involvement in Behcet's disease. *Yonsei Med. J.* 43: 457–460.

Hruban, R.H., Yardley, J.H., Donehower, R.C. et al. (1989). Taxol toxicity, Epithelial necrosis in the gastrointestinal tract associated with polymerized microtubule accumulation and mitotic arrest. *Cancer* 63: 1944–1950.

Huppmann, A.R. and Orenstein, J.M. (2010). Opportunistic disorders of the gastrointestinal tract in the age of highly active antiretroviral therapy. *Hum. Pathol.* 41: 1777–1787.

Isaacson, P. (1982). Biopsy appearances easily mistaken for malignancy in gastrointestinal endoscopy. *Histopathology* 6: 377–389.

Jain, S.K., Jain, S., J.M., and Yaduvanshi, A. (2002). Esophageal tuberculosis: is it so rare? Report of 12 cases and review of the literature. *Am. J. Gastroenterol.* 97: 287–291.

Kahrilas, P.J. (2003). GERD pathogenesis, pathophysiology, and clinical manifestations. *Cleve. Clin. J. Med.* 70 (Suppl. 5): S4–S19.

Kahrilas, P.J. (2008). Clinical practice. Gastroesophageal reflux disease. *N. Engl. J. Med.* 359: 1700–1707.

Katzka, D.A., Smyrk, T.C., Bruce, A.J. et al. (2010). Variations in presentations of esophageal involvement in lichen planus. *Clin. Gastroenterol. Hepatol.* 8: 777–782.

Kaye, P., Abdulla, K., Wood, J. et al. (2008). Iron-induced mucosal pathology of the upper gastrointestinal tract: a common finding in patients on oral iron therapy. *Histopathology* 53: 311–317.

Keate, R.F., Williams, J.W., and Connolly, S.M. (2003). Lichen planus esophagitis: report of three patients treated with oral tacrolimus or intraesophageal corticosteroid injections or both. *Dis. Esophagus* 16: 47–53.

Kephart, G.M., Alexander, J.A., Arora, A.S. et al. (2010). Marked deposition of eosinophil-derived neurotoxin in adult patients with eosinophilic esophagitis. *Am. J. Gastroenterol.* 105: 298–307.

Kikendall, J.W. (1999). Pill esophagitis. *J. Clin. Gastroenterol.* 28: 298–305.

Kikendall, J.W. (2007). Pill-induced esophagitis. *Gastroenterol. Hepatol.* 3: 275–276.

Krugmann, J., Neumann, H., Vieth, M., and Armstrong, D. (2013). What is the role of endoscopy and oesophageal biopsies in the management of GERD? *Best Pract. Res. Clin. Gastroenterol.* 27: 373–385.

Kurihara, K., Mizuseki, K., Ichikawa, M. et al. (2001). Esophageal inflammatory pseudotumor mimicking malignancy. *Intern. Med.* 40: 18–22.

Lamps, L.W. (2008). Infectious disorders of the upper gastrointestinal tract (excluding *Helicobacter pylori*). *Diagn. Histopathol.* 14: 427–436.

Lamps, L.W., Lai, K.K.T., and Milner, D.A. Jr. (2014). Fungal infections of the gastrointestinal tract in the immunocompromised host: an update. *Adv. Anat. Pathol.* 21: 217–227.

Larner, A.J. and Lendrum, R. (1992). Oesophageal candidiasis after omeprazole therapy. *Gut* 33: 860–861.

Lemonovich, T.L. and Watkins, R.R. (2012). Update on cytomegalovirus infections of the gastrointestinal system in solid organ transplant recipients. *Curr. Infect. Dis. Rep.* 14: 33–40.

Leung, J., Beukema, K.R., and Shen, A.H. (2015). Allergic mechanisms of eosinophilic esophagitis. *Best Pract. Res. Clin. Gastroenterol.* 29: 709–720.

Lewin, D.N.B. (2015). Systemic illness involving the GI tract. In: *Surgical Pathology of the GI Tract, Liver Biliary Tract and Pancreas*, 2e (eds. R.D. Odze and J.R. Goldblum), 116–118. Philadelphia: Saunders Elsevier.

Liacouras, C.A., Furuta, G.T., Hirano, I. et al. (2011). Eosinophilic esophagitis: updated consensus recommendations for children and adults. *J. Allergy Clin. Immunol.* 128: 3–20.

Lin, J., McKenna, B.J., and Appelman, H.D. (2010). Morphologic findings in upper gastrointestinal biopsies of patients with ulcerative colitis. *Am. J. Surg. Pathol.*: 1672–1677.

Ma, C., Limketai, B.N., and Montgomery, E.A. (2014). Recently highlighted non-neoplastic pathologic entities of the upper GI tract and their clinical significance. *Gastrointest. Endosc.* 80: 960–969.

Maguire, A. and Sheahan, K. (2012). Pathology of oesophagitis. *Histopathology* 60: 864–879.

Maharshak, N., Sagi, M., Santos, E. et al. (2013). Oesophageal involvement in bullous pemphigoid. *Clin. Exp. Dermatol.* 38: 274–275.

Maiorana, A., Baccarini, P., Foroni, M. et al. (2003). Human cytomegalovirus infection of the gastrointestinal tract in apparently immunocompetent patients. *Hum. Pathol.* 34: 1331–1336.

Manapov, F., Sepe, S., Niyazi, M. et al. (2013). Dose-volumetric parameters and prediction of severe acute esophagitis in patients with locally-advanced non small-cell lung cancer treated with neoadjuvant concurrent hyperfractionated-accelerated chemoradiotherapy. *Radiat. Oncol.* 8: 122–125.

McBane, R.D. and Gross, J.B. Jr. (1991). Herpes esophagitis: clinical syndrome,endoscopic appearance, and diagnosis in 23 patients. *Gastrointest. Endosc.* 37: 600–603.

Medlicott, S.A.C., Ma, M. et al. (2013). Vascular wall degeneration in dosxycycline-related esophagitis. *Am. J. Surg. Pathol.* 37: 1114–1115.

Mihas, A.A., Slaughter, R.L., Goldman, L.N. et al. (1976). Double lumen esophagus due to reflux esophagitis with fibrous septum formation. *Gastroenterology* 71: 136–137.

Misdraji, J. Drug induced pathology of the upper gastrointestinal tract. *Diag. Histopath.* 14 (9): 411–418.

Mohan, P., Srinivas, C.R., and Leelakrishnan, V. (2013). A rare initial presentation of esophageal involvement in pemphigus. *Dis. Esophagus* 26 (3): 351.

Monkemuller, K., Neumann, H., and Fry, L.C. (2010). Esophageal blebs and blisters. *Gastroenterology* 138: e3–e4.

Montgomery, E.A. and Voltaggio, L. (2012). Esophagus. In: *Biopsy Interpretation of the Gastrointestinal Tract Mucosa. Volume 1: Non-neoplastic*, 2e (ed. E.A. Montgomery), 1–54. Philadelphia: Lippincott Williams and Wilkins.

Moretti, F., Uberti-Foppa, C., Quiros-Roldan, E. et al. (2002). Oesophagobronchial fistula caused by varicella zoster virus in a patient with AIDS: a unique case. *J. Clin. Pathol.* 55: 397–398.

Murro, D. and Jakate, S. (2015). Radiation esophagitis. *Arch. Pathol. Lab. Med.* 139: 827–830.

Nakshabendi, I.M., Maldonado, M.E., Coppola, D. et al. (2000). Esophageal cast: a manifestation of graft-versus-host disease. *Dig. Dis.* 18: 103–105.

Nguyen, T., Park, J.Y., Scudiere, J.Y. et al. (2009). Mycophenolic acid (cellcept and myofortic) induced injury of the upper GI tract. *Am. J. Surg. Pathol.* 33: 1355–1363.

Noffsinger, A.E. (2009). Update on esophagitis. Controversial and underdiagnosed causes. *Arch. Pathol. Lab. Med.* 133: 1087–1095.

Ntoumazios, S.K., Voulgari, P.V., Potsis, K. et al. (2006). Esophageal involvement in scleroderma: gastroesophageal reflux, the common problem. *Semin. Arthritis Rheum.* 36: 173–181.

Odze, R.D. (2009). Pathology of eosinophilic esophagitis: what the clinician needs to know. *Am. J. Gastroenterol.* 104: 485–490.

Pantanowitz, L., Gelrud, A., Apstein, M., and Nasser, I. (2004). Crohn's disease of the esophagus. *Ear NoseThroat J.* 83 (420): 422–423.

Parfitt, J.R. and Driman, D.K. (2007). Pathological effects of drugs on the gastrointestinal tract. *Hum. Pathol.* 38: 527–536.

Parfitt, J.R., Gregor, J.C., Suskin, N.G. et al. (2006). Eosinophilic esophagitis in adults: distinguishing features from gastroesophageal reflux disease: a study of 41 patients. *Mod. Pathol.* 19: 90–96.

Parfitt, J.R., Jayakumar, S., and Driman, D.K. (2008). Mycophenolate mofetil-related gastrointestinal mucosal injury: variable injury patterns, including graft-versus-host disease-like changes. *Am. J. Surg. Pathol.* 32: 1367–1372.

Polydorides, A.D. (2010). Gastroesophageal reflux disease. In: *Diagnostic Pathology: Gastrointestinal, Section 1* (ed. J.K. Greenson), 22–25. Salt Lake City, UT: Amirsys.

Potter, J.W., Saeian, K., Staff, D. et al. (2004). Eosinophilic esophagitis in adults: an emerging problem with unique esophageal features. *Gastrointest. Endosc.* 59: 355–361.

Pugh, J.L., Moore, R.J., Wilcox, C.M. et al. (2005). Soughing Esophagitis: a newly recognized clinicopathologic entitiy. *Gastroenterology* 128: A636–A637.

Purdy, J.K., Appelman, H.D., Golembeski, C.P. et al. (2006). Lymphocytic esophagitis: a chronic or recurring pattern of esophagitis resembling allergic contact dermatitis. *Am. J. Clin. Pathol.* 125: 432–437.

Purdy, J.K., Appelman, H.D., and McKenna, B.J. (2012). Sloughing esophagitis is associated with chronic debilitation and medications that injure the esophageal mucosa. *Mod. Pathol.* 25: 767–775.

Qiao, W.-B., Zhao, Y.-H., Zhao, Y.-B. et al. (2005). Clinical and dosimetric factors of radiation-induced esophageal injury: radiation-induced esophageal toxicity. *World J. Gastroenterol.* 11: 2626–2629.

Radhi JM, Schweiger F. Bacterial oesophagitis in an immunocompromised patient. *Postgrad. Med. J.* 1994;70:233–234.

Ramaswamy, K., Jacobson, K., Jevon, G. et al. (2003). Esophageal Crohn disease in children: a clinical spectrum. *J. Pediatr. Gastroenterol. Nutr.* 36: 454–458.

Reggiani Bonetti, L., Losi, L., DiGregorio, C. et al. (2011). Cytomegalovirus infection of the upper gastrointestinal tract: a clinical and pathological study of 30 cases. *Scand. J. Gastroenterol.* 46: 1228–1235.

Reissmann, A., Hahn, E.G., Faller, G. et al. (2006). Sole treatment of lichen planus-associated esoph-ageal stenosis with injection of corticosteroids. *Gastrointest. Endosc.* 63: 168–169.

Remmelts, H.H., van den Brink, J.W., Laan, R., and BacDJ (2011). Herpes simplex viruso esophagitis in a pregnant woman. *Neth. J. Med.* 69: 76–78.

Roman, S., Savarino, E., Savarino, V., and Mion, F. (2013). Eosinophilic oesophagitis: from physiopathology to treatment. *Dig. Liver Dis.* 45: 871–878.

Ronkainen, J., Walker, M.M., Aro, P. et al. (2012). Lymphocytic oesophagitis, a condition in search of a disease? *Gut* 61: 1776.

Rothenberg, M.E. (2015). Molecular, genetic and cellular bases for treating eosinophilic esophagitis. *Gastroenterology* 148: 1143–1157.

Rubenstein, J.H. and Chen, J.W. (2014). Epidemiology of gastroesophageal reflux disease. *Gastroenterol. Clin. N. Am.* 43: 1–14.

Rubio, C.A., Sjodahl, K., and Lagergren, J. (2006). Lymphocytic esophagitis: a histologic subset of chronic esophagitis. *Am. J. Clin. Pathol.* 125: 432–437.

Rudolph, I., Goldstein, F., and DiMarino, A.J. Jr. (2001). Crohn's disease of the esophagus: three cases and a literature review. *Can. J. Gastroenterol.* 15: 117–122.

Ruuska, T., Vaajalahti, P., Arajarvi, P. et al. (1994). Prospective evaluation of upper gastrointes-tinal mucosal lesions in children with ulcerative colitis and Crohn's disease. *J. Pediatr. Gastroenterol. Nutr.* 19: 181–186.

Salaria, S.N., Abu Alfa, A.K., Cruise, M.W. et al. (2013). Lichenoid esophagitis: clinicopathologic overlap with established esophageal lichen planus. *Am. J. Surg. Pathol.* 37: 1889–1994.

Schneider, N.I., Plieschnegger, W., Geppert, M. et al. (2014). Validation study of the Esohisto consensus guidelines for the recognition of microscopic esophagitis (histoGERD trial). *Hum. Pathol.* 45: 994–1002.

Schoepfer, A. (2015). Diagnostic approach to eosinophilic oesophagitis: pearls and pitfalls. *Best Pract. Res. Clin. Gastroenterol.* 29: 783–792.

Schwartz, M.P., Sigurdsson, V., Vreuls, W. et al. (2006). Two siblings with lichen planus and squamous cell carcinoma of the oesophagus. *Eur. J. Gastroenterol. Hepatol.* 18: 1111–1115.

Shields, M.H., Shaffer, K., O'Farrell, R.P. et al. (2007). Gastrointestinal manifestations of dermatologic disorders. *Clin. Gastroenterol. Hepatol.* 5: 1010–1017.

Shih, A.R., Lauwers, G.Y., Mattia, A. et al. (2017). Vascular injury characterizes doxycycline-induced upper gastrointestinal tract mucosal injury. *Am. J. Surg. Pathol.* 41: 374–381.

Shulman, H.M., Kleiner, D., Lee, S.J. et al. (2006). Histopathologic diagnosis of chronic graft-versus-host disease: national institutes of health consensus development project on criteria for clinical trials in chronic graft-versus-host disease: II. pathology working group report. *Blood Marrow Transplant* 12 (1): 31–47.

Sodhi, S.S., Srinivasan, R., and Thomas, R.M. (2000). Esophageal graft versus host disease. *Gastrointest. Endosc.* 52: 235.

Squires, K.A.G., Cameron, D.J., Oliver, M. et al. (2009). Herpes simplex and eosinophilic oesophagitis: the chicken or the egg? *J. Pediatr. Gastroenterol. Nutr.* 49: 246–250.

Stewart, M.I., Woodley, D.T., and Briggaman, R.A. (1991). Epidermolysis bullosa acquisita and associated symptomatic esophageal webs. *Arch. Dermatol.* 127: 373–377.

Sutton, L.M., Heintz, D.D., Patel, A.S. et al. (2014). Lymphocytic esophagitis in children. *Inflamm. Bowel Dis.* 20: 1324–1328.

Takubo, K. (2009). Esophageal manifestations of collagen vascular and other systemic diseases. In: *Pathology of the Esophagus: An Atlas and Textbook*, 2e, 70–83. Tokyo: Springer.

Takubo, K., Honma, N., Aryal, G. et al. (2005). Is there a set of histologic changes that are invariably reflux associated? *Arch. Pathol. Lab. Med.* 129: 159–163.

Tian, X.P. and Zhang, X. (2013). Gastrointestinal complications of systemic sclerosis. *World J. Gastroenterol.* 19: 7062–7068.

Tobey, N.A., Carson, J.L., Alkiek, R.A., and Orlando, R.C. (1996). Dilated intercellular spaces: a morphological feature of acid reflux–damaged human esophageal epithelium. *Gastroenterology* 111: 1200–1205.

Tobin, J.M., Sinha, B., Ramani, P. et al. (2001). Upper gastrointestinal mucosal disease in pediatric Crohn disease and ulcerative colitis: a blinded, controlled study. *J. Pediatr. Gastroenterol. Nutr.* 32: 443–448.

Tummala, V., Barwick, K.W., Sontag, S.J. et al. (1987). The significance of intraepithelial eosinophils in the histologic diagnosis of gastroesophageal reflux. *Am. J. Clin. Pathol.* 87: 43–48.

Vanagunas, A., Jacob, P., and Olinger, E. (1990). Radiation-induced esophageal injury: a spectrum from esophagitis to cancer. *Am. J. Gastroenterol.* 85: 808–812.

Vidal-Casariego, A., Calleja-Fernandez, A., Ballesteros-Pomar, M.D. et al. (2013). Efficacy of glutamine in the prevention of oral mucositis and acute radiation-induced esophagitis: a retrospective study. *Nutr. Cancer* 65: 424–429.

Walsh, T.J., Belitsos, N.J., and Hamilton, S.R. (1986). Bacterial esophagitis in immunocompromised patients. *Arch. Intern. Med.* 146: 1345–1348.

Wang, H.H., Mangano, M.M., and Antonioli, D.A. (1994). Evaluation of T-lymphocytes in esophageal mucosal biopsies. *Mod. Pathol.* 7: 55–58.

Washington, K. and Jagasia, M. (2009). Pathology of graft-versus-host disease in the gastrointestinal tract. *Hum. Pathol.* 40: 909–917.

Wen, T., Stucke, E.M., Grotjan, T.M. et al. (2013). Molecular diagnosis of eosinophilic esophagitis by gene expression profiling. *Gastroenterology* 145: 1289–1299.

Werner-Wasik, M., Yorke, E., Deasy, J. et al. (2010). Radiation dose-volume effects in the esophagus. *Int. J. Radiat. Oncol. Biool. Phys.* 76: S86–S93.

Wilcox, C.M. and Schwartz, D.A. (1996). Endoscopic-pathologic correlates of Candida esophagitis in acquired immunodeficiency syndrome. *Dig. Dis. Sci.* 41 (7): 1337–1345.

Winter, H.S., Madara, J.L., Stafford, R.J. et al. (1982). Intraepithelial eosinophils: a new diagnostic criterion for reflux esophagitis. *Gastroenterology* 83: 818–823.

Wise, J.L. and Murray, J.A. (2002). Esophageal manifestations of dermatologic disease. *Curr. Gastroenterol. Rep.* 4: 205–212.

Xue, Y., Suriawinata, A., Liu, X. et al. (2015). Lymphocytic esophagitis with CD4 T-cell-predominant intraepithelial lyphocytes and primary esophageal motility abnormalities: a potential novel clinicopathologic entity. *Am. J. Surg. Pathol.* 39: 1558–1567.

Yerian, L., Fiocca, R., Mastracci, L. et al. (2011). Refinement and reproducibility of histologic criteria for the assessment of microscopic lesions in patients with gastroesophageal reflux disease: the Esohisto Project. *Dig. Dis. Sci.* 56: 2656–2665.

Yi, S.W., Cheon, J.H., Kim, J.H. et al. (2009). The prevalence and clinical characteristics of esophageal involvement in patients with Behçet's disease: a single center experience in Korea. *J. Korean Med. Sci.* 24: 52–56.

Zografos, G.N., Georgiadou, D., Thomas, D. et al. (2009). Drug-induced esophagitis. *Dis. Esophagus* 22: 633–637.

Zukerberg, L., Mahadevan, K., Selig, M., and Deshpande, V. (2016). Esophageal intrasquamous IgG4 deposits: an adjunctive marker to distinguish eosinophilic esophagitis from reflux esophagitis. *Histopathology.* 68: 968–976.

3

Epithelial Metaplastic, Polypoid, and Neoplastic Conditions of the Esophagus

Till S. Clauditz[1], Gregory Y. Lauwers[2], Michael B. Wallace[3] and Anthony R. Mattia[4]

[1] Department of Pathology, University-Medical-Center, Hamburg, Germany
[2] Moffitt Cancer Center, Tampa, Florida, USA
[3] Mayo Clinic, Jacksonville, Florida, USA
[4] Department of Pathology, Salem, Massachusetts, USA

Barrett's Esophagus

Definition, General Features, Predisposing Factors

Barrett's esophagus (BE) represents the replacement of the lower esophageal squamous mucosa by metaplastic columnar mucosa. It arises as a complication of chronic gastrointestinal reflux disease (GERD) and is a precursor to esophageal adenocarcinoma. Recent decades have shown a dramatic rise in the incidence of BE and adenocarcinoma, particularly in western populations, which may be reaching a plateau. In western countries, the prevalence of BE is estimated between 0.5 and 1.5% of the general population, and up to 5–10% of symptomatic GERD patients who undergo endoscopy. Other risk factors include age older than 50 years, male sex, Caucasian race, hiatal hernia, and central/visceral obesity.

The definition of BE encompasses both endoscopic and histologic abnormalities and varies depending on the requirement of the presence of intestinal metaplasia (IM) for diagnosis. The American College of Gastroenterology (ACG) currently defines BE as the extension of salmon-colored mucosa into the tubular esophagus ≥1 cm proximal to the gastroesophageal junction (GEJ) with biopsy confirmation of intestinal metaplasia. The designation of a ≥1 cm endoscopic abnormality represents a change from prior guidelines. Shorter segments are classified as "specialized columnar mucosa of the gastroesophageal junction" rather than BE, due to high interobserver variability and the low risk for adenocarcinoma. The continued requirement of intestinal metaplasia for the diagnosis of BE is based on data supporting that this type of epithelium predisposes to an increased risk of adenocarcinoma.

In the United Kingdom and Japan, the diagnosis of BE can be established by the presence of columnar mucosa without goblet cells. The 2014 guidelines of the British Society of Gastroenterology (BSG), although not requiring the presence of intestinal metaplasia, have also established a minimum visible length of columnar mucosa of >1 cm above the GEJ. The BSG recognizes that intestinal metaplasia is the mucosal type most closely associated with cancer risk, and that the risk associated with other types of columnar mucosa may be, in part, related to the patchy nature of intestinal metaplasia within the columnar metaplasia and sampling error for its detection, depending on the number of biopsy samples that are obtained, which has been factored into current diagnostic biopsy recommendations (see below).

There is evidence that nonspecialized columnar epithelium may contain similar molecular abnormalities to intestinal metaplasia and predispose to neoplastic transformation, although the magnitude of that risk remains undefined. As more data are accumulated, the definition of BE may continue to evolve. For now, the presence or absence of intestinal metaplasia can be taken into account in the determination of clinical management.

Once diagnosed, BE is further classified as long-segment (>3 cm) and short-segment (1–3 cm) based on endoscopic measurement. The longer the segment, the more likely goblet cells are identified on biopsy. Under current guidelines, the former designation of ultrashort-segment BE (<1 cm) is now encompassed under intestinal metaplasia of the GEJ region.

Clinical Features and Endoscopic Characteristics

Barrett's esophagus, although associated with GERD, is paradoxically associated with resolution of GERD symptoms. The primary reason to screen for BE is due to the increased risk of esophageal adenocarcinoma. Screening for BE may be considered in men with chronic (>5 years) and/or

Gastrointestinal Pathology: Correlative Endoscopic and Histologic Assessment, First Edition. Edited by Gregory Y. Lauwers and Michael B. Wallace.

frequent (weekly or more) symptoms of gastroesophageal reflux (heartburn or acid regurgitation) and two or more risk factors as described above.

The endoscopist must carefully identify landmarks of the GEJ, as noted by the top of the visible gastric folds on slight deflation of the esophagus. If present, BE is described based on the Prague classification, which connotes the circumferential length (C) and maximal length (M). The presence of visible nodules or irregular mucosa and surface blood vessels raises suspicion for neoplasia and should prompt targeted tissue sample.

To maximize the yield of intestinal metaplasia on histology, both the ACG and BSG guidelines recommend that in patients with suspected BE, at least eight random biopsies should be taken. In patients with short segments of suspected BE in whom eight biopsies are unattainable, at least four biopsies per cm of circumferential BE, and one biopsy per cm in tongues of BE, should be obtained. In patients with suspected BE and lack of intestinal metaplasia on histology, a repeat endoscopy should be considered in one to two years to rule out BE. The ACG recommends that endoscopic biopsy should not be performed in the presence of a normal Z-line or a Z-line with <1 cm of variability.

For established BE, current surveillance biopsy protocols call for four-quadrant biopsy every 1–2 cm of length and targeted sampling of visible focal abnormalities. Endoscopic mucosal resection (EMR), which is performed with a suction cap and ligating snare or rubber band, has been shown to be superior to biopsy for histological evaluation of visible nodules in BE and is not recommended as standard of care.

Advanced imaging modalities such as chromoendoscopy (acetic acid) and optical enhancements (e.g. narrow band imaging) have been shown to significantly increase the yield for neoplasia (Figure 3.1).

Microscopic Features

The goals of biopsies are to determine (i) whether the findings are consistent with BE, and (ii) if there is evidence of neoplastic progression (i.e. dysplasia, see Section "Barrett's Esophagus–Dysplasia—Esophageal Adenocarc").

The three main types of mucosa that are encountered in BE include cardia, fundic (oxyntic), and intestinal, often in a patchwork appearance juxtaposed with squamous mucosa. Intestinal metaplasia occurs in a background of

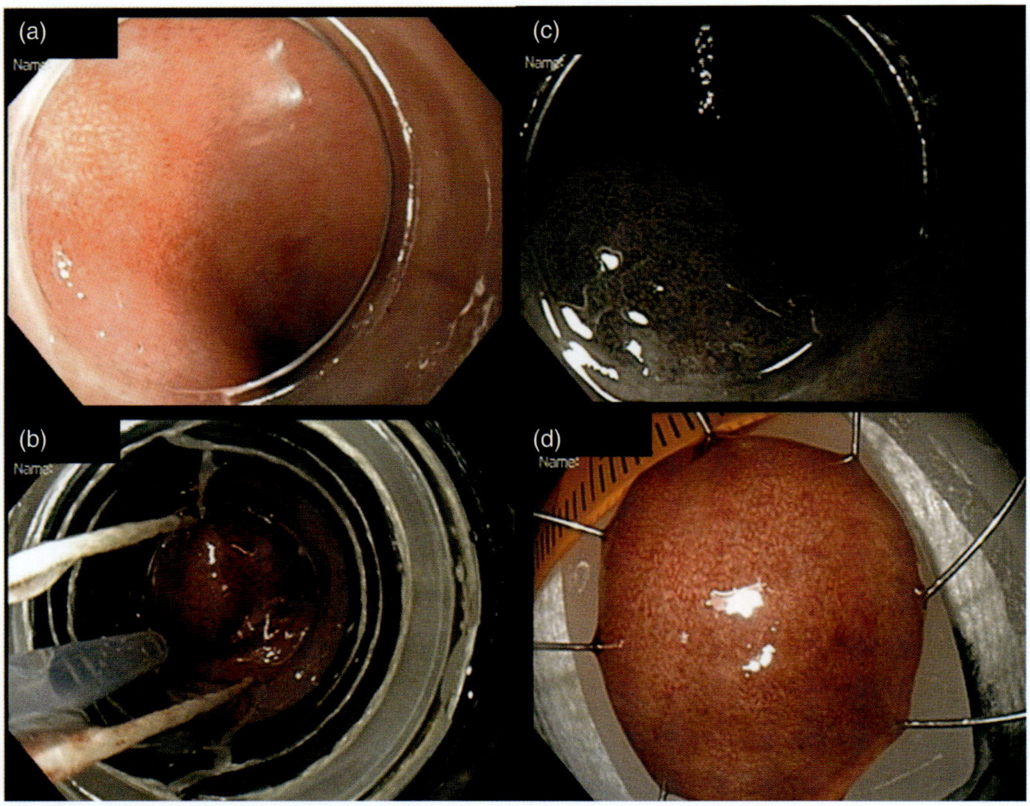

Figure 3.1 Endoscopic view of Barrett's esophagus. From upper left and clockwise you see (a) white light view, (b) NBI view showing subtle vascular dilation on the surface of the nodule, (c) endoscopic mucosal resection of nodule (d) gross specimen pinned for histology.

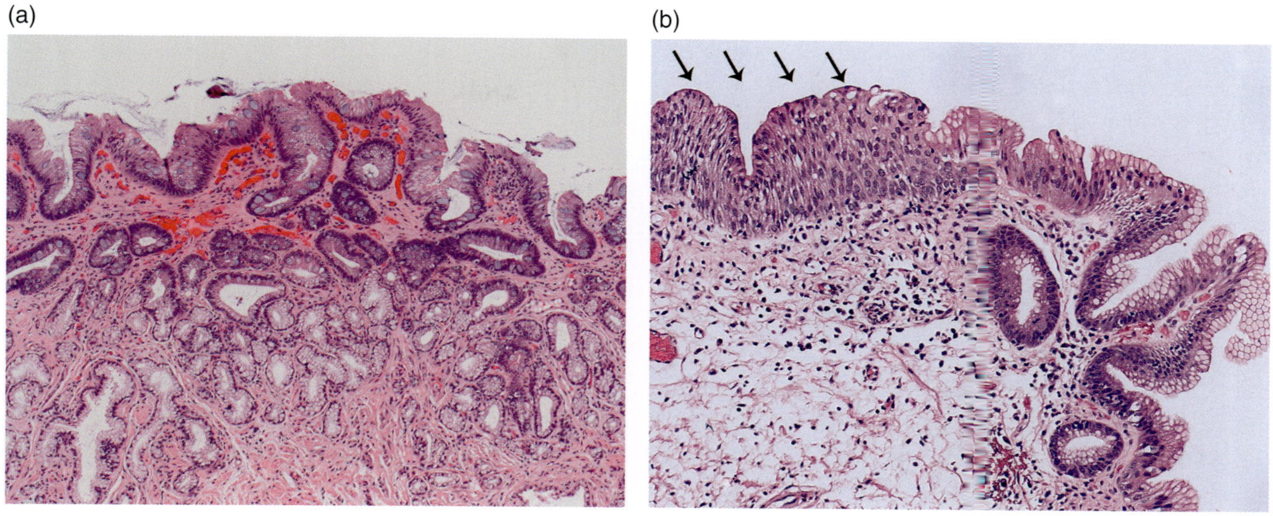

Figure 3.2 (a) Typical appearance of Barrett's esophagus with numerous goblet cells; (b) Multilayered epithelium. This hybrid epithelium with squamous and columnar features is believed to represent a precursor of Barrett's esophagus.

cardia-type or oxyntocardia-type gastric mucosa. Goblet cells are readily detected on hematoxylin and eosin stained slides, containing blue staining acid mucin vacuoles, which compress the nuclei and laterally displace the membranes of adjacent cells (Figure 3.2a). Distinguishing true goblet cells from a variety of goblet cell mimics can be challenging (see Section "Differential diagnosis"). Pure fundic-type mucosa is inversely associated with BE.

The presence of multilayered epithelium (Figure 3.2b), a composite epithelium of abortive acid mucin-containing glandular cells and immature, basally located squamous cells, has been proposed as a precursor epithelium to intestinal metaplasia and BE, although its specificity in identifying BE is debated.

Interpretation of the histologic findings may be problematic when there is endoscopic uncertainty regarding the location of the squamocolumnar junction, or biopsies are taken from an "irregular Z-line" or GEJ. In addition to multilayered epithelium, morphologic features that that are useful in determining the esophageal origin of metaplastic columnar mucosa without IM, as well as the distinction of BE with IM from IM of the gastric cardia (CIM) or GEJ, include the presence of esophageal glands/gland ducts, squamous epithelium overlying crypts with IM, hybrid glands, gland disarray and atrophy, and diffuse intestinal metaplasia affecting >50% of the biopsy (Table 3.1). These features are typically seen in BE but not CIM. However, native structures such as esophageal gland ducts are only seen in a minority of biopsy samples (10–15%), limiting their utility in establishing esophageal origin. In such cases, CIM cannot be confidently ruled out.

Table 3.1 Histologic features of columnar mucosa suggesting esophageal origin.

Multilayered epithelium
Esophageal glands and/or gland ducts
Squamous epithelium overlying crypts with IM
Hybrid glands
Gland disarray and atrophy
Diffuse IM (>50% of the biopsy)

Importantly, there is a certain level of baseline or metaplastic atypia in BE that must be recognized in order to avoid misinterpretation as dysplasia. Intestinalized crypts often exhibit enlarged, pencillate, and hyperchromatic nuclei with some stratification. In contrast to dysplasia, surface maturation is typically present.

Another unique feature of BE is the presence of a double muscularis mucosae that should not misdiagnosed as evidence of invasion on biopsy and can pose challenges in staging of early adenocarcinoma.

Immunohistochemical Studies and Molecular Features

Immunohistochemical staining plays a limited role in the diagnosis of BE. The markers reported to date, such as CK7/CK20 staining pattern, MUC antigens (MUC-1, MUC-2, MUC-6) Das1, CDX2, Hepar-1, and CD10 lack adequate sensitivity and/or specificity for routine clinical use in the identification of intestinal metaplasia.

The molecular mechanisms underlying the progression from normal esophagus to BE and subsequent neoplastic transformation are numerous. P16 inactivation, p53 loss of heterozygosity, and DNA ploidy abnormalities have been shown to be significant molecular events. Epigenetic mechanisms involving CpG island methylation also regulate several genes involved in protection from oxidative DNA damage, tumor suppression, Wnt pathway, apoptosis, and cytokine signaling. The exact sequence and clinical significance of these molecular changes during malignant progression remains uncertain.

The application of IHC and molecular biomarkers to non-dysplastic Barrett mucosal biopsies is not currently recommended (see Section "Barrett's Esophagus–Dysplasia—Esophageal Adenocarcinoma").

Differential Diagnosis

Clinical

BE may occasionally be diagnosed erroneously when the gastric cardia is sampled in error. It is critical that the endoscopist carefully samples tissue from the tubular esophagus after proper location of the anatomic landmarks. This can be challenging in a patient with a dilated lower esophagus and hiatal hernia, where the exact transition from esophagus to cardia is unclear.

Microscopic

It is important to recognize goblet cell mimics in order to avoid a false positive diagnosis of BE (Table 3.2). Alcian Blue (pH 2.5) or Alcian Blue/periodic acid–Schiff stains may be used to highlight goblet cells, although they are not recommended for routine use. Diagnostic pitfalls include other cell types that can exhibit blue staining, such as globoid-shaped reactive foveolar cells (pseudo-goblet cells). Columnar cells of gastric foveolar type may contain blue-tinged mucin ("columnar blues"), but lack a goblet cell shape. Other Alcian Blue positive goblet cell mimics include surface mucous cells of multilayered epithelium, columnar cells lining mucosal and submucosal gland ducts, and submucosal mucinous glands. None of these mimics have been shown to confer a risk of malignant progression and should not be considered to represent specialized epithelium.

Table 3.2 Goblet cell mimics.

Reactive, globoid-shaped foveolar cells (pseudo-goblet cells)
Foveolar cells with blue-tinged mucin ("columnar blues")
Surface mucous cells of multilayered epithelium
Columnar cells lining mucosal and submucosal gland ducts
Submucosal mucinous glands

Inflammation and IM in the region of the GEJ is etiologically related to either GERD or chronic gastritis (e.g. *Helicobacter pylori*-associated). IM can occur in approximately 5–18% of patients with an endoscopically normal gastroesophageal junction. Distinction of BE from CIM is important because endoscopic surveillance is generally not recommended in patients with IM at the cardia or in those with an irregular Z-line regardless of the presence of IM. There is evidence that individuals with IM at the cardia or GEJ have a significantly lower cancer risk than patients with Barrett's esophagus.

Ancillary Studies

As noted, most immunohistochemical stains studied to date are of limited practical value in distinguishing Barrett's esophagus from intestinal metaplasia of the cardia.

Prognosis, Evolution, and Clinical Management

Once BE is diagnosed, either through screening or as a result of an investigation for upper GI symptoms, patients with BE should receive once-daily PPI therapy for control of reflux symptoms or esophagitis. Surveillance is generally recommended followed by intervention at the point at which low- or high-grade dysplasia (HGD) or adenocarcinoma is detected. Available data suggest that surveillance correlates with earlier staging and improved survival from cancer, and endoscopic monitoring with histopathological assessment of dysplasia remains the gold standard for identification of high-risk patients most likely to benefit from close surveillance (see Section "Barrett's Esophagus–Dysplasia—Esophageal Adenocarcinoma"). The cost-effectiveness of this approach to surveillance remains controversial, and more reliable methods are needed to identify those patients who are at higher risk of cancer progression in order to tailor more focused management. Surveillance regimens should take into account the presence of IM and length of the Barrett's segment.

Endoscopic surveillance biopsy protocols call for four-quadrant biopsies at 2-cm intervals in patients without dysplasia and 1-cm intervals in patients with prior dysplasia. Mucosal abnormalities should be sampled separately, preferably with endoscopic mucosal resection.

Current guidelines outline standard methods for screening, surveillance, and treatment of BE. Recent changes include limiting screening only to those individuals with multiple risk factors (e.g. male, obese, chronic GERD), increasing the interval between surveillance to three to five years when no dysplasia is found, and endoscopic treatment when definite dysplasia is present. The later issue is a major change over the past decade.

Barrett's Esophagus–Dysplasia–Esophageal Adenocarcinoma

Definition, General Features, Predisposing Factors

Barrett's esophagus is the only established precursor to esophageal adenocarcinoma, and is the single strongest risk factor. Most adenocarcinomas occur in middle-aged white males, and in the United States the incidence of esophageal adenocarcinoma and associated mortality has risen dramatically over the past several decades. Progression occurs via a metaplasia–dysplasia–adenocarcinoma sequence, and despite the association with BE, adenocarcinoma is often diagnosed at a late stage.

Historically, the annual incidence of adenocarcinoma in patients with BE was reported between 0.5 and 1% per year; however, more recent studies quote a lower risk of approximately 0.12–0.38% per year. The risk of developing dysplasia is also limited. The overall annual incidence of low-grade dysplasia is 4.3% and that of high-grade dysplasia is 0.9%. However, the risk of cancer increases with extent of disease, and patients with long-segment BE (≥3 cm) are at higher risk for progression. In addition, identification of dysplasia selects a group of patients with BE who are at an even higher risk, and dictates the need for more frequent surveillance and early intervention.

Clinical Features and Endoscopic Characteristics

For low-grade dysplasia, with no visible nodules, ablation with radiofrequency energy has been shown to reduce progression to high-grade dysplasia and cancer. An important caveat is that most samples diagnosed as low-grade dysplasia in the community are subsequently downgraded to indefinite or no dysplasia when reviewed by experts in GI pathology. Thus, ablation should only be considered after at least two pathologists, including a GI expert, confirm low-grade dysplasia.

High-grade dysplasia, which is often seen as a focal visible nodule as well as low-risk T1a cancers and superficial T1b (differentiated, no lymphovascular invasion, invasion depth <500 microns below muscularis mucosa) can be effectively treated with endoscopic resection of the visible nodule, followed by ablation of flat BE. In this area, collaboration between endoscopist and pathologist is critical. Specific issues include careful preparation of the tissue specimen with pinning of the tissue in the endoscopy lab to allow precise staging and margin assessment, as well as measurement of the depth of invasion.

Microscopic Features

The morphologic diagnosis of dysplasia remains the basis for current management guidelines. Surveillance biopsies are categorized as negative for dysplasia, indefinite for dysplasia, low-grade dysplasia (LGD), high-grade dysplasia (HGD), and adenocarcinoma (encompassing intramucosal or deeper invasion). The diagnostic categories represent points on a spectrum, and there is well-documented inter- and intraobserver diagnostic variability, particularly in the categories of negative, indefinite, and low-grade dysplasia.

Histologic features useful in the assessment of mucosal biopsies for dysplasia include: (i) lack of epithelial surface maturation compared to deep glands, (ii) gland architecture, (iii) cytologic features, and (iv) inflammation and erosions/ulcers (Table 3.1). Intestinal-type dysplasia represents the most common type of dysplasia arising in BE, and resembles the epithelium of usual colonic adenomas.

Negative for Dysplasia

Negative biopsies generally show surface maturation characterized by a greater amount of cytoplasm in the surface epithelial cells compared to the deep glands. Glands architecture is preserved, with rounded glands evenly dispersed in the mucosa and surrounded by lamina propria. Cytologic features are bland with polarized basally located nuclei, small nucleoli, and evenly dispersed chromatin. Mitotic figures are confined to the deep glands. Non-dysplastic BE exhibits a degree of mild baseline or metaplastic atypia, particularly at the base, in comparison with adjacent non-metaplastic gastric fundic or cardiac-type glands, characterized by mildly enlarged pencillate nuclei with hyperchromasia and some stratification. Inflammation is variable and, if present, generally located in the superficial mucosa. Associated reparative features may be present, including loss of surface mucin, nuclear enlargement, small nucleoli, and some mitoses. However, in baseline atypia and reparative changes, smooth nuclear contours, nuclear polarity, and surface maturation are maintained. In contrast, true morphologic dysplasia, of any grade, has two main characteristics at low-power examination: loss of surface maturation and abrupt transition from background non-dysplastic epithelium to dysplasia, associated with the acquisition of additional cytologic abnormalities described under low-grade and high-grade dysplasia below.

Indefinite for Dysplasia

Some biopsies may be categorized as indefinite for dysplasia when there is diagnostic uncertainty between *true* dysplasia and regenerative/inflammatory atypia. This category is considered a provisional or interim diagnosis used in specific situations. This categorization is indicated in the

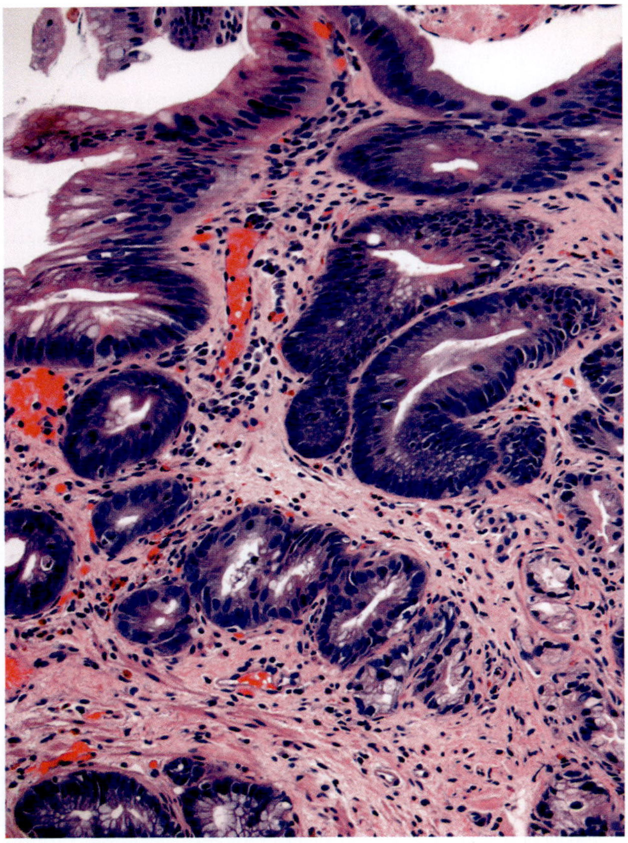

Figure 3.3 Barrett's esophagus indefinite for dysplasia. Nuclear hyperchromasia is limited to the glandular elements. Inflammation and maturation toward the surface epithelium are clues for the diagnosis.

setting of significant active inflammation or ulcer with associated marked epithelial atypia, and when it is unclear whether inflammation can account for the cytological changes (Figure 3.4). Technical issues may also be a factor, such as poor staining, denuded surface epithelium, significant cautery artifact, or mal-oriented biopsies with tangential sectioning. Gradual resolution of atypia toward the periphery of the inflamed focus in contrast to abrupt transition is also a useful morphologic clue favoring a reactive process instead of dysplasia. However, high-grade cytologic atypia that exceeds what can be explained by reactive or regenerative atypia should be considered to represent dysplasia.

This categorization may also be used when cytologic atypia in deep glands overlaps with that of low-grade dysplasia, with maturation of the overlying surface epithelium (Figure 3.4). This finding, also reported by some authors as crypt dysplasia (see subsequent discussion), shows properties similar to low-grade dysplasia and it may represent an early stage or precursor lesion; however, in practice a designation of indefinite for dysplasia is currently preferred.

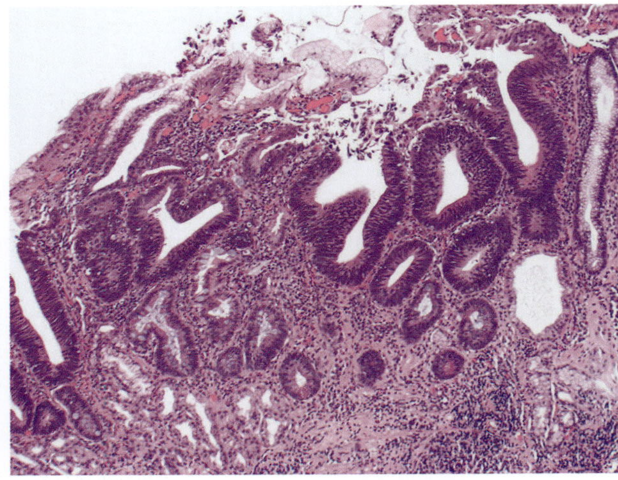

Figure 3.4 Low-grade dysplasia. Note the sharp transition between nuclear hyperchromasia and limited stratification.

Notably, patients with a diagnosis of indefinite for dysplasia show similar progression-free survival to those with low-grade dysplasia, and both groups are managed similarly for surveillance purpose. Explicit mention in the pathology report of the reason justifying this diagnosis is useful to aid patient management.

Low-Grade Dysplasia

Low-grade intestinal-type dysplasia demonstrates a lack of surface maturation. The cells exhibit mild cytologic abnormalities characterized by nuclear enlargement, elongation, hyperchromasia, and increased mitotic activity, although there is a minimal loss of nuclear polarity (Figure 3.4). Mild nuclear stratification up to 3/4 of the cell height may be present, not extending to the luminal surface. An abrupt transition from adjacent non-dysplastic epithelium can be a helpful clue to the diagnosis. Because inflammation-related cytologic atypia shows substantial overlap with the features of low-grade dysplasia, it is generally unwise to make a diagnosis of low-grade dysplasia in the presence of marked epithelial inflammation. Finally, architectural abnormalities consist of mild glandular crowding, but complex glands are lacking.

The estimated risk of progression to HGD or esophageal adenocarcinoma varies widely among patients with low-grade dysplasia, reflecting inconsistent diagnostic criteria and interobserver variability. However, the predictive value of a diagnosis of LGD for progression increases substantially when at least two pathologists agree on the diagnosis. The extent of low-grade dysplasia is also associated with an increased risk for adenocarcinoma, and quantifying the number of biopsies involved by dysplasia may be helpful in assessing risk of progression.

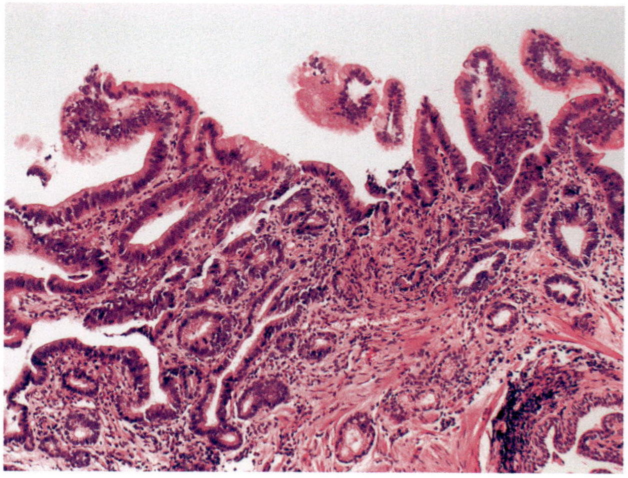

Figure 3.5 High-grade dysplasia. The architectural features with back to back, small neoplastic glands are diagnostic features.

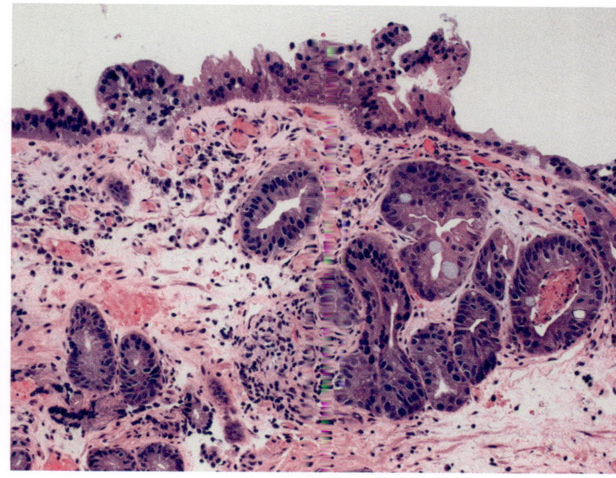

Figure 3.6 Crypt dysplasia. This lesion is characterized by neoplastic features limited to the glands with negative mucosal surface.

High-Grade Dysplasia (Incorporating Carcinoma In Situ)

The distinction between intestinal-type HGD and LGD is largely based on the presence of architectural changes in conjunction with increased nuclear atypia (Figure 3.5), although the distinction between the upper end of LGD and HGD can be subjective. Surface maturation is lacking. Architectural abnormalities, including gland crowding, fused glands, and micropapillae, may be striking. Nuclear polarity is lost and full-thickness nuclear stratification is common. Hyperchromasia, nuclear membrane irregularities, and prominent nucleoli are generally present. Numerous mitotic figures, including atypical ones, are frequent. Marked cytologic abnormalities associated with lesser architectural distortion are also acceptable. The presence of HGD in any amount is sufficient to report that diagnosis. HGD can be accompanied by active inflammation, but the degree of atypia exceeds that which can be explained by reactive changes, and the diagnosis should not be downgraded in its presence.

Certain pathological features, when present in biopsies showing high-grade dysplasia, may predict synchronous or underlying invasive carcinoma. These features include dilated glands containing necrotic debris, cribriform/solid growth, ulceration, prominent neutrophils within dysplastic glands, and invasion of dysplastic glands or Pagetoid cells into overlying squamous epithelium. The risk of synchronous adenocarcinoma is high (up to 80%), if two or more of these features are present.

Variants of Dysplasia

Crypt Dysplasia Crypt dysplasia (also called basal gland dysplasia or basal crypt dysplasia-like atypia) is a term proposed for cases of cytologic atypia that meets criteria for either low- or high-grade dysplasia that is limited to the deep glands, which is noted in up to 7.3% of cases of BE (Figure 3.6).

These foci show overexpression of p53 and Ki67, loss of heterozygosity at 17p (TP53), and aneuploidy, suggesting that this may be early form of dysplasia confined to the crypt base. Crypt dysplasia has also been reported to be associated with a higher prevalence of concurrent conventional dysplasia and adenocarcinoma. When present in isolation, serial sectioning is warranted to exclude surface involvement.

Since the predictive value of crypt dysplasia is uncertain, it may be to classify cases with low-grade abnormalities as indefinite for dysplasia to ensure surveillance. However, the presence of high-grade cytologic abnormalities in deep glands that cannot be explained by regenerative atypia should be considered to represent dysplasia with a risk for progression to cancer. Such cases may be placed into an "at least low grade" category. Presently, cases of isolated crypt dysplasia are probably best managed as low grade until further data become available.

Non-adenomatous Dysplasia (Foveolar Dysplasia) In addition to the more common intestinal-type of dysplasia, other distinct morphologic subtypes of dysplasia have been described recently in BE. Non-adenomatous dysplasia, also termed foveolar dysplasia, accounts for approximately 6–8% of dysplasia cases and is characterized by back-to-back glands composed of cuboidal cells with round to ovoid nuclei; a variable nuclear-to-cytoplasmic ratio; nuclear pleomorphism; prominent nucleoli; and clear, mucin-containing cytoplasm (Figures 3.7a and 3.8b). The nuclei may form a monolayer.

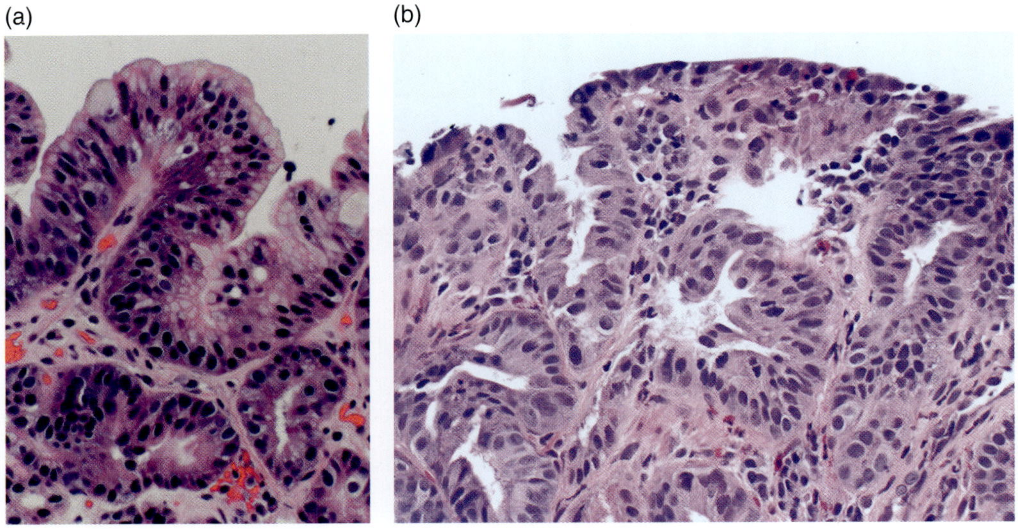

Figure 3.7 (a) Foveolar dysplasia, low grade. This lesion is characterized by tall mucin-rich cytoplasm with basally located round hyperchromatic nuclei; (b) Foveolar dysplasia—high grade. This example shows marked nuclear and architectural atypia. Low columnar/cuboidal cells with ground glass cytoplasm are consistent with the diagnosis.

The grading of this variant is not well characterized, and proposed criteria for high-grade dysplasia in this subtype include high nuclear cytoplasmic ratios (>50%), nuclear enlargement, and complex glandular architecture. However, the high rate of DNA abnormalities and greater prevalence of associated conventional high-grade dysplasia and adenocarcinoma support the concept that foveolar dysplasia is biologically a high-grade lesion. There is evidence that foveolar dysplasia is more likely to arise in a goblet cell-depleted background and carcinomas arising in this setting more often show a gastric phenotype. These findings support the concept of two pathways of malignant transformation in BE: (i) an intestinal pathway associated with intestinal metaplasia and type 1 (intestinal/classical) dysplasia, and (ii) a gastric pathway associated with the development of type 2 (foveolar) dysplasia.

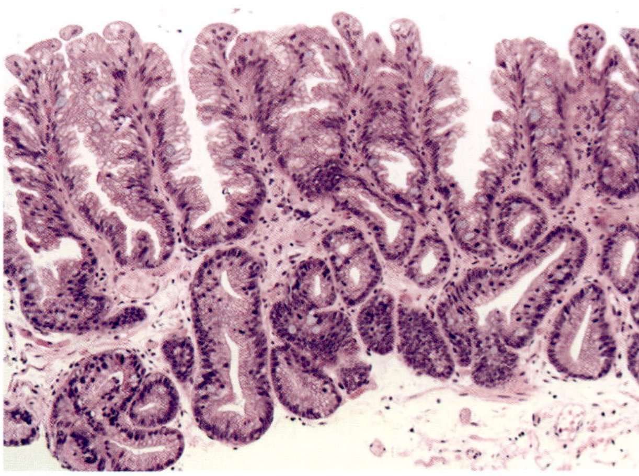

Figure 3.8 Serrated dysplasia—note the serrated profile of the glands with limited nuclear atypia.

Serrated Dysplasia Serrated dysplasia is rare, seldom occurs in pure form, and resembles traditional serrated adenoma of the colorectum. The glands exhibit serrated architecture and the cells show elongated and stratified nuclei, dense eosinophilic cytoplasm, and luminal secretions (Figure 3.8).

Serrated dysplasia, like foveolar dysplasia, appears to have natural history similar to conventional high-grade dysplasia, and it too should be regarded as a high-grade dysplastic phenotype.

Polypoid Dysplasia Polypoid dysplastic lesions exhibit architectural similarities to tubular or tubulovillous adenomas of the colorectum, and polypoid dysplasia has been formerly regarded as an adenoma arising in BE, although the term adenoma is not recommended. A polyp or nodule noted endoscopically that demonstrates high-grade dysplasia on biopsy is associated with a high risk for synchronous adenocarcinoma.

Intramucosal and Invasive Adenocarcinoma in Barrett's Esophagus

Intramucosal adenocarcinoma is defined as invasion of the lamina propria or muscularis mucosae, but without invasion into the submucosa. Lamina propria invasion is often difficult and subjective due to the lack of associated desmoplasia. It can be recognized by the presence of complex glandular patterns such as sheets of neoplastic cells, complex

(a) (b)

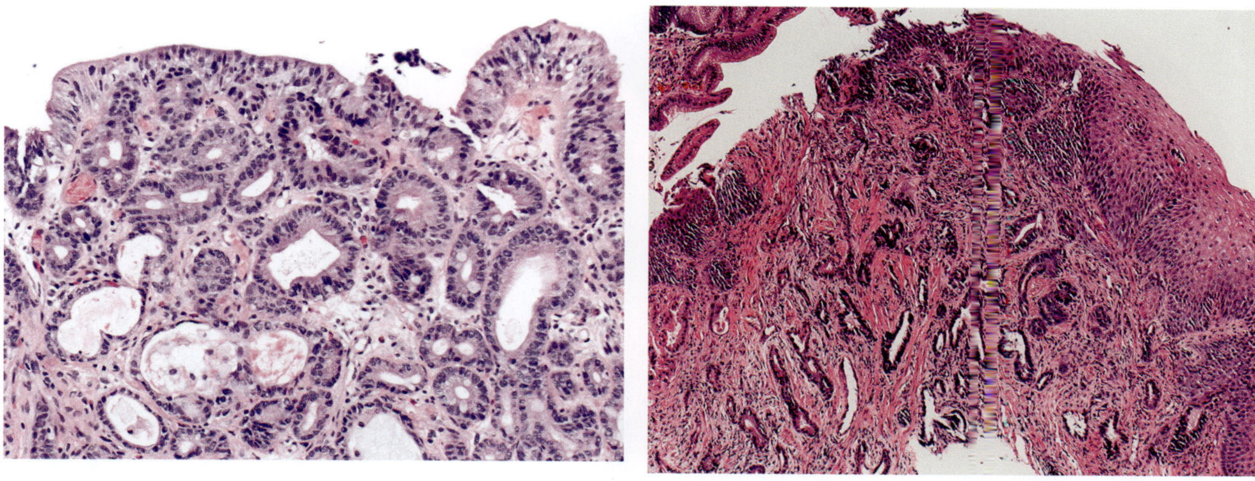

Figure 3.9 (a) Intramucosal adenocarcionma—the lesion is characterized by disorganized and withering neoplastic glands lined by markedly atypical nuclei. Additionally, the glands show necrotic debris. (b) Invasive adenocarcinoma with infiltrating glands surrounded by desmoplastic stroma.

tubular or cribriform glands, abortive angulated glands, confluent and fused glands, dilated glands with intraluminal necrotic debris, and single cell infiltration or neoplastic glands infiltrating the muscularis mucosae (Figures 3.9a, b and 3.12). As previously noted, pagetoid spread of tumor cells is a manifestation of invasive adenocarcinomas. Unequivocal invasion of submucosa or deeper structures is often accompanied by a desmoplastic response. If definitive submucosal invasion is in question, the term "suspicious for invasive carcinoma" can be used.

Musculofibrous anomalies, such as duplication of the muscularis mucosae, prolapse changes, and/or gland entrapment, are frequent in BE with or without neoplasia, and can present a diagnostic pitfall (Figure 3.10). Entrapped atrophic cardiac-type glands and "misplaced" dysplastic glands within and between this musculature may mimic submucosal invasion. In this setting, unequivocal cyto-architectural atypia should be present identified for a diagnosis of invasive adenocarcinoma.

In practice, given the important management implications and the well-recognized inter- and intraobserver variability in the diagnosis of dysplasia, current guidelines recommend that all cases of dysplasia and suspected dysplasia be reviewed by a second pathologist with GI pathology expertise.

Pathologic Features of Endoscopic Mucosal Resection (EMR)

Endoscopic mucosal resection and submucosal dissection (EMR/ESD) have become standard management for localized neoplasia in BE, especially for high-grade dysplasia and intramucosal carcinoma. These specimens can also provide more accurate and reproducible diagnostic and staging information for superficial lesions compared to biopsy specimens and endoscopic ultrasound. EMR and ESD specimens allow evaluation of the duplicated muscularis mucosae, and do not (usually) include muscularis propria. The deepest muscle represents the original muscularis mucosae, and adenocarcinoma extending deep to that

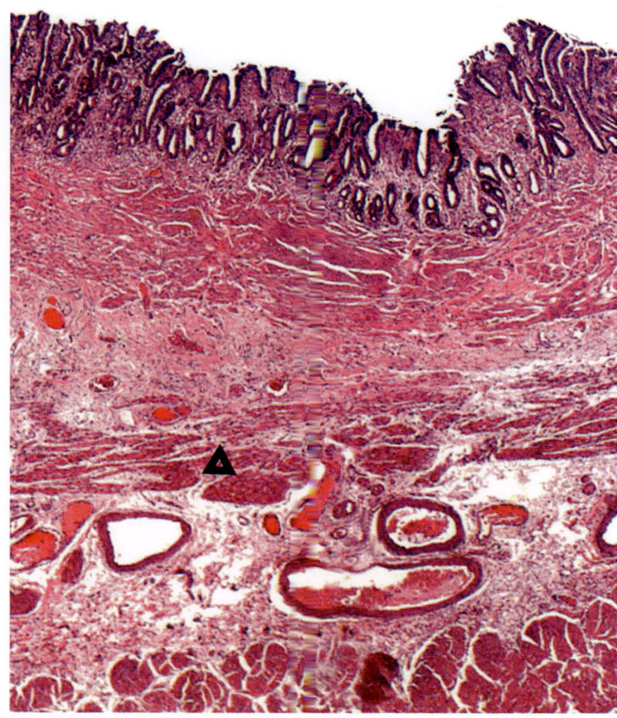

Figure 3.10 Duplicated muscularis mucosae—note the inner and outer (duplicated; triangle) muscular layer.

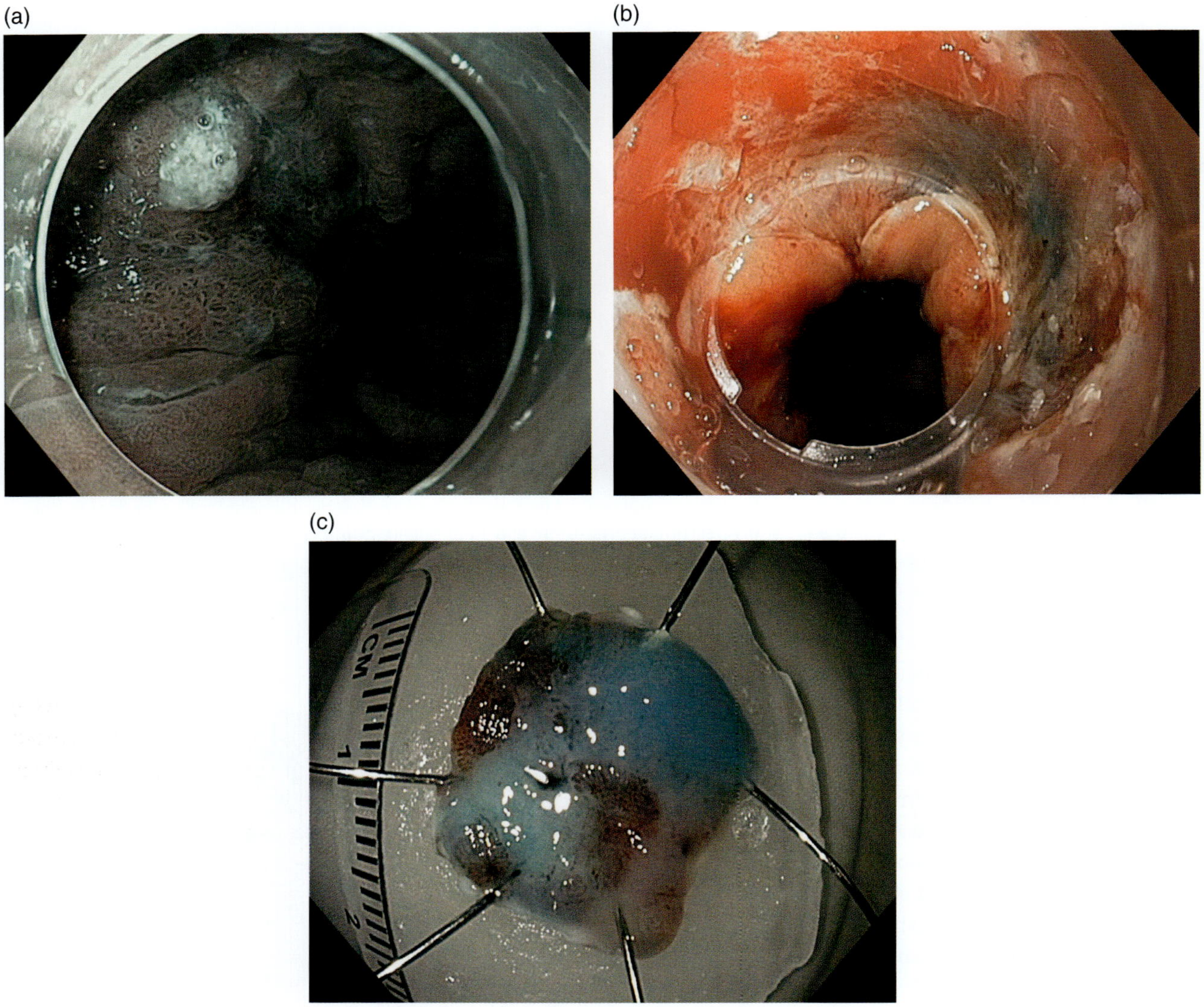

Figure 3.11 (a) Barrett's esophagus with high-grade dysplasia in the 8–12 o'clock region. The image is obtained with narrow-band imaging (blue light) to highlight surface vessels. Note the surface nodularity and hypertrophy and irregularity of surface blood vessels. (b) Appearance of the esophagus after endoscopic mucosal resection. The entire mucosa and part of the submucosa have been resected from 9 to 4 o'clock. (c) The resected specimen is pinned flat to facilitate localization of the lateral and deep margins.

musculature represents submucosal invasion. Additional clues for submucosal invasion include juxtaposition of the malignant glands to submucosal structures, such as esophageal glands/ducts, or large arterioles and venules.

The evaluation of EMR and ESD specimens involves accurate staging and the assessment of margin status. The specimens are typically mounted to a wax block when submitted, which allows for proper orientation and specimen photography. The deep and circumferential margins are inked, and following fixation, tissue sections are obtained at 2-mm intervals. Depending on the specimen size, the ends may be submitted en face or via radial sections. Piecemeal excisions or technical artifacts such as hemorrhage and electrocautery effects may lead to more difficult evaluation for staging and margins.

Great care should be given in the reporting of endoscopic resection specimens. The status of the tissue margins is an important predictor of a relatively high risk of recurrence and lateral and deep margins should be reported separately. Lymphovascular invasion (LVI) is a common finding, noted in 10% of intramucosal carcinomas involving the space between the duplicated layers of muscularis mucosae. It is associated with an increased risk of nodal metastasis. Nodal involvement is demonstrated in 17% of cases with invasion of the duplicated muscularis mucosae, and invasion into the outer muscularis mucosae shows a similar survival rate to invasion of superficial third of the submucosa. Therefore, comprehensive reporting should include a comment on the depth of invasion into the thickened and duplicated muscularis mucosae (Figure 3.11).

Pathologic Features of Ablative Therapy

A variety of ablative therapies (see Section "Prognosis, Evolution, and Clinical Management") are used to manage both non-neoplastic and neoplastic epithelium in BE, with the goal of ablation of BE mucosa and squamous reepithelialization. These techniques may not remove all glandular epithelium, which can persist as hidden or buried epithelium beneath surface squamous epithelium, not visible to the endoscopist (Figure 3.12). Evaluation of these buried glands can be difficult, due to the lack of surface glandular epithelium for the assessment of maturation. Associated desmoplasia and extension of neoplastic glands into the squamous epithelium are features of invasion.

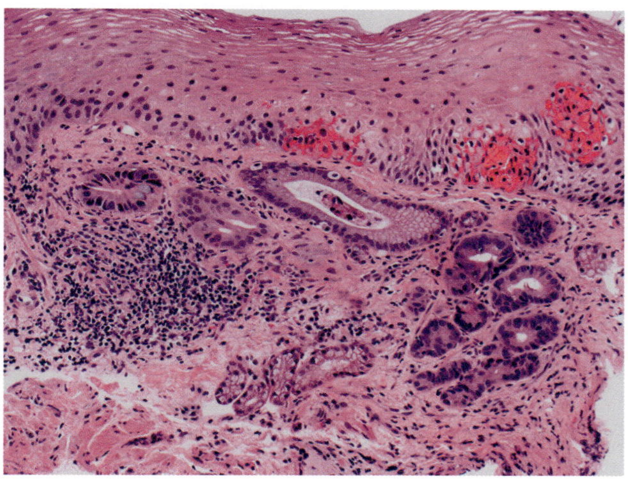

Figure 3.12 Buried BE glands with low-grade dysplasia. This phenomenon can be observed after PPI therapy or radiofrequency ablation.

Immunohistochemical Studies and Molecular Features

Given the overall low risk of neoplastic progression in BE, there is considerable interest in the development of reliable diagnostic and predictive biomarkers. Multiple studies have evaluated the role of immunohistochemical and molecular biomarkers in the classification of dysplasia, as well as risk stratification for neoplastic progression. No single biomarker has shown sufficient utility for routine diagnostic practice, and a panel of biomarkers may ultimately be required for risk stratification. Prospective validation data are lacking, and ACG guidelines state that the use of additional biomarkers or biomarker panel is currently not recommended. The BSG guidelines suggest that addition of p53 immunohistochemistry may improve the diagnostic reproducibility of dysplasia in Barrett's esophagus and should be considered as an adjunct to routine clinical diagnosis.

Immunohistochemistry Immunohistochemistry for nuclear p53, which represents a surrogate marker of underlying *TP53* mutations, has been the most extensively studied marker. The evolving role of p53 IHC includes utility as an adjunct to the diagnosis of dysplasia (particularly HGD), improved diagnostic reproducibility, and as a predictive biomarker for increased risk of progression in both dysplastic and non-dysplastic mucosa. A low level of background wild-type p53 expression is often seen in non-dysplastic BE, which can be a useful baseline. Aberrant expression is defined as either p53 overexpression or a complete loss of p53 expression (Figure 3.13).

A higher risk of neoplastic progression has been reported in LGD with p53 overexpression. A recent study showed that aberrant p53 IHC was a powerful predictor of progression, and the pattern of complete loss of p53 staining was

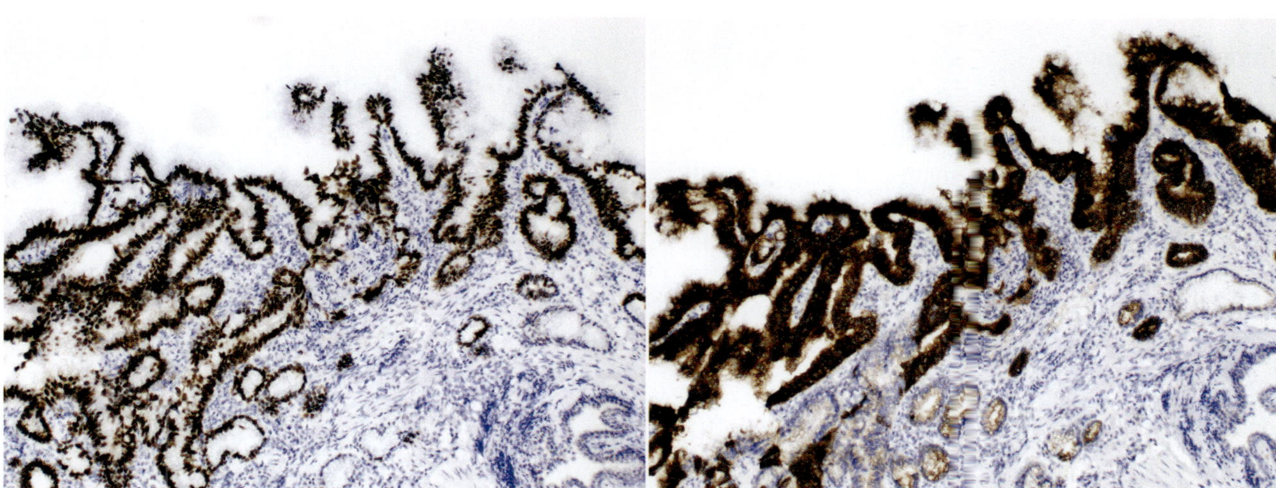

Figure 3.13 Barrett's esophagus with high-grade dysplasia showing p53 (left) and IMP3 (right) overexpression.

associated with a higher risk of neoplastic progression than overexpression. However, false positive and false negative results may be encountered in up to 10–20% of cases.

Alpha-methylacyl-CoA racemase (AMACR) immunoreactivity has been reported as a marker of high-grade dysplasia and carcinoma and as a predictor of progression, but its low sensitivity limits the clinical utility. Alternatively, insulin like growth factor II mRNA-binding protein 3 (IMP3) has been noted as a more specific marker for the diagnosis of high-grade dysplasia. The protein is a member of the IMP family, which appears to play a role in stabilization, binding, and trafficking during embryogenesis. It is generally undetectable or weakly expressed in benign tissue.

Molecular Techniques Flow cytometric DNA content analysis using a panel combining aneuploidy and tetraploidy with 9p LOH (p16) and 17p LOH (p53) has been shown to be a strong predictor of progression to adenocarcinoma. The technical requirements have limited widespread use in clinical practice. Cytometric DNA analysis of Feulgen-stained, formalin-fixed, paraffin embedded tissue samples may be a means to improve the feasibility of clinical implementation. Fluorescence in situ hybridization (FISH) panels, such as those utilizing probes for CDKN2A, CMYC, erbB-2, and 20q13.2, may increase sensitivity of detecting abnormal DNA content.

A recent whole-genome sequencing study unexpectedly showed that the majority of recurrently mutated genes in esophageal adenocarcinoma were also mutated in non-dysplastic Barrett mucosa. Only p53 and SMAD4 mutations occurred in a stage-specific manner, with p53 confined to HGD in high frequency (86%) and SMAD4 found in adenocarcinoma in low frequency (13%). Other molecular markers, such as those detecting BE neoplasia-related gene methylation abnormalities, remain experimental.

Differential Diagnosis

Microscopic

The microscopic features distinguishing the spectrum of non-dysplastic, dysplastic, and malignant changes in BE are discussed in Section "Barrett's Esophagus–Dysplasia—Esophageal Adenocarc." The major differential diagnostic considerations are summarized in Table 3.3.

Ancillary studies (if applicable)—see Section "Immunohistochemical Studies and Molecular Features."

Prognosis, Evolution, and Clinical Management

Management of neoplasia in Barrett's esophagus has been transformed in the past 15 years from one of surveillance vs. surgery to endoscopic therapy in many cases. The current threshold for endoscopic treatment is low-grade dysplasia or worse. It is critical to have low-grade dysplasia confirmed by a second expert pathologist given the marked variability in interpretation of LGD. Once any degree of dysplasia is confirmed, the Barrett's epithelium should be eradicated until all dysplasia and intestinal metaplasia is absent.

Focal nodular or depressed regions should be resected endoscopically, typically by band-mucosectomy. This involves suctioning the target lesion into a modified variceal banding cap, followed by snare resection. This may be repeated multiple times ("multiband mucosectomy") until all nodular areas are removed. It is important to note that the true lateral margins can only be assessed with single, en bloc resections; however, the deep margins can be assessed in all specimens.

Following EMR and pathological staging, lesions that are confined to the mucosa or superficial lesions (typically <500 micron invasion below muscularis mucosa) are further treated with radiofrequency ablation until all visible Barrett's epithelium is eradicated. This may require two to three or more sessions, spaced two to three months apart. Complete eradication of intestinal metaplasia (CRIM) is confirmed both endoscopically (no visible salmon-colored mucosa) and histologically, by biopsy of the distal neo-squamous epithelium and GE junction.

Following CRIM, endoscopic surveillance should continue since there is a small but real recurrence rate. For HGD or CIS, this is typically every three months for one year, followed by less intensive surveillance afterward. For LGD, this is typically every six months for one year, then less intensive.

Recent studies suggest that it is only necessary to biopsy the distal 2 cm of neo-squamous epithelium above the new squamocolumnar junction in addition to visible islands of Barrett's epithelium.

Squamous Cell Dysplasia and Carcinoma

Definition, General Features, Predisposing Factors

Esophageal squamous cell carcinoma remains the predominant type of esophageal carcinoma worldwide. The vast majority of cases occur in Asia, Africa, and South America. In the West, particularly in white males, squamous cell carcinomas have been eclipsed by adenocarcinomas arising in Barrett's esophagus. However, in North America, squamous carcinoma still predominates among African American males. It has a male predominance and the risk increases with age, particularly beyond the age of 60 years, and an association with low socioeconomic status.

Table 3.3 Histological features in the assessment of mucosal biopsies for dysplasia and carcinoma in Barrett's esophagus.

	Surface maturation	Gland architecture	Cytologic features	Inflammation erosions ulcers
Negative reactive	Present	Preserved	Uniform, vesicular chromatin Small nucleoli Gradual transition in morphology as they move away from focus of inflammation	Variable
LGD	Absent	Mild gland crowding Serrated architecture in serrated dysplasia	Intestinal: Pencillate, hyperchromatic, stratified nuclei limited to basal portion of cytoplasm Minimal loss of polarity Abrupt transition Foveolar: Few or no goblet cells Cuboidal cells with round-oval nuclei N/C ratio <50% Mucinous cytoplasm Serrated: Eosinophilic cytoplasm Small, oval nuclei with mild stratification	Variable
HGD	Absent	Marked gland crowding Fused glands Villiform pattern serrated architecture in serrated dysplasia	Intestinal: Loss of nuclear polarity Full thickness stratification Hyperchromasia, irregular nuclear membranes, prominent nucleoli Atypical mitosis Foveolar: Nuclear enlargement and pleomorphism High N/C ratio Serrated: Nuclear enlargement, stratification, pleomorphism, loss of polarity Atypical mitoses	Variable, may be prominent
IMCa	Absent	Complex—sheets, cribriform glands, confluent and fused glands, abortive and angulated glands, single-cell infiltration, dilated crypts with necrosis Lack of desmoplasia	Similar to HGD	Variable
SMCa	Absent	Desmoplastic response present	Similar to HGD/IMCa	

IMCa, intramucosal carcinoma; SMCa, submucosal carcinoma; LED, low-grade dysplasia; HGD, high-grade dysplasia.
Source: Modified from Naini, B.V., Souza, R.F., and Odze, R.D. (2016). Barrett's esophagus: a comprehensive and contemporary review for pathologists. *Am. J. Surg. Pathol.* 40: e45–e66.

Squamous dysplasia, or squamous intraepithelial neoplasia, represents the important precursor lesion. The concept of early squamous cell carcinoma encompasses intramucosal carcinoma regardless of the nodal status.

Environmental factors that cause chronic irritation and inflammation of the esophageal mucosa play a major role in pathogenesis. Major risk factors include alcohol and smoking, particularly in combination, similar to other aerodigestive malignancies. The risk of synchronous or metachronous esophageal cancer in a patient with a primary head and neck squamous cell carcinoma is between 3 and 9%. A synergistic affect has also been demonstrated with chewing tobacco, ingesting or smoking pipe stem residues, and chewing betel quid. In a subset of Asian patients, a genetic polymorphism in the aldehyde dehydrogenase (ALDH2) gene enhances the risk for esophageal squamous cancer with alcohol use. Dietary factors also play a role, such as ingestion of N-nitroso compounds and consumption of foods and beverages at very high temperatures (e.g. strong tea in northeastern China and hot maté in southern Brazil).

To date, the pathogenetic role of human papillomavirus remains inconclusive, although it may be a cofactor in certain high-incidence regions, or in groups whose behavior exposes them to a high risk of esophageal HPV infections.

Achalasia, esophageal diverticula, and caustic injury, which lead to stasis of food or saliva and to chronic mucosal irritation, are also associated with an increased risk. Patients with a history of corrosive esophageal strictures should also be monitored closely for the late development of carcinoma. The occurrence of squamous carcinoma arising in chronic lichen planus esophagitis has been reported, as well as after ablative therapy or endoscopic mucosal resection (EMR) for Barrett neoplasia.

A higher incidence of squamous carcinoma is associated with Plummer–Vinson syndrome (iron deficiency anemia, dysphagia, and upper esophageal webs) and tylosis (a rare autosomal-dominant disorder characterized by hyperkeratosis of the squamous epithelium of the palmar and plantar surfaces as well as oral and esophageal mucosa).

An association between high-grade dysplasia and/or squamous cell carcinoma has been reported in patients with esophageal leukoplakia or epidermoid metaplasia, a rare lesion predominantly involving the mid-distal esophagus in middle-aged to elderly females, and associated with smoking and excessive alcohol consumption.

Clinical Features and Endoscopic Characteristics

Squamous cell carcinomas are most common in the middle third of the esophagus, but may also occur in the distal or proximal esophagus.

Microscopic Features

Squamous Dysplasia

Squamous dysplasia (intraepithelial neoplasia), the principle precursor lesion, is commonly found adjacent to the invasive carcinomas and is frequently multifocal. Carcinomas associated with dysplasia are also more likely to be multifocal in origin.

A two-tier classification scheme is currently recommended, i.e. low-grade and high-grade dysplasia. The 2010 WHO classification uses the term "intraepithelial neoplasia" for dysplasia and CIS. "Low-grade intraepithelial neoplasia" encompasses mild or moderate dysplasia, while "high-grade intraepithelial neoplasia" is used for severe dysplasia and carcinoma in situ (CIS), two lesions that have the same clinical implications. Once invasion of the lamina propria is observed, the lesion is diagnosed as invasive carcinoma.

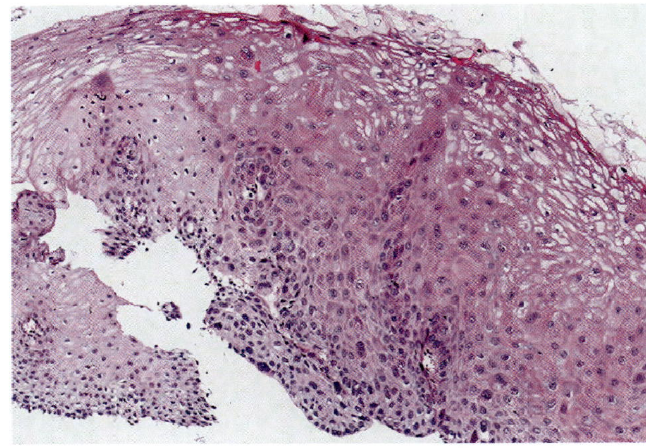

Figure 3.14 Squamous low-grade dysplasia/intraepithelial neoplasia. Note the sharp oblique line of demarcation between benign and neoplastic epithelium.

Dysplasia is characterized by both architectural and cytological abnormalities that vary in extent and severity. Architectural abnormalities include loss of normal cell polarity, overlapping nuclei, and lack of surface maturation. Diagnostic cytologic features include enlarged, hyperchromatic nuclei with irregular nuclear membranes, increased nuclear-to-cytoplasmic ratio, increased mitotic activity, and abnormal mitotic figures. At low magnification, a sharp demarcation forming an oblique line or front commonly delineates the neoplastic epithelium from the surrounding epithelium (Figure 3.14). In low-grade dysplasia/low-grade intraepithelial neoplasia, the diagnostic features are confined to the basal half of the epithelium, whereas they involve the full thickness of the epithelium in high-grade dysplasia/CIS (Figure 3.15a, b). It is important to recognize that the dysplastic epithelium may extend into the submucosal ducts and glands, a feature that should not be misdiagnosed for invasion.

There are interpretive differences between Japanese and western pathologists. For example, lesions diagnosed as high-grade IN, and some lesions categorized as low-grade IN in the West would be diagnoses as squamous cell carcinoma in situ in Japan. Japanese pathologists recognize a lesion reported as "basal layer type squamous cell carcinoma in situ," in which the basal half of the epithelium is replaced by carcinoma cells that have the cytologic appearance similar to that of the cells of an invasive squamous cell carcinoma, with loss of polarity but somewhat preserved surface maturation (Figure 3.16).

Squamous Cell Carcinoma

Squamous cell carcinomas may be separated into early (superficial) and late (advanced) types. *Superficial* or *early carcinomas* are synonyms relating to carcinoma involving either the mucosa or submucosa regardless of the presence

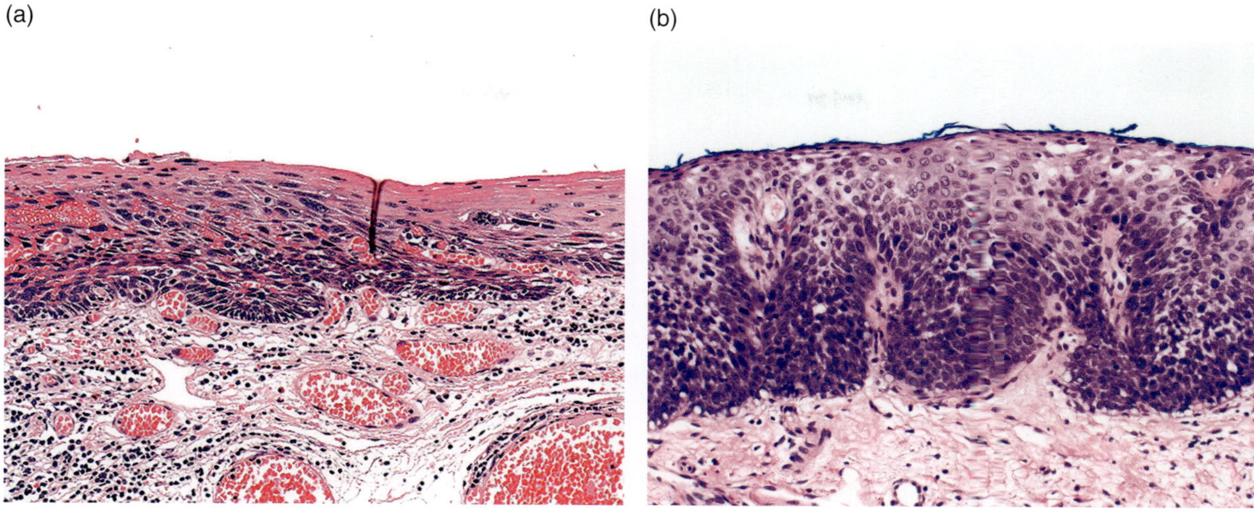

Figure 3.15 (a) Squamous high-grade dysplasia/intraepithelial neoplasia with hyperchromatic angulated nuclei reaching the upper layers of the mucosa. (b) Squamous high-grade dysplasia extending the entire thickness of the epithelium.

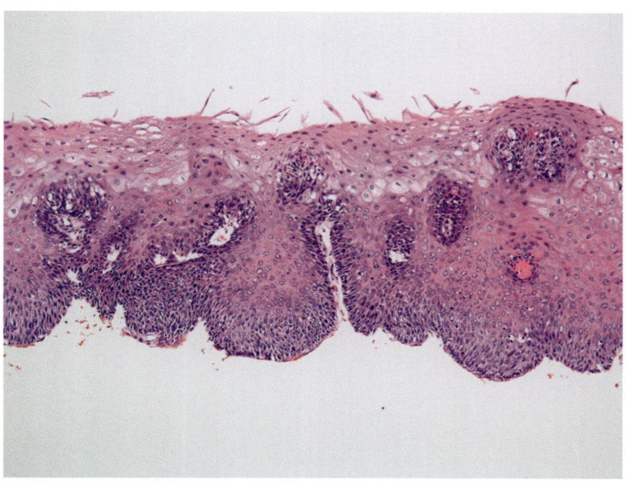

Figure 3.16 Basal layer dysplasia/intraepithelial neoplasia—note the basal atypical cells with increased mitotic activity, hyperchromatic angulated nuclei, and high N/C ratio.

of lymph node metastasis. Superficial carcinomas comprise 15–20% of all invasive squamous cell carcinomas, with higher prevalence rates in populations routinely undergoing endoscopic surveillance (Figure 3.17).

Superficial carcinoma can be further divided into six groups according to the depth of invasion (Figure 3.18). M1–M3 represent in situ and intramucosal carcinoma, and SM1–SM3 represent invasion of submucosa (divided into thirds). In ESD specimens, SM1 is distinguished from SM2 at a depth of 200 microns from the muscularis mucosa. In this subclassification, M1–M3 carcinomas are considered to be early squamous cell carcinoma regardless of nodal metastases; M1 and M2 carcinomas with essentially no risk of nodal metastases are considered to be curable by endoscopic mucosal resection alone.

Superficially invasive tumors are more commonly multicentric (up to 20% of cases) compared with advanced tumors. Multicentric tumors may represent synchronous primary tumors occurring in a dysplastic field or reflect satellite tumor nodules resulting from intramural metastases.

The diagnosis of invasion is established by the presence of single-cell infiltration, irregular discontinuous nests of cells, and a desmoplastic stromal response, which may be challenging in small or poorly oriented biopsy specimens. In superficial invasion, the tumor cells extend into the lamina propria, muscularis mucosae, or submucosa as isolated cells or clusters of cells. The desmoplastic response may be minimal at this stage. Mucosal and submucosal lymphatic invasion is common and may account for intramural metastasis. Advanced carcinomas invade the muscularis propria and beyond, exhibiting either an infiltrative or expansile (pushing) growth pattern.

Well to moderately differentiated tumors display nests of polygonal epithelioid cells with ample eosinophilic cytoplasm, intercellular bridges, and keratinization (Figure 3.19). Poorly differentiated tumors show no keratinization and grow in solid sheets or as single cells, which may be large and pleomorphic. Focal glandular differentiation occurs in up to 20% of cases. When the glandular and squamous components are comparable in volume and admixed, a diagnosis of adenosquamous carcinoma is warranted. Prominent tumor budding at the invasive front has been reported as an adverse prognostic indicator in early (pT1) carcinoma.

In small, poorly oriented biopsy specimens, distinguishing between squamous dysplasia and invasive carcinoma

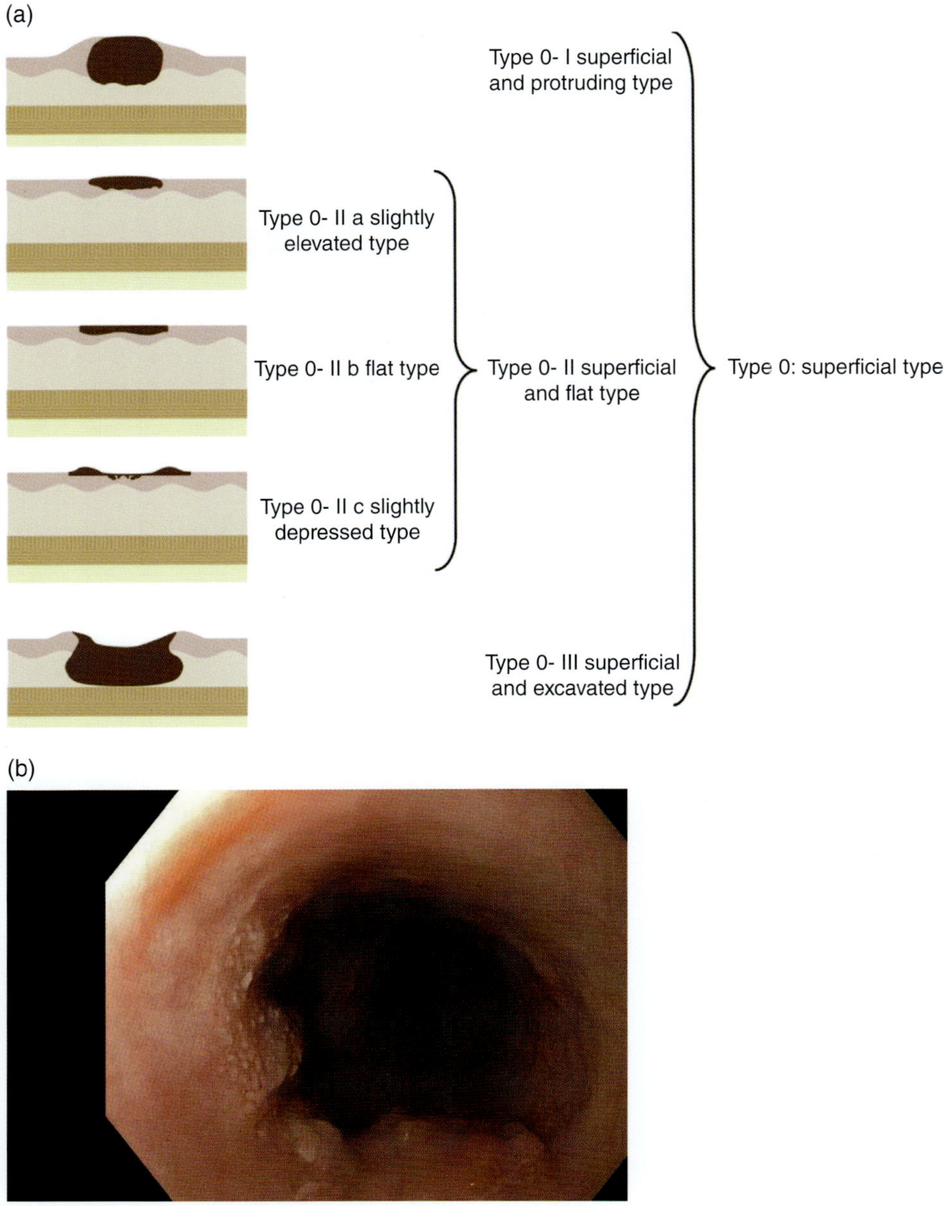

Figure 3.17 (a) Schema of endoscopic and macroscopic classification of superficial carcinoma of the esophagus. (b) Squamous T1a carcinoma from 6 to 10 o'clock. The mucosa appears nodular and reddish. *Source:* From Shimizu M, Zaninotto G, Nagata K, et al. Esophageal squamous cell carcinoma with special reference to its early stage. Best Prac Res Clin Gastroenterol, 27:171–186. © 2013 Elsevier.

may be challenging. Dysplasia, unlike invasive carcinoma, displays smooth-edged papillations with a continuous basement membrane and a connection to the surface epithelium. It lacks single-cell infiltration, the presence of irregular discontinuous cellular nests of cells and desmoplasia. Repeat biopsies and endoscopic correlation may be necessary to establish a diagnosis in difficult cases.

Variants of esophageal squamous cell carcinoma include basaloid carcinoma (Figure 3.20), verrucous carcinoma (Figure 3.21), sarcomatoid carcinoma, and lymphoepithelial carcinoma (Figure 3.22). These entities may be difficult to diagnose in small mucosal biopsy specimens, or confused with other tumor types. The sarcomatoid subtype (spindle cell carcinoma, carcinosarcoma) often presents as an exophytic, polypoid mass with obstruction. Notably, the squamous component may be focal and peripheral or absent in the biopsy sampling. Extensive sampling of the resected tumor and cytokeratin stains may be necessary to confirm the diagnosis.

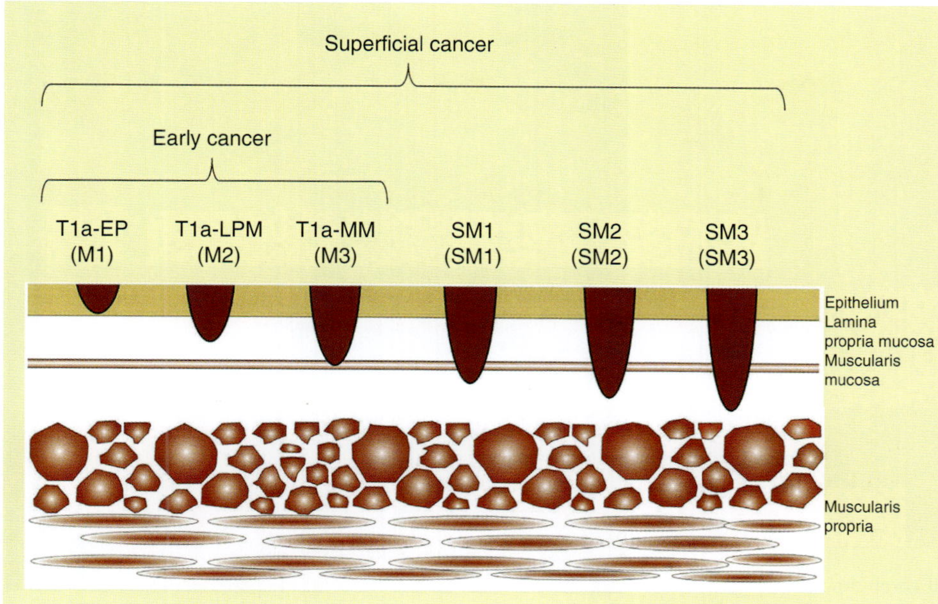

Figure 3.18 Schematic presentation of early and superficial esophageal cancer. **T1a** is designated as an early cancer and divided into three groups: epithelial (EP), lamina propria muscularis (LPM), and muscularis mucosae (MM) on the basis of the depth of invasion. **T1b** is also divided into three groups according to tumor invasion of the submucosa: (i) into the upper third (SM1); (ii) middle third (SM2); (iii) lower third (SM3). *Source:* Japanese classification of esophageal cancer, 7th edition. © Japan Esophageal Society.

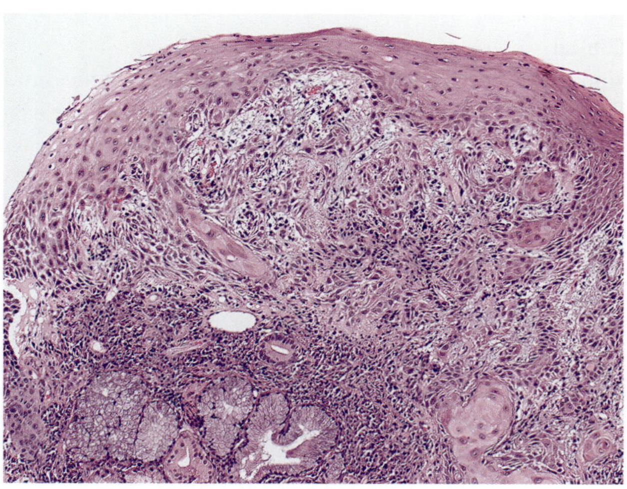

Figure 3.19 Well-differentiated squamous cell carcinoma showing nests of atypical squamous cells with abortive keratinization surrounded by stroma with desmoplastic changes, characterized by the mucoid background.

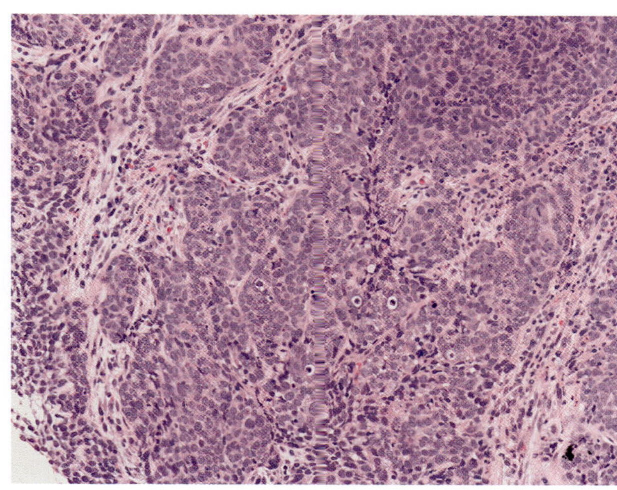

Figure 3.20 Basaloid squamous cell carcinoma characteristically showing pleomorphic hyperchromatic nuclei, scant cytoplasm, and high rate of single cell necrosis.

Immunohistochemical Studies and Molecular Features

In conventional squamous dysplasia and invasive squamous cell carcinoma, special studies are not required to establish a diagnosis. For invasive carcinoma, immunostains may be useful in small biopsy specimens, poorly differentiated tumors, or when rare tumor cells are present, e.g. post neoadjuvant therapy. Malignant squamous cells are positive for p63, p40, CK 5/6, and broad-spectrum cytokeratin stains. Most cases are negative for CK7 and CK20, although CK7 expression in a subset of cases has been reported to be a useful biomarker for predicting a worse outcome of stage I/IIA/IIB patients. Focal positivity for chromogranin and synaptophysin may occur in a minority of tumor cells in otherwise typical squamous carcinomas. Altered expression of various molecular markers

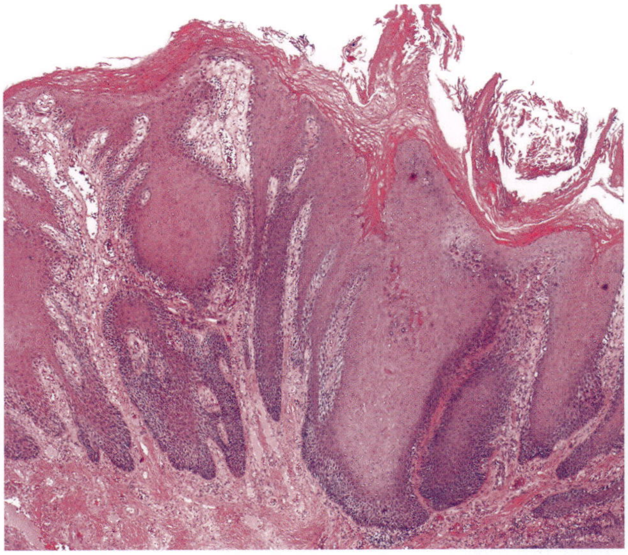

Figure 3.21 Verrucous squamous cell carcinoma showing hyper- and parakeratosis and pushing invasive boarders at the base.

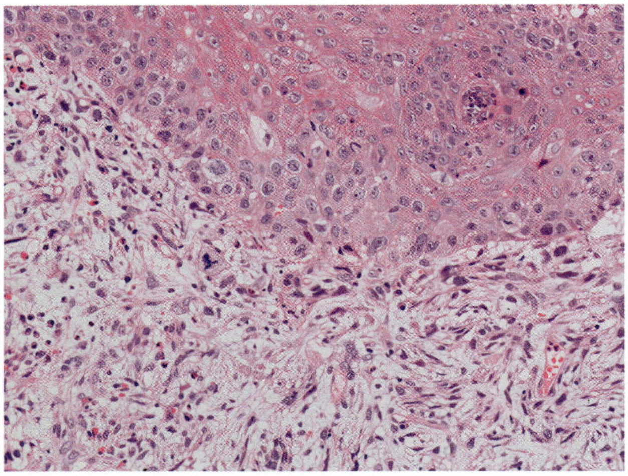

Figure 3.22 Sarcomatoid squamous cell carcinoma. This picture shows atypical squamous epithelium with a high-grade spindle cell neoplasm underneath. Note the tripolar atypical mitosis on the left side of the picture. Detection of high-grade dysplasia/CIS is necessary for a reliable diagnosis of sarcomatoid squamous cell carcinoma.

such as p53, p16, cyclin D1, EGFR, E-cadherin, p27 (a CDK inhibitor), p21, bcl-2, and Rb have associated with the development and progression of esophageal squamous cell carcinoma but currently have a limited role in routine practice. Other markers reported to be associated with adverse prognosis include aberrant methylation of the Fragile Histidine Triad (FHIT) gene, high expression of phosphorylated 4E-BP-1 (a regulator of cell signaling pathways), and hypermethylation of E-cadherin (CDH1) and integrin $\alpha 4$ genes.

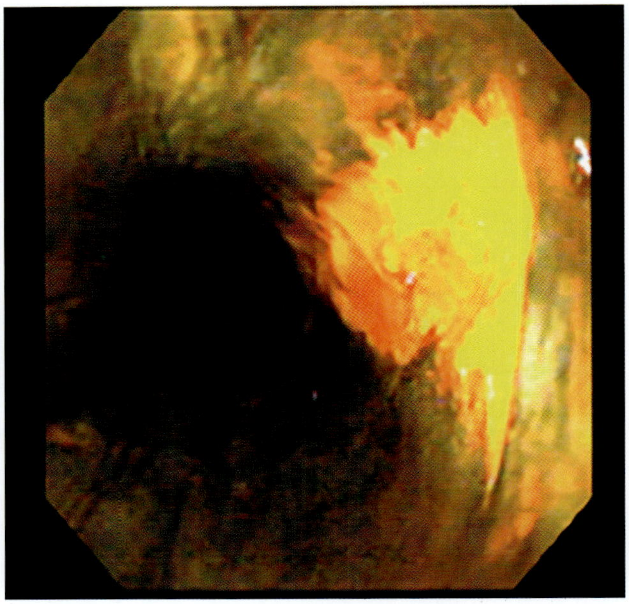

Figure 3.23 Lugol's iodine staining in vivo of an early squamous cell carcinoma. The malignant lesion appears pale amid the background of darkly stained normal epithelium.

Differential Diagnosis

Clinical

Squamous neoplasia may present as subtle plaques and color change in the esophageal mucosal. These can be easily confused with esophagitis. High-resolution narrow-band imaging as well as Lugol's iodine staining (Figure 3.27) is helpful for detection of early dysplastic lesions. Iodine is taken up by the normal esophageal cells but not dysplastic cells. Under NBI imaging, there are dilated intrapapillary capillary loops (IPCLs) (Figure 3.23).

Microscopic

The most frequent differential diagnosis is distinguishing squamous dysplasia from esophagitis-associated reactive atypia (Table 3.4), which may also exhibit mild nuclear enlargement, hyperchromasia, and expansion of the basal cell layer (Figure 3.16). However, unlike dysplasia, the nuclear chromatin is generally fine and homogeneous and nucleoli are small. The reactive cells also lack irregular nuclear membranes, nuclear hyperchromasia and pleomorphism, nuclear overlapping, increased nuclear-to-cytoplasmic ratio, eosinophilic nucleoli, increased mitotic activity, and abnormal mitoses. Architecturally, reactive epithelium often displays surface maturation and maintained cellular polarity. Mucosal inflammation, spongiosis, and vascular congestion are frequently present. In some cases, a definitive diagnosis of dysplasia may be difficult, and a diagnosis of "indefinite for dysplasia" is appropriate. Follow-up biopsies

Table 3.4 Histologic features of reactive squamous epithelium vs. dysplasia.

Feature	Reactive change	Dysplasia/intraepithelial neoplasia
Basal cell hyperplasia	Uniform cells	Highly atypical cells
Surface maturation	Present	Usually absent (HGD)
Demarcation with normal epithelium	Indistinct	Sharp demarcation, oblique line
Keratinization	Usually absent	Usually present
Nuclear chromatin	Fine and homogenous	Hyperchromasia
Nuclear overlapping	Absent	Present
Nuclear pleomorphism	Mild	Prominent
Nuclear membranes	Smooth contour	Irregular contour
Nuclear polarity	Maintained	Abnormal
Nucleoli	Present, small and uniform	Prominent, eosinophilic
Mitoses	Present, typical	Increased, atypical
Inflammation	Present	Variable

Source: Modified from Arai, T., Matsuda, Y., Nishimura, M. et al. (2015). Histopathological diagnoses of squamous intraepithelial neoplasia, carcinoma in situ and early invasive cancer of the oesophagus: the Japanese viewpoint. *Diagnostic Histopathology* 21 (8): 303–311.

after treatment of the underlying esophagitis may be necessary to resolve the diagnostic uncertainty. Immunostains for Ki67 and p53 have been reported to assist in some cases in distinguishing dysplasia from reactive changes.

Squamous cell carcinoma must also be distinguished from pseudoepitheliomatous hyperplasia and pseudodiverticulosis. The former is an exuberant reactive process lacking significant nuclear pleomorphism, loss of polarity, or overlapping of nuclei, lacks desmoplasia, and maintains a connection to the surface epithelium. Pseudodiverticulosis is rare and caused by extensive squamous metaplasia of the esophageal ducts and glands that may be irregular in shape, simulating a carcinoma. An infiltrative growth pattern and other histologic features of neoplastic epithelium are lacking.

Squamous epithelial atypia due to chemotherapy and/or radiation is also a diagnostic challenge in the setting of treated squamous cell carcinoma. The squamous epithelium may contain atypical cells with enlarged hyperchromatic nuclei, but these cells do not exhibit an increased nuclear-to-cytoplasmic ratio and often show distinctive cytoplasmic vacuolization. In addition, underlying mesenchymal cells in the lamina propria show similar changes, as well as other features of radiation effect. Distinguishing between residual neoplastic cells and reactive mesenchymal cells can be difficult and may require cytokeratin immunostains.

The differential diagnosis of spindle cell squamous carcinomas may include leiomyosarcoma, GIST and melanoma, particularly in small biopsies. Appropriate immunohistochemical markers include cytokeratins, melanoma markers (S100, HMB-45, MART-1), and GIST markers (CD117, DOG1). Primary sarcomas and GIST of the esophagus are rare.

Prognosis, Evolution, and Clinical Management

Endoscopic screening in high-risk individuals has led to detection of squamous dysplasia and superficial carcinoma. Endoscopic resection has been curative for early stage (T1a and superficial, <500 micron invasion T1b) lesions. Two techniques have been described including endoscopic mucosal resection, typically with a suction cap device, and endoscopic submucosal dissection (ESD). ESD is technically more challenging but allows wide-field endoscopic resection of lesions of almost any size. Practically, ESD is used for lesions 1–3 cm in size as lesions larger than this are frequently more deeply invasive.

Stage T2N0 lesions can be resected with surgery alone; however, T3 or N1 disease is typically treated with neoadjuvant chemoradiotherapy followed by resection. Advanced, T4 or M1 disease is treated with palliative measures including stenting.

Epithelial Polyps

Inflammatory and Hyperplastic Polyps

Definition, General Features, Predisposing Factors

Inflammatory polyps are a localized exaggerated response to mucosal injury. Most occur in adult males in the distal esophagus and at the gastroesophageal junction, and are associated with gastroesophageal reflux disease (GERD). Some may represent healed ulcer sites. Proximal to the gastroesophageal junction, inflammatory polyps may be associated with mucosal injury caused by pill fragments, infection, or surgical anastomoses.

Clinical Features and Endoscopic Characteristics

Inflammatory polyps of the esophagus are rare, perhaps surprisingly so given the frequency of GERD. Hyperplasia typically occurs at the gastroesophageal junction and is associated with erosive esophagitis. Raised sessile tissue and hypertrophied esophageal folds are much more frequently encountered than true polyps. Endoscopically, they appear as inflamed, reddish folds, usually with associated erosive esophagitis.

Microscopic Features

Squamous lined inflammatory polyps have a smooth, rounded surface and consist of irregular tongues of squamous epithelium that extend into the inflamed lamina propria. These polyps represent an endophytic subtype of squamous papilloma (see Section "Squamous Papilloma"). At the gastroesophageal junction, GERD-associated hyperplastic polyps may also be composed of hyperplastic gastric foveolar epithelium, with or without adjacent hyperplastic and regenerative squamous epithelium. In about 1/3 of cases, these gastric-type hyperplastic polyps are associated with short-segment Barrett's esophagus.

Differential Diagnosis

Clinical The main differential diagnosis is to distinguish from nodular Barrett's esophagus as well as carditis with hypertrophied gastric folds.

Microscopic Pseudoepitheliomatous hyperplasia in squamous lined inflammatory polyps may need to be differentiated from invasive squamous cell carcinoma, which shows cytologic atypia, abnormal deep keratinization, and a desmoplastic stromal reaction.

Prognosis, Evolution, and Clinical Management

Once Barrett's esophagus is excluded, treatment is aimed at the management of GERD, typically with proton pump inhibitors and lifestyle modifications. In cases of bleeding, the polyps can be removed with standard polypectomy or ablated with thermal or cryogenic devices.

Squamous Papilloma

Definition, General Features, Predisposing Factors

Esophageal squamous papillomas are benign epithelial polyps composed of hyperplastic squamous epithelium. They are rare lesions with an incidence in patients undergoing upper endoscopy ranging from 0.01 to 0.45%. They typically occur in adults in their 50's, and are more common in men. They are rare in children unless associated with laryngeal papillomatosis.

The pathogenesis of esophageal papillomas is uncertain, although most appear to represent post-inflammatory lesions. Approximately 70% of papillomas occur in the distal esophagus, and are associated with reflux or other forms of esophageal mucosal injury. The role of human papilloma virus (HPV) in the pathogenesis of esophageal papillomas is inconclusive, with geographic variation. Most squamous papillomas are not associated with HPV, although rare lesions (<10%) may be HPV related. Both low-risk and high-risk subtypes (e.g. types 6/11 and 16, respectively) have been reported. A subset of patients with laryngeal papillomatosis may have HPV-associated esophageal papillomas. They can be seen more frequently in patients with tylosis and acanthosis nigricans, and there is an association with Goltz syndrome.

Clinical Features and Endoscopic Characteristics

Esophageal papillomas are an uncommon, often incidental finding at endoscopy. They are generally small, 1–3 mm, verrucous growths and benign. Their clinical significance is unknown. They can be removed by biopsy forceps or snare to confirm the diagnosis (Figure 3.24).

Microscopic Features

Grossly, esophageal squamous papillomas are usually small, discrete, sessile, soft, tan lesions that range in size from 0.5 to 3 cm. As much as 20% of cases are multiple, and rare cases of diffuse papillomatosis have also been reported.

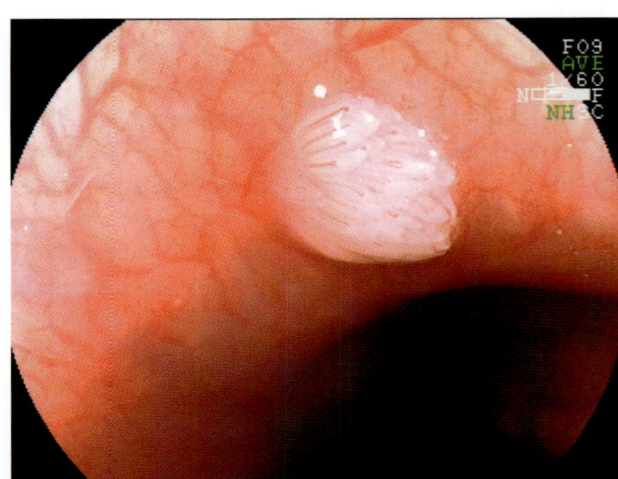

Figure 3.24 Endoscopic appearance of an esophageal papilloma appearing as a whitish nodule composed of papillary projection with thin vascular cores.

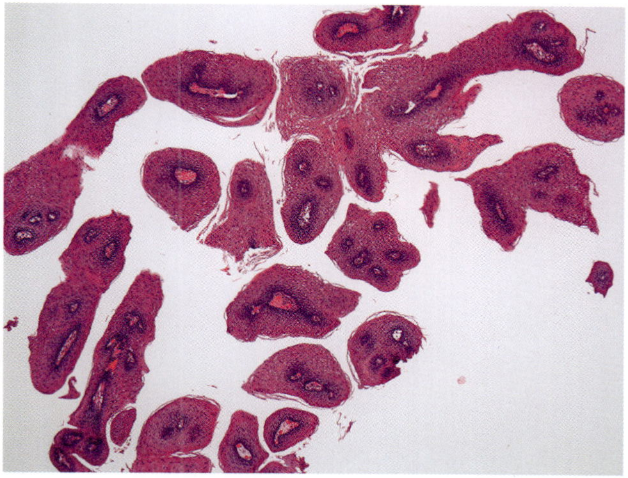

Figure 3.25 Exophytic squamous papilloma showing delicate fibro-vascular cores being covered by mature squamous epithelium.

Histologic growth patterns include exophytic, endophytic, and spiked (verrucous). The most common exophytic type is characterized by finger-like projections of squamous papillae with delicate fibrovascular cores (Figure 3.25). Well-developed features of koilocytosis are usually absent. The endophytic type of papilloma has a round, smooth surface and an inverted appearance, indistinguishable from some inflammatory squamous polyps. Uncommon spiked squamous papillomas have a verrucous appearance, hyperkeratosis, and a prominent granular cell layer. This subtype may more commonly harbor HPV (40% in one study).

Immunohistochemical Studies and Molecular Features

In most lesions, ancillary studies for detecting the presence of HPV are not indicated. If suspected, in situ hybridization may be utilized to demonstrate HPV serotypes.

Differential Diagnosis

Squamous papillomas may all be confused clinically with squamous carcinoma, glycogenic acanthosis, or granular cell tumors (although these typically have a smooth surface).

Microscopic The bland and benign appearance of esophageal squamous papillomas rarely leads to difficulty in distinguishing these lesions from dysplastic or malignant squamous proliferations. Rarely, large lesions may need to be distinguished from verrucous carcinoma (see Section "Squamous Cell Carcinoma").

Prognosis, Evolution, and Clinical Management

Squamous papillomas are benign lesions that may recur. Rare cases of possible malignant transformation have been reported.

Heterotopias

Definition, General Features, Predisposing Factors

Several types of heterotopic tissue may present as nodular or polypoid lesions in the esophagus, most commonly gastric, sebaceous, and pancreatic. These deposits are presumed to be congenital anomalies, although in some cases a possible relationship with GERD and BE has been proposed.

Gastric heterotopia ("inlet patch") is the most common type, with a reported prevalence of 2–11% of patients undergoing upper endoscopy. These lesions are usually located in the proximal esophagus, and have been reported in all ages, most commonly in middle-aged adults.

Heterotopic sebaceous glands are the second most common form of heterotopia in the esophagus. They may occur at any level of the esophagus and are frequently multiple. Pancreatic acinar tissue may be also discovered in the distal esophagus and gastroesophageal junction, although it typically is an incidental finding and not visible endoscopically. The nature of whether these foci of pancreatic tissue represent congenital heterotopic lesions or metaplastic phenomena due to GERD is uncertain.

Clinical Features and Endoscopic Characteristics

Gastric heterotopia/inlet patches are seen in the very proximal esophagus, just below the upper esophageal sphincter. They have an appearance of typical gastric-type mucosa (Figure 3.26). They have recently been associated with globus sensation and their ablation led to resolution of globus sensation. Progression to cancer, as is seen in classical Barrett's esophagus, is extremely rare. The other forms of heterotopia are very rare (Figure 3.27).

Microscopic Features

In gastric heterotopia, biopsies show corpus or fundic-type gastric mucosa (Figure 3.28), usually with parietal cells. These inlet patches may also exhibit evidence of injury due to acid secretion, such as associated inflammation, ulceration, fibrotic stricture, or perforation. Patients with *H. pylori* gastritis frequently show concurrent colonization of the heterotopic mucosa. Intestinal metaplasia may be identified, and some studies have found a correlation with concomitant distal Barrett's esophagus, but others have not confirmed this correlation. There are also reports of adenocarcinoma arising from gastric heterotopia in the upper esophagus.

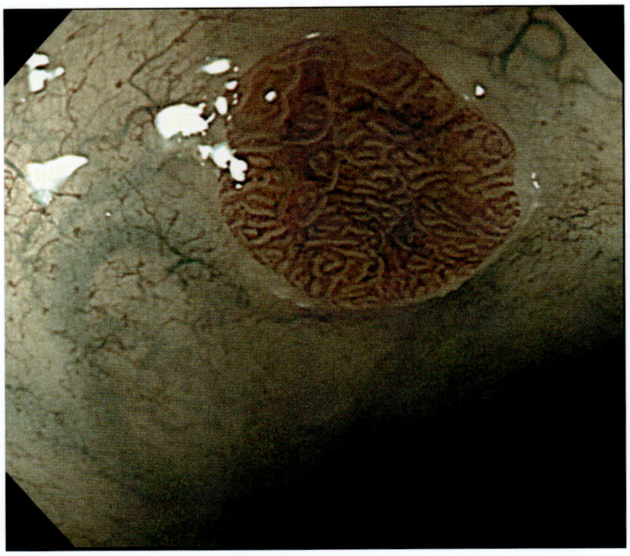

Figure 3.26 Gastric heterotopia "inlet patch." The salmon-colored mucosa is similar to Barrett's esophagus but is detected as an isolated patch in the proximal esophagus.

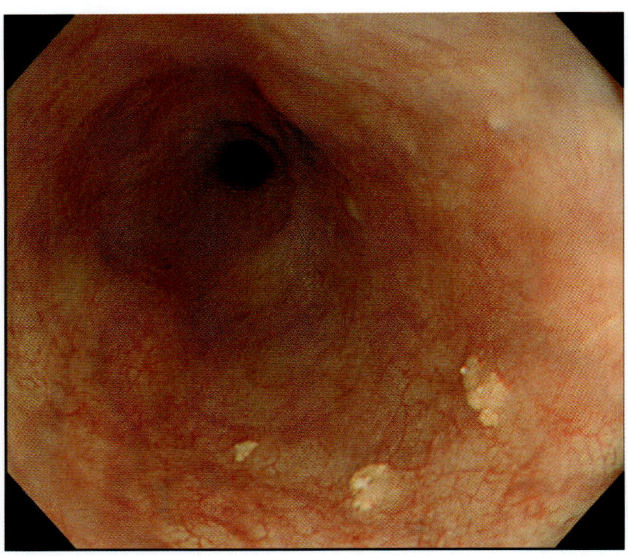

Figure 3.27 Typical endoscopic image of heterotopic sebaceous glands in mid-upper esophagus, appearing as multiple yellowish mucosal plaques.

Heterotopic sebaceous glands are characterized by small lobules of sebaceous cells with microvesicular, vacuolated cytoplasm within the epithelium or lamina propria (Figure 3.29). Hyperkeratosis of the adjacent squamous epithelium may be present. There is no known malignant potential.

In pancreatic heterotopia/metaplasia, tightly packed lobules of pancreatic acini are present, without ducts, or islet cells.

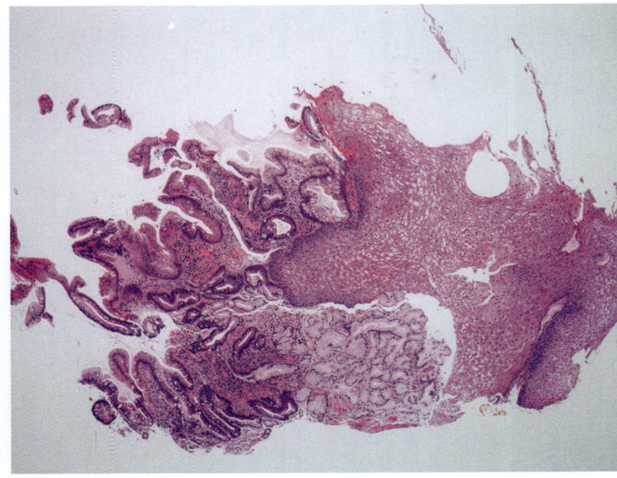

Figure 3.28 Common histomorphological appearance of "inlet patch."

Immunohistochemical Studies and Molecular Features

H. pylori immunohistochemistry of inlet patches is suggested if inflamed or concomitant *H. pylori* gastritis is present.

Differential Diagnosis

Clinical

Focal erythema of the proximal esophagus should raise suspicion of squamous neoplasia. In this case, the erythema is due to dilation of the squamous intrapapillary capillary loops (IPCL) but the surface pattern otherwise has a squamous, flat appearance, unlike inlet patch, which has a gastric appearance with small visible pits.

Prognosis, Evolution, and Clinical Management

Inlet patch was traditionally considered a benign, incidental finding without clinical correlation. The recent association with globus sensation and resolution with ablation of the patch suggests there may be a role in endoscopic therapy in symptomatic patients. In asymptomatic patients, there is no well-established association with adenocarcinoma and thus there is no indication for surveillance or ablation.

Glycogenic Acanthosis

Definition, General Features, Predisposing Factors

Glycogenic acanthosis represents focal nodular thickening of the squamous mucosa with cells that contain prominent intracytoplasmic glycogen. It is typically an incidental

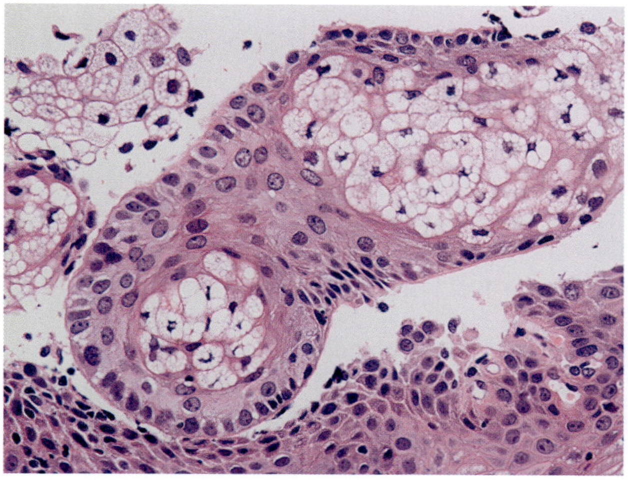

Figure 3.29 Heterotopic sebaceous glands. Note the typical vacuolated cytoplasm of the sebaceous glands similar to adnexal structures of the skin.

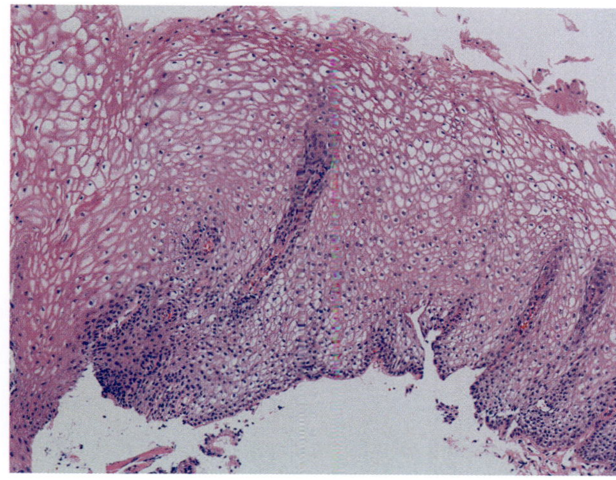

Figure 3.30 Glycogenic acanthosis characterized by thickening of the epithelium with glycogen packed squamous cells.

finding in adults, described in 3.5–15% of all upper endoscopies. The pathogenesis is unclear. Numerous or diffuse foci of glycogenic acanthosis may be a manifestation of Cowden syndrome (PTEN hamartoma-tumor syndrome). There is also some evidence suggesting an association with celiac disease, especially in children.

Clinical Features and Endoscopic Characteristics

Glycogenic acanthosis appears as small, incidental verrucous lesions in the esophagus similar to papilloma. They are clinically benign and do not require therapy. Biopsy should be performed to confirm the entity and exclude other pathologies.

Microscopic Features

Biopsies show nodular hyperplasia of the squamous epithelium, with prominent accumulation of cytoplasmic glycogen, usually involving >50% of the luminal mucosal thickness (Figure 3.30). The lesion is best appreciated when adjacent non-lesional, normal mucosa is included in the biopsy.

Differential Diagnosis

Clinical

These lesions have a similar appearance to papillomas and can occasionally be confused with granular cell tumors.

Microscopic

This histological differential diagnosis includes normal esophageal squamous mucosa, which may be partially glycogenated, particularly if adjacent non-lesional tissue is not identified. Acanthosis due to *Candida* esophagitis should be considered if surface neutrophils are present, and should be evaluated by PAS–Diastase or GMS stains.

Prognosis, Evolution, and Clinical Management

These are benign lesions. When diffuse, the diagnosis of Cowden syndrome should be considered.

Mesenchymal Polyps

Granular Cell Tumor

Definition, General Features, Predisposing Factors

Granular cell tumors (GCT) are benign, mesenchymal tumors of Schwann cell origin that can arise in any part of the body, most commonly the tongue, skin, and subcutaneous tissue. GCTs involving the gastrointestinal (GI) tract are uncommon (approximately 4–6% of all GCTs), and the esophagus is the most frequent location, followed by the colon. These tumors occur in adults (median age 49 years), with a slight predominance in females and blacks in the United States. Some Asian studies have shown a male predominance. Most tumors are solitary and located in the distal esophagus, although they may rarely be discovered in more proximal locations or be multicentric. Malignant GCT is exceedingly rare at any site, including the esophagus.

Clinical Features and Endoscopic Characteristics-GI

Most granular cell tumors are benign with rare reports of malignant conversion. They appear as whitish lesion in the esophagus with overlying normal mucosa.

Microscopic Features

Most esophageal granular cell tumors are small (<0.5 cm) and are located in the lamina propria or submucosa. They are unencapsulated and typically exhibit a well-marginated growth pattern, although some tumors may be infiltrative. The tumors are composed of sheets or nests of closely packed plump, rounded neoplastic cells with abundant eosinophilic granular cytoplasm and small, hyperchromatic, or pyknotic nuclei (Figure 3.31). The cytoplasmic granules are positive for PAS-diastase stain. Lymphoid cuffing may be observed at the periphery of some GCTs, a feature more frequently observed colonic tumors.

Prominent reactive (pseudoepitheliomatous) hyperplasia in the overlying squamous epithelium is common, and may mimic squamous cell carcinoma on superficial biopsies. Atypical cytologic features, including large nuclei, prominent nucleoli, and mitotic figures and an infiltrative growth pattern may be signify the potential for more aggressive behavior, although determination malignancy is best confirmed by identification of metastasis.

Immunohistochemical Studies and Molecular Features

Most GCTs are immunoreactive for S-100 protein, SOX10, CD56, and CD68 (Figure 3.32). They may also show reactivity for alpha-inhibin, myelin basic protein, and nestin, but lack expression of muscle and other melanoma markers.

Differential Diagnosis

Clinical The whitish nature of the lesion can be confused with mucosal polyps such as glycogenic acanthosis or papilloma; however, the overlying squamous epithelium in GCT is intact.

Microscopic Histologic differential diagnostic considerations include tumors such as leiomyoma, melanoma, rhabdomyoma, and alveolar soft part sarcoma. The spindle cells of leiomyoma are immunoreactive for actin, desmin, and caldesmon. Melanomas often exhibit more prominent cytologic atypia with macronucleoli, inclusions, and pigment deposition. S-100 is also positive, and expression of other melanoma markers allows distinction (HMB-45, MART-1/Melan-A, MITF). Rhabdomyomas lack S-100 staining, and show positivity for skeletal muscle markers (desmin, myoD1, myogenin). Alveolar soft part sarcoma (ASPS) is distinguished by its prominent nucleoli, alveolar pattern, vascularity, and PAS-positive crystals. Both ASPS and GCT are immunoreactive for TFE3.

In superficial biopsy specimens, overlying reactive pseudoepitheliomatous hyperplasia may raise a concern for squamous cell carcinoma.

Prognosis, Evolution, and Clinical Management

Esophageal granular cell tumors typically behave in a benign fashion, and malignancy is extremely rare. Endoscopic local excision is both diagnostic and curative. In the setting of small lesions in comorbid patients, observation is also reasonable.

Leiomyoma and Leiomyosarcoma

Definition, General Features, Predisposing Factors

Leiomyomas are the most common mesenchymal tumor of the esophagus, representing 10% of all gastrointestinal tract leiomyomas. They occur equally in men and women and are usually solitary. Large tumors tend to be symptomatic. Multiple small tumors may be encountered, which are typically small and incidental (so-called seedling leiomyoma). Large multifocal leiomyomas (leiomyomatosis) have been described in young adult females and in association with Alport syndrome or MEN-1.

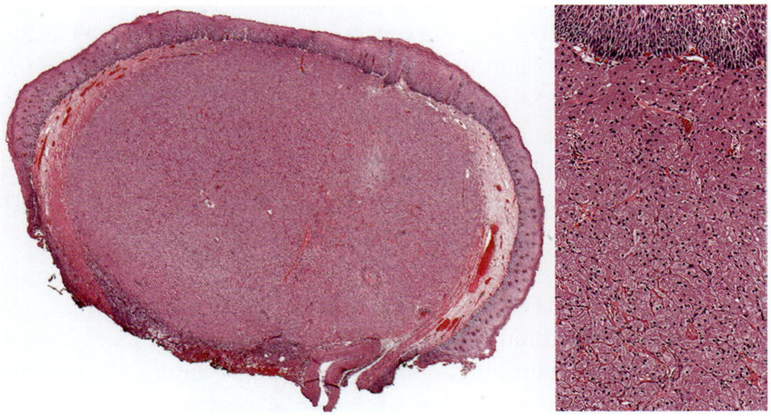

Figure 3.31 Submucosal granular cell tumor showing a sharp demarcation to the submucosal stroma. The tumor cells typically show an eosinophilic granulated cytoplasm with small hyperchromatic nuclei.

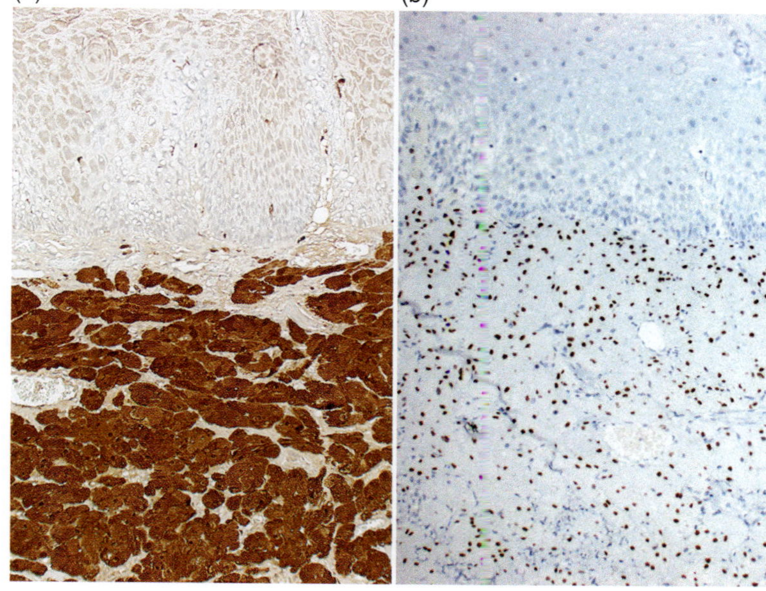

Figure 3.32 Granular cell tumors are typically immunohistochemically positive for (a) S100 and (b) SOX10 and demonstrate the neural origin of the neoplasia.

Most leiomyomas arise within the inner layer of muscularis propria. However, nearly 20% occur within the muscularis mucosae. In one large study, 79% were located in the distal esophagus, 18% in the mid-esophagus, and 3% in the proximal esophagus.

In contrast, leiomyosarcoma arising in the esophagus is an exceedingly rare tumor that has been reported in the distal and mid-esophagus in adults.

Clinical Features and Endoscopic Characteristics

Esophageal leiomyomas are endoscopically indistinguishable from leiomyosarcomas and GI stromal tumors. All are subepithelial, round, oval or irregular, and typically arise from the muscularis propria or muscularis mucosae layer. Endoscopic ultrasound is required to make a definitive diagnosis. They appear as dark/hypo-echoic lesions. Sarcomas and advanced stromal tumors are typically larger, associated with irregular shape, and heterogenous internal echoes (Figure 3.33).

Microscopic Features

Esophageal leiomyomas are firm, circumscribed tumors that exhibit a whorled cut surface appearance similar to leiomyomas in other sites. Histologically, leiomyomas are paucicellular and comprised of eosinophilic spindle cells with elongated nuclei, minimal cytologic atypia and no or minimal mitotic activity (Figure 3.34).

Leiomyosarcomas typically are large and necrotic with highly atypical eosinophilic spindle cells and frequent mitoses (Figure 3.35).

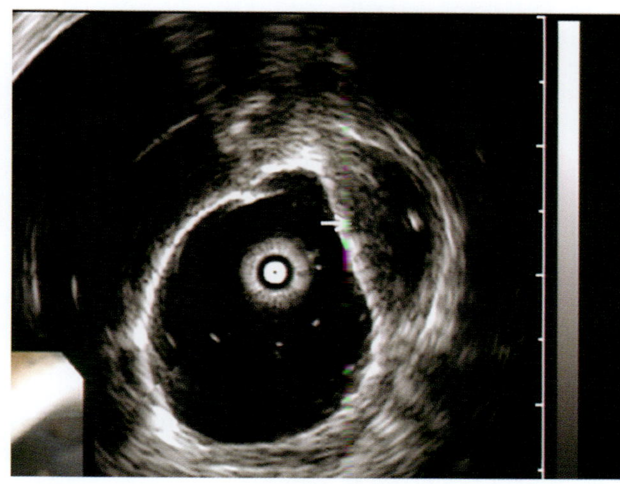

Figure 3.33 Esophageal leiomyoma (arrow) arising from the muscularis propria. Image obtained with endoscopic ultrasound.

Immunohistochemical Studies and Molecular Features

Leiomyomas and leiomyosarcomas are immunoreactive for actin, desmin, and caldesmon.

Differential Diagnosis

Clinical

The differential diagnosis of subepithelial tumors of the esophagus includes leiomyoma, sarcoma, GIST, lipoma, cyst, and extrinsic compression. These are best resolved by endoscopic ultrasound.

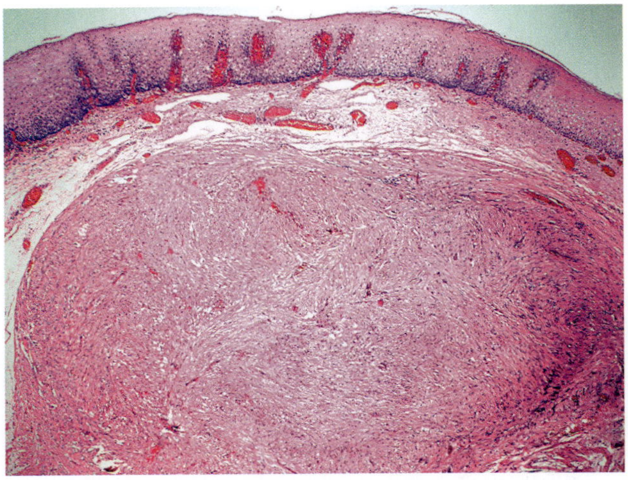

Figure 3.34 Well-defined submucosal leiomyoma with typical whorled fascicular growth pattern, fibrillar cytoplasm, and elongated rounded "cigar"-shaped nuclei.

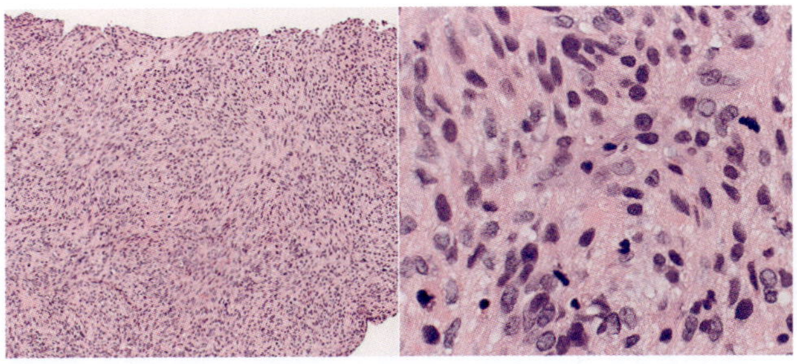

Figure 3.35 Leiomyosarcoma—fascicles of high cellularity with marked nuclear pleomorphism and high mitotic rate.

Microscopic

Leiomyomas may need to be distinguished from other mesenchymal tumors (e.g. GIST or granular cell tumor), as well as sarcomatoid (spindle cell) carcinoma or melanoma. GIST is distinguished by immunoreactivity for CD117, DOG1 and CD34, and GCT stains for S100 protein. Sarcomatoid carcinomas show positivity for cytokeratin immunostains. Melanoma is immunoreactive for S100, HMB-45, MART-1 (Melan-A), and MITF.

Prognosis, Evolution, and Clinical Management

Small leiomyomas that are asymptomatic are generally benign and can be followed by endoscopic ultrasound. Larger or symptomatic leiomyomas arising from the muscularis mucosa are treated by enucleation, endoscopic mucosal resection, or endoscopic submucosal dissection. Those tumors arising from the muscularis propria require surgical resection or peroral submucosal tunnel endoscopic resection (STER). The tumors typically do not recur.

Esophageal leiomyosarcomas have a good prognosis with radical resection.

Giant Fibrovascular Polyp

Definition, General Features, Predisposing Factors

Giant fibrovascular polyps (GFPs) are rare benign lesions of adults that affect men and women equally. In one series, the mean age at presentation was 56 years. These polyps typically occur in the proximal esophagus at the level of the cricopharyngeus muscle.

The pathogenesis of fibrovascular polyps is unknown, although they are generally considered a reactive, non-neoplastic tumor-like condition that may result from mucosal prolapse injury. Alternatively, some authors suggest that some fibrovascular polyps may represent lipomas with features of secondary prolapse injury.

Clinical Features and Endoscopic Characteristics

Patients typically present with dysphagia. At endoscopy, a massive polypoid structure may be found that fills the esophageal lumen, making full endoscopic inspection challenging. Dramatic presentations include prolapse of the polyp via the mouth. Endoscopic or surgical resection is indicated for large lesions.

Microscopic Features

Fibrovascular polyps are elongated tubular structures that can range up to 15 cm in length. They are covered by benign, reactive squamous epithelium that may exhibit surface erosion or ulceration. The fibrovascular core of these polyps consists of loose, edematous, myxoid, or hyalinized fibrous tissue with variable amounts of adipose tissue, smooth muscle fibers, and scattered inflammatory cells. Enlarged, reactive fibroblasts and myofibroblasts are typical. The stroma is also highly vascular, with numerous dilated arteries and veins.

Differential Diagnosis

Microscopic

Atypical lipomatous tumor (ALT) is a rare tumor that may mimic GFP both grossly and microscopically. ALT contains pleomorphic adipocytes, multivacuolated lipoblasts, and nuclear atypia in adipocytes and spindle cells. Unlike ALT, GFP lacks immunoreactivity for MDM2 and CDK4, or MDM2 amplification by FISH.

Prognosis, Evolution, and Clinical Management

Most lesions are symptomatic and require resection. Endoscopic polypectomy can be done but requires special techniques such as prophylactic strangulation with a detachable endoscopic loop followed by snare resection.

Gastrointestinal Stromal Tumor (GIST)

Definition, General Features, Predisposing Factors

In contrast to other gastrointestinal sites, gastrointestinal stromal tumors (GISTs) rarely arise in the esophagus, accounting for only 2% of all reported GISTs. Esophageal GISTs occur in older patients (median age 63 years), more commonly in males. They typically involve lower third of the esophagus, in a predominantly intramural location, although a subset may present as an intraluminal polypoid mass.

Clinical Features and Endoscopic Characteristics

The clinical and endoscopic features of GIST lesions are identical to those of leiomyoma. These are only distinguished by biopsy and histological evaluation.

Microscopic Features

Most esophageal GISTs exhibit spindle cell morphology with variable combinations of solid, myxoid, and perivascular growth patterns. Approximately 25% show an epithelioid morphology. A high proportion (more than 50%) of esophageal GISTs show features of high risk or malignant behavior, such as size >5 cm, a high mitotic rate, and necrosis.

Immunohistochemical Studies and Molecular Features

GIST diagnosis is established by immunoreactivity for KIT/CD117 and DOG1 antibodies. As in other sites, KIT and PDGFRA mutational analysis may be important for prognosis and targeted therapy considerations.

Differential Diagnosis

Clinical

The differential diagnosis of subepithelial tumors of the esophagus includes leiomyoma, sarcoma, GIST, lipoma, cyst, and extrinsic compression. These are best resolved by endoscopic ultrasound.

Microscopic

The differential diagnosis of esophageal GISTs includes leiomyoma, schwannoma, inflammatory fibroid polyp, granular cell tumor, Kaposi's sarcoma, and spindle cell carcinoma.

Ancillary Studies

A panel of immunohistochemical stains including CD117/KIT and DOG1, as well as smooth muscle, neural and/or epithelial markers may be necessary for diagnosis.

Prognosis, Evolution, and Clinical Management

Most reported esophageal GISTs have exhibited malignant behavior. Currently most require resection due to the concern for malignant potential. These lesions are resected surgically or endoscopically similar to leiomyoma (see above).

Hemangioma

Definition, General Features, Predisposing Factors

Hemangiomas are rare in the esophagus. They may occur at any level, although the most common location is the lower esophagus (approximately 50%), followed by the middle and upper esophagus. They are typically solitary, and affect both males and females equally with a wide age range from neonates to the eighth decade. For unknown reasons, these tumors have been more commonly reported from Japan. Multiple lesions are associated with hereditary vascular disorders such as Osler–Weber–Rendu disease, Klippel–Trénaunay syndrome, or the blue rubber bleb nevus syndrome.

Clinical Features and Endoscopic Characteristics

Hemangiomas may present as lobulated or polypoid intraluminal lesions but have a reddish/blue appearance indicative of their vascular nature. Most are asymptomatic, although they can rarely cause bleeding or dysphagia.

Microscopic Features

Polypoid hemangiomas typically involve the submucosa or lamina propria. Both capillary and cavernous-type growth patterns have been described. Histologically, the capillary hemangioma is characterized by a well-circumscribed, unencapsulated, lobular proliferation of small capillary-sized blood vessels lined by plump or flattened endothelial cells. Depending on the lesion's age, variable amounts of fibrous stroma may develop. Cavernous hemangiomas exhibit larger, blood-filled vascular spaces.

Immunohistochemical Studies and Molecular Features

The endothelial cells of hemangiomas are immunoreactive for vascular markers, such as CD31, CD34, and Factor VIII.

Differential Diagnosis

Microscopic

Polypoid granulation tissue or pyogenic granuloma, resulting from localized mucosal injury may resemble hemangioma histologically. The overlying mucosa of these lesions may be ulcerated.

Prognosis, Evolution, and Clinical Management-GI

When suspected, the lesions should be confirmed by endoscopic ultrasound (including Doppler flow studies) and/or contrast enhanced CT. Resection or vascular therapy is only required for symptomatic lesions. Treatment options include endoscopic resection (for small lesions), surgical resection, vascular embolization, or ligation.

Kaposi Sarcoma

Definition, General Features, Predisposing Factors

Kaposi sarcoma (KS) is a low-grade vascular tumor associated with Kaposi sarcoma herpesvirus/human herpesvirus 8 (KSHV/HHV8) infection, which may involve the skin, mucosa, and viscera. Gastrointestinal involvement occurs in Classic (Mediterranean), HIV/AIDS-associated and iatrogenic-immunosuppressed forms. Esophageal involvement is rare.

Clinical Features and Endoscopic Characteristics

KS lesions of the esophagus are similar to KS lesions elsewhere in the GI tract. They consist of hard, blue, nodular protruding lesions, typically in deeply immunosuppressed patients with late-stage AIDS. Biopsy is confirmatory.

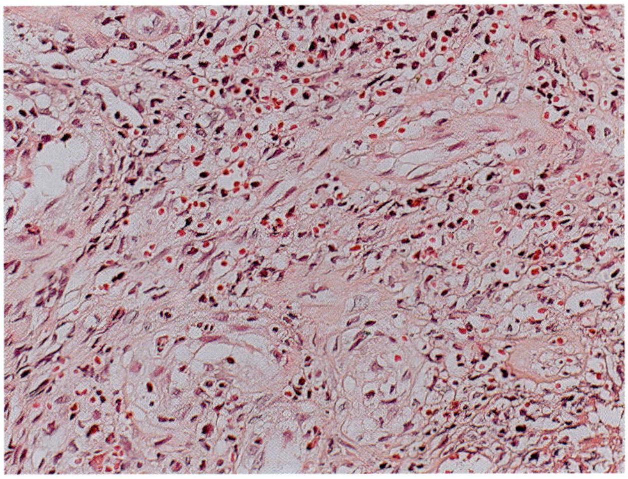

Figure 3.36 Kaposi sarcoma with characteristic slit-like spaces filled with erythrocytes as well as extravasated erythrocytes. Immunohistochemical stains for HHV8 and vascular markers (e.g. ERG) are useful to confirm the diagnosis.

Microscopic Features

Esophageal plaque or nodular lesions exhibit an infiltrative proliferation of spindle cells with thin-walled, slit-like vascular spaces lined by flattened endothelial cells (Figure 3.36). Extravasated red blood cells, hemosiderin-laden macrophages, and mixed inflammatory cells are present in the background. Eosinophilic and PAS-positive hyaline globules are a common finding in advanced lesions. There is minimal cytologic atypia and mitoses are few.

Immunohistochemical Studies and Molecular Features

Nuclear staining for HHV8 LNA-1 (LANA-1) is the most diagnostically useful immunohistochemical marker for KS. Lesional cells are also immunoreactive for endothelial markers (factor VIII-related antigen, CD31, CD34, and FLI1); lymphatic markers (D2-40, LYVE-1, and VEGFR-3); and Bcl-2. PCR may also be used to detect HHV8.

Differential Diagnosis

Microscopic

KS lesions may resemble granulation tissue. Other spindle cell tumors such as leiomyomas, GIST, or other sarcomas may be considered in the differential diagnosis, which must be distinguished by appropriate immunohistochemical analysis.

Prognosis, Evolution, and Clinical Management

The management of esophageal KS is similar to systemic KS and is beyond the scope of this article.

Miscellaneous Tumors

Melanoma

Definition, General Features, Predisposing Factors

Both primary and metastatic melanoma may present as polypoid esophageal masses. Primary malignant melanoma of the esophagus is a rare but aggressive tumor, with an estimated frequency of 0.1–0.2% of all esophageal malignancies, totaling 300–400 reported cases. The average age at diagnosis is 60.5 years, with a male predominance (male-to-female ratio of 2 : 1). Approximately 90% of these tumors occur in the distal or middle thirds of the esophagus, usually as a solitary lesion, although multiple tumors have been reported. There is a greater concentration of melanocytes in this location. Proliferation of these basal melanocytes (esophageal melanocytosis) has been demonstrated to be associated with melanoma in 25–30% of cases, and has been proposed as a predisposing factor.

Clinical Features and Endoscopic Characteristics

The mucosal lesions of melanoma anywhere in the GI tract, primary of metastatic, have a dark appearance and may be raised, often with heaped up margins and an irregular surface pattern

Microscopic Features

These melanomas may or may not be pigmented, grossly or microscopically. The histologic features are similar to melanomas of other sites, consisting of a range of patterns including both epithelioid and spindle cell components. Tumors often exhibit a sheet-like growth pattern comprised of large polygonal or spindle-shaped cells. Nuclei are large and round, with prominent nucleoli and occasional intranuclear pseudo-inclusions. The cytoplasm may contain fine black-brown melanin granules. Admixed pigment containing macrophages may also be present. The presence of associated in situ melanoma, radial growth phase, melanocytosis, and/or a mixed epithelioid and spindle cell morphology is helpful to establish the diagnosis of primary esophageal melanoma in the absence of a history of melanoma elsewhere.

Immunohistochemical Studies and Molecular Features

Immunohistochemical stains useful in confirming the diagnosis of melanoma include SOX10, S100, HMB-45, MART-1 (Melan-A), and MITF, particularly in nonpigmented or spindle cell tumors. BRAF V600E immunostaining and mutational analysis is also important for determining targeted therapy in cases of advanced tumors.

Differential Diagnosis

Clinical Dark stained nodular lesions are rare. Other entities with a similar appearance include foreign body reactions, fecaliths within a diverticulum, and blood clot on the surface of an ulcer.

Microscopic Distinguishing primary from metastatic melanoma is established by demonstrating the presence of an associated radial growth phase in the adjacent mucosa, and clinical exclusion of a primary melanoma elsewhere.

Given the protean morphology of malignant melanoma, the differential diagnosis includes poorly differentiated tumors of many types, such as squamous cell carcinoma, spindle cell carcinoma, adenocarcinoma but also lymphoma, GIST, or sarcoma. Confirmatory immunohistochemical stains are crucial, along with appropriate studies to exclude other tumor types. Granular cell tumor may also be challenging given the shared S100 positivity but notably fail to express other melanoma markers.

Prognosis, Evolution, and Clinical Management

Metastatic melanoma is typically late stage and managed per oncological protocols. In rare cases with local complications such as bleeding or obstruction, surgical resection or debulking can be considered.

Esophageal Lymphoma

Definition, General Features, Predisposing Factors

Although GI tract lymphoma is fairly common, esophageal lymphoma is rare, accounting for less than 1% of all gastrointestinal lymphomas. Esophageal involvement is most often secondary to contiguous spread from the proximal stomach (distal esophagus), adjacent mediastinal lymph nodes (mid-esophagus), or cervical lymph nodes (proximal esophagus). Primary esophageal lymphoma is exceedingly uncommon, and HIV infection/immunosuppression is a recognized risk factor. Age of presentation is highly variable, and it has been more commonly reported in males. Patients with primary esophageal lymphoma associated with HIV infection/AIDS tend to be middle-aged adults, and younger than non-HIV associated tumors.

Clinical Features and Endoscopic Characteristics

Primary esophageal lymphoma is exceedingly rare although mucosal-associated lymphoid tissue (MALT)

Table 3.5 Miscellaneous esophageal polyps and polypoid lesions.

Epithelial lesions	Location	Microscopic features	Ancillary studies
Inflammatory polyp	GEJ, distal	Endophytic tongues of benign squamous mucosa	N/A
Hyperplastic polyp	GEJ, distal	Polypoid foveolar hyperplasia	N/A
Squamous papilloma	70% distal	Exophytic, endophytic, spiked/verrucous patterns	Rarely HPV associated (in situ hybridization)
Heterotopias	Gastric—proximal ("inlet patch")	Gastric body-type mucosa	*H. pylori* IHC for inflamed gastric tissue
	Sebaceous—any	Sebaceous glands	
	Pancreatic—GEJ, distal	Pancreatic acinar tissue	
Glycogenic acanthosis	Any; multifocal assoc. with Cowden Syndrome	Focally thickened mucosa, enlarged squamous cells with clear cytoplasm	N/A (PAS positive)
Mesenchymal lesions			
Granular cell tumor	Distal predominant	Sheets of rounded cells, eosinophilic granular cytoplasm, pyknotic nuclei; pseudo-epitheliomatous hyperplasia	PASD+ S100, CD68, CD56, SOX10+
Leiomyoma (leiomyosarcoma rare)	Distal predominant	Circumscribed, paucicellular, eosinophilic spindle cells, elongated nuclei, minimal atypia; atypia, mitoses, necrosis in LMSA	Actin, desmin, caldesmon+
Giant fibrovascular polyp	Proximal	Elongated tubular structure, squamous lining, fibrovascular core with adipose tissue, smooth muscle, inflammatory cells	N/A
GIST	Distal	Spindle or epithelioid cells	CD117/KIT, DOG1+ KIT, PDGFRA mutations
Hemangioma	Any (50% distal)	Capillary or dilated/cavernous vascular proliferation	CD31, CD34, Factor VIII+
Kaposi's sarcoma	Any	Slit-like vascular spaces, spindle cells, extravasated RBC, hemosiderin	LNA-l (LANA-1), CD31, CD34, Factor VIII, FLI1, D2-40+ (and others, see text)
Misc lesions			
Melanoma (primary or metastatic)	90% distal or mid	Atypical epithelioid or spindle cell melanocytic tumor, ± pigment, junctional component in primary melanoma	S100, HMB-45, MART1/ Melan-A, MITF+
Lymphoma	Any	Large B-cell lymphoma most common	IHC for lymphoid markers, flow cytometry, molecular genetics, FISH

lymphoma as well as traditional lymphomas occasionally manifest as esophageal subepithelial nodules or thickening. Endoscopic biopsy may be diagnostic; however, in deep submucosal lesions, EUS with deep fine-needle biopsy may be necessary.

Microscopic Features

Biopsies of polypoid or ulcerated lesions show a proliferation of atypical, rounded, discohesive lymphoid cells. Most reported cases of primary esophageal lymphoma are diffuse large B-cell lymphomas. There have been rare reports of several other histologic types, such as MALT lymphoma (Figure 3.46), and anaplastic large cell lymphoma.

Ulcers are commonly superinfected with *Candida* species, which may obscure the underlying neoplastic lymphoid cells.

Immunohistochemical Studies and Molecular Features

Specimens submitted with a suspected diagnosis of lymphoma may require special handling in order to optimize the histologic diagnosis and to prepare the tissue for molecular and other ancillary special studies. Formalin fixation, particularly with limited tissue samples, is suitable for many ancillary tests such as molecular/genetic studies, FISH, and immunophenotyping by immunohistochemistry. Flow cytometry requires fresh tissue samples.

Differential Diagnosis

Microscopic

Conditions to be considered in the differential diagnosis of esophageal lymphoma include infections (e.g. CMV, HSV, *Candida*) as well as other poorly differentiated nonlymphoid malignant tumors. Rarely, focal lymphoid hyperplasia may also mimic lymphoma.

Ancillary Studies

A panel of immunohistochemical stains including lymphoid markers, epithelial markers, and sarcoma markers may be necessary to distinguish a high-grade lymphoma from a poorly differentiated carcinoma or sarcoma.

Prognosis, Evolution, and Clinical Management

Subepithelial lesions of the esophagus including lymphoma are best evaluated by endoscopic ultrasound and core biopsy. Endoscopist's and pathologist's collaboration on appropriate tissue sampling (in cytological preservative) and special processing for flow cytometry and staining are needed to confirm a diagnosis. Treatment is based on management of the systemic disease.

Further Reading

Abraham, S.C., Singh, V.K., Yardley, J.H. et al. (2001). Hyperplastic polyps of the esophagus and esophagogastric junction: histologic and clinicopathologic findings. *Am. J. Surg. Pathol.* 25: 1180–1187.

Abraham, S.C., Krasinskas, A.M., Correa, A.M. et al. (2007). Duplication of the muscularis mucosae in Barrett esophagus: an underrecognized feature and its implication for staging of adenocarcinoma. *Am. J. Surg. Pathol.* 31: 1719–1725.

Agaimy, A. (2013). Risk assessment and pathological reporting of gastrointestinal stromal tumour. *Diagn. Histopathol.* 19: 191–197.

Ahmed, K., Timmerman, G., Meyer, R. et al. (2013). Verrucous carcinoma of the esophagus: a potential diagnostic dilemma. *Case Rep. Gastroenterol.* 7: 498–502.

Allan, E.A. and Miller, G.J.J. (2015). Aneusomy detected by fluorescence in-situ hybridization has high positive predictive value for Barrett's dysplasia. *Histopathology* 67: 451–456.

Allende, D., Dumot, J., and Yerian, L. (2013). Esophageal squamous cell carcinoma arising after endoscopic ablation therapy of Barrett's esophagus with high-grade dysplasia. Report of a case. *Dis. Esophagus* 26: 314–318.

Alrawi, S.J., Winston, J., Tan, D. et al. (2005). Primary adenocarcinoma of cervical esophagus. *J. Exp. Clin. Cancer Res.* 24: 325–330.

An, S., Jang, J., Min, K. et al. (2015). Granular cell tumor of the gastrointestinal tract: histologic and immunohistochemical analysis of 98 cases. *Hum. Pathol.* 46: 813–819.

Anaparthy, R., Gaddam, S., Kanakadandi, V. et al. (2013). Association between length of Barrett's esophagus and risk of high-grade dysplasia or adenocarcinoma in patients without dysplasia. *Clin. Gastroenterol. Hepatol.* 11: 1430–1436.

Arai, T., Matsuda, Y., Nishimura, M. et al. (2015). Histopathological diagnoses of squamous intraepithelial neoplasia, carcinoma in situ and early invasive cancer of the oesophagus: the Japanese viewpoint. *Diagn. Histopathol.* 8: 303–311.

Arora, M. and Goldberg, E.M. (2010). Kaposi sarcoma involving the gastrointestinal tract. *Gastroenterol. Hepatol.* 6: 459–462.

Avezzano, E.A., Fleischer, D.E., Merida, M.A., and Anderson, D.L. (1990). Giant fibrovascular polyps of the esophagus. *Am. J. Gastroenterol.* 85: 299–302.

Belafsky, P., Amedee, R., and Zimmerman, J. (1999). Giant fibrovascular polyp of the esophagus. *South. Med. J.* 92: 428–431.

Bennett, C., Vakil, N., Bergman, J. et al. (2012). Consensus statements for management of Barrett's dysplasia and early-stage esophageal adenocarcinoma, based on a Delphi process. *Gastroenterology* 143: 336–346.

Bhat, S., Coleman, H.G., Yousef, F. et al. (2011). Risk of malignant progression in Barrett's esophagus patients: results from a large population-based study. *J. Natl. Cancer Inst.* 103: 1049–1057.

Bird-Lieberman, E.L., Dunn, J.M., Coleman, H.G. et al. (2012). Population-based study reveals new risk-stratification biomarker panel for Barrett's esophagus. *Gastroenterology* 143: 927–935.

Bisceglia, M., Perri, F., Tucci, A. et al. (2011). Primary malignant melanoma of the esophagus. *Adv. Anat. Pathol.* 18: 235–252.

Blum, M.G., Bilimoria, K.Y., Wayne, J.D. et al. (2007). Surgical considerations for the management and resection of esophageal gastrointestinal stromal tumors. *Ann. Thorac. Surg.* 84: 1717–1723.

Bohn, O.L., Navarro, L., Saldivar, J., and Sanchez-Sosa, S. (2008). Identification of human papillomavirus in esophageal squamous papillomas. *World J. Gastroenterol.* 14: 7107–7111.

Boni, A., Lisovsky, M., Dal Cin, P. et al. (2013). Atypical lipomatous tumor mimicking giant fibrovascular polyp of the esophagus: report of a case and a critical review of literature. *Hum. Pathol.* 44: 1165–1170.

Brinson, R.R., Schuman, B.M., Mills, L.R. et al. (1987). Multiple squamous papillomas of the esophagus associated with Goltz syndrome. *Am. J. Gastroenterol.* 82: 1177–1179.

Brown, L.M., Hoover, R., Silverman, D. et al. (2001). Excess incidence of squamous cell esophageal cancer among US black men: role of social class and other risk factors. *Am. J. Epidemiol.* 153: 114–122.

Brown, I.S., Whiteman, D.C., and Lauwers, G.Y. (2010). Foveolar type dysplasia in Barrett esophagus. *Mod. Pathol.* 23: 834–843.

Burdelski, C., Jakani-Karimi, N., Jacobsen, F. et al. (2018). IMP3 overexpression occurs in various important cancer types and is linked to aggressive tumor features: a tissue microarray study on 8,877 human cancers and normal tissues. *Oncol. Rep.* 39 (1): 3–12. https://doi.org/10.3892/or.2017.6072. Epub 2017 Nov.

Carr, N.J., Monihan, J.M., and Sobin, L.H. (1994). Squamous cell papilloma of the esophagus. A clinicopathologic and follow-up study of 25 cases. *Am. J. Gastroenterol.* 89: 245–248.

Carr, N.J., Bratthauer, G.L., Lichy, J.H. et al. (1994). Squamous cell papillomas of the esophagus: a study of 23 lesions for human papillomavirus by in situ hybridization and the polymerase chain reaction. *Hum. Pathol.* 25: 536–540.

Chadha, K.S., Hernandez-Ilizaliturri, F.J., and Javle, M. (2006). Primary esophageal lymphoma: case series and review of the literature. *Dig. Dis. Sci.* 51: 77–83.

Chandrasoma, P.T., Der, R., Dalton, P. et al. (2001). Distribution and significance of epithelial types in columnar lined esophagus. *Am. J. Surg. Pathol.* 25: 1188–1193.

Chandrasoma, P., Wijetunge, S., Demeester, S. et al. (2012). Columnar-lined esophagus without intestinal metaplasia has no proven risk of adenocarcinoma. *Am. J. Surg. Pathol.* 36: 1–7.

Chang, F. and Deere, H. (2006). Esophageal melanocytosis: morphologic features and review of the literature. *Arch. Pathol. Lab. Med.* 130: 552–557.

Chatelain, D., de Lajarte-Thirouard, A.S., Tiret, E., and Flejou, J.F. (2002). Adenocarcinoma of the upper esophagus arising in heterotopic gastric mucosa: common pathogenesis with Barrett's adenocarcinoma? *Virchows Arch.* 441: 406–411.

Chen, S.B., Weng, H.R., Wang, G. et al. (2013). Primary adenosquamous carcinoma of the esophagus. *World J. Gastroenterol.* 19: 8382–8390.

Choi, S.E. and Hur, C. (2012). Screening and surveillance for Barrett's esophagus: current issues and future directions. *Curr. Opin. Gastroenterol.* 28: 377–381.

Choi, H., Kim, S., Moon, J.H. et al. (2008). Multiple endocrine neoplasia type 1 with multiple leiomyomas linked to a novel mutation in the MEN1 gene. *Yonsei Med. J.* 49: 655–661.

Chong, V.H. (2013). Clinical significance of heterotopic gastric mucosal patch of the proximal esophagus. *World J. Gastroenterol.* 19: 331–338.

Coco, D.P., Goldblum, J.R., Hornick, J.L. et al. (2011). Interobserver variability in the diagnosis of crypt dysplasia in Barrett esophagus. *Am. J. Surg. Pathol.* 35: 45–54.

Cotton, C.C., Wolf, W.A., Overholt, B.F. et al. (2017). Late recurrence of Barrett's esophagus after complete eradication of intestinal metaplasia is rare: final report from ablation in intestinal metaplasia containing dysplasia trial. *Gastroenterology* 153: 681–688.e2.

Croyle, P., Nikaidoh, H., and Currarino, G. (1981). Inflammatory esophagogastric junction polyp. *Am. J. Gastroenterol.* 76: 438–440.

Curvers, W.L., ten Kate, F.J., Krishnadath, K.K. et al. (2010). Low-grade dysplasia in Barrett's esophagus: overdiagnosed and underestimated. *Am. J. Gastroenterol.* 105: 1523–1530.

Desai, T.K., Krishnan, K., Samala, N. et al. (2012). The incidence of oesophageal adenocarcinoma in non-dysplastic Barrett's oesophagus: a meta-analysis. *Gut* 61 (7): 970–976.

Downs-Kelly, E., Mendelin, J.E., Bennett, A.E. et al. (2008). Poor interobserver agreement in the distinction of high grade dysplasia and adenocarcinoma in pre-treatment Barrett's esophagus biopsies. *Am. J. Gastroenterol.* 103: 2333–2340.

Doyle, L.A. and Hornick, J.L. (2014). Gastrointestinal stromal tumours: from KIT to succinate dehydrogenase. *Histopathology* 64: 53–67.

Eguchi, T., Nakanishi, Y., Shimoda, T. et al. (2006). Histopathological criteria for additional treatment after endoscopic mucosal resection for esophageal cancer: analysis of 464 surgically resected cases. *Mod. Pathol.* 19: 475–480.

Estrella, J.S., Hofstetter, W.L., Correa, A.M. et al. (2011). Duplicated muscularis mucosae invasion has similar risk of lymph node metastasis and recurrence-free survival as intramucosal esophageal adenocarcinoma. *Am. J. Surg. Pathol.* 35: 1045–1053.

Fang, M., Lew, E., Klein, M. et al. (2004). DNA abnormalities as marker of risk for progression of Barrett's esophagus to adenocarcinoma: image cytometric DNA analysis in formalin-fixed tissues. *Am. J. Gastroenterol.* 99: 1887–1894.

Fei, B.Y., Yang, J.M., and Zhao, Z.S. (2014). Differential clinical and pathological characteristics of esophageal stromal tumors and leiomyomata. *Dis. Esophagus* 24: 30–35.

Fitzgerald, R.C., di Pietro, M., Ragunath, K. et al. (2014). British Society of Gastroenterology guidelines on the diagnosis and management of Barrett's oesophagus. *Gut* 63: 7–42.

Flaherty, K.T., Infante, J.R., Daud, A. et al. (2012). Combined BRAF and MEK inhibition of melanoma with BRAF V600 mutations. *N. Engl. J. Med.* 367: 1694–1703.

Gaskin, C.M., Low, V.H., and Ho, L.M. (2001). Isolated primary non-hodgkin's lymphoma of the esophagus. *AJR Am. J. Roentgenol.* 176: 551–552.

Geddert, H., Kiel, S., Heep, H.J. et al. (2003). The role of p63 and deltaNp63 (p40) protein expression and gene amplification in esophageal carcinogenesis. *Hum. Pathol.* 34 (9): 850–856.

Glickman, J.N., Chen, Y.Y., Wang, H.H. et al. (2001). Phenotypic characteristics of a distinctive multilayered epithelium suggests that it is a precursor in the development of Barrett's esophagus. *Am. J. Surg. Pathol.* 25: 569–578.

Gorospe, E.C., Gupta, M., Prasad, G.A. et al. (2012). Double trouble: two cases of squamous carcinoma arising from Barrett's dysplasia after endoscopic mucosal resection. *Am. J. Gastroenterol.* 107: 1595–1596.

Gray, N.A., Odze, R.D., and Spechler, S.J. (2011). Buried metaplasia after endoscopic ablation of Barrett's esophagus: a systematic review. *Am. J. Gastroenterol.* 106: 1899–1908.

Gupta, V., Lal, A., Sinha, S.K. et al. (2009). Leiomyomatosis of the esophagus: experience over a decade. *J. Gastrointest. Surg.* 13: 206–211.

Hirota, W.K., Loughney, T.M., Lazas, D.J. et al. (1999). Specialized intestinal metaplasia, dysplasia, and cancer of the esophagus and esophagogastric junction: prevalence and clinical data. *Gastroenterology* 116: 277–285.

Hirst, N.G., Gordon, L.G., Whiteman, D.C. et al. (2011). Is endoscopic surveillance for nondysplastic Barrett's esophagus cost-effective? Review of economic evaluations. *J. Gastroenterol. Hepatol.* 26: 247–254.

Hopcroft, S.A. and Shepherd, N.A. (2014). The changing role of he pathologist in the management of Barrett's oesophagus. *Histopathology* 65: 441–455.

Hosaka, S., Nakamura, N., Akamatsu, T. et al. (2002). A case of primary low grade mucosa associated lymphoid tissue (MALT) lymphoma of the oesophagus. *Gut* 51: 281–284.

Hricak, H., Thoeni, R.F., Margulis, A.R. et al. (1980). Extension of gastric lymphoma into the esophagus and duodenum. *Radiology* 135: 309–312.

Hvid-Jensen, F., Pedersen, L., Drewes, A.M. et al. (2011). Incidence of adenocarcinoma among patients with Barrett's esophagus. *N. Engl. J. Med.* 365 (15): 1375–1383.

Iwanuma, Y., Tomita, N., Amano, T. et al. (2012). Current status of primary malignant melanoma of the esophagus: clinical features, pathology, management and prognosis. *J. Gastroenterol.* 47: 21–28.

Jacobs, E. and Dehou, M.F. (1997). Heterotopic gastric mucosa in the upper esophagus: a prospective study of 33 cases and review of literature. *Endoscopy* 29: 710–715.

Jakowski, J.D. and Wakely, P.E. Jr. (2009). Rhabdomyomatous well-differentiated liposarcoma arising in giant fibrovascular polyp of the esophagus. *Ann. Diagn. Pathol.* 13: 263–268.

John, B.K., Dang, N.C., Hussain, S.A. et al. (2008). Multifocal Granular Cell Tumor Presenting as an Esophageal Stricture. *J. Gastrointest. Cancer* 39: 107–113.

de Jonge, P.J.F., van Blankenstein, M., Grady, W.M. et al. (2014). Barrett's oesophagus: epidemiology, cancer risk and implications for management. *Gut* 63: 191–202.

Kahl, P., Buettner, R., Friedrichs, N. et al. (2007). Kaposi's sarcoma of the gastrointestinal tract: report of two cases and review of the literature. *Pathol. Res. Pract.* 203: 227–231.

Kalogeropoulos, I.V., Chalazonitis, A.N., Tsolaki, S. et al. (2009). A case of primary isolated non-Hodgkin's lymphoma of the esophagus in an immunocompetent patient. *World J. Gastroenterol.* 15: 1901–1903.

Kaneshiro, D.K., Post, J.C., Rybicki, L. et al. (2011). Clinical significance of the duplicated muscularis mucosae in Barrett esophagus-related superficial adenocarcinoma. *Am. J. Surg. Pathol.* 35: 697–700.

Kastelein, F., Biermann, K., Steyerberg, E.W. et al. (2013). Aberrant p53 protein expression is associated with an increased risk of neoplastic progression in patients with Barrett's oesophagus. *Gut* 62: 1676–1683.

Kastelstein, F., Biermann, K., Steyerberg, E.W. et al. (2013). Value of α-methylacyl-CoA racemase immunohistochemistry for predicting neoplastic progression in Barrett's oesophagus. *Histopathology* 63 (5): 630–639.

Kay, P.S., Soetikno, R.M., Mindelzun, R., and Young, H.S. (1997). Diffuse esophageal glycogenic acanthosis: an endoscopic marker of Cowden's disease. *Am. J. Gastroenterol.* 92: 1038–1040.

Kaye, P.V., Haider, S.A., Ilyas, M. et al. (2009). Barrett's dysplasia and the Vienna classification: reproducibility, prediction of progression and impact of consensus reporting and p53 immunohistochemistry. *Histopathology* 54: 699–712.

Kaye, P.V., Haider, S.A., James, P.D. et al. (2010). Novel staining pattern of p53 in Barrett's dysplasia – the absent pattern. *Histopathology* 57: 933–935.

Kelty, C.J., Gough, M.D., Van Wyk, Q. et al. (2007). Barrett's oesophagus: intestinal metaplasia is not essential for cancer risk. *Scand. J. Gastroenterol.* 42: 1271–1274.

Kerkhof, M., van Dekken, H., Steyerberg, E.W. et al. (2007). Grading of dysplasia in Barrett's oesophagus: substantial interobserver variation between general and gastrointestinal pathologists. *Histopathology* 50: 920–927.

Khor, T.S., Alfaro, E.E., Ooi, E.M. et al. (2012). Divergent expression of MUC5AC, MUC6, MUC2, CD10, and CDX-2 in dysplasia and intramucosal adenocarcinomas with intestinal and foveolar morphology: is this evidence of distinct gastric and intestinal pathways to carcinogenesis in Barrett esophagus? *Am. J. Surg. Pathol.* 36: 331–342.

Klare, P., Meining, A., von Delius, S. et al. (2013). Argon plasma coagulation of gastric inlet patches for the treatment of globus sensation: it is an effective therapy in the long term. *Digestion* 88: 165–171.

Kobayashi, M., Kawachi, H., Takizawa, T. et al. (2006). p53 Mutation analysis of low-grade dysplasia and high-grade dysplasia/carcinoma in situ of the esophagus using laser capture microdissection. *Oncology* 71: 237–245.

Lack, E.E., Worsham, G.F., Callihan, M.D. et al. (1980). Granular cell tumor: a clinicopathologic study of 110 patients. *J. Surg. Oncol.* 13: 301–316.

Langer, R., Becker, K., Feith, M. et al. (2011). Genetic aberrations in primary esophageal melanomas: molecular analysis of c-KIT, PDGFR, KRAS, NRAS and BRAF in a series of 10 cases. *Mod. Pathol.* 24: 495–501.

Lauwers, G.Y., Grant, L.D., Scott, G.V. et al. (1998). Spindle cell squamous carcinoma of the esophagus: analysis of ploidy and tumor proliferative activity in a series of 13 cases. *Hum. Pathol.* 29: 863–868.

Li, B., Lei, W., Shao, K. et al. (2007). Characteristics and prognosis of primary malignant melanoma of the esophagus. *Melanoma Res.* 17: 239–242.

Lisovsky, M. and Srivastava, A. (2013). Barrett esophagus evolving concepts in diagnosis and neoplastic progression. *Surg. Pathol.* 6: 475–496.

Liu, W., Hahn, H., Odze, R.D. et al. (2009). Metaplastic esophageal columnar epithelium without goblet cells shows DNA content abnormalities similar to goblet cell-containing epithelium. *Am. J. Gastroenterol.* 104: 816–824.

Liyanage, S.S., Segelov, E., Garland, S.M. et al. (2013). Role of human papillomaviruses in esophageal squamous cell carcinoma. *Asia Pac. J. Clin. Oncol.* 9: 12–28.

Lo, O.S., Law, S., Wei, W.I. et al. (2008). Esophageal cancers with synchronous or antecedent head and neck cancers: a more formidable challenge? *Ann. Surg. Oncol.* 15: 1750–1756.

Lomo, L.C., Blount, P.L., Sanchez, C.A. et al. (2006). Crypt dysplasia with surface maturation: a clinical, pathologic, and molecular study of a Barrett's esophagus cohort. *Am. J. Surg. Pathol.* 30: 423–435.

Long, K. and Odze, R. (2011). Gastroesophageal junction hyperplastic (inflammatory) polyps: a clinical and pathologic study of 46 cases. *Am. J. Surg. Pathol.* 35: 1038–1044.

Long, G.V., Menzies, A.M., Nagrial, A.M. et al. (2011). Prognostic and clinicopathologic association of oncogenic BRAF in metastatic melanoma. *J. Clin. Oncol.* 29: 1239–1246.

Mahajan, D., Bennett, A.E., Liu, X. et al. (2010). Grading of gastric foveolar-type dysplasia in Barrett's esophagus. *Mod. Pathol.* 23: 1–11.

Mandal, R.V., Forcione, D.G., Brugge, W.R. et al. (2009). Effect of tumor characteristics and duplication of the muscularis mucosae on the endoscopic staging of superficial Barrett esophagus-related neoplasia. *Am. J. Surg. Pathol.* 33: 620–625.

McGarrity, T.J., Wagner Baker, M.J., Ruggiero, F.M. et al. (2003). GI polyposis and glycogenic acanthosis of the esophagus associated with PTEN mutation positive Cowden syndrome in the absence of cutaneous manifestations. *Am. J. Gastroenterol.* 98: 1429–1434.

Miettinen, M. and Lasota, J. (2006). Gastrointestinal stromal tumors: review on morphology, molecular pathology, prognosis, and differential diagnosis. *Arch. Pathol. Lab. Med.* 130: 1466–1478.

Miettinen, M., Sarlomo-Rikala, M., Sobin, L.H. et al. (2000). Esophageal stromal tumors: a clinicopathologic, immunohistochemical, and molecular genetic study of 17 cases and comparison with esophageal leiomyomas and leiomyosarcomas. *Am. J. Surg. Pathol.* 24: 211–222.

Mino-Kenudson, M., Hull, M.J., Brown, I. et al. (2007). EMR for Barrett's esophagus-related superficial neoplasms offers better diagnostic reproducibility than mucosal biopsy. *Gastrointest. Endosc.* 66: 660–666.

Montgomery, E., Field, J.K., Boffetta, P. et al. (2010). Squamous cell carcinoma of the oesophagus. In: WHO Classification of Tumours of the Digestive System (eds. F.T. Bosman, F. Carneiro, R.H. Hruba and N.D. Theise), 18–24. Lyon: IARC.

Morita, F.H.A., Ribiero, U., Sollum, A.A.S. et al. (2013). Primary malignant melanoma of the esophagus: a rare and aggressive disease. *World J. Surg. Oncol.* 11: 210–216.

Mosca, S., Manes, G., Monaco, R. et al. (2001). Squamous papilloma of the esophagus: long-term follow up. *J. Gastroenterol. Hepatol.* 16: 857.

Murray, L., Sedo, A., Scott, M. et al. (2006). TP53 and progression from Barrett's metaplasia to oesophageal adenocarcinoma in a UK population cohort. *Gut* 55: 1390–1397.

Mutrie, C.J., Donahue, D.M., Wain, J.C. et al. (2005). Esophageal leiomyoma: a 40-year experience. *Ann. Thorac. Surg.* 79: 1122–1125.

Naini, B.V., Souza, R.F., and Odze, R.D. (2016). Barrett's esophagus: a comprehensive and contemporary review for pathologists. *Am. J. Surg. Pathol.* 40: e45–e66.

Nakanishi, Y., Ochiai, A., Shimoda, T. et al. (1999). Heterotopic sebaceous glands in the esophagus: histopathological and immunohistochemical study of a resected esophagus. *Pathol. Int.* 49: 364–368.

Neumann, W.L., Luján, G.M., and Genta, R.M. (2012). Gastric heterotopia in the proximal oesophagus ("inlet patch"): association with adenocarcinomas arising in Barrett mucosa. *Dig. Liver Dis.* 44: 292–296.

Odze, R.D. and Lauwers, G.Y. (2008). Histopathology of Barrett's esophagus after ablation and endoscopic mucosal resection therapy. *Endoscopy* 40: 1008–1015.

Odze, R., Antonioli, D., Shocket, D. et al. (1993). Esophageal squamous papillomas. A clinicopathologic study of 38 lesions and analysis for human papillomavirus by the polymerase chain reaction. *Am. J. Surg. Pathol.* 17: 803–812.

Ohmori, T., Arita, N., Uraga, N. et al. (1987). Malignant granular cell tumor of the esophagus. A case report with light and electron microscopic, histochemical, and immunohistochemical study. *Acta Pathol. Jpn.* 37: 775–783.

Omar, M., Thaker, A.M., Wani, S. et al. (2019). Anatomic location of Barrett's esophagus recurrence after endoscopic eradication therapy: development of a simplified surveillance biopsy strategy. *Gastrointest. Endosc.* 90: 395–403.

Orvidas, L.J., McCaffrey, T.V., Lewis, J.E. et al. (1994). Lymphoma involving the esophagus. *Ann. Otol. Rhinol. Laryngol.* 103: 843–848.

Owonikoko, T., Loberg, C., Gabbert, H.E., and Sarbia, M. (2001). Comparative analysis of basaloid and typical squamous cell carcinoma of the oesophagus: a molecular biological and immunohistochemical study. *J. Pathol.* 193: 155–161.

Panarelli, N.C. and Yantiss, R.K. (2016). Do ancillary studies aid detection and classification of Barrett esophagus? *Am. J. Surg. Pathol.* 40 (8): e83–e93. https://doi.org/10.1097/PAS.598.

Patil, D.T., Goldblum, J.R., Rybicki, L. et al. (2012). Prediction of adenocarcinoma in esophagectomy specimens based upon analysis of preresection biopsies of Barrett esophagus with at least high-grade dysplasia: a comparison of 2 systems. *Am. J. Surg. Pathol.* 36: 134–141.

Phoa, K.N., van Vilsteren, F.G., Weusten, B.L. et al. (2014). Radiofrequency ablation vs endoscopic surveillance for patients with Barrett esophagus and low-grade. *JAMA* 311: 1209–1217.

di Pietro, M. and Fitzgerald, R. (2013). Screening and risk stratification for Barrett's esophagus: how to limit the clinical impact of the increasing incidence of esophageal adenocarcinoma. *Gastroenterol. Clin. N. Am.* 42: 155–173.

Poljak, M., Orlowska, J., and Cerar, A. (1995). Human papillomavirus infection in esophageal squamous cell papillomas. A study of 29 lesions. *Anticancer Res.* 15: 965–969.

Qi, Z., Jiang, Q., Chen, X. et al. (2013). Human papillomavirus (HPV) infection and the risk of esophageal squamous cell carcinoma. *Dis. Esophagus* 26: 61–67.

Rabin, M.S., Bremner, C.G., and Botha, J.R. (1980). The reflux gastroesophageal polyp. *Am. J. Gastroenterol.* 73: 451–452.

Radu, O. and Pantanowitz, L. (2013). Kaposi sarcoma. *Arch. Pathol. Lab. Med.* 137: 289–294.

Rasalkar, D.D., Chiu, P.W.Y., Teoh, A.Y.B. et al. (2010). Oesophageal haemangioma: imaging characteristics of this rare condition. *Hong Kong Med. J.* 16: 230–231.

Rasheed, A., Vasudevan, V., Virk, M. et al. (2012). A rare case of esophageal Kaposi's sarcoma (KS) presenting with massive hematemesis. *Chest* 142: 570A.

Reid, B.J., Levine, D.S., Longton, G. et al. (2000). Predictors of progression to cancer in Barrett's esophagus: baseline histology and flow cytometry identify low- and high-risk patient subsets. *Am. J. Gastroenterol.* 95: 1669–1676.

Reynoso, J., Davis, R.E., Daniels, W.W. et al. (2004). Esophageal papillomatosis complicated by squamous cell carcinoma in situ. *Dis. Esophagus* 17: 345–347.

Riddell, R.H. and Odze, R.D. (2009). Definition of Barrett's esophagus: time for a rethink – is intestinal metaplasia dead? *Am. J. Gastroenterol.* 104: 2588–2594.

Risk, J.M., Mills, H.S., Garde, J. et al. (1999). The tylosis esophageal cancer (TOC) locus: more than just a familial cancer gene. *Dis. Esophagus* 12: 173–176.

Robertson, E.V. and Jankowski, J.A. (2008). Genetics of gastroesophageal cancer: paradigms, paradoxes, and prognostic utility. *Am. J. Gastroenterol.* 103: 443–449.

Roehrl, M.H.A. and Farraye, F.A. (2012). Capillary hemangioma of the esophagus in a patient with systemic sclerosis and gastric antral vascular ectasia. *Gastrointest. Endosc.* 76: 418–419.

Rucker-Schmidt, R.L., Sanchez, C.A., Blount, P.L. et al. (2009). Nonadenomatous dysplasia in Barrett esophagus: a clinical, pathologic, and DNA content flow cytometric study. *Am. J. Surg. Pathol.* 33: 886–893.

Rustgi, A.K. and El-Serag, H.B. (2014). Esophageal carcinoma. *N. Engl. J. Med.* 371: 2499–2509.

Sa, M.J., Fieremans, N., de Brouwer, A.P. et al. (2013). Deletion of the 5'exons of COL4A6 is not needed for the development of diffuse leiomyomatosis in patients with Alport syndrome. *J. Med. Genet.* 50: 745–753.

Sanchez, A.A., Wu, T.T., Prieto, V.G. et al. (2008). Comparison of primary and metastatic malignant melanoma of the esophagus: clinicopathologic review of 10 cases. *Arch. Pathol. Lab. Med.* 132: 1623–1629.

Schlemper, R.J., Riddell, R.H., Kato, Y. et al. (2000). The Vienna classification of gastrointestinal neoplasia. *Gut* 47: 251–255.

Shaheen, N.J., Falk, G.W., Iyer, P.G. et al. (2016). ACG clinical guideline: diagnosis ans management of Barrett's esophagus. *Am. J. Gastroenterol.* 111: 30–50.

Sharma, P., Morales, T.G., and Sampliner, R.E. (1998). Short segment Barrett's esophagus – the need for standardization of the definition and of endoscopic criteria. *Am. J. Gastroenterol.* 93: 1033–1036.

Sharma, P., Weston, A.P., Morales, T. et al. (2000). Relative risk of dysplasia for patients with intestinal metaplasia in the distal oesophagus and in the gastric cardia. *Gut* 46: 9–13.

Sharma, P., Falk, G.W., Weston, A.P. et al. (2006). Dysplasia and cancer in a large multicenter cohort of patients with Barrett's esophagus. *Clin. Gastroenterol. Hepatol.* 4: 566–572.

Shimizu, M., Nagata, K., Yamaguchi, H., and Kita, H. (2009). Squamous intraepithelial neoplasia of the esophagus: past, present, and future. *J. Gastroenterol.* 44: 103–112.

Shimizu, M., Zaninotto, G., Nagata, K. et al. (2013). Esophageal squamous cell carcinoma with special reference to its early stage. *Best Pract. Res. Clin. Gastroenterol.* 27: 171–186.

Sikkema, M., Kerkhof, M., Steyerberg, E.W. et al. (2009). Aneuploidy and overexpression of Ki67 and p53 as markers for neoplastic progression in Barrett's esophagus: a case–control study. *Am. J. Gastroenterol.* 104: 2673–2680.

Singhi, A.D., Arnold, C.A., Crowder, C.D. et al. (2014). Esophageal leukoplakia or epidermoid metaplasia: a clinicopathological study of 18 patients. *Mod. Pathol.* 27: 38–43.

Smith, J., Garcia, A., Zhang, R. et al. (2016). Intestinal metaplasia is present in most if not all patients who have undergone endoscopic mucosal resection for esophageal adenocarcinoma. *Am. J. Surg. Pathol.* 40: 537–543.

Sonwalkar, S.A., Rotimi, O., Scott, N. et al. (2010). A study of indefinite for dysplasia in Barrett's oesophagus: reproducibility of diagnosis, clinical outcomes and predicting progression with AMACR (alpha-methylacyl-CoA-racemase). *Histopathology* 56: 900–907.

Spechler, S.J. and Souza, R.F. (2014). Barrett's esophagus. *N. Engl. J. Med.* 371: 836–845.

Spechler, S.J., Sharma, P., Souza, R.F. et al. (2011). American Gastroenterological Association medical position statement on the management of Barrett's esophagus. *Gastroenterology* 140: 1084–1091.

Srivastava, A., Odze, R.D., Lauwers, G.Y. et al. (2007). Morphologic features are useful in distinguishing Barrett esophagus from carditis with intestinal metaplasia. *Am. J. Surg. Pathol.* 31: 1733–1741.

Srivastava, A., Hornick, J.L., Li, X. et al. (2007). Extent of low-grade dysplasia is a risk factor for the development of esophageal adenocarcinoma in Barrett's esophagus. *Am. J. Gastroenterol.* 102: 483–493.

Srivastava, A., Sanchez, C.A., Cowan, D.S. et al. (2010). Foveolar and serrated dysplasia are rare high-risk lesions in Barrett's esophagus: a prospective outcome analysis of 214 patients. *Mod. Pathol.* 23: 168a.

Suoglu, O.D., Emiroglu, H.H., Sokucu, S. et al. (2004). Celiac disease and glycogenic acanthosis: a new association? *Acta Paediatr.* 93: 568–570.

Sweetser, S., Jacobs, N.L., and Song, L.M. (2014). Endoscopic diagnosis and treatment of esophageal verrucous squamous cell cancer. *Dis. Esophagus* 27: 452–456.

Swerdlow, S., Campo, E., Harris, N. et al. (eds.) (2008). WHO Classification of Tumours of Haematopoietic and Lymphoid Tissues. Geneva: WHO Press.

Szántó, I., Szentirmay, Z., Banai, J. et al. (2005). Squamous papilloma of the esophagus. Clinical and pathological observations based on 172 papillomas in 155 patients. *Orv. Hetil.* 146: 547.

Taal, B.G., Van Heerde, P., and Somers, R. (1993). Isolated primary oesophageal involvement by lymphoma: a rare cause of dysphagia: two case histories and a review of other published data. *Gut* 34: 994–998.

Takubo, K. (2009). Pathology of the Esophagus. An Atlas and Textbook, 191–190. Tokyo: Springer.

Takubo, K., Nakagawa, H., Tsuchiya, S. et al. (1981). Seedling leiomyoma of the esophagus and esophagogastric junction zone. *Hum. Pathol.* 12: 1006–1010.

Takubo, K., Sasajima, K., Yamashita, K. et al. (1991). Double muscularis mucosae in Barrett's esophagus. *Hum. Pathol.* 22: 1158–1161.

Takubo, K., Aida, J., Sawabe, M. et al. (2007). Early squamous cell carcinoma of the oesophagus: the Japanese viewpoint. *Histopathology* 51: 733–742.

Tarapore, R. and Katz, J. (2013). Molecular pathology of squamous carcinomas of the esophagus. In: Molecular Pathology of Neoplastic Gastrointestinal Diseases (eds. A.R. Sepulveda and J.P. Lynch), 53–66. New York: Springer Science+Business Media.

Taylor, P.R., Abnet, C.C., and Dawsey, S.M. (2013). Squamous dysplasia – the precursor lesion for esophageal squamous cell carcinoma. *Cancer Epidemiol. Biomark. Prev.* 22: 540–552.

Thurberg, B.L., Duray, P.H., and Odze, R.D. (1999). Polypoid dysplasia in Barrett's esophagus: a clinicopathologic, immunohistochemical, and molecular study of five cases. *Hum. Pathol.* 30: 745–752.

Vadva, M.D. and Triadafilopoulos, G. (1993). Glycogenic acanthosis of the esophagus and gastroesophageal reflux. *J. Clin. Gastroenterol.* 17: 79–83.

Van Cutsem, E., Geboes, K., and Vantrappen, G. (1992). Malignant degeneration of esophageal squamous papilloma associated with the human papillomavirus. *Gastroenterology* 103: 1119–1120.

Varghese, S., Lao-Sirieix, P., and Fitzgerald, R.C. (2012). Identification and clinical implementation of biomarkers for Barrett's esophagus. *Gastroenterology* 142: 435–441. e2.

Vogt, N., Schonegg, R., Gschossmann, J.M. et al. (2010). Benefit of baseline cytometry for surveillance of patients with Barrett's esophagus. *Surg. Endosc.* 24: 1144–1150.

Wang, H.H., Zeroogian, J.M., Spechler, S.J. et al. (1996). Prevalence and significance of pancreatic acinar metaplasia at the gastroesophageal junction. *Am. J. Surg. Pathol.* 20: 1507–1510.

Weeratunge, C.N., Bolivar, H.H., Anstead, G.M., and Lu, D.H. (2004). Primary esophageal lymphoma: a diagnostic challenge in acquired immunodeficiency syndrome – two case reports and review. *South. Med. J.* 97: 383–387.

Weickert, U., Wolf, A., Schröder, C. et al. (2011). Frequency, histopathological findings, and clinical significance of cervical heterotopic gastric mucosa (gastric inlet patch): a prospective study in 300 patients. *Dis. Esophagus* 24: 63–68.

Wu, N., Pang, L., Chen, Z. et al. (2011). Primary esophageal CD30-positive ALK-positive anaplastic large cell lymphoma: a case report and literature review. *J. Gastrointest. Cancer* 42: 57–60.

Yamada, A., Sasaki, H., Aoyagi, K. et al. (2008). Expression of cytokeratin 7 predicts survival in stage I/IIA/IIB squamous cell carcinoma of the esophagus. *Oncol. Rep.* 20: 1021–1027.

Ye, L.P., Zhang, Y., Mao, X.L. et al. (2013). Submucosal tunnelling endoscopic resection for the treatment of esophageal submucosal tumours originating from the muscularis propria layer: An analysis of 15 cases. *Dig. Liver Dis.* 45: 119–123.

Yong, F., Xudong, N., and Lijie, T. (2013). Human papillomavirus types 16 and 18 in esophagus squamous cell carcinoma: a meta-analysis. *Ann. Epidemiol.* 23: 726–734.

Yoshimura, N., Mukaida, H., Kaneko, M. et al. (2013). Primary esophageal gastrointestinal stromal tumor with PDGFRA mutation. *Esophagus* 10: 95–98.

Yoshizawa, A., Ota, H., Sakaguchi, N. et al. (2004). Malignant granular cell tumor of the esophagus. *Virchows Arch.* 444: 304–306.

Younes, M., Ertan, A., Ergun, G. et al. (2007). Goblet cell mimickers in esophageal biopsies are not associated with an increased risk for dysplasia. *Arch. Pathol. Lab. Med.* 131 (4): 571–575.

Younes, M., Lauwers, G.Y., Ertan, A. et al. (2011). The significance of indefinite for dysplasia grading in Barrett metaplasia. *Arch. Pathol. Lab. Med.* 135: 430–432.

Zagari, R.M., Fuccio, L., Wallander, M.A. et al. (2008). Gastro-oesophageal reflux symptoms, oesophagitis and Barrett's oesophagus in the general population: the Loiano-Monghidoro study. *Gut* 57 (10): 1354–1359.

Zendehdel, K., Nyrén, O., Edberg, A. et al. (2011). Risk of esophageal adenocarcinoma in achalasia patients, a retrospective cohort study in Sweden. *Am. J. Gastroenterol.* 106: 57–61.

Zhang, X., Huang, Q., Goyal, R.K. et al. (2008). DNA ploidy abnormalities in basal and superficial regions of the crypts in Barrett's esophagus and associated neoplastic lesions. *Am. J. Surg. Pathol.* 32: 1327–1335.

Zhang, B.H., Zhang, H.T., and Wang, Y.G. (2014). Esophageal leiomyosarcoma: clinical analysis and surgical treatment of 12 cases. *Dis. Esophagus* 27: 547–551.

Zhu, X., Zhang, X.Q., Li, B.M. et al. (2007). Esophageal mesenchymal tumors: endoscopy, pathology and immunohistochemistry. *World J. Gastroenterol.* 13: 768–773.

Zhu, Q., Xu, B., Xu, K. et al. (2008). Primary non-Hodgkin's lymphoma in the esophagus. *J. Dig. Dis.* 9: 241–244.

4

Inflammatory Disorders of the Stomach

Till S. Clauditz[1], Michael B. Wallace[2] and Gregory Y. Lauwers[3]

[1] Department of Pathology, University-Medical-Center Hamburg-Eppendorf, Hamburg, Germany
[2] Mayo Clinic, Jacksonville, Florida, USA
[3] Moffitt Cancer Center, Tampa, Florida, USA

One of the main reasons for upper GI endoscopy is gastric discomfort. Although the recognition of *Helicobacter pylori* gastritis remains important when evaluating chronic gastritis, a decrease in the prevalence of the infection and the enhanced quality of endoscopic evaluation have led to the recognition of new patterns of gastritis.

In this chapter we will to present a broad clinicopathological overview of well-known but also more recently characterized entities that may be challenging in daily practice.

Helicobacter-Associated Gastritis and Peptic Ulcer Disease

Definition, General Features, Predisposing Factors

Helicobacter pylori (*HP*) gastritis is a worldwide infection that predominantly takes place during childhood and is transmitted from human to human. HP gastritis has a wide range of prevalence, affecting less than 15% of the western population and over 80% of the population in low- and middle-income countries. In the United States, African and Asian Americans as well as Hispanics have a higher prevalence than Caucasians (70 vs. 35%).

H. pylori organism is a 3.5-μm long and generally comma-shaped or slightly spiral in form, microaerophilic Gram-negative bacteria. It is motile, using single polar flagellum. This organism has a tropism for gastric mucosa or metaplastic gastric mucosa in organs such as the duodenum. The pathogenesis of the bacterium depends on its ability to colonize gastric epithelium via adhesins such as BabA, SabA, and urease and virulence factors such as Cag A, Vac A, and urease, which in turn generates cytokines such as interleukin-8 to attract neutrophils.

Clinical Features and Endoscopic Characteristics

HP infection is commonly devoid of clinical symptoms or associated with mild dyspepsia. Severe gastritis with variable symptoms such as abdominal pain, nausea, vomiting, dyspepsia, weight loss, and iron deficiency anemia may appear, whereas some patients may develop duodenal ulcer disease. The symptoms of peptic ulcer disease are comparable with those of severe gastritis with exacerbation after food intake.

However, peptic ulcer disease may also be caused by corticosteroids, NSAIDs or syncromic diseases as Zollinger–Ellison syndrome.

Hematemesis, melena, and strictures of the gastric outlet may occur with deep ulceration.

It is important to underscore that *H. pylori* infection is associated with several coincidental benign and malignant conditions such as peptic ulcer disease, gastric MALT lymphoma, and adenocarcinoma.

Endoscopy examination can reveal a wide range of mucosal changes including erythema with/without erosive changes (Figure 4.1). Nodular mucosal irregularity may be observed, possibly caused by follicular hyperplasia.

Gastric ulcer disease is commonly found on the lesser curvature with round to oval ulceration showing a smooth base and regular, perpendicular edges. Characteristically, the borders are unlikely to be irregular in comparison to malignant ulcerations.

Microscopic Features

HP infection is characterized by the presence *of* comma-shaped or slightly spiral in form bacteria found in the antral and fundic body mucosa depending on the extent of infection (Figure 4.2). Mononuclear and lymphoplasmacytic

Gastrointestinal Pathology: Correlative Endoscopic and Histologic Assessment, First Edition. Edited by Gregory Y Lauwers and Michael B. Wallace.

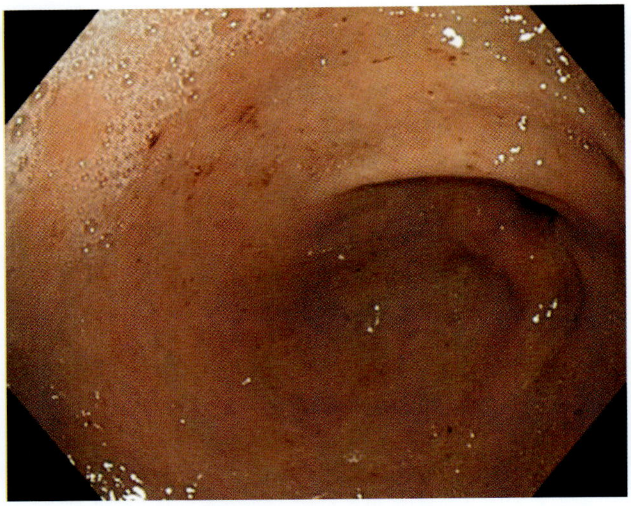

Figure 4.1 Endoscopic appearance of acute gastritis with superficial erosions of the antrum. Note the small, 1–2 mm erosions with erythema.

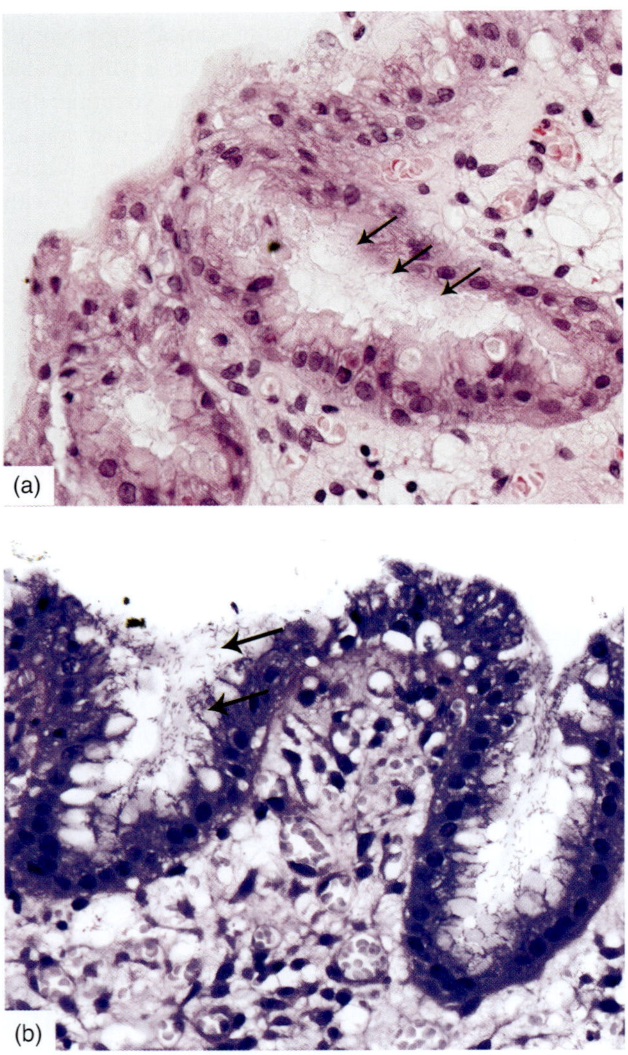

Figure 4.2 HP. Gastric antral biopsy with a severe population *of Helicobacter pylori* on the mucosal surface and the pits (a; arrows), highlighted in the Giemsa stain (b).

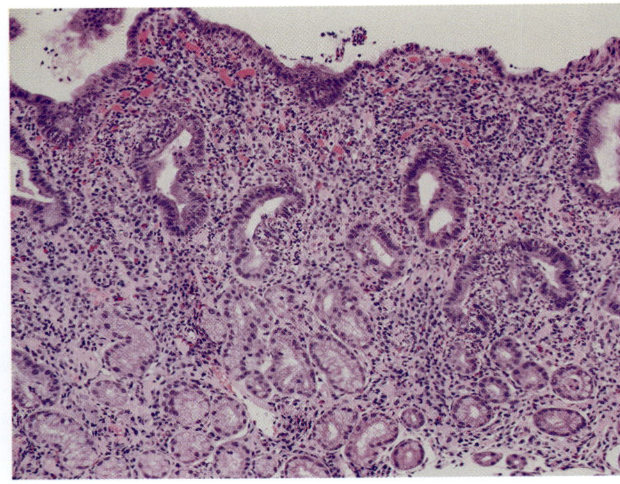

Figure 4.3 HP inflammation. H.E. stain of a punch biopsy with typical inflammatory pattern of HP infection characterized by a dense infiltrate of lymphoplasmacellular component as well as active inflammation, here with infiltration of the epithelium.

infiltrates cause an expansion of the lamina propria. Variable degrees of neutrophilic infiltrate ("activity") can affect the stroma, surface epithelium, and/or gastric pits with or without variably crypt abscesses. A pattern of lymphocytic gastritis can be seen (Figure 4.3). Additionally, foveolar hyperplasia, erosion, and reactive epithelial changes may be present.

In case of long-term use of proton pump inhibitor (PPI), pH microenvironmental changes may lead to the detection of *H. pylori* in the body and fundus, while the antrum mucosa is free of bacteria. Gastroenterologists should be aware of these changes and optimally PPIs should be discontinued two weeks before endoscopy to prevent possible false negative biopsies.

In chronic infection, atrophy (i.e. loss of glandular epithelium) as well as intestinal metaplasia may develop.

Depending on the bacterial load, *H. pylori* may be detected on hematoxylin and eosin stain but can be easily highlighted with special stains like Giemsa and Warthin–Starry.

Ulcer disease is defined by the presence of mucosal defects reaching at least the submucosa or even the muscularis propria. Early changes show acute inflammation with fibrinoid necrosis and granulation tissue. The adjacent epithelium may display reactive changes. A chronic ulcer additionally goes along with fibrosis and scaring.

Immunohistochemical Studies and Molecular Features

In case of negative hematoxylin and eosin as well as histochemical stains, immunohistochemistry and/or polymerase chain reaction can be helpful in detecting HP infection.

Differential Diagnosis

- *Helicobacter heilmannii* gastritis is caused by a spiral shaped bacterium that is nearly double in size that of *H. pylori* (measuring up to 6 microns in size). It has been detected in cats and dogs, raising the possibility of a zoonosis. The corkscrew bacteria can be detected in gastric mucous or pits without epithelial contact. *Helicobacter heilmannii* are reactive when *H. pylori* immunohistochemistry is applied.
- Marginal zone B-cell lymphoma (MALT) lymphoma: Benign follicular hyperplasia can be misdiagnosed as low-grade lymphoma. Immunohistochemistry is useful to underscore the reactive infiltrate using CD20 (positive germinal center and mantle cuff) and CD3 (positive interfollicular T-cells). MALT lymphoma is characterized by monomorphic lymphocytes extending below the muscularis mucosae and destructive lymphoepithelial lesions. *Helicobacter* gastritis causes only superficial inflammation and lacking destructive lesions. A caveat to underscore is that lymphoepithelial lesions and dense B-cell aggregates may also be seen in cases of severe gastritis.
- Crohn's disease should be distinguished in *HP*-negative cases with focally enhanced gastritis.
- Autoimmune gastritis: The characteristic changes affect the oxyntic mucosa with atrophy (and ultimately absence of oxyntic glands), pseudopyloric, pancreatic, and/or intestinal metaplasia along with hyperplasia of the enterochromaffin-like (ECL) cells. The antral mucosa may show mild chemical gastritis. Serology usually confirms anti-parietal cell or anti-intrinsic factor antibodies.
- Non-*H. pylori* infection: The biopsies may demonstrate colonies of bacteria commonly of oral origin. They can be detected in areas of ulceration and are easily recognized. The bacteria are not spiral shaped and may have a coccoid or rod-shaped appearance and are arranged in clusters. Furthermore, the gastric mucosa does not show HP-related changes.

Prognosis, Evolution, and Clinical Management

Optimally, biopsies from three regions (antrum, incisura angularis, and body/fundus) submitted separately will allow the precise assessment of HP infection and mucosal atrophy (using for example the Sydney system as well as the operative link for gastritis assessment [OLGA] classification)

HP infection is treated with antibiotics ("quadruple" therapy: bismuth, tetracycline, nitroimidazole, and proton pump inhibitor, or "triple" therapy: metronidazole, clarithromycin, and tetracycline or amoxicillin) for two weeks. Clarithromycin resistance is increasingly problematic and warrants quadruple therapy with non-macrolide agents when patients have prior macrolide exposure or known resistance. The cure rate reaches up to 95%. Cure should be confirmed by either urease breath test, stool antigen, or, if endoscopy is otherwise warranted, biopsy. Anti-*H. pylori* serology is inaccurate for confirmation of eradication due to persistence of Ab after eradication.

In case of gastric ulcer disease, *H. pylori* eradication but also PPIs are used in addition to stopping NSAIDs and prostaglandin analogues. Quitting smoking, and limiting or stopping alcohol are also helpful steps. In case of bleeding, endoscopic mechanical closure with clips or coagulation of visible vessels with or without epinephrine injection is the preferred therapy. Recent innovations include topically hemostatic/desiccant sprays delivered via endoscopes. In case of perforation or severe hemorrhage, surgical management may be required.

Acute (Erosive/Hemorrhagic) Gastritis

Definition, General Features, Predisposing Factors

Acute (erosive/hemorrhagic) gastritis is defined as severe and frequently acute mucosal injury. Typically, large alcohol consumption, iatrogenic injury, drugs (steroids, NSAIDs), and major stress are causative.

Clinical Features and Endoscopic Characteristics

Symptoms are usually and include sensation of burning, epigastric pain, nausea, vomiting, and gastrointestinal bleeding. The bleeding can be occult but life-threatening hematemesis may occur. Alcohol and NSAID-induced cases recover much faster than hypoperfusion-related cases (stress ulcers), which are associated with greater morbidity and mortality.

Multifocal erosions presenting as rounded dark superficial lesions can be endoscopically detected, measuring 2–5 mm in size (see Figure 4.1). The adjacent mucosa is edematous with hyperemia and petechiae. Notably, fundic and body ulcers are often stress related, whereas NSAID-related lesions are more commonly antral in location.

Microscopic Features

The morphology of erosive/hemorrhagic-type gastritis is varied and in part depends on the interval between the insult and biopsy sampling. On *H&E* stained slides, the changes can range from hemorrhage of the lamina propria

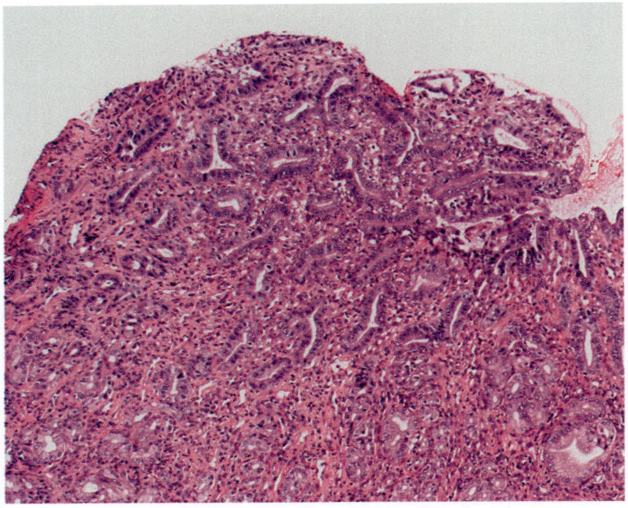

Figure 4.4 Acute erosive changes. Antral biopsy with superficial erosion and prominent reactive epithelial changes.

to mucosal sloughing and necrosis with or without neutrophil infiltration. Erosive changes can be limited to the mucosa or may affect the submucosa and superficial muscularis propria (Figure 4.4). Healing regenerative epithelial changes, granulation tissue can be detected as well. It is worth underscoring that marked reactive atypia can closely mimic a neoplastic lesion with increased mitosis, enlarged hyperchromatic nuclei with prominent nucleoli and amphophilic cytoplasm.

Differential Diagnosis

- Iatrogenic injury: Placement of nasogastric tube can elicit mucosal injury with focal erosion and hemorrhage. Diagnostic clues include the unremarkable surrounding mucosa, whereas the clinical information is obviously cardinal.
- Chemical gastropathy: It is commonly caused by NSAIDs and bile reflux, histologically characterized by foveolar hyperplasia and hyperplasia of muscle fibers. Reactive mucin depletion may be present.
- Biopsy forceps trauma: The biopsy site can show mucosal superficial congestion without evidence of epithelial injury and/or inflammation and should not be mistaken for evidence of mucosal hemorrhage.

Prognosis, Evolution, and Clinical Management

Most patients recover within a short time period when the inciting agent is removed. The management may consist of supportive care such as intravenous fluids and/or blood transfusion depending on the hemodynamic status. Supportive measures including prescription of H_2 blockers, proton pump inhibitors or prostaglandin analogues may be necessary as well.

Chemical (Reactive) Gastritis/ Gastropathy

Definition, General Features, Predisposing Factors

Chemical (reactive) gastritis/gastropathy is characterized by chemically induced mucosal damage. Alternative terminology such as type C gastritis, alkaline or bile reflux gastritis has also been used. The histologic diagnosis is rarely associated with a specific clinical presentation.

Clinical Features and Endoscopic Characteristics

The patients, more frequently female, are usually asymptomatic, but complaints of vague abdominal pain, nausea, and vomiting can be reported. Bleeding occur rarely. Various medications such aspirin or other NSAID, ferrous sulfate can be associated. Bile reflux either related to surgery (post gastroenterostomies, vagotomy, and pyloroplasty) or not (associated to a low pyloric sphincter tone or gastric dysmotility) maybe related to this type of gastritis. Again, alcohol intake and smoking may affect the disease.

The gastric mucosa may appear normal or display nonspecific changes such as erythema and focal erosion. The endoscopic detection of bile may be helpful in establishing an etiologic diagnosis.

Microscopic Features

The characteristic features include foveolar hyperplasia, usually detected in antral mucosa with elongated gastric pits that may adopt a serrated (corkscrew-like) profile. The epithelium may show regenerative/reactive changes with uniform cuboidal cells, depleted mucin, and high N : C ratio (Figure 4.5). Smooth muscle proliferation and vascular congestion and limited inflammation complete the histologic picture. Erosion can be detected, usually associated with neutrophils as well as intestinal metaplasia.

In patients with previous gastric surgery and bile reflux-related gastropathy, the changes affect the body and fundic mucosa.

Differential Diagnosis

See Table 4.1.

Prognosis, Evolution, and Clinical Management

Treatment of chemical gastritis is aimed at removing the offending agent (NSAID, ethanol) where possible. In cases of NSAID gastritis, co-administration with a proton pump inhibitor reduces gastric injury and may be necessary when continued therapy with aspirin (e.g. in severe coronary/vascular disease) or NSAID (in severe inflammatory arthritis) is necessary. In cases of bile reflux, topical, mucosal protecting agents such as sucralfate are helpful.

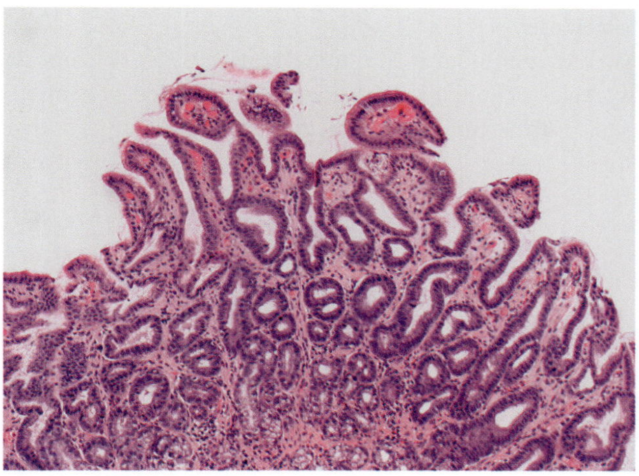

Figure 4.5 Reactive gastropathy. Antral mucosa showing foveolar hyperplasia covered by typically cuboid-shaped regenerative epithelium with hyperchromatic round to ovoid nuclei.

Granulomatous Gastritis

Definition, General Features, Predisposing Factors

Granulomatous gastritis is a rare entity representing less than 1% of all types of gastritides.

The granuloma(s) usually is/are detected in the submucosa, possibly presenting variant several morphologic patterns (with admixed granulocytes, necrosis, giant cells, lymphoid cuff, foreign bodies, etc.)

Determining the etiology requires the evaluation of clinical, endoscopic, and radiologic characteristics with, in some cases, possibly microbiological confirmation since the morphology may not be diagnostic.

A controversial diagnosis of *idiopathic granulomatous gastritis* (isolated granulomatosis of condition) has been proposed as a diagnosis after exclusion of entities such as Crohn's disease and sarcoidosis have been ruled out. It has also been reported that granulomatosis may appear after successful *H. pylori* eradication therapy or in the setting of vasculitis.

Clinical Features and Endoscopic Characteristics

In case of Crohn's disease, granulomatosis gastritis can be detected in 30–50% of the cases, whereas upper GI involvement is only reported in about 10% of patients affected by systemic sarcoidosis. Although patients with upper GI involvement in the setting of Crohn's or sarcoidosis are usually young, Crohn's disease is more often diagnosed in the pediatric age group and sarcoidosis in young adults.

Furthermore, patients with Crohn's disease may present with lower GI symptoms such as chronic diarrhea and

Table 4.1 Overview of differential diagnoses to be considered in the setting of reactive gastropathy.

Lesion	Features
• Polypoid foveolar hyperplasia/hyperplastic polyp	• Share morphologic features with reactive gastritis • Endoscopy distinguishes the conditions
• Gastric epithelial dysplasia	• Irregular nuclear membrane and macronucleoli • Atypical mitoses • Sharp transition with surrounding epithelium (normal or intestinal metaplasia)
• Gastric antral vascular ectasia	• Endoscopic appearance, i.e. watermelon stomach • Vascular ectasia with fibrin thrombi
• Portal hypertension gastropathy	• Prominent dilated and congested capillaries lacking fibrin thrombi • Perivascular stromal fibrosis and lamina propria edema • Surface foveolar epithelium can show associated reactive changes • Clinical history and endoscopic appearance

weight loss. However, upper GI manifestations may precede lower GI Crohn's disease by months to years.

Endoscopically, the mucosal appearance is quite variable and ranges from completely normal mucosa to findings that include erythema, erosions, superficial or deep ulcers, nodules, thickened folds (so-called bamboo stomach), and even gastric outlet stenosis. Findings are usually predominant in the antrum. For sarcoidosis, a linitis plastica-like appearance was described.

Gastric Tuberculosis B

Gastrointestinal tuberculosis (TB) classically affects the terminal ileum and may mimic Crohn's disease, however isolated gastric or multiorgan infection can rarely occur. Manifestations include, most commonly, nonhealing gastric ulcer with or without perforation, submucosal tumors, and gastric outlet obstruction. Treatment is similar to other systemic TB with prolonged multidrug therapy.

Microscopic Features

Crohn's Disease

The changes range from focally enhanced gastritis (Figure 4.6a) to the presence of granulomas to essentially any pattern of active and chronic gastritis. Epithelioid granulomas are present in only 7–34% of cases and usually consist of small clusters of epithelioid histiocytes (Figure 4.6b). Detected frequently in younger age group, they often correspond to mucosal nodules or aphthoid erosions. They can also be been found in normal mucosa.

Commonly, gastric involvement shows a spectrum of inflammatory changes ranging from normal to *HP*-negative mild inflammatory changes. Furthermore, patchy chronic active gastritis is usually related to focally enhanced gastritis, which is defined as a patchy inflammatory process composed of a focal lymphohistiocytic cluster with admixed acute inflammation. For Crohn's disease typical other histologic findings include pit abscesses and focal active gastritis. Focally enhanced gastritis is a good indicator for Crohn's disease, especially the pediatric population, but it is not specific. It can also be associated with ulcerative colitis, graft versus host disease (GvHD) as well as incompletely treated *H. pylori* gastritis. It is important that *HP* infection is always excluded in these patients.

The diagnosis of Crohn's in resection specimens is more straightforward, as the findings are comparable to the colonic changes (e.g. fissures, undermining ulcers, transmural inflammation, lymphoid follicles, granulomas, etc.).

Sarcoidosis

Sarcoid granulomas are noncaseating with a compact aggregate of epithelioid histiocytes surrounded by lymphocytes. Furthermore, the detection of involvement of other organ(s) being diagnosed (e.g. lung) is highly suggestive of the diagnosis.

Differential Diagnosis

Several other diseases can mimic granulomatous gastritis including gastric adenocarcinoma, chronic granulomatous disease, common variable immunodeficiency, Langerhans cell histiocytosis, Whipple's disease, vasculitis (including granulomatosis with polyangiitis) and xanthogranulomatous gastritis.

(a)

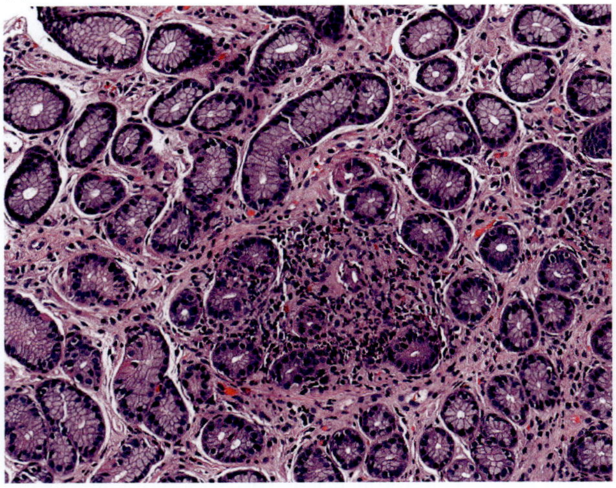

(b)

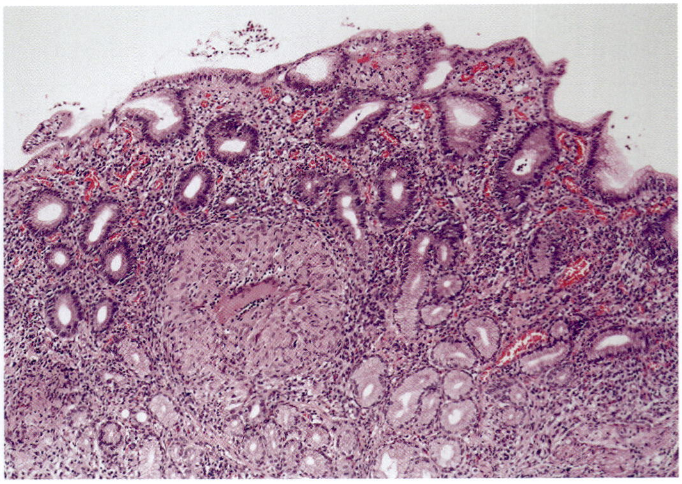

Figure 4.6 (a) Focally enhanced gastritis. Gastric antral mucosa with a small round focus of active inflammation affecting only a few foveolae, whereas the other parts of the biopsy appear normal. (b) Granulomatous gastritis. Superficial gastric mucosa with an mixed inflammatory infiltrate and an epithelioid granuloma with prominent giant-cells (center of granuloma).

Besides other diseases, foreign body reactions caused by food, surgical material, or drugs (e.g. magnesium, aluminum, silicon) can appear as granulomatous gastritis.

When granuloma is seen on H.E. infectious conditions (e.g. TBC, Mucor) and additional stains as AFB, GMS, and PAS are obligatory part of the diagnostic assessment.

Prognosis, Evolution, and Clinical Management

Sarcoidosis may present in the GI tract or liver either in combination with systemic sarcoidosis or as a first manifestation. Diagnosis is based on luminal or liver biopsy using the criteria discussed above. The symptoms are not specific, and may include dysphagia (esophagus), dyspepsia (stomach), or malabsorption/diarrhea (small bowel/colon). There is occasional co-occurrence with inflammatory bowel disease. Treatment is similar to systemic sarcoidosis including immunosuppressive agents such as prednisone although the response, like systemic response, is limited.

Gastritides with Prominent Lympho(plasma)cytic Infiltrate

Definition, General Features, Predisposing Factors

Autoimmune gastritis (type A gastritis) is the most common type of gastritis with a prominent lymphocytic infiltrate. It is defined as an immune-mediated chronic injury of the body and fundus caused by antibodies targeting oxyntic mucosa (esp. parietal cells). As a result, hypochlorhydria and vitamin B_{12} deficiency can develop.

Compared to type A gastritis, lymphocytic gastritis (varioliform or chronic erosive verrucous gastritis) is uncommon. It is defined by marked intraepithelial lymphocytosis of the superficial mucosa including the pits. Deeper glands are usually less affected.

Other rare entities with predominant lymphocytic infiltrate are associated to *Treponema pallidum* (syphilis), EBV infection, and NK-cell enteropathy.

Clinical Features and Endoscopic Characteristics

Autoimmune gastritis is responsible for about 4% of chronic gastritides and affects nearly 2% of the population over 60 years of age. Commonly, females in the fifth and sixth decade are affected with a female-to-male ratio of 3 : 1.

The range of symptoms is wide from asymptomatic to abdominal pain, weight loss, diarrhea, malabsorption, and vitamin B_{12} deficiency. As result of long-standing B_{12} deficiency, neurologic complications such as peripheral neuropathy and degenerative changes of the spinal cord can develop. Several antibodies can be identified (anti-parietal cell antibodies 60–85%; anti-intrinsic factor antibodies 30–50%). As a result of reduced gastric acid, iron deficiency-related anemia is found in up to 40% of affected patients. Pernicious anemia, resulting from a decrease in intrinsic factor, is found in up to 25% of the patients and may appear after more than 20 years of history. Other manifestations such as insulin-dependent diabetes mellitus, Hashimoto's thyroiditis, adrenal insufficiency, Graves' disease, vitiligo, and/or myasthenia gravis may be present.

Endoscopically, the mucosa of the body and fundus appear flattened. As a result of flattened mucosal folds, submucosal vessels are prominent. Coincidentally hyperplastic polyps, pyloric adenomas, low-grade neuroendocrine tumors, and even adenocarcinoma can occur.

Lymphocytic gastritis is a rare condition with a reported prevalence between 1 and 4%. Symptoms are not specific and similar to those detected in autoimmune gastritis. Older adults are the main group of patients afflicted, but children can also be affected, whereas a slight female predominance is also reported.

Lymphocytic gastritis can be found in gastric biopsies of patients with celiac disease (33%) and *HP* gastritis (4%). Celiac disease patients with lymphocytic gastritis may also show lymphocytic colitis in approximately 38% of the cases. Less common are associations with Crohn's disease, HIV infection, esophageal carcinoma, and gastric lymphoma.

A wide spectrum of mucosal alterations can be seen endoscopically reaching from normal mucosa to nodular (sometimes with central depression), erosive/ulcerative appearance and/or prominent Ménétrier's-like gastric folds. The mucosal changes can mimic neoplasia endoscopically, reminiscent of the patterns seen in poorly cohesive type adenocarcinoma or gastric lymphoma.

Clinical symptoms as well as endoscopic appearance of syphilis and EBV-associated cases as well as NK-cell enteropathy are comparable with the findings mentioned above. Furthermore, obstruction and markedly thickened rugal folds mimicking linitis plastica can be seen in EBV gastritis.

NK-cell gastropathy is a rare condition that regresses spontaneously without any therapy.

NK-cells are rarely found in inflammatory disorders of the GI tract, and a misdiagnosis as malignant lymphoma can be rendered, especially extranodal NK/T-cell lymphoma and intestinal enteropathy-associated T-cell lymphoma.

Microscopic Features

Autoimmune Pattern

Autoimmune gastritis is characterized by limited lymphoplasmacytic infiltrate of the lamina propria of the body and fundic mucosa while sparing the antrum. Over time, paucity and/or loss of oxyntic glands with pseudopyloric gland metaplasia will develop. In addition, intestinal, Paneth cell and pancreatic acinar metaplasia commonly appear. Early stages of the disease may only show inflammatory widening of the stroma between the oxyntic glands with loose fibrotic stromal changes (Figure 4.7).

At a late stage, the diseased oxyntic mucosa resembles the mucosa of the antrum or even small intestine. Nucleomegaly or megaloblastoid changes may occur in the foveolar epithelium.

Changes of antral mucosa are unspecific showing foveolar hyperplasia, sparse chronic inflammation, and G-cell hyperplasia, caused by loss of the parietal cells and secondary decrease of HCL production. The development of neuroendocrine or enterochromaffin-like (ECL) cells hyperplasia is a characteristic feature of autoimmune gastritis, usually presenting a linear or nodular pattern. The cutoff for the diagnosis of adenomatous hyperplasia/dysplasia and well-differentiated neuroendocrine tumor (NET) is 0.5 mm or an endoscopically visible lesion. Microscopically, an infiltrative growth may be present.

Other lesions that can develop in the setting of autoimmune gastritis include gastric hyperplastic polyps, pyloric gland adenomas, multiple well-differentiated neuroendocrine tumors, as well as gastric adenocarcinoma.

Lymphocytic Pattern

Microscopically, marked intraepithelial lymphocytosis of foveolar and pit epithelium is a characteristic feature the glands are usually spared. The intraepithelial lymphocytes may show a clear halo. The number of lymphocytes may reach more than 25 per 100 epithelial cells (Figure 4.8). Comparatively, *HP* gastritis may show approximately 5 lymphocytes per 100 epithelial cells. Elongated hyperplastic pits may be observed. Chronic inflammatory expansion of the lamina propria can be seen as well. Neutrophils can be seen associated to erosive changes.

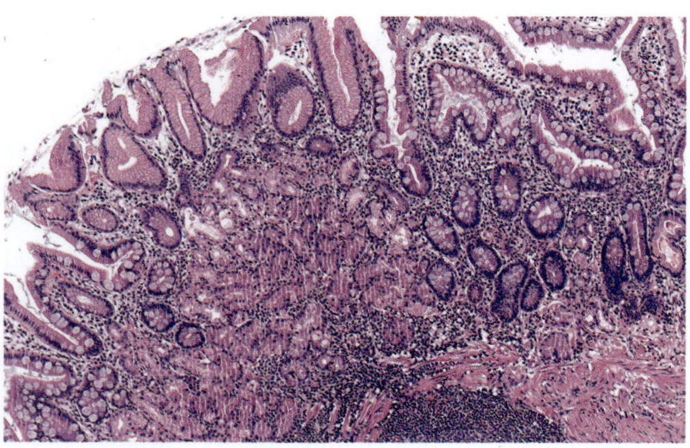

Figure 4.7 Autoimmune gastritis. Typical changes of mucosa of the body in the setting of autoimmune gastritis with pyloric and intestinal metaplasia as well as proliferation of ECL cells at the bottom foveolae.

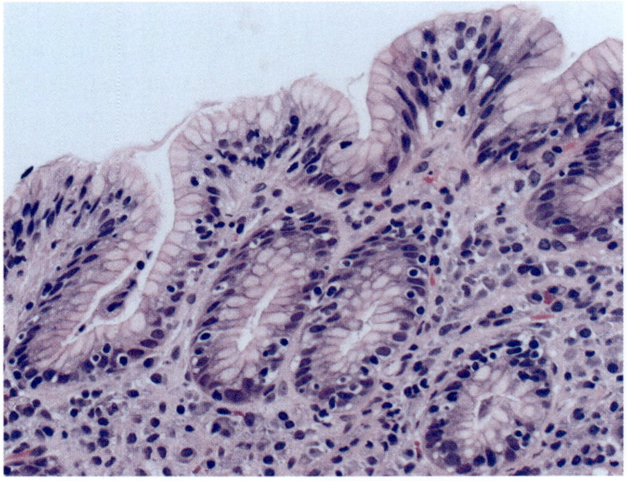

Figure 4.8 Lymphocytic gastritis. Superficial high magnification of a gastric mucosa showing a dense lymphoplasmocytic infiltrate affecting the epithelium.

Lymphocytic gastritis can involve the entire gastric mucosa or may predominantly involve the antrum or the body and fundic region. Studies have shown that antrum-predominant disease is more commonly associated with celiac disease, whereas *H. pylori*-associated lymphocytic gastritis has a predilection to involve the body/fundus.

Treponema Pallidum (Syphilitic)

The condition is characterized by a dense lymphoplasmacytic infiltrate. The detection of proliferative endarteritis, gland destruction, and/or ill-formed granulomas are hints for suspecting syphilitic gastritis (Figure 4.9). Spirochetes can be highlighted with silver stains like Warthin–Starry or modified Steiner or immunohistochemistry. Concurrent *HP* infection is common.

EBV

A diffuse, polymorphic lymphocytic infiltrate limited to the lamina propria is the main finding and can mimic several other forms of chronic gastritis (*HP* gastritis, AIG, lymphocytic gastritis). Plasma cells and neutrophils are commonly not present. Lymphoepithelial lesions may occur as well.

NK-Cell Enteropathy

This benign condition is characterized by a diffuse infiltrate of medium- to large-sized atypical cells with NK-cell immunophenotype (positivity: CD3, CD56, T-cell-restricted

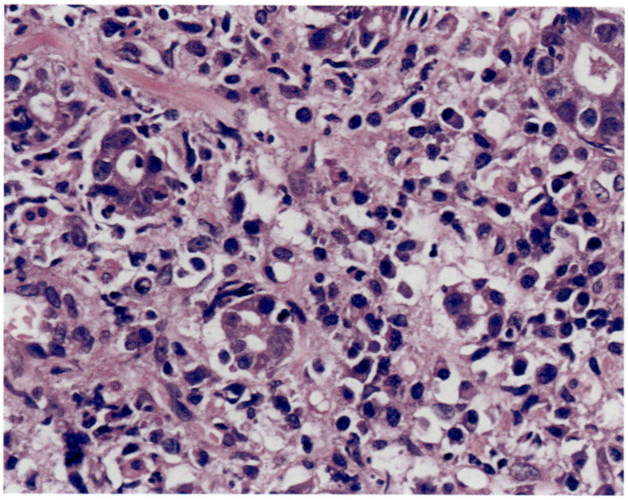

Figure 4.9 Syphilitic gastritis. Higher magnification of a corpus biopsy showing a dense infiltrate of plasma cells as well as a depletion of glandular structures. Furthermore, residual glands show prominent reactive atypia.

intracellular antigen 1, granzyme B). T-cell receptor-γ gene rearrangement shows no evidence of a clonal process, a differentiating feature from EATL.

Immunohistochemical Studies and Molecular Features

Gastrin immunohistochemical stain can be helpful to distinguish antral biopsies from biopsies of the body/fundus displaying atrophy with pseudo-pyloric gland metaplasia. It is negative in atrophic oxyntic mucosa and positive in antral mucosa. Gastrin can also highlight antral the G-cell hyperplasia. Using immunohistochemical stains for chromogranin A and synaptophysin is helpful to highlight linear or micronodular ECL cell hyperplasia.

In cases of NK-cell enteropathy, the intraepithelial lymphocytes are CD3- and CD8-positive cytotoxic/suppressor T-lymphocytes and can easily be distinguished from CD20-positive B-cells excluding an extranodal marginal zone lymphoma (MALT lymphoma). The cells also show reactivity to CD56, T-cell-restricted intracellular antigen 1 and granzyme B.

EBV can be detected using in situ hybridization (ISH) for EBV-encoded RNA (EBER).

Syphilitic gastritis can be identified by immunohistochemistry, immunofluorescence staining for *Treponema pallidum* and/or polymerase chain reaction (PCR).

Differential Diagnosis

Main differential diagnoses for lymphocytic predominant gastritides include MALT lymphoma and *H. pylori* infection.

MALT lymphoma shows a vast expansion of the lamina propria caused by a uniform monocytoid lymphocellular infiltrate. The lymphocytes are of small to medium size and lymphoepithelium may be observed destroying surrounding epithelial structures.

Immunohistochemical may be needed to differentiate between lymphoma and lymphocytic gastritis.

HP gastritis can occur with intraepithelial lymphocytosis, but it classically shows also active gastritis with neutrophils and plasma cells. Furthermore, the intraepithelial count is much less than in lymphocytic gastritis (up to 5 lymphocytes per 100 epithelial cells).

Prognosis, Evolution, and Clinical Management

About 9% of autoimmune gastritis patients will develop well-differentiated neuroendocrine tumors. Additionally, in the same population the prevalence of gastric adenocarcinoma is three times higher than in normal stomach. Autoimmune gastritis-associated NET is mostly less than 10 mm in size and minimally invasive. Compared with sporadic cases, NETs in background of autoimmune gastritis have a better prognosis.

Multiple NETs can be treated with endoscopic polypectomy or EMR followed by close surveillance. It was shown that reduced gastrin levels after antrectomy led to reduction of the size of NETs.

In case of vitamin B_{12} deficiency, supplemental therapy may be indicated.

Infectious Gastritis

Definition, General Features, Predisposing Factors

Infectious gastritis is caused by bacterial and/or virus infection and can arise in several settings. Immunocompromised patients seem to be the most affected group. Gastritis caused by bacterial infection is more common and is distinguished between the phlegmonous and the emphysematous type. They are both characterized by focal or disseminated bacterial spread with or without evidence of intramural air.

Virus-associated gastritis is uncommon. In the event of occurrence it is more likely associated to CMV than to HSV infection.

Clinical Features and Endoscopic Characteristics

Clinical symptoms of bacterial or virus infection are overlapping and nonspecific (e.g. epigastric pain, nausea, vomiting, bleeding, hematemesis, etc.). Bacterial and viral gastritis can occur in different settings, whereas immunosuppression (e.g. cause by alcoholism, diabetes, HIV, iatrogenic) is one of the major risk factors. Several bacteria (non- and/or gas-forming types) can cause phlegmonous or emphysematous gastritis (e.g. *Streptococcus* and *Staphylococcus* species as well as *Haemophilus influenza*, *Klebsiella pneumoniae*, *Enterococcus* spp., and *Clostridium* spp., *Enterobacter* spp. and *Pseudomonas aeruginosa*).

Besides immunodeficiency, phlegmonous and emphysematous gastritis may occur in context with endoscopic mucosal resection (EMR) or submucosal dissection (ESD), corrosive substances, dialysis or after surgery.

Mortality for phlegmonous and emphysematous gastritis is high and was reported to be 27 and 61%, respectively.

Endoscopic findings for phlegmonous-type gastritis show enlarged gastric folds with edematous as well as erythematous changes and fibrinopurulent deposits.

Emphysematous gastritis is an escalation of phlegmonous-type gastritis and shows intramural gas formation.

Viral gastritis is predominantly caused by CMV and HSV infection. *Pediatric Ménétrier's disease* has been reported to be associated with CMV infection in 70% of children. Therefore, viral infection should always be excluded in cases of protein-loss paired with hypertrophic gastropathy in pediatric patients. Contraty, HP was found in approximately 90% of adults diagnosed with Ménétrier's disease.

Endoscopic findings in virus-affected gastritides vary and can show erythema, ulceration (single, multiple), plaques, nodules, and mucosal necrosis. For CMV, friability of the mucosa was reported, whereas polypoid lesions as well as thickened folds were described for HSV-associated cases.

Microscopic Features

Phlegmonous

Diagnostic features include acute purulent inflammation with neutrophilic abscesses and bacterial organisms in the submucosa. Mucosal and mural necrosis can be detected.

Emphysematous

Microscopic evaluation reveals cystic glandular dilatation with diffuse neutrophilic infiltrate. Clusters of bacteria, mucosal ulcers, bleeding, and/or necrosis may be observed.

CMV

CMV-infected cells are up to four times larger than normal cells and display eosinophilic intranuclear inclusions surrounded by a white halo (Figure 4.10). Additionally, basophilic intracytoplasmic granules can be seen. The background mucosa can show a broad spectrum of inflammation ranging from mild chronic to active erosive/ulcerative changes.

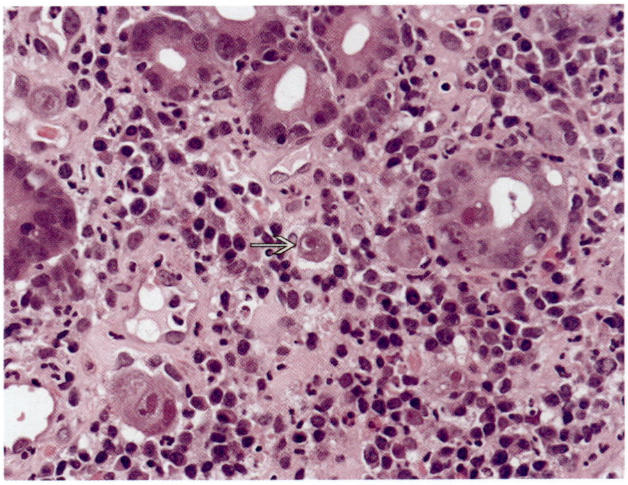

Figure 4.10 High magnification of CMV gastritis with typical cherry red nuclei and paranuclear halo (arrow). Furthermore, severe reactive atypia and a dense lymphoplasmocytic inflammatory infiltrate are present.

HSV

HSV-infected cells can be single or form clusters. The nuclei have a ground-glass appearance with eosinophilic intranuclear inclusion as well as a perinuclear halo. The number of inclusions may be scant. Mucosal changes, i.e. reactive foveolar hyperplasia may occur.

Immunohistochemical Studies and Molecular Features

Virus-related infections can be highlighted with immunohistochemical stains for CMV, HSV1&2.

Differential Diagnosis

- Chronic active *HP* gastritis: It is uncommonly presenting with an acute onset. The detection of a dense stromal lymphoplasmocytic infiltrate as well as cryptitis may be helpful. Additional stains (Giemsa, immunohistochemistry) may be helpful.
- Chemical gastropathy: It is mainly caused by NSAIDs and bile reflux. It is characterized by foveolar hyperplasia and hyperplasia of muscle fibers. Reactive mucin depletion is common.

Prognosis, Evolution, and Clinical Management

In cases of phlegmonous and emphysematous gastritis, an early initiation of broad-spectrum antibiosis is indicated to prevent an exacerbation. In refractory cases or in the setting of clinical complication (bleeding, necrosis, perforation), gastrectomy may be indicated.

If viral disease (CMV/HSV) is confirmed, specific antiviral therapy is warranted.

Eosinophilic Gastritis

Definition, General Features, Predisposing Factors

Eosinophilic gastritis is defined by dense eosinophilic mucosal infiltrate. Etiologic associations are numerous including manifestation of eosinophilic gastroenteritis, a rare inflammatory condition characterized by intense eosinophilic infiltration of the gastrointestinal tract.

Clinical Features and Endoscopic Characteristics

Eosinophilic gastroenteritis can affect every race and age group. Main groups are adults between second and fifth decade but pediatric involvement is reported in up to 20% of cases. No sex predominance is reported.

To diagnose eosinophilic gastritis, several criteria have to be fulfilled as follows:

1) Gastrointestinal symptoms: abdominal pain, nausea, vomiting, diarrhea, weight loss, malabsorption, protein-losing enteropathy, and anemia caused by bleeding.
2) Histological evidence of eosinophilic infiltration of the gastrointestinal tract.
3) Absence of eosinophilic infiltration in extraintestinal organs.
4) Exclusion of other eosinophilia causing etiologies like parasites and drugs.

The entire GI tract can be affected by eosinophilia whereas antrum is the most common in the stomach.

Patients with eosinophilia often show history of allergy, asthma, food intolerance, and have elevated IgG E levels in the blood serum.

Radiographic studies may show edema and thickening of gastric mucosal folds and/or obstruction.

Endoscopically gastric mucosal changes range from normal to erythema with erosion/ulceration as well as nodular changes.

Microscopic Features

Eosinophilic gastritis is defined by increased eosinophilic infiltrate limited to the stomach (Figure 4.11). No consensus diagnostic criteria exist. Some authors have suggested that ≥30 peak eosinophils in a minimum of five separate high-power fields (400× magnification) and absence of known causes of eosinophilia (parasites, drugs). The distribution of eosinophils can be patchy and multiple biopsies are required for a reliable diagnosis.

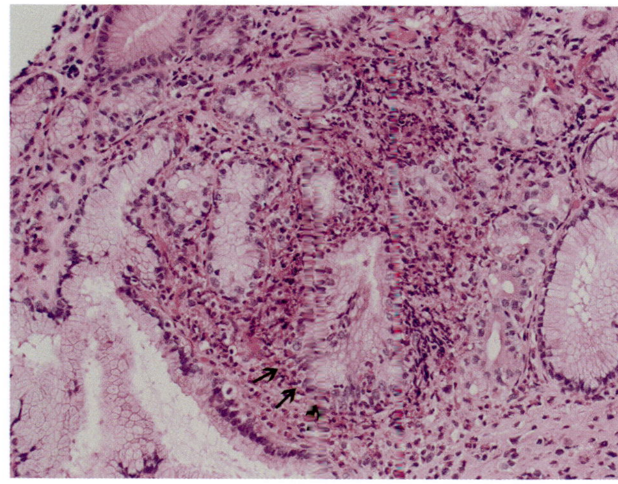

Figure 4.11 Eosinophilic gastritis. Superficial biopsy of the antrum with a dense infiltrate of eosinophils affecting the mucosal epithelium (arrows).

Epithelial damage, regenerative changes, and marked edema may be observed. Scattered neutrophils or lymphocytes can be found in the inflammatory background. Small submucosal muscular or serosal clusters of eosinophils are abnormal. Therefore, transmural biopsies and/or open biopsies may be necessary for diagnosis.

Differential Diagnosis

Parasitic Infestation

Parasites in the GI tract are mostly associated with severe eosinophilia in areas where ova, larvae, or nematodes (e.g. anisakiasis, strongyloides, Ascaris) are deposited. Cautious histologic evaluation is required, especially in case of stool specimen.

Drugs

Gold, azathioprine, carbamazepine, enalapril, and co-trimoxazole have been associated with eosinophilia of the GI tract.

Systemic Mastocytosis

Mucosal involvement of systemic mastocytosis can be masked by eosinophils. Ancillary studies like tryptase, CD117, and CD25 are useful to detect mast cells. Clinical information like the presence of urticaria can be helpful.

Langerhans Cell Histiocytosis

This condition is usually detected in the pediatric population. The eosinophils are intermixed with Langerhans histiocytes. The histiocytes are immunoreactive for CD1a and S-100.

Other conditions can cause eosinophilia like hypereosinophilic syndrome, inflammatory bowel disease, gastric carcinomas, lymphomas, connective tissue disorders, vasculitis (e.g. Churg–Strauss disease), and peptic ulcer disease. Thus, clinicopathological assessment is essential to make the right diagnosis.

Prognosis, Evolution, and Clinical Management

Eosinophilic gastroenteritis shows an excellent response to steroids. Recess can be followed by relapse and in case of obstructive changes or therapy refractory cases surgery may be needed.

Collagenous Gastritis

Definition, General Features, Predisposing Factors

Collagenous gastritis is defined by the deposition of subepithelial collagen bands in the superficial gastric mucosa. The collagen deposits exceed 10 μm in thickness. Epithelial damage, lymphoplasmacytic inflammation, and intraepithelial lymphocytosis may be present. The pathophysiology of collagenous gastritis is not well established. It was entertained that the collagenous deposition may be related to a reparative processes following previous mucosal damage and chronic inflammation or as a result of autoimmune, toxic, or infectious agents. The collagen deposition may be caused by abnormal pericryptal fibroblasts or as result of leakage of plasma proteins and fibrinogen replaced by collagen.

Clinical Features and Endoscopic Characteristics

Females show a slight predominance, whereas children and adults are affected (range from first to eightieth decade). Broad clinical symptoms can appear such as abdominal pain, weight loss, bleeding, diarrhea, anorexia, nausea, and vomiting. Clinically affected patients fall in two subgroups as follows:

1) Pediatric patients and young adults presenting anemia limited disease to the gastric mucosa.
2) Adults with chronic watery diarrhea in association with collagen colitis.

Several other inflammatory conditions like collagenous colitis, lymphocytic colitis, celiac disease, collagenous sprue, lymphocytic gastritis, and inflammatory bowel disease may be found additionally.

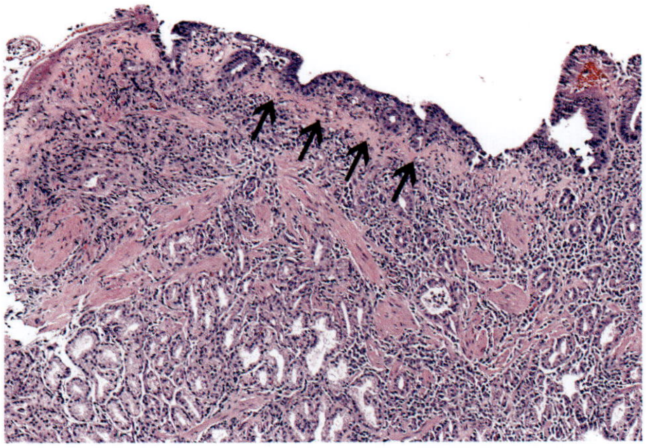

Figure 4.12 Collagenous gastritis. Antral mucosa showing a prominent submucosal thick collagenous band (arrows) entrapping small capillaries. Common findings in a prolonged stage are erosion (upper left) and reactive atypia of the mucosal epithelium.

Endoscopically diffuse mucosal nodularity, erythema, and erosions may be present. Especially, children and young adults show nodular mucosal changes in endoscopy.

Microscopic Features

Typical histologic findings include the deposition of diffuse or patchy thickened discontinuous subepithelial collagen band (Figure 4.12). The collagen band is thicker than 10 μm (normally less than 2–3 μm) with an average thickness of 30–40 μm (and reported to measure up to 120 μm in some rare cases). Capillaries and inflammatory cells are also entrapped in the collagen band. The epithelium shows various degenerative changes (mucin depletion and epithelial stripping).

Lymphoplasmacytic inflammation with intermixed eosinophils can be seen in the lamina propria. Active inflammation is rarely observed. Increased intraepithelial lymphocytosis (>20 lymphocytes/100 epithelial cells) may be recognized. Mostly, HP infection is absent.

Histo- and Immunohistochemical Studies

To highlight collagen deposits, Masson's trichrome or tenascin immunohistochemical stains may be useful for diagnosis. Amyloid stains like Congo red or thioflavin T are negative.

Differential Diagnosis

- Gastric amyloidosis is the main differential of collagenous gastritis. Typically, amyloid is not only located in the lamina propria but also affects the submucosa as well as vessel

walls. Congo red stain is useful to highlight amyloid, which also shows apple-green birefringence upon polarization.
- Lamina propria fibrosis may be a differential diagnosis in small specimens, but commonly it shows strong hyalinization. Further, the fibrosis involves diffusely the mucosa. It is typically found in different clinical settings like radiation, ischemia as well as scleroderma. Especially scleroderma may also show submucosa, muscularis propria and (sub-)serosa. In case of radiation-related changes, thickened vessels as well as severe epithelial and stromal atypia may be present.

Prognosis, Evolution, and Clinical Management

The current treatment is still empirical using steroids, salicylates as well as nutritional supplements or dietary procedures like gluten-free diet. It was reported that a combination of steroids and gluten-free diet led to improvement of symptoms. However, follow-up biopsies still showed collagen deposits. Because of frequent association to other collagenous enterocolitides, evaluation of duodenum and colon should be provided in patients with diagnosed collagenous gastritis.

Iatrogenic Gastritis

Definition, General Features, Predisposing Factors

Many drugs and chemical agents can cause gastritis, producing various morphologic patterns of injury. In some cases, given the absence of specific histopathological features, the diagnosis often relies upon thorough clinicopathological correlation. In others, a specific etiologic diagnosis can be achieved. Common causative agents include NSAIDs, oral iron therapy (approximately 15% of treated patients can be affected). Furthermore antibiotics (tetracycline, doxycyclin), chemotherapeutics (e.g. colchicine, taxol), or conditions like bone marrow transplants can be associated with gastric inflammatory changes with or without erosive or ulceration. A complete review of this subject is beyond the scope of this chapter and we will only discuss the best recognized entities.

Clinical Features and Endoscopic Characteristics

Clinical presentation varies, from asymptomatic to abdominal/epigastric pain, nausea, and vomiting. Melena can also develop, whereas others such colchicine and taxol may lead to multiorgan failure. The clinical context and timing are important to recognize and implicate some etiologies. For example, GvHD can be detected approximately one to two months after bone marrow transplantation.

Endoscopically iatrogenic gastritis reaches from normal up to erythematous and erosive or ulcerative changes as well as bleeding. Furthermore, brown-greenish mucosal deposits may be present in cases of iron pill intake. GMC shows white plaques and/or mucosal nodules (<5 mm).

Microscopic Features

Iron Pill Gastritis

On H.E., the biopsy shows crystalline deposits of golden brown color. It is mostly found in the superficial portion of the lamina propria and may be surrounded by macrophages and stromal elements. It can also appear as an exogenous layer or encrustation or be found in vessel walls. Background mucosa or affected areas may show erosion and or regenerative atypia with foveolar hyperplasia. Prussian blue can be helpful to highlight the iron deposition (Figure 4.13).

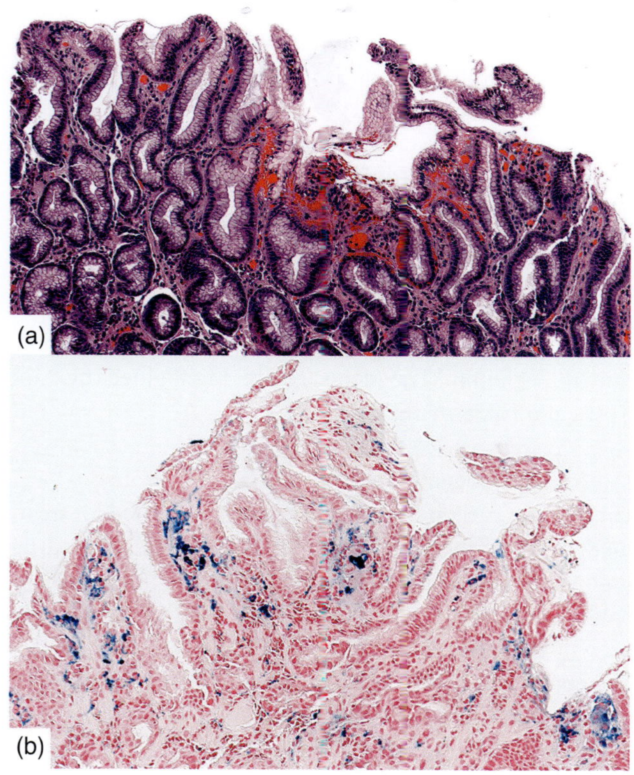

Figure 4.13 Iron pill induced gastritis. Superficial antral mucosa with appearance of reactive atypia of the mucosal epithelium and barely recognizable brownish material in the lamina propria (a) being highlighted in the Prussian blue stain (b).

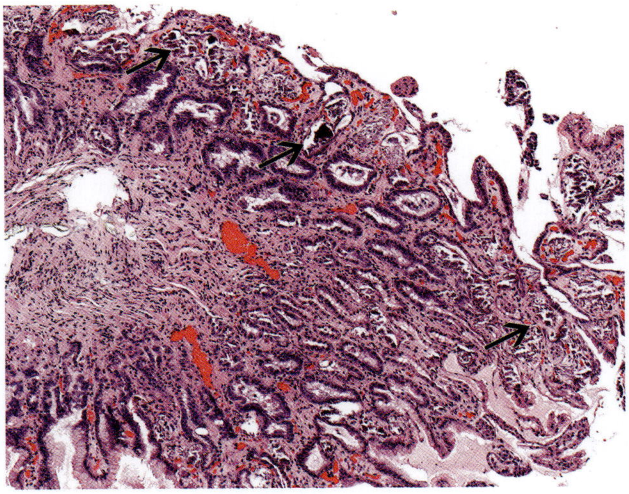

Figure 4.14 Calcifying gastritis. Antral punch biopsy with erosive and reactive inflammatory changes showing dense deposits of bluish calcifications in the lamina propria (see arrows).

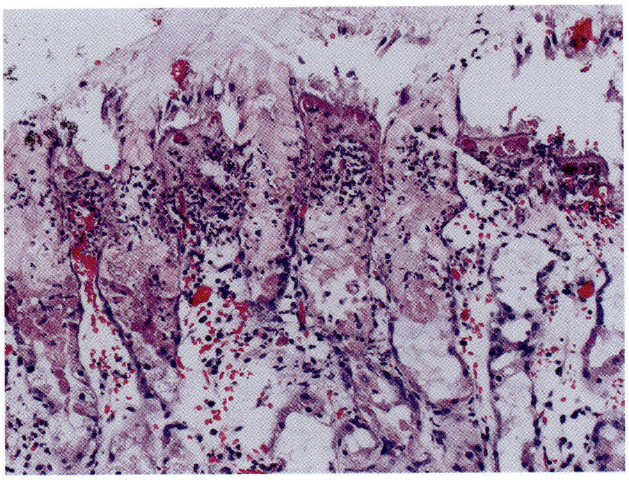

Figure 4.15 Doxycycline erosive gastritis. The classic appearance is composed of fibrinoid degeneration of the superficial capillaries accompanied by necrosis of the mucosa accompanied by neutrophilic infiltrate.

Mucosal Calcinosis

Gastric mucosal calcinosis develops in patients with renal failure after intake of antacids containing aluminum and in the setting of organ transplant. Other conditions leading to hypercalcemia and hyperphosphatemia such as hyperparathyroidism, sarcoidosis, multiple myeloma, tumor lysis syndrome, hypervitaminosis D, hypervitaminosis A, milk-alkali syndrome, and isotretinoin use can cause gastric mucosal calcinosis.

The diagnosis is established when purple/bluish deposits (50–500 μm in size) are found in the superficial mucosal layers (Figure 4.14). They are usually located beneath the lining foveolar epithelium but can also be found in deeper portions of the biopsy. A peripheral rim of histiocytes and giant cells may be present. Background mucosal changes are comparable with iron pill gastritis and may also show mucin depletion. The deposits are highlighted by Von Kossa and Alizarin red stains.

Lanthanum Carbonate

Lanthanum carbonate is a phosphate binder used for treatment of hyperphosphatemia in dialysis patients. The drug is poorly absorbed and reported to be present in over 80% of patients treated with Lanthanum carbonate. The deposits present as granular intracytoplasmic deposits within stromal histiocytes. The granular deposits are PAS negative but positive for Prussian blue stain.

Doxycyclin

The main finding is mucosal necrosis and erosion, with various degrees of neutrophilic infiltrate and regenerative epithelium. Degeneration of the capillaries with ring-like eosinophilic structures is observed on the superficial mucosa, sometimes with fibrin microthrombi. The background mucosa may show foveolar hyperplasia (Figure 4.15).

Graft Versus Host Disease

In case of GvHD, the epithelial neck region is predominantly affected with various degrees of necrosis and apoptosis of single epithelial cells (while sparing the surface foveolar epithelium). Furthermore, attenuated dilated glandular structures with eosinophilic granular debris can be seen (Figure 4.16a). Significant acute inflammation is not a typical feature.

In cases of severe GvHD, marked glandular destruction and/or complete mucosal effacemnet as well as fibrotic changes is observed. These changes should also lead to consider (and exclude) radio-chemotherapy mucosal damage and CMV infection. To avoid any misinterpretation, a diagnosis of GvHD should (usually) not be rendered within 20 days following the last cycle of pre-transplant chemotherapeutic induction. Furthermore, an important mimicker every pathologist has to be aware of in GvHD is a severe apoptotic frequency caused by PPI therapy (Figure 4.16b).

Colchicine and Taxol-Induced Gastritis

The most prominent finding related to colchicine and Taxol on H.E. stains is the presence of numerous mitotic figures showing an M-phase arrest (characteristic "ring" appearance). It is associated with nuclear pseudo-stratification and loss of nuclear polarity. Furthermore, severe apoptosis is commonly present in the pits or glands (commonly in the antrum).

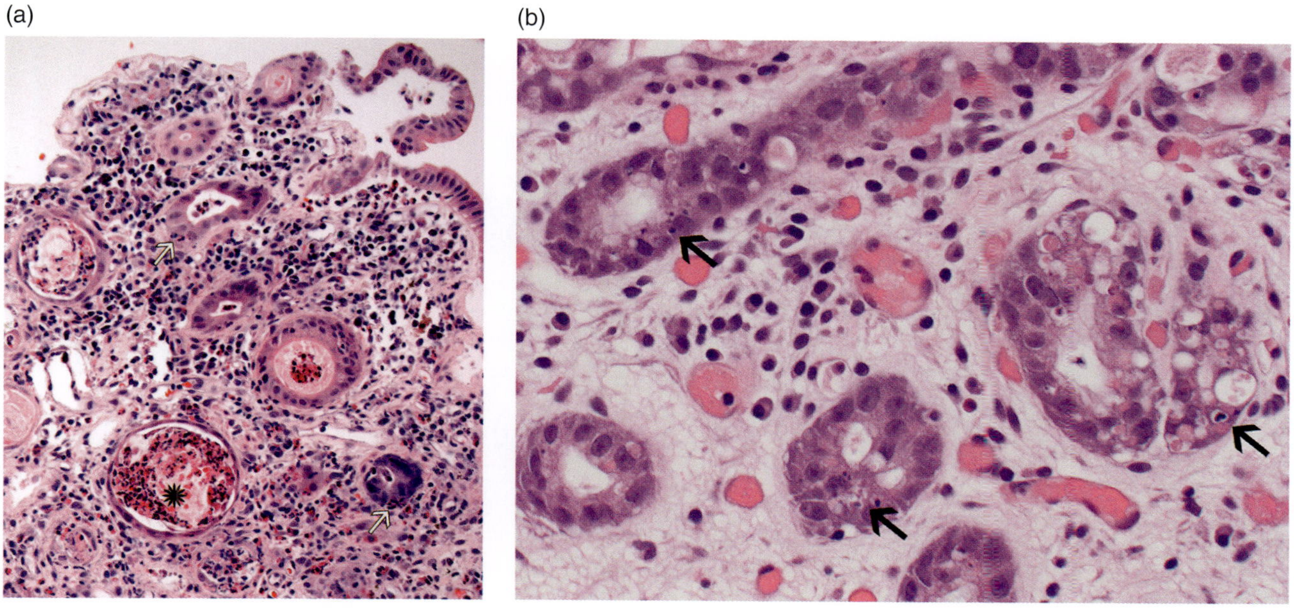

Figure 4.16 (a) GvHD. Typical changes in longstanding GvHD showing multiple apoptotic bodies (arrows) as well as crypt explosions (star). Background mucosa shows epithelial reactive changes as well as an eosinophil-rich lymphoplasmocytic infiltrate. (b) PPI apoptosis. High magnification of a body biopsy with multiple apoptotic figures (arrows) caused by longstanding proton pump inhibitor therapy.

The mitotic arrest is present within 11 days of receiving Taxol therapy and may not be present for more than two weeks after drug intake.

Chemoradiation

Several chemotherapeutic agents (e.g. mitomycin C, 5-fluoro-2-deoxyuridine, and floxuridine) have been described to elicit severe nuclear atypia with or without increased mitotic activity and apoptosis (Figure 4.17). Contrary to neoplastic atypia, nuclear atypia in the setting of chemoradiation is characteristically found at the base of glands, as well as in endothelial and stromal cells. Additionally, reactive epithelium, necrosis, and/or ulcerative changes are present. Mucosal changes caused by radiation alone are comparable and fibrinoid necrosis of the vessel walls may be detected while inflammation is commonly insignificant.

Kayexalate

Sodium polystyrene sulfonate (sorbitol) contains kayexalate and is used for treatment of hyperkalemia in the setting of renal failure. On H&E stained slides (Figure 4.18), kayexalate is characteristically present as basophilic, rhomboid, or triangular crystals with a mosaic pattern (that allows distinction from cholestyramine crystals). The crystals appear red on periodic acid–Schiff and acid-fast stains and blue when Diff-Quick stain is performed.

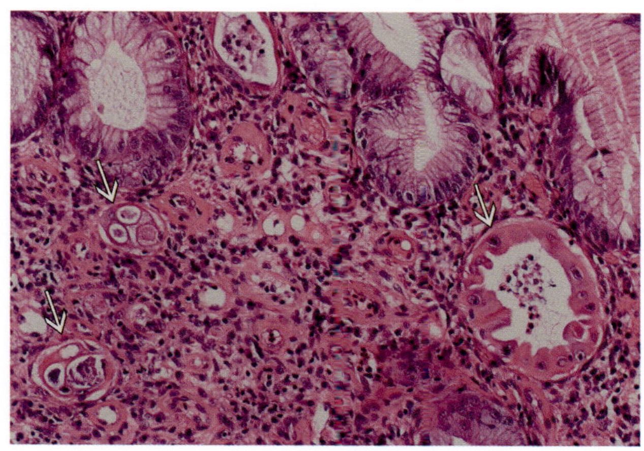

Figure 4.17 Chemoradiation. High magnification of a gastric mucosal biopsy with severe cytological changes caused by chemoradiation. Typically affected areas show severe atypia with bizarre nuclei, vacuolation, and eosinophilia of the cytoplasm as well as degenerative changes.

Prognosis, Evolution, and Clinical Management

In case of drug-associated gastritis, the offending medication should be discontinued or less corrosive medication should be chosen. In cases where these agents cannot be discontinued, PPI or other mucosal protectants such as sucralfate may be used.

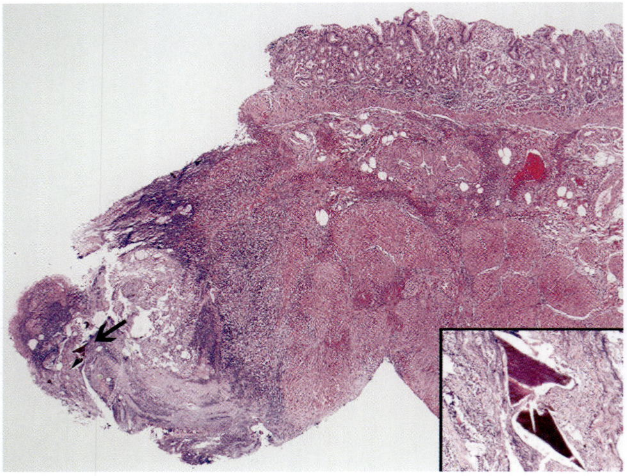

Figure 4.18 Kayaxylate. Example of a chronic gastric ulcer caused by Kayaxalate, showing the typical violet sharp deposits, leading to a perforation of the stomach in this case.

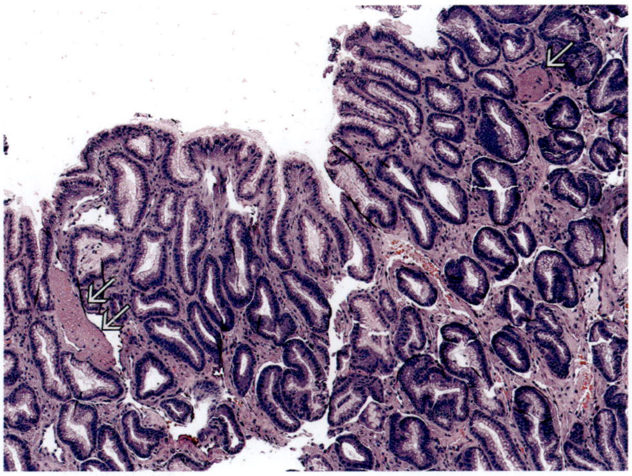

Figure 4.19 GAVE. Antral mucosa with dilation changes of the capillaries and prominent thrombi in the marked vessels (arrows).

Vascular Gastropathy

Gastral Antral Vascular Ectasia (GAVE)

The mucosa may endoscopically show the characteristic "watermelon stomach" appearance. Microscopically, GAVE is characterized by foveolar hyperplasia, dilated mucosal capillaries with or without fibrin thrombi (Figure 4.19). The presence of fibrin thrombi is characteristic of the diagnosis and CD61 can be useful to highlight platelets within the microthrombi. In addition, the lamina propria may show fibromuscular hyperplasia with or without inflammation. Reactive epithelial changes may be present. GAVE is treated effectively with endoscopic ablation. This may be accomplished by thermal therapy (argon plasma coagulation), radiofrequency ablation, or endoscopic band ligation. In some cases, the vascular ectasia may affect the cardia, which suggests that both are due to hypercontractile/mechanical causes. Cardia vascular ectasia is managed similarly to GAVE.

Portal Hypertensive Gastropathy (PHG)

The patients may clinically present with limited bleeding and anemia. Transfusion requirement is less common than for GAVE patients. In these individuals, hemodynamic alterations and increased splenic circulation cause an increased gastric mucosal blood flow associated with portal hypertension. In contrast to GAVE, portal hypertensive gastropathy commonly affects the proximal stomach. Endoscopic findings are varied, including fine pinkish speckles, mosaic pattern (snake skin appearance), cherry-red spots, and diffuse hemorrhage. Microscopically, dilated mucosal capillaries and venules with marked congestion, thickened intima, and perivascular fibrosis are present. Edematous stromal changes are common but inflammation is scant or absent. Microvascular thrombi are not seen. Deep mucosal biopsies are optimal to best detect the diagnostic features of portal hypertensive gastropathy.

Although pathophysiologically different than GAVE, there is overlap in appearance and management when PHG is isolated to the antrum or cardia. In this case, management is similar to GAVE. Most PHG is a diffuse process and not amenable to local endoscopic therapies. Treatment is aimed at reducing portal pressure with Beta blockers or transhepatic intrahepatic portosystemic shunts (TIPSs). In severe/refractory cases, liver transplant is warranted.

Hypertrophic Gastropathy

Definition, General Features, Predisposing Factors

Hyptertrophic gastropathy can be caused by different conditions, including amyloidosis, Zollinger–Ellison Syndrome, and Ménétrier's disease.

Clinical Features and Endoscopic Characteristics

Ménétrier's disease is a rare acquired disorder defined by hypoproteinemia and hypochlorhydria, as well as rugal hypertrophy. It is also known as giant hypertrophic gastritis and hypoproteinemic hypertrophic gastropathy.

Ménétrier's disease is mainly found in adults (fourth to sixth decade) but has also been described in children. Coinfection of CMV and HP has been described in 70 and 90%, respectively. Whereas children are most likely affected by CMV and adults by HP infections. In adults, it is a chronic disease with clinical presentation of loss of immunoglobulins, albumin, and transferrin. Vomiting, abdominal pain, dyspepsia, anorexia, and peripheral edema are common. Mucosal bleeding may lead to iron deficiency. Furthermore, overexpression of TGF-α was discussed to be involved in the pathogenesis of Ménétrier's disease.

Zollinger–Ellison syndrome is defined by the triad of hypergastrinemia (cause by gastrinoma), increased gastric acid, and peptic ulcer disease. It can be diagnosed in children and adults, whereas the average age of diagnosis is 50 years. Most gastrinomas (8% sporadic, 20% as part of MEN-I-syndrome) are diagnosed in duodenal specimens, but can also be present in pancreas and common bile duct. Pathophysiologically, hypergastrinemia leads to increased levels of gastric acid and pepsin causing multiple erosions and ulcer of the gastric mucosa. Common clinical presentation includes esophagitis, duodenitis and epigastric pain. Diarrhea and weight loss may also be present. Serum gastrin levels of more than 1000 pg/ml are diagnostic of Zollinger–Ellison syndrome.

On CT or MRI scans, thickened gastric folds can be seen, whereas the thickness ranges from 0.6 to 4.5 cm. Additionally, somatostatin receptor scintigraphy and endosonography are helpful in finding gastrinoma.

Amyloidosis represents diffuse deposits of insoluble fibrillary protein sheets as well as non-fibrillar components (e.g. proteoglycans serum amyloid P etc.). Amyloid is classified based on the fibril precursor protein (see Table 4.2), whereas the AL form is most commonly found in the GI-tract. The amyloidosis is most commonly diagnosed in the sixth decade of life, except the familial form. The patients can present with hemorrhage, nausea, vomiting, weight loss, malabsorption, gastric outlet obstruction, and gastroparesis sometimes associated with bacterial overgrowth. Tumor forming amyloidosis is rare. Imaging studies show thickened gastric walls.

Table 4.2 Overview of different types of amyloidosis and associated conditions.

Type	Associated conditions
AL–amyloid light chain	Plasma cell dyscrasias
AA–amyloid	Infectious, inflammatory or neoplastic disorders
Aβ2M – β2 microglobulin related	Long-term renal dialysis
ATTR—amyloid transthyretin	Hereditary systemic amyloidosis
Wild-type transthyretin deposition	Senile systemic amyloidosis

Endoscopically, the mucosa shows erosion/ulceration, thickened folds, and as already mentioned rarely a mass lesion.

Microscopic Features

Zollinger–Ellison Syndrome

High levels of gastrin cause proliferative changes of the oxyntic mucosa with hypertrophy and hyperplasia of the parietal cells reaching out to the foveolar neck region. An extension of parietal cells into the antrum can be seen. Linear or nodular hypertrophy of the enterochromaffin-like cells (ECL cells) of the oxyntic mucosa is also a characteristic feature. Subsequently, low-grade neuro-endocrine tumors (NETs) may develop. In the setting of MEN-I, up to 37% of patients with Zollinger–Ellison syndrome show NETs, while they are rarely seen in sporadic ZES.

Gastrinomas as well as ECL cells are positive for chromogranin and synaptophysin. Additionally, ECL cells may show positivity for isoform 2 of vesicular monoamine transporter (VMAT-2) whereas gastrin, somatostatin, and serotonin are negative.

Ménétrier's Disease

Biopsies of gastric mucosa affected by Ménétrier's disease show prominent elongated and tortuous foveolae lined by mucous cells. Cystic dilatation of the pits may also develop, sometimes protrude into the submucosa (i.e. gastritis cystica profunda). Absence of parietal and chief cells is also a characteristic feature. Marked eosinophilia can be detected but chronic inflammation is commonly sparse or absent. Intraepithelial lymphocytosis may be present.

Full thickness biopsies are more reliable than conventional biopsies in evaluating and establishing the diagnosis of foveolar hyperplasia.

Amyloidosis

Deposits of amyloid can be diffuse or patchy. It presents mainly in the lamina propria as a homogenous, dense, amorphous extracellular deposit (Figure 4.20a). It can be found throughout the stomach wall (mucosa, lamina propria, submucosa, muscularis) as well as in vessels and nerves. Deposits of amyloid can be highlighted by histochemical and immunohistochemical stains. The most commonly used stain is Congo red (Figure 4.20b), which reveals amyloid as deep orange deposit with apple-green birefringence in

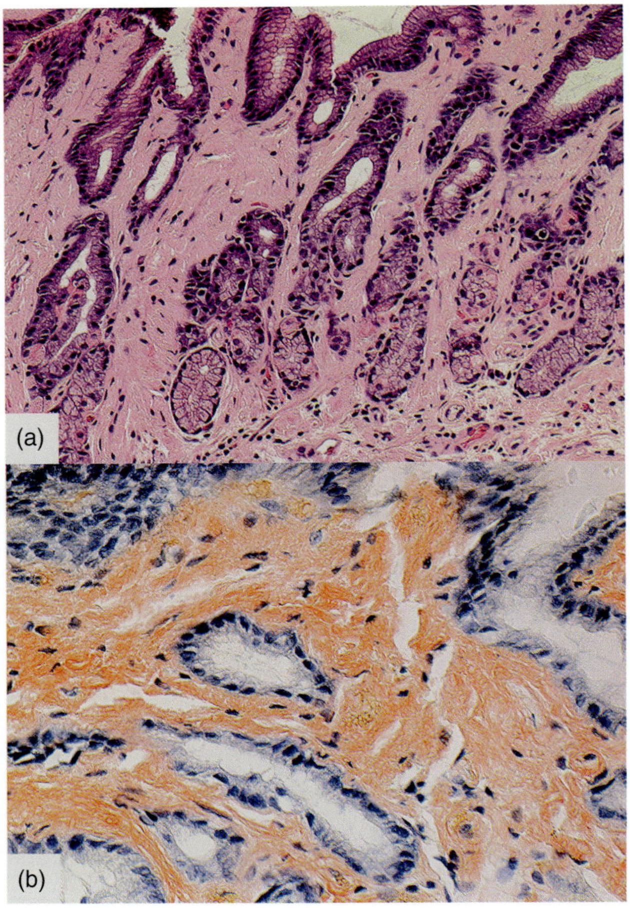

Figure 4.20 Amyloidosis. Superficial gastric mucosa showing dense homogenous eosinophilic deposits of amyloid expanding the lamina propria (a) and showing a positive Congo red stain (b).

polarized light. Immunostains may be used to subtype amyloidosis (e.g. κ- and λ-light chain, anti-AA, transthyretin [TTR], and β_2 microglobulin, anti-apo AI).

Differential Diagnosis

Enlarged gastric folds can be caused by several entities (Table 4.3) although most fail to show a severe foveolar hyperplasia as in Ménétrier's disease.

- **Hyperplastic hypersecretory gastropathy** is defined by hyperplasia of parietal and chief cells. Compared to ZES, the gastrin levels are normal. Furthermore, normal to increased acid production may be present. Protein loss is uncommon.
- **Cronkhite–Canada syndrome** is defined by diffuse gastrointestinal polyposis with morphologic overlap with hyperplastic polyps. Abnormal skin pigmentation, nail dystrophy, and colon polyposis are also commonly detected.
- **Arteriosclerosis of vessels or systemic sclerosis** (connective tissue disorder) may mimic amyloid deposits, which can be distinguished using histochemical stains like Masson's trichrome or Elastic van Gieson to highlight the collagen (while Congo red is negative).
- **Ischemic and radiation gastritis** may result with hyalinization and fibrosis of the lamina propria. The findings include mucosal erosion and architectural distortion of the gastric glands with associated ischemic features and/or radiation associated atypia of stromal and epithelial cells.

Prognosis, Evolution, and Clinical Management

Ménétrier's disease can show different courses in children and adults. In children, Ménétrier presents as a self-limited transient disease resolving within few months. On the contrary, adults show a chronic course with poor prognosis. As CMV and *H. pylori* coinfections may be present, they should be ruled out and treated. Development of neoplasia has been discussed to have a 2–15% lifetime risk.

Symptoms can improve using a wide spectrum of agents such as antibiotics, antacid therapeutics (H_2-blocker, PPI), corticosteroids, or anticholinergic agents to reduce protein loss.

Cases with complications like bleeding, obstruction, or refractory protein loss may lead to surgical intervention.

ZES patients require long-term medical therapy to control hypersecretion. Therefore PPI is the first-line therapy. In some, surgical intervention (partial or total gastrectomy) may be needed. Gastrinomas are commonly multiple,

Table 4.3 Showing several nonneoplastic and neoplastic conditions causing giant folds.

Systemic and syndromic conditions	Neoplastic conditions	Benign conditions
Ménétrier's disease	Gastric lymphoma	*H. pylori* gastritis
Zollinger–Ellison syndrome (ZES)	Diffusely infiltrative, signet ring carcinoma	CMV gastritis
Polyposis as Cronkhite–Canada syndrome	Metastasis to stomach	Granulomatous gastritis
		Eosinophilic gastritis

whereas 50% of cases reveal to be malignant. In the setting of metastatic gastrinomas, chemotherapy, hormonal therapy, or surgery may occur. The reported 10 years' survival shows a wide range between 60 and 100%. In unresectable cases, five years' survival rate reaches 40%. In ZES patients with MEN-I, lifelong antacidic therapy and family screening are indicated, whereas this group shows a better survival than the patients with sporadic ZES.

Prognosis of patients with gastric amyloidosis is influenced by several factors (e.g. extent, severity, number of involved organs). Therapy of amyloidosis includes reduction of precursor proteins, improvement of gastric motility as well as prevention of bleeding. In hereditary transthyretin-related amyloidosis, liver transplantation is curative, because mutated transthyretin is synthesized by the liver itself.

Further Reading

Abraham, S.C., Yardley, J.H., and Wu, T.T. (1999). Erosive injury to the upper gastrointestinal tract in patients receiving iron medication: an underrecognized entity. *Am. J. Surg. Pathol.* 23: 1241–1247.

Abraham, S.C., Bhagavan, B.S., Lee, L.A. et al. (2001). Upper gastrointestinal tract injury in patients receiving kayexalate (sodium polystyrene sulfonate) in sorbitol: clinical, endoscopic, and histopathologic findings. *Am. J. Surg. Pathol.* 25: 637–644.

Ajibe, H., Osawa, H., Yoshizawa, M. et al. (2008). Phlegmonous gastritis after endoscopic submucosal dissection for early gastric cancer. *Ther. Adv. Gastroenterol.* 1: 91–95.

Akbayir, N., Alkim, C., Erdem, L. et al. (2002). A case report of doxycycline induced esophageal and gastric ulcer. *Turk. J. Gastroenterol.* 13: 232–235.

Alcántara, M., Rodriguez, R., Potenciano, J.L. et al. (1993). Endoscopic and bioptic findings in the upper gastrointestinal tract in patients with Crohn's disease. *Endoscopy* 25: 282–286.

Allan, K., Barriga, J., Afshani, M. et al. (2005). Emphysematous gastritis. *Am. J. Med. Sci.* 329: 205–207.

American Thoracic Society (1999). Statement on sarcoidosis. Joint Statement of the American Thoracic Society (ATS). *Am. J. Respir. Crit. Care Med.* 160: 736–755.

Amieva, M.R. and El-Omar, E.M. (2008). Host-bacterial interactions in *Helicobacter pylori* infection. *Gastroenterology* 134 (1): 306–323. https://doi.org/10.1053/j.gastro.2007.11.009.

Anagnostopoulos, I. and Hummel, M. (1996). Epstein–Barr virus in tumours. *Histopathology* 29: 297–315.

Anderson, R.D., Patel, R., Kent Hamilton, J., and Richard Boland, C. (2006). Cronkhite–Canada syndrome presenting as eosinophilic gastroenteritis. *Proc. (Baylor Univ. Med. Cent.)* 19 (3): 209–212.

Annibale, B., Azzoni, C., Corleto, V.D. et al. (2001). Atrophic body gastritis patients with enterochromaffin-like cell dysplasia are at increased risk for the development of type I gastric carcinoid. *Eur. J. Gastroenterol. Hepatol.* 13: 1449–1456.

Arnason, T., Brown, I.S., Goldsmith, J.D. et al. (2015). Collagenous gastritis: a morphologic and immunohistochemical study of 40 patients. *Mod. Pathol.* 28: 533–544.

Barreiros, A.P., Galle, P.R., and Otto, G. (2013). Familial amyloid polyneuropathy. *Dig. Dis.* 31 (1): 170–174.

Barreiros, A.P., Otto, G., Kahlen, B. et al. (2015). Familial amyloidosis: great progress for an orphan disease. *J. Hepatol.* 62 (2): 483–485.

Bayerdörffer, E., Ritter, M.M., Hatz, R. et al. (1994). Healing of protein losing hypertrophic gastropathy by eradication of *Helicobacter pylori* – is *Helicobacter pylori* a pathogenic factor in Ménétrier's disease? *Gut* 35: 701–704.

Bellan, L., Semelka, R., and Warren, C.P. (1988). Sarcoidosis as a cause of linitis plastica. *Can. Assoc. Radiol. J.* 39: 72–74.

Berna, M.J., Annibale, B., Marignani, M. et al. (2008). A prospective study of gastric carcinoids and enterochromaffin-like cell changes in multiple endocrine neoplasia type 1 and Zollinger–Ellison syndrome: identification of risk factors. *J. Clin. Endocrinol. Metab.* 93 (5): 1582–1591.

Berthrong, M. and Fajardo, L.F. (1981). Radiation injury in surgical pathology. Part II. Alimentary tract. *Am. J. Surg. Pathol.* 5: 153–178.

Bettington, M. et al. (2014). The challenging diagnosis of Cronkhite–Canada syndrome in the upper gastrointestinal tract: a series of 7 cases with clinical follow-up. *Am. J. Surg. Pathol.* 38 (2): 215–223.

Bhansali, S.K. (1977). Abdominal tuberculosis. Experiences with 300 cases. *Am. J. Gastroenterol.* 67: 324–337.

Billiémaz, K., Robles-Medranda, C., Le Gall, C. et al. (2009). A first report of collagenous gastritis, sprue, and colitis in a 9-month-old infant: 14 years of clinical, endoscopic, and histologic follow-up. *Endoscopy* 41: E233–E234.

Blonski, W.C., Katzka, D.A., Lichtenstein, G.R., and Metz, D.C. (2005). Idiopathic gastric acid hypersecretion presenting as a diarrheal disorder and mimicking both Zollinger–Ellison syndrome and Crohn's disease. *Eur. J. Gastroenterol. Hepatol.* 17 (4): 441–444.

Bordi, C., D'Adda, T., Azzoni, C. et al. (1995). Hypergastrinemia and gastric enterochromaffin-like cells. *Am. J. Surg. Pathol.* 19 (Suppl 1): S8–S19.

Brain, O., Rajaguru, C., Warren, B. et al. (2009). Collagenous gastritis: reports and systematic review. *Eur. J. Gastroenterol. Hepatol.* 21: 1419–1424.

Caldwell, J.M., Collins, M.H., Stucke, E.M. et al. (2014). Histologic eosinophilic gastritis is a systemic disorder associated with blood and extragastric eosinophilia, TH2 immunity, and a unique gastric transcriptome. *J. Allergy Clin. Immunol.* 134: 1114–1124.

Campbell, D.A., Piercey, J.R., Shnitka, T.K. et al. (1977). Cytomegalovirus-associated gastric ulcer. *Gastroenterology* 72: 533–535.

Canan, O., Ozçay, F., and Bilezikçi, B. (2008). Ménétrier's disease and severe gastric ulcers associated with cytomegalovirus infection in an immunocompetent child: a case report. *Turk. J. Pediatr.* 50: 291–295.

Cary, E.R., Tremaine, W.J., Banks, P.M., and Nagorney, D.M. (1989). Isolated Crohn's disease of the stomach. *Mayo Clin. Proc.* 64: 776–779.

Chalasani, N., Wilcox, C.M., Hunter, H.T., and Schwartz, D.A. (1997). Endoscopic features of gastroduodenal cryptococcosis in AIDS. *Gastrointest. Endosc.* 45: 315–317.

Chamberlain, C.E. (1993). Acute hemorrhagic gastritis. *Gastroenterol. Clin. N. Am.* 22: 843–873.

Chang, K.W., Lin, S.J., Hsueh, C., and Kong, M.S. (2000). Menetrier's disease associated with cytomegalovirus infection in a child. *Acta Paediatr. Taiwan.* 41: 339–340.

Chao, C.J. et al. (2013). Endoscopic features of radiation gastritis after irradiation of hepatocellular carcinoma. *Endoscopy* 45 (Suppl 2): E280–E281.

Chazan, B.I. and Aitchison, J.D. (1960). Gastric tuberculosis. *Br. Med. J.* 2: 1288–1290.

Chen, C.Y., Chi, K.H., George, R.W. et al. (2006). Diagnosis of gastric syphilis by direct immunofluorescence staining and real-time PCR testing. *J. Clin. Microbiol.* 44: 3452–3456.

Chen, Z.M., Shah, R., Zuckerman, G.R., and Wang, H.L. (2007). Epstein–Barr virus gastritis: an underrecognized form of severe gastritis simulating gastric lymphoma. *Am. J. Surg. Pathol.* 31: 1446–1451.

Choi, H.Y. and Takeda, M. (1985). Gastric epithelial atypia following hepatic arterial infusion chemotherapy. *Diagn. Cytopathol.* 1: 241–244.

Chuang, J.Y., Brown, I., Conway, L., and Singh, M. (2016). Doxycycline induced gastritis and oesophageal ulcer. *Pathology* 48: S121.

Cianferoni, A. and Spergel, J.M. (2015). Eosinophilic esophagitis and gastroenteritis. *Curr Allergy Asthma Rep* 15: 58.

Coati, I., Fassan, M., Farinati, F. et al. (2015). Autoimmune gastritis: pathologist's viewpoint. *World J. Gastroenterol.* 21: 12179–12189.

Cockburn, A.N., Morgan, C.J., and Genta, R.M. (2013). Neuroendocrine proliferations of the stomach: a pragmatic approach for the perplexed pathologist. *Adv. Anat. Pathol.* 20: 148–157.

Coffey, R.J. Jr. and Tanksley, J. (2012). Pierre Menetrier and his disease. *Trans. Am. Clin. Climatol. Assoc.* 123: 126–133. discussion 133-124.

Collins, M.H. (2009). Histopathology associated with eosinophilic gastrointestinal diseases. *Immunol. Allergy Clin. N. Am.* 29: 109–117.

Côté, J.F., Hankard, G.F., Faure, C. et al. (1998). Collagenous gastritis revealed by severe anemia in a child. *Hum. Pathol.* 29: 883–886.

Cox, G.J., Matsui, S.M., Lo, R.S. et al. (1994). Etiology and outcome of diarrhea after marrow transplantation: a prospective study. *Gastroenterology* 107: 1398–1407.

Cui, I., Chen, Z., Panarelli, N., and Yantiss, R.K. (2016). Patterns of lymphocytic gastritis may reflect the underlying etiology. *Mod. Pathol.* 29: 109–117.

Curvêlo, L.A., Brabosa, W., Rhor, R. et al. (2009). Underlying mechanism of portal hypertensive gastropathy in cirrhosis: a hemodynamic and morphological approach. *J. Gastroenterol. Hepatol.* 24 (9): 1541–1546.

Danzi, J.T., Farmer, R.G., Sullivan, B.H.J., and Rankin, G.B. (1976). Endoscopic features of gastroduodenal Crohn's disease. *Gastroenterology* 70: 9–13.

DeLuca, R.F., Morton, R., Kafka, E.C., and Raskin, J.B. (1975). Early luetic gastritis presenting as an antral mass. *Gastrointest. Endosc.* 22: 95.

Dixon, M.F., O'Connor, H.J., Axon, A.T. et al. (1986). Reflux gastritis: distinct histopathological entity? *J. Clin. Pathol.* 39: 524–530.

Doria, M.I.J., Doria, L.K., Faintuch, J., and Levin, B. (1994). Gastric mucosal injury after hepatic arterial infusion chemotherapy with floxuridine. A clinical and pathologic study. *Cancer* 73: 2042–2047.

Ectors, N.L., Dixon, M.F., Geboes, K.J. et al. (1993). Granulomatous gastritis: a morphological and diagnostic approach. *Histopathology* 23: 55–61.

Eisenstat, D.D., Griffiths, A.M., Cutz, E. et al. (1995). Acute cytomegalovirus infection in a child with Ménétrier's disease. *Gastroenterology* 109: 592–595.

Ellison, E.C. and Johnson, J.A. (2009). The Zollinger–Ellison syndrome: a comprehensive review of historical, scientific, and clinical considerations. *Curr. Probl. Surg.* 46 (1): 13–106.

Elta, G., Turnage, R., Eckhauser, F.E. et al. (1986). A submucosal antral mass caused by cytomegalovirus infection in a patient with acquired immunodeficiency syndrome. *Am. J. Gastroenterol.* 81: 714–717.

Elwir, S. et al. (2016). Ischemic gastritis: a multicenter case series of a rare clinical entity and a review of the literature. *J. Clin. Gastroenterol.* 50 (9): 722–726.

Epstein, R.J., McDonald, G.B., Sale, G.E. et al. (1980). The diagnostic accuracy of the rectal biopsy in acute graft-versus-host disease: a prospective study of thirteen patients. *Gastroenterology* 78: 764–771.

Farman, J., Ramirez, G., Rybak, B. et al. (1997). Gastric sarcoidosis. *Abdom. Imaging* 22: 248–252.

Ferreira, R.M., Machado, J.C., and Figueiredo, C. (2014). Clinical relevance of *Helicobacter pylori* vacA and cagA genotypes in gastric carcinoma. *Best Pract. Res. Clin. Gastroenterol.* 28 (6): 1003–1015. https://doi.org/10.1016/j.bpg.2014.09.004.

Fireman, Z., Sternberg, A., Yarchovsky, Y. et al. (1997). Multiple antral ulcers in gastric sarcoid. *J. Clin. Gastroenterol.* 24: 97–99.

Fong, T.L., Dooley, C.P., Dehesa, M. et al. (1991). *Helicobacter pylori* infection in pernicious anemia: a prospective controlled study. *Gastroenterology* 100: 328–332.

Franzin, G., Manfrini, C., Musola, R. et al. (1984). Chronic erosions of the stomach – a clinical, endoscopic and histological evaluation. *Endoscopy* 16: 1–5.

Freudenthaler, S., Hegenbart, U., Schönland, S. et al. (2016). Amyloid in biopsies of the gastrointestinal tract-a retrospective observational study on 542 patients. *Virchows Arch.* 468 (5): 569–577.

Fung, W.P., Foo, K.T., and Lee, Y.S. (1975). Gastric sarcoidosis presenting with haematemesis. *Med. J. Aust.* 2: 47–49.

García Díaz, E., Castro Fernández, M., Romero Gómez, M., and Castilla Higuero, L. (2001). Upper gastrointestinal tract injury caused by ingestion of caustic substances. *Gastroenterol. Hepatol.* 24: 191–195.

Gleeson, F.C. et al. (2008). Endoscopic ultrasound and endoscopic mucosal resection features of a non-protein losing form of Menetrier's disease. *Clin. Gastroenterol. Hepatol.* 6 (5): e24–e25.

Glickman, J. and Antonioli, D. (2001). Gastritis. *Gastrointest. Endosc. Clin. N. Am.* 11: 717–740.

Goldenring, J.R., Nam, K.T., Wang, T.C. et al. (2010). Spasmolytic polypeptide-expressing metaplasia and intestinal metaplasia: time for reevaluation of metaplasias and the origins of gastric cancer. *Gastroenterology* 138: 2207–2210.

Goldman, H. and Proujansky, R. (1986). Allergic proctitis and gastroenteritis in children. Clinical and mucosal biopsy features in 53 cases. *Am. J. Surg. Pathol.* 10: 75–86.

Gómez, B., Tabar, A.I., Tuñón, T. et al. (1998). Eosinophilic gastroenteritis and Anisakis. *Allergy* 53: 1148–1154.

Goto, K. and Ogawa, K. (2016). Lanthanum deposition is frequently observed in the gastric mucosa of dialysis patients with lanthanum carbonate therapy: a clinicopathologic study of 13 cases, including 1 case of lanthanum granuloma in the colon and 2 nongranulomatous gastric cases. *Int. J. Surg. Pathol.* 24: 89–92.

Greenson, J.K., Trinidad, S.B., Pfeil, S.A. et al. (1993). Gastric mucosal calcinosis. Calcified aluminum phosphate deposits secondary to aluminum-containing antacids or sucralfate therapy in organ transplant patients. *Am. J. Surg. Pathol.* 17: 45–50.

Greenstein, D.B., Wilcox, C.M., and Schwartz, D.A. (1994). Gastric syphilis. Report of seven cases and review of the literature. *J. Clin. Gastroenterol.* 18: 4–9.

Groisman, G.M., Rosh, J.R., and Harpaz, N. (1994). Langerhans cell histiocytosis of the stomach. A cause of granulomatous gastritis and gastric polyposis. *Arch. Pathol. Lab. Med.* 118: 1232–1235.

Groisman, G.M., Meyers, S., and Harpaz, N. (1996). Collagenous gastritis associated with lymphocytic colitis. *J. Clin. Gastroenterol.* 22: 134–137.

Guarner, J. (2004). The spectrum of gastric disease associated with *Helicobacter pylori* and other infectious gastritides. *Curr. Gastroenterol. Rep.* 6: 441–446.

Gutierrez, O., Cantalapiedra, A., Tabuyo, M.I. et al. (2003). Emphysematous gastritis and severe aplastic anemia. *Hematol. J.* 4: 82–84.

Haber, M.M. and Lopez, I. (1999). Gastric histologic findings in patients with nonsteroidal anti-inflammatory drug-associated gastric ulcer. *Mod. Pathol.* 12: 592–598.

Hage, E. et al. (2003). Histopathology of the gastric oxyntic mucosa in two different patient groups during long-term treatment with omeprazole. *Eur. J. Gastroenterol. Hepatol.* 15 (7): 781–789.

Haig, A. and Driman, D.K. (2006). Iron induced mucosal injury to the upper gastrointestinal tract. *Histopathology* 48: 808–812.

Han, S., Chaudhary, N., and Wassef, W. (2015). Portal hypertensive gastropathy and gastric antral vascular ectasia. *Curr. Opin. Gastroenterol.* 31 (6): 506–512.

Haot, J., Hamichi, L., Wallez, L., and Mainguet, P. (1988). Lymphocytic gastritis: a newly described entity: a retrospective endoscopic and histological study. *Gut* 29: 1258–1264.

Haot, J., Jouret, A., Willette, M. et al. (1990). Lymphocytic gastritis – prospective study of its relationship with varioliform gastritis. *Gut* 31: 282–285.

Haot, J., Bogomoletz, W.V., Jouret, A., and Mainguet, P. (1991). Ménétrier's disease with lymphocytic gastritis: an unusual association with possible pathogenic implications. *Hum. Pathol.* 22: 379–386.

Heilmann, K.L. and Borchard, F. (1991). Gastritis due to spiral shaped bacteria other than *Helicobacter pylori*: clinical, histological, and ultrastructural findings. *Gut* 32 (2): 137–140.

Hinnant, K.L., Rotterdam, H.Z., Bell, E.T., and Tapper, M.L. (1986). Cytomegalovirus infection of the alimentary tract: a clinicopathological correlation. *Am. J. Gastroenterol.* 81: 944–950.

Hisamatsu, A., Nagai, T., Okawara, H. et al. (2010). Gastritis associated with Epstein–Barr virus infection. *Intern. Med.* 49: 2101–2105.

Ho, V. et al. (2008). Hyperpigmentation, nail dystrophy and alopecia with generalised intestinal polyposis: Cronkhite–Canada syndrome. *Australas. J. Dermatol.* 49 (4): 223–225.

Hosoe, N., Imaeda, H., Okamoto, S. et al. (2011). A case of beef tapeworm (Taenia saginata) infection observed by using video capsule endoscopy and radiography (with videos). *Gastrointest. Endosc.* 74: 690–691.

Howell, J. and Brown, G. (2008). Education and imaging. Gastrointestinal: beef tapeworm (Taenia saginata). *J. Gastroenterol. Hepatol.* 23: 1769.

Hruban, R.H., Yardley, J.H., Donehower, R.C., and Boitnott, J.K. (1989). Taxol toxicity. Epithelial necrosis in the gastrointestinal tract associated with polymerized microtubule accumulation and mitotic arrest. *Cancer* 63: 1944–1950.

Hsing, A.W., Hansson, L.E., McLaughlin, J.K. et al. (1993). Pernicious anemia and subsequent cancer. A population-based cohort study. *Cancer* 71: 745–750.

Huang, C.T. and Liao, W.Y. (2009). Emphysematous gastritis: a deadly infectious disease. *Scand. J. Infect. Dis.* 41: 317–319.

Huh, W.J., Coffej, R.J., and Washington, M.K. (2016). Menetrier's disease: its mimickers and pathogenesis. *J. Pathol. Transl. Med.* 50 (1): 10–16.

Hungermann, D., Müller, S., Spieker, T. et al. (2001). Low prevalence of latently Epstein–Barr virus-infected cells in chronic gastritis. *Microsc. Res. Tech.* 53: 409–413.

Iacobuzio-Donahue, C.A., Lee, E.L., Abraham, S.C. et al. (2001). Colchicine toxicity: distinct morphologic findings in gastrointestinal biopsies. *Am. J. Surg. Pathol.* 25: 1067–1073.

Ito, T. et al. (2013). Zollinger–Ellison syndrome: recent advances and controversies. *Curr. Opin. Gastroenterol.* 29 (6): 650–661.

Jehangir, A., Rettew, A., Shaikh, B. et al. (2015). A case report of emphysematous gastritis in a diabetic patient: favorable outcome with conservative measures. *J. Community Hosp. Intern. Med. Perspect.* 5: 28010.

Jimenez-Rivera, C., Ngan, B., Jackson, R., and Ahmed, N. (2005). Gastric pseudopolyps in eosinophilic gastroenteritis. *J. Pediatr. Gastroenterol. Nutr.* 40: 83–86.

Johnstone, J.M. and Morson, B.C. (1978). Eosinophilic gastroenteritis. *Histopathology* 2: 335–348.

Jun, D.W., Kim, D.H., Kim, S.H. et al. (2007). Ménétrier's disease associated with herpes infection: response to treatment with acyclovir. *Gastrointest. Endosc.* 65: 1092–1095.

Kagawa, M., Fujino, Y., Muguruma, N. et al. (2016). Localized amyloidosis of the stomach mimicking a superficial gastric cancer. *Clin. J. Gastroenterol.* 9 (3): 109–113.

Kajino, Y., Kushima, R., Koyama, S. et al. (2003). Collagenous gastritis in a young Japanese woman. *Pathol. Int.* 53: 174–178.

Kakizoe, S., Kakizoe, H., Kakizoe, K. et al. (1995). Endoscopic findings and clinical manifestation of gastric anisakiasis. *Am. J. Gastroenterol.* 90: 761–763.

Kamimura, K., Kobayashi, M., Narisawa, R. et al. (2007). Collagenous gastritis: endoscopic and pathologic evaluation of the nodularity of gastric mucosa. *Dig. Dis. Sci.* 52: 995–1000.

Kamimura, K., Kobayashi, M., Sato, Y. et al. (2015). Collagenous gastritis: review. *World J. Gastrointest. Endosc.* 7: 265–273.

Kaneki, T., Koizumi, T., Yamamoto, H. et al. (2001). Gastric sarcoidosis – a single appearance in the involvement. *Hepato-Gastroenterology* 48: 1209–1210.

Khilnani, M.T. and Keller, R.J. (1971). Roentgen and pathological changes in the gastrointestinal tract in herpes zoster generalizata: a unique case and brief review. *Mt Sinai J. Med.* 38: 303–310.

Kim, G.Y., Ward, J., Henessey, B. et al. (2005). Phlegmonous gastritis: case report and review. *Gastrointest. Endosc.* 61: 168–174.

Kim, K.H., Kim, C.G., Kim, Y.W. et al. (2016). Phlegmonous gastritis with early gastric cancer. *J. Gastric Cancer* 16: 195–199.

Krasinskas, A.M., Abraham, S.C., Metz, D.C., and Furth, E.E. (2003). Oxyntic mucosa pseudopolyps: a presentation of atrophic autoimmune gastritis. *Am. J. Surg. Pathol.* 27: 236–241.

Lagorce-Pages, C., Fabiani, B., Bouvier, R. et al. (2001). Collagenous gastritis: a report of six cases. *Am. J. Surg. Pathol.* 25: 1174–1179.

Laine, L. (1996). Nonsteroidal anti-inflammatory drug gastropathy. *Gastrointest. Endosc. Clin. N. Am.* 6: 489–504.

Lauwers, G.Y., Furman, J., Michael, L.E. et al. (2001). Cytoskeletal and kinetic epithelial differences between NSAID gastropathy and *Helicobacter pylori* gastritis: an immunohistochemical determination. *Histopathology* 39: 133–140.

Lauwers, G.Y., Fujita, H., Nagata, K., and Shimizu, M. (2010). Pathology of non-*Helicobacter pylori* gastritis: extending the histopathologic horizons. *J. Gastroenterol.* 45: 131–145.

Lavery, E.A. and Coyle, W.J. (2008). Herpes simplex virus and the alimentary tract. *Curr. Gastroenterol. Rep.* 10: 417–423.

Leber, A. and Stal, J. (2012). Simultaneous esophageal and gastric ulceration due to doxycycline ingestion: case report and review of the literature. *Gastroenterol. Res.* 5: 236–238.

Lee, B.S., Kim, S.M., Seong, J.K. et al. (2005). Phlegmonous gastritis after endoscopic mucosal resection. *Endoscopy* 37: 490–493.

Liu, H., Ruskon-Fourmestraux, A., Lavergne-Slove, A. et al. (2001). Resistance of t(11;18) positive gastric mucosa-associated lymphoid tissue lymphoma to *Helicobacter pylori* eradication therapy. *Lancet* 357: 39–40.

Liu, Y., Patel, A.A., Shaw, J.C. et al. (2013). Gastroduodenal cryptococcus in an AIDS patient presenting with melena. *Gastroenterol. Res.* 6: 26–28.

Ma, C., Park, J.Y., Montgomery, E.A. et al. (2015). A comparative clinicopathologic study of collagenous gastritis in children and adults: the same disorder with associated immune-mediated diseases. *Am. J. Surg. Pathol.* 39: 802–812.

Makino, M., Kawaguchi, K., Shimojo, H. et al. (2015). Extensive lanthanum deposition in the gastric mucosa: the first histopathological report. *Pathol. Int.* 65: 33–37.

Malfertheiner, P., Venerito, M., and Schulz, C. (2018). *Helicobacter pylori* infection: new facts in clinical management. *Curr. Treat Options Gastroenterol.* 16 (4): 605–615. https://doi.org/10.1007/s11938-018-0209-8.

Mansoor, A., Pittaluga, S., Beck, P.L. et al. (2011). NK-cell enteropathy: a benign NK-cell lymphoproliferative disease mimicking intestinal lymphoma: clinicopathologic features and follow-up in a unique case series. *Blood* 117: 1447–1452.

Marginean, E.C., Bennick, M., Cyczk, J. et al. (2006). Gastric siderosis: patterns and significance. *Am. J. Surg. Pathol.* 30: 514–520.

Marshall, J.B. (1993). Tuberculosis of the gastrointestinal tract and peritoneum. *Am. J. Gastroenterol.* 88: 989–999.

Matsukuma, K., Gui, D., Olson, K.A. et al. (2016). OsmoPrep-associated gastritis: a histopathologic mimic of iron pill gastritis and mucosal Calcinosis. *Am. J. Surg. Pathol.* 40: 1550–1556.

Matsunaga, M., Fujii, T., Ushijima, T., and Miwa, K. (2015). Emphysematous gastritis in a patient with breast cancer. *Intern. Med.* 54: 1667–1668.

Mercky, P., Gonzalez, J.M., and Ah-Soune, P. (2014). An unusual gastric encounter: a beef tapeworm diagnosed by gastroscopy. *Endoscopy* 46: E36–E37.

Mino-Kenudson, M., Tomita, S., and Lauwers, G.Y. (2007). Mucin expression in reactive gastropathy: an immunohistochemical analysis. *Arch. Pathol. Lab. Med.* 131: 86–90.

Mitchell, R.M. and Bradlow, S.P. (1964). Acute erosive gastritis due to early syphilis. *Ann. Intern. Med.* 61: 933–938.

Moosvi, A.R., Saravolatz, L.D., Wong, D.H., and Simms, S.M. (1990). Emphysematous gastritis: case report and review. *Rev. Infect. Dis.* 12: 848–855.

Moustafellos, P., Hadjianastasiou, V., and Gray, D. (2006). Postural epigastric pain as a sign of CMV gastritis: a case report. *Transplant. Proc.* 38: 1357–1358.

Muraoka, A., Suehiro, I., Fujii, M. et al. (1996). Acute gastric anisakiasis: 28 cases during the last 10 years. *Dig. Dis. Sci.* 41: 2362–2365.

Novak, J.M., Collins, J.T., Donowitz, M. et al. (1979). Effects of radiation on the human gastrointestinal tract. *J. Clin. Gastroenterol.* 1: 9–39.

Oberhuber, G., Püspök, A., Oesterreicher, C. et al. (1997). Focally enhanced gastritis: a frequent type of gastritis in patients with Crohn's disease. *Gastroenterology* 112: 698–706.

Oi, R.H. (1978). The microscopic appearance of a sodium-potassium exchange resin in histologic sections. *Am. J. Clin. Pathol.* 69: 359–361.

Ona, F.V. (1981). Gastric sarcoid: unusual cause of upper gastrointestinal hemorrhage. *Am. J. Gastroenterol.* 75: 286–288.

O'Toole, P.A. and Morris, J.A. (1988). Acute phlegmonous gastritis. *Postgrad. Med. J.* 64: 315–316.

O'Toole, D., Delle Fave, G., and Jensen, R.T. (2012). Gastric and duodenal neuroendocrine tumours. *Best Pract. Res. Clin. Gastroenterol.* 26 (6): 719–735.

Owen, D.A. (2003). Gastritis and carditis. *Mod. Pathol.* 16: 325–341.

Owens, S.R., Walls, A., Krasinskas, A.M., and Rund, C.R. (2011). Epstein–Barr virus gastritis: rare or rarely sampled? A case report. *Int. J. Surg. Pathol.* 19: 196–198.

Palmer, E.D. (1950). Tuberculosis of the stomach and the stomach in tuberculosis; a review with particular reference to gross pathology and gastroscopic diagnosis. *Am. Rev. Tuberc.* 61: 116–130.

Papadopoulos, A.A., Tzathas, C., Polymeros, D., and Ladas, S.D. (2005). Symptomatic eosinophilic gastritis cured with *Helicobacter pylori* eradication. *Gut* 54: 1822.

Parfitt, J.R. and Driman, D.K. (2007). Pathological effects of drugs on the gastrointestinal tract: a review. *Hum. Pathol.* 38: 527–536.

Parrado, R.H., Lemus, H.N., Coral-Alvarado, P.X., and Quintana, L.G. (2015). Gastric antral vascular ectasia in systemic sclerosis: current concepts. *Int. J. Rheumatol.* 2015: 762546.

Paul, M., John, S., Menon, M.C. et al. (2010). Successful medical management of emphysematous gastritis with concomitant portal venous air: a case report. *J. Med. Case Rep.* 19: 140.

Petras, R.E., Hart, W.R., and Bukowski, R.M. (1985). Gastric epithelial atypia associated with hepatic arterial infusion chemotherapy. Its distinction from early gastric carcinoma. *Cancer* 56: 745–750.

Poley, J.W., Steyerberg, E.W., Kuipers, E.J. et al. (2004). Ingestion of acid and alkaline agents: outcome and prognostic value of early upper endoscopy. *Gastrointest. Endosc.* 60: 372–377.

Polydorides, A.D. (2014). Pathology and differential diagnosis of chronic, noninfectious gastritis. *Semin. Diagn. Pathol.* 31: 114–123.

Pulimood, A.B., Ramakrishna, B.S., Kurian, G. et al. (1999). Endoscopic mucosal biopsies are useful in distinguishing granulomatous colitis due to Crohn's disease from tuberculosis. *Gut* 45: 537–541.

Pulimood, A.B., Amarapurkar, D.N., Ghoshal, U. et al. (2011). Differentiation of Crohn's disease from intestinal tuberculosis in India in 2010. *World J. Gastroenterol.* 17: 433–443.

Quinn, C.M., Bjarnason, I., and Price, A.B. (1993). Gastritis in patients on non-steroidal anti-inflammatory drugs. *Histopathology* 23: 341–348.

Rada-Palomino, A., Muñoz-Duyos, A., Pérez-Romero, N. et al. (2014). Phlegmonous gastritis: a rare entity as a differential diagnostic of an acute abdomen. Description of a case and a bibliographic review. *Rev. Esp. Enferm. Dig.* 106: 418–424.

Rank, E.L., Goldenberg, S.A., Hasson, J. et al. (1992). Treponema pallidum and *Helicobacter pylori* recovered in a case of chronic active gastritis. *Am. J. Clin. Pathol.* 97: 116–120.

Rappel, S., Rindi, G., Bordi, C. et al. (1996). Carcinoid tumors of the stomach in atrophic autoimmune gastritis: classification, differential diagnosis and prognosis. *Verh. Dtsch. Ges. Pathol.* 80: 199–207.

Rashid, A. and Hamilton, S.R. (1997). Necrosis of the gastrointestinal tract in uremic patients as a result of sodium polystyrene sulfonate (Kayexalate) in sorbitol: an underrecognized condition. *Am. J. Surg. Pathol.* 21: 60–69.

Ripoll, C. and Garcia-Tsao, G. (2011). The management of portal hypertensive gastropathy and gastric antral vascular ectasia. *Dig. Liver Dis.* 43 (5): 345–351.

Rothenberg, M.E. (2004). Eosinophilic gastrointestinal disorders (EGID). *J. Allergy Clin. Immunol.* 113: 11–28.

Rothenberg, M.E., Araya, H., Longacre, T.A., and Pasricha, P.J. (2015). Lanthanum-induced gastrointestinal histiocytosis. *ACG Case Rep. J.* 2: 187–189.

Roy, J., Snover, D., Weisdorf, S. et al. (1991). Simultaneous upper and lower endoscopic biopsy in the diagnosis of intestinal graft-versus-host disease. *Transplantation* 51: 642–646.

Ruiz, A.R.J. and Borum, M.L. (2001). Cytomegalovirus hemorrhagic gastritis. *AIDS Patient Care STDs* 15: 1–5.

Rutgeerts, P., Onette, E., Vantrappen, G. et al. (1980). Crohn's disease of the stomach and duodenum: a clinical study with emphasis on the value of endoscopy and endoscopic biopsies. *Endoscopy* 12: 288–294.

Saab, S., Venkataramani, A., Behling, C.A., and Savides, T.J. (1996). Gastric mucosal calcinosis in a patient with dyspepsia. *J. Clin. Gastroenterol.* 22: 156–164.

Sandya, P., Baste Balaji, D., Umap Pradeep, S., and Shrivastava Alok, C. (2015). Isolated gastric tuberculosis masquerading as chronic peptic ulcer: a case report. *Int. J. Med. Res. Health Sci.* 4: 896–898.

Sattianayagam, P.T., Hawkins, P.N., and Gillmore, J.D. (2009). Systemic amyloidosis and the gastrointestinal tract. *Nat. Rev. Gastroenterol. Hepatol.* 6 (10): 608–617.

Schultz, M.J., van der Hulst, R.W., and Tytgat, G.N. (1996). Acute phlegmonous gastritis. *Gastrointest. Endosc.* 44: 80–83.

Settle, S.H. et al. (2005). Chronic treatment of Menetrier's disease with Erbitux: clinical efficacy and insight into pathophysiology. *Clin. Gastroenterol. Hepatol.* 3 (7): 654–659.

Sève, P., Stankovic, K., Michalet, V. et al. (2005). Carbimazole induced eosinophilic granulomatous vasculitis localized to the stomach. *J. Intern. Med.* 258: 191–195.

Shapiro, J.L., Goldblum, J.R., and Petras, R.E. (1993). A clinicopathologic study of 42 patients with granulomatous gastritis. Is there really an "idiopathic" granulomatous gastritis? *Am. J. Surg. Pathol.* 20: 462–470.

Sharif, F., McDermott, M., Dillon, M. et al. (2002). Focally enhanced gastritis in children with Crohn's disease and ulcerative colitis. *Am. J. Gastroenterol.* 97: 1415–1420.

Sherman, A. and Bini, E.J. (1999). Pill-induced gastric injury. *Am. J. Gastroenterol.* 94: 511–513.

Shin, J.K., Jung, Y.H., Bae, M.N. et al. (2013). Successful treatment of protein-losing enteropathy due to AA amyloidosiswith octreotide in a patient with rheumatoid arthritis. *Mod. Rheumatol.* 23 (2): 406–411.

Shuster, L.D., Cox, G., Bhatia, P., and Miner, P.B.J. (1989). Gastric mucosal nodules due to cytomegalovirus infection. *Dig. Dis. Sci.* 34: 103–107.

Singhal, A.V. and Sepulveda, A.R. (2005). *Helicobacter heilmannii* gastritis: a case study with review of literature. *Am. J. Surg. Pathol.* 29 (11): 1537–1539. Review.

Snover, D.C., Sibley, R.K., Freese, D.K. et al. (1984). Orthotopic liver transplantation: a pathological study of 63 serial liver biopsies from 17 patients with special reference to the diagnostic features and natural history of rejection. *Hepatology* 4: 1212–1222.

Snover, D.C., Weisdorf, S.A., Vercellotti, G.M. et al. (1985). A histopathologic study of gastric and small intestinal graft-versus-host disease following allogeneic bone marrow transplantation. *Hum. Pathol.* 16: 387–392.

Sobala, G.M., King, R.F., Axon, A.T., and Dixon, M.F. (1990). Reflux gastritis in the intact stomach. *J. Clin. Pathol.* 43: 303–306.

Sobala, G.M., O'Connor, H.J., Dewar, E.P. et al. (1993). Bile reflux and intestinal metaplasia in gastric mucosa. *J. Clin. Pathol.* 46: 235–240.

Solcia, E., Fiocca, R., Villani, L. et al. (1991). Morphology and pathogenesis of endocrine hyperplasias, precarcinoid lesions, and carcinoids arising in chronic atrophic gastritis. *Scand. J. Gastroenterol. Suppl.* 180: 146–159.

Sperling, H.V. and Reed, W.G. (1977). Herpetic gastritis. *Am. J. Dig. Dis.* 22: 1033–1034.

Srivastava, A. and Lauwers, G.Y. (2007). Pathology of non-infective gastritis. *Histopathology* 50: 15–29.

Stewart, C.A. and Sanyal, A.J. (2003). Grading portal gastropathy: validation of a gastropathy scoring system. *Am. J. Gastroenterol.* 98 (8): 1758–1765.

Stolte, M., Ritter, M., Borchard, F., and Koch-Scherrer, G. (1990). Collagenous gastroduodenitis on collagenous colitis. *Endoscopy* 22: 186–187.

Strickland, R.G. and Mackay, I.R. (1973). A reappraisal of the nature and significance of chronic atrophic gastritis. *Am. J. Dig. Dis.* 18: 426–440.

Stroehlein, K.B., Stroehlein, J.R., Kahan, B.D., and Gruber, S.A. (1999). Gastric mucosal calcinosis in renal transplant patients. *Transplant. Proc.* 31: 2124–2126.

Sugawa, C. and Lucas, C.E. (1989). Caustic injury of the upper gastrointestinal tract in adults: a clinical and endoscopic study. *Surgery* 106: 802–806.

Sugimachi, K., Inokuchi, K., Ooiwa, T. et al. (1985). Acute gastric anisakiasis. Analysis of 178 cases. *JAMA* 253: 1012–1013.

Szuchmacher, M., Bedford, T., Sukharamwala, P. et al. (2013). Is surgical intervention avoidable in cases of emphysematous gastritis? A case presentation and literature review. *Int. J. Surg. Case Rep.* 4: 456–459.

Takano, Y., Yamamura, E., Gomi, K. et al. (2015). Successful conservative treatment of emphysematous gastritis. *Intern. Med.* 54: 195–198.

Takata, K., Noujima-Harada, M., Miyata-Takata, T. et al. (2015). Clinicopathologic analysis of 6 lymphomatoid gastropathy cases: expanding the disease spectrum to CD4-CD8+ cases. *Am. J. Surg. Pathol.* 39: 1259–1266.

Takeuchi, K., Yokoyama, M., Ishizawa, S. et al. (2010). Lymphomatoid gastropathy: a distinct clinicopathologic entity of self-limited pseudomalignant NK-cell proliferation. *Blood* 116: 5631–5637.

Talley, N.J., Shorter, R.G., Phillips, S.F., and Zinsmeister, A.R. (1990). Eosinophilic gastroenteritis: a clinicopathological study of patients with disease of the mucosa, muscle layer, and subserosal tissues. *Gut* 31: 54–58.

Tanaka, M., Kimura, K., Sakai, H. et al. (1986). Long-term follow-up for minute gastroduodenal lesions in Crohn's disease. *Gastrointest. Endosc.* 32: 206–209.

Tanaka, T., Mori, Y., Morishita, Y. et al. (1991). Gastric antral vascular ectasia. *Hum. Pathol.* 22 (10): 1053–1055.

Tapan, U., Kutlugun, A.A., Arici, M., and Altun, B. (2012). Postural epigastric pain: a challenging symptom for cytomegalovirus (CMV) gastritis. *Ren. Fail.* 34: 235–236.

Tarnawski, A.S. and Ahluwalia, A. (2018). Increased susceptibility of aging gastric mucosa to injury and delayed healing: clinical implications. *World J. Gastroenterol.* 24 (42): 4721–4727. https://doi.org/10.3748/wjg.v24.i42.4721.

Tierney, L.M.J., Gooding, G., Bottles, K. et al. (1987). Phlegmonous gastritis and *Hemophilus influenzae* peritonitis in a patient with alcoholic liver disease. *Dig. Dis. Sci.* 32: 97–101.

Toh, B.H., van Driel, I.R., and Gleeson, P.A. (1997). Pernicious anemia. *N. Engl. J. Med.* 337: 1441–1448.

Torbenson, M., Abraham, S.C., Boitnott, J. et al. (2002). Autoimmune gastritis: distinct histological and immunohistochemical findings before complete loss of oxyntic glands. *Mod. Pathol.* 15: 102–109.

Uygur-Bayramiçli, O., Yavuzer, D., Dolapçioğlu, C. et al. (1998). Granulomatous gastritis due to taeniasis. *J. Clin. Gastroenterol.* 27: 351–352.

Vakiani, E., Arguelles-Grande, C., Mansukhani, M.M. et al. (2010). Collagenous sprue is not always associated with dismal outcomes: a clinicopathological study of 19 patients. *Mod. Pathol.* 23: 12–26.

Van Allan, R.J., Krebs, T.L., Henzie, G.M. et al. (1995). Emphysematous gastritis in an immunocompromised host. *Clin. Imaging* 19: 129–130.

Van Spreeuwel, J.P., Lindeman, J., Van der Wal, A. et al. (1982). Morphological and immunohistochemical findings in upper gastrointestinal biopsies of patients with Crohn's disease of the ileum and colon. *J. Clin. Pathol.* 35: 934–940.

Vanderhulst, J. (2015). Gastric sarcoidosis: rare presentation of a rare disease. *Acta Clin. Belg.* 70: 58–60.

Vannella, L., Lahner, E., and Annibale, B. (2012). Risk for gastric neoplasias in patients with chronic atrophic gastritis: a critical reappraisal. *World J. Gastroenterol.* 18: 1279–1285.

Vesoulis, Z., Lozanski, G., Ravichandran, P., and Esber, E. (2000). Collagenous gastritis: a case report, morphologic evaluation, and review. *Mod. Pathol.* 13: 591–596.

Wallace, J.L. (1997). Nonsteroidal anti-inflammatory drugs and gastroenteropathy: the second hundred years. *Gastroenterology* 112: 1000–1016.

Warshaw, A.L. (1979). Bile gastritis without prior gastric surgery: contributing role of cholecystectomy. *Am. J. Surg.* 137: 527–531.

Washington, K., Gottfried, M.R., and Wilson, M.L. (1991). Gastrointestinal cryptococcosis. *Mod. Pathol.* 4: 707–711.

Washington, K., Bentley, R.C., Green, A. et al. (1997). Gastric graft-versus-host disease: a blinded histologic study. *Am. J. Surg. Pathol.* 21: 1037–1046.

Waters, H.M., Dawson, D.W., Howarth, J.E., and Geary, C.G. (1993). High incidence of type II autoantibodies in pernicious anaemia. *J. Clin. Pathol.* 46: 45–47.

Watson, A., Bul, V., Staudacher, J. et al. (2016). The predictors of mortality and secular changes in management strategies in emphysematous gastritis. *Clin. Res. Hepatol. Gastroenterol.* 41: e1–e7.

Weisdorf, D.J., Snover, D.C., Haake, R. et al. (1990). Acute upper gastrointestinal graft-versus-host disease: clinical significance and response to immunosuppressive therapy. *Blood* 76: 624–629.

Westerhoff, M., Tretiakova, M., Hovan, L. et al. (2010). CD61, CD31, and CD34 improve diagnostic accuracy in gastric antral vascular ectasia and portal hypertensive gastropathy: an immunohistochemical and digital morphometric study. *Am. J. Surg. Pathol.* 34 (4): 494–501.

Winslow, J.L., Trainer, T.D., and Colletti, R.B. (2001). Collagenous gastritis: a long-term follow-up with the development of endocrine cell hyperplasia, intestinal metaplasia, and epithelial changes indeterminate for dysplasia. *Am. J. Clin. Pathol.* 116: 753–758.

Winters, H.A., Notar-Francesco, V., Bromberg, K. et al. (1992). Gastric syphilis: five recent cases and a review of the literature. *Ann. Intern. Med.* 116: 314–319.

Wolber, R.A., Owen, D.A., Anderson, F.H., and Freeman, H.J. (1991). Lymphocytic gastritis and giant gastric folds associated with gastrointestinal protein loss. *Mod. Pathol.* 4: 13–15.

Wolfe, M.M., Lichtenstein, D.R., and Singh, G. (1999). Gastrointestinal toxicity of nonsteroidal antiinflammatory drugs. *N. Engl. J. Med.* 340: 1888–1899.

Wolfsen, H.C., Carpenter, H.A., and Talley, N.J. (1993). Menetrier's disease: a form of hypertrophic gastropathy or gastritis? *Gastroenterology* 104: 1310–1319.

Wong, Y.Y. and Chu, W.C. (2002). Emphysematous gastritis associated with gastric infarction in a patient with adult polycystic renal disease: CT diagnosis. *AJR Am. J. Roentgenol.* 178: 1291.

Wright, C.L. and Riddell, R.H. (1998). Histology of the stomach and duodenum in Crohn's disease. *Am. J. Surg. Pathol.* 22: 383–390.

Wu, T.T. and Hamilton, S.R. (1999). Lymphocytic gastritis: association with etiology and topology. *Am. J. Surg. Pathol.* 23: 153–158.

Xin, W. and Greenson, J.K. (2004). The clinical significance of focally enhanced gastritis. *Am. J. Surg. Pathol.* 28: 1347–1351.

Yalamanchili, M. and Cady, W. (2003). Emphysematous gastritis in a hemodialysis patient. *South. Med. J.* 96: 84–88.

Ye, H., Liu, H., Attygalle, A. et al. (2003). Variable frequencies of t(11;18)(q21;q21) in MALT lymphomas of different sites: significant association with CagA strains of H pylori in gastric MALT lymphoma. *Blood* 102: 1012–1018.

Zhang, Y. and Molot, R. (2003). Severe gastritis secondary to Epstein-Barr viral infection. Unusual presentation of infectious mononucleosis and associated diffuse lymphoid hyperplasia in gastric mucosa. *Arch. Pathol. Lab. Med.* 127: 478–480.

Zhang, L., Huang, X., and Li, J. (1992). Xanthogranuloma of the stomach: a case report. *Eur. J. Surg. Oncol.* 18: 293–295.

5

Polyps of the Stomach

K. Kim[1], *Till S. Clauditz*[2], *Jun Haeng Lee*[1] *and Gregory Y. Lauwers*[3]

[1] *Samsung Medical Center, Sungkyunkwan University School of Medicine, Seoul, South Korea*
[2] *Department of Pathology, University-Medical-Center Hamburg-Eppendorf, Hamburg, Germany*
[3] *Moffitt Cancer Center, Tampa, Florida, USA*

Gastric polyps represent a heterogeneous group of lesions with an overall prevalence of 6.3% of upper endoscopies. Their epidemiology has changed over the years, in parallel with the decrease in prevalence of *Helicobacter pylori* infection and the increased use of proton pump inhibitors. Nowadays, fundic gland polyps represent 77% of gastric polyps, followed by hyperplastic polyps at 14.4%.

Most gastric polyps are asymptomatic and discovered incidentally during an upper endoscopy performed for unrelated reasons. Some characteristics may allow a diagnosis based on the endoscopic appearance; however, in many cases the histology is necessary to determine the type.

Fundic Gland Polyps (FGPs)

Definition and General Features

The prevalence of FGPs has been increasing in the last 10 years, with rates from 3.2 to 11% of patients. Today, FGPs are the most common polyps detected by endoscopists and represent as many as 50% of resected gastric polyps.

These polyps develop exclusively in an otherwise normal acid-secreting oxyntic mucosa. In most instances, FGPs are typically multiple, developing after the use of proton pump inhibitors (PPIs) in a time- and dose-dependent manner. Not surprisingly, most regress after the cessation of PPI therapy. Interestingly, there is a negative association with *H. pylori* infection and FGPs, disappearing upon infection, and recurring after eradication of the bacteria.

Sporadic lesions can also develop and are usually diagnosed in middle-aged, predominantly female, patients. FGPs can be observed in the context of familial adenomatous polyposis (FAP). In that setting, their prevalence approaches 90%. They are detected at a younger age, and in both genders.

Clinical and Endoscopic Features

Most FGPs are discovered in the context of upper endoscopy performed during exploration of gastroesophageal reflux disease or for unrelated reasons.

They appear as small (1–20 mm), rounded, sessile, translucent lesions covered by benign-looking mucosa (Figure 5.1a). As previously noted, they can be single, but tend to be multiple (Figure 5.1b). In sporadic cases, there are usually fewer than 10 polyps, compared to larger numbers (>50 polyps, Figure 5.2) in syndromic cases, where they also may become confluent. The term fundic gland polyposis has been used for such cases. "Giant" FGPs measuring as much as 5 or 8 cm have been reported as well.

Microscopic Features

FGPs are formed by cystically dilated oxyntic glands lined by compressed parietal cells, chief cells, and mucous neck epithelium (Figures 5.3 and 5.4). In patients taking PPIs, parietal cell hyperplasia presenting as a protrusion of the parietal cells into the lumen is common in the surrounding mucosa.

Dysplasia is noted in 25–46% of FAP-associated FGPs, but is uncommon in sporadic FGPs. In most cases, low grade is detected (Figure 5.5), high-grade dysplasia is rarely observed, and association with gastric adenocarcinoma is even rarer. The risk of developing dysplastic FGP appears to correlate with increased severity of concurrent duodenal polyposis, larger size, and the presence of antral gastritis.

In practice, if multiple polyps are detected, especially in young patients without prior acid suppression therapy, evaluation of FAP should be suggested. This is even more true if dysplasia is present.

In the early stage of autoimmune atrophic gastritis, hyperplastic patches of preserved oxyntic mucosa can be

Gastrointestinal Pathology: Correlative Endoscopic and Histologic Assessment, First Edition. Edited by Gregory Y. Lauwers and Michael B. Wallace.

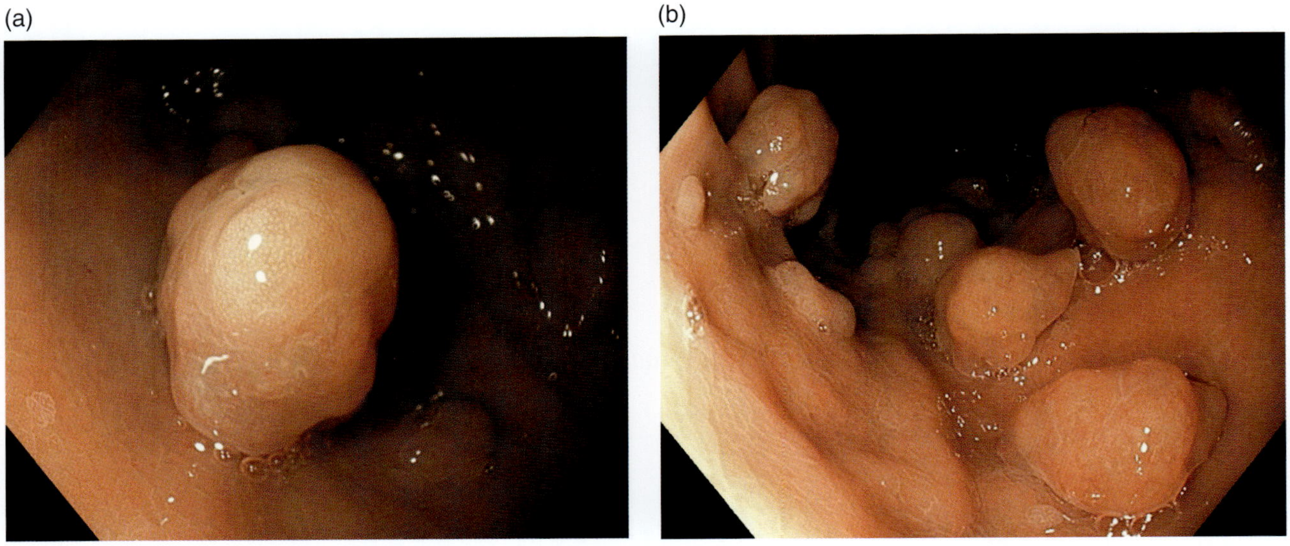

Figure 5.1 Single (a) or multiple (b) small translucent lesions covered by benign-looking mucosa.

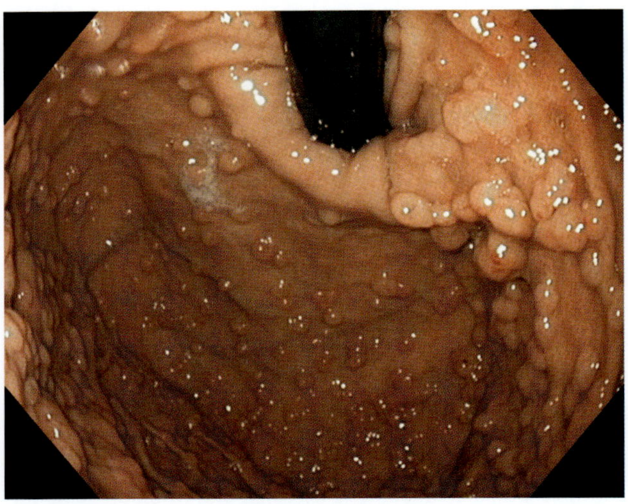

Figure 5.2 Fundic gland polyposis in familial adenomatous polyposis. There are numerous sessile polyps in the proximal stomach. Most of the polyps are less than 1 cm in diameter.

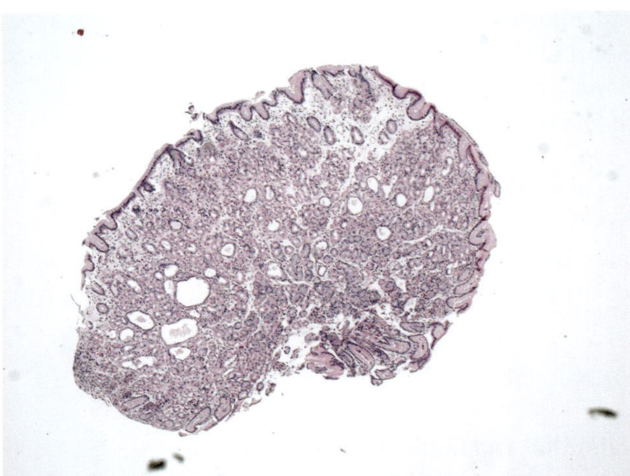

Figure 5.3 Low-power photomicrograph of fundic gland polyp with multiple cystical dilated oxyntic glands structures.

misinterpreted as fundic gland polyp. However, cystic glandular elements are absent.

Molecular analyses have suggested the neoplastic nature of FGP, with the *β-catenin/Wnt* signaling pathway implicated in both syndromic and sporadic lesions. In FAP-associated FGPs, a somatic second-hit mutation of the *APC* gene leads to inactivation of both copies of the tumor suppressor gene. This mutation is observed in up to 75% of cases, independently of the presence of dysplasia. Instead, sporadic FGPs display a somatic mutation in the *β-catenin* gene in up to–90% of cases or methylation of tumor suppressor genes in 21% of cases. Multiple polyps will present different *β-catenin* mutations, confirming their somatic nature. Interestingly, the rare cases of sporadic dysplastic FGP harbor *APC* mutations similar to those observed in syndromic cases, while being negative for *β-catenin* gene mutations. Epigenetic alterations involving methylation of CpG islands might have a role in the development of some FGPs, particularly those with a PPI effect.

Prognosis, Evolution, and Clinical Management

The management will depend on the clinical setting. Since both the sporadic and PPI-related FGPs have an extremely low malignant potential (<1%) and PPI-related lesions may regress once the drug is discontinued. Larger polyps

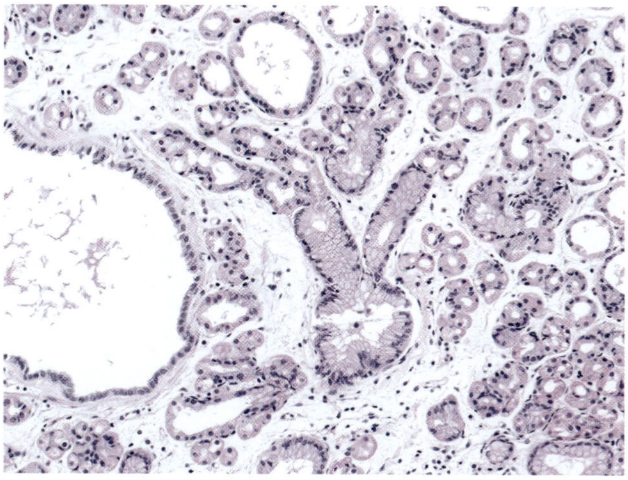

Figure 5.4 Higher magnification of Figure 5.3 showing cystically dilated glands lined by parietal cells, chief cells, and mucous neck epithelium.

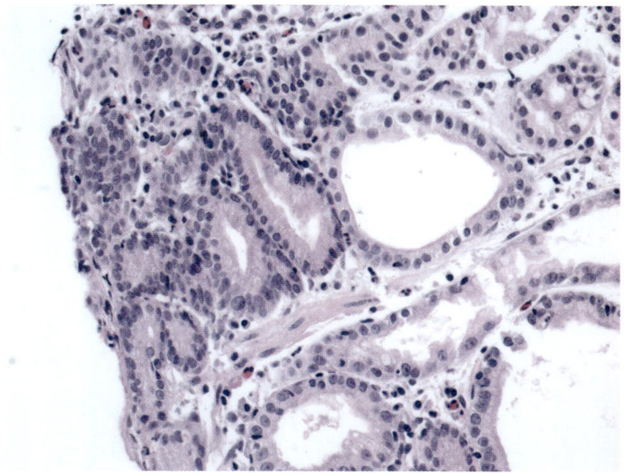

Figure 5.5 Low-grade (foveolar type) dysplasia in a sporadic fundic gland polyp characterized by nuclear rounding and glandular disarray.

(>1 cm) can be removed endoscopically. In patients with FAP, there is a role for surveillance of FGP because of the 30–50% risk of developing dysplasia. FGP dysplasia is associated with larger polyp size, increased severity of duodenal polyposis, and antral gastritis. Acid-suppressive therapy use appears protective against dysplasia in FGPs.

Hyperplastic Polyps

Definition and General Features

Hyperplastic polyps are usually detected in adults (mean age: 60 years). Most are single, but multiple polyps are found in up to 20% of all cases. They are believed to represent a hyperproliferative foveolar response to mucosal injury. Hyperplastic polyps once represented approximately 75% of all gastric polyps, but currently they represent only 14% of the cases in North America. Over the last decade, the increasing use of PPIs and the simultaneous decrease in the prevalence of *H. pylori* infection have explained the decrease in incidence.

These polyps commonly arise in a background of chronic gastritis, either related to *H. pylori* infection or autoimmune gastritis. The predisposing role of *H. pylori* has been indirectly proven by the disappearance or regression of the polyps after eradication of the bacteria and their resurgence when *H. pylori* reinfection occurs. Mucosal atrophy, particularly in the gastric corpus, is also important in the genesis of the polyps. Bile reflux is also implicated as an etiologic factor. Some authors have also shown that up to 15% of hyperplastic polyps arise in solid organ transplant patients.

Clinical Features and Endoscopic Characteristics

Hyperplastic polyps commonly present as round, sessile polyps measuring between 0.5 and 1.5 cm in size (Figure 5.6). Those measuring over 2 cm in size may become pedunculated, presenting a lobulated, frequently eroded surface. Most hyperplastic polyps are asymptomatic. However, blood loss, iron deficiency anemia, and abdominal pain can be associated with large and eroded cases. Gastric outlet obstruction has complicated large antral polyps.

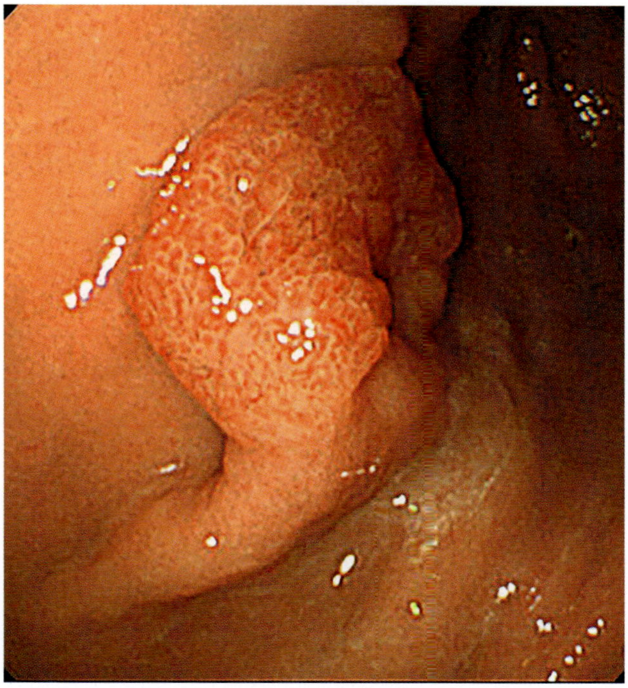

Figure 5.6 Endoscopic appearance of a large hyperplastic polyp covered by eroded mucosal surface.

Microscopic Features

Hyperplastic polyps are composed of exuberant and elongated foveolae embedded in an expanded, edematous, and inflammatory stroma (Figure 5.7a; low magnification of hyperplastic polyp). The foveolae frequently show intraluminal infolding and branching. Cystic dilatation of the pits is also common (Figure 5.7b). The lining epithelium consists of a single layer of variably hypertrophied foveolar epithelium, but regenerative cuboidal cells with an eosinophilic cytoplasm may be seen focally. Parietal and chief cells are uncommon, even in polyps found in the body mucosa, since the basal aspect of the mucosa is not a component of these polyps. Intestinal metaplasia can be seen, and is usually focal and incomplete. Small pyloric type glands can be found beneath the proliferating foveolae (Figure 5.8). Sparse, thin bundles of smooth muscle fibers are commonly seen in an expanded and variably edematous lamina propria that is infiltrated by plasma cells and lymphocytes. Lymphoid aggregates can be detected.

Large polyps are frequently eroded, and reactive atypical cells with mucin depletion and high N : C ratio mimicking dysplasia may be seen (Figure 5.9). In those, the cuff of fibrinopurulent exudate over the granulation tissue despite the presence of mitotically active, bizarre-appearing, reactive stromal cells with hyperchromatic nuclei and prominent nucleoli is key to the diagnosis.

Practically, reporting the size of the hyperplastic polyp and a comment on the absence or presence of dysplasia is helpful. The quality of the resection margin, if present, should be commented upon.

Hamartomatous polyps and Menetrier's disease represent the two main differential diagnoses. The difficulty in diagnosing these lesions stems from two pitfalls: (i) lack of appropriate clinical data and/or access to endoscopic information and (ii) the limited sampling allowed by superficial pinch biopsies. The latter diagnosis cannot be made based on histology alone; an endoscopic correlation must be made. In Menetrier's disease, the gastric lamina propria is generally devoid of inflammation. Hamartomatous polyps are associated with various syndromes such as Cowden's syndrome, Peutz–Jeghers syndrome, juvenile polyposis, or Cronkhite–Canada syndrome. These lesions are characterized by dilated glands and splaying of smooth muscle fibers with a villous appearance differing from that of hyperplastic polyps.

Evaluation of Ki-67, COX2, and p21 reveals increased expression, consistent with increased cellular turnover. TP53 mutations and, less commonly, K-ras mutations can be identified in dysplastic or malignant foci.

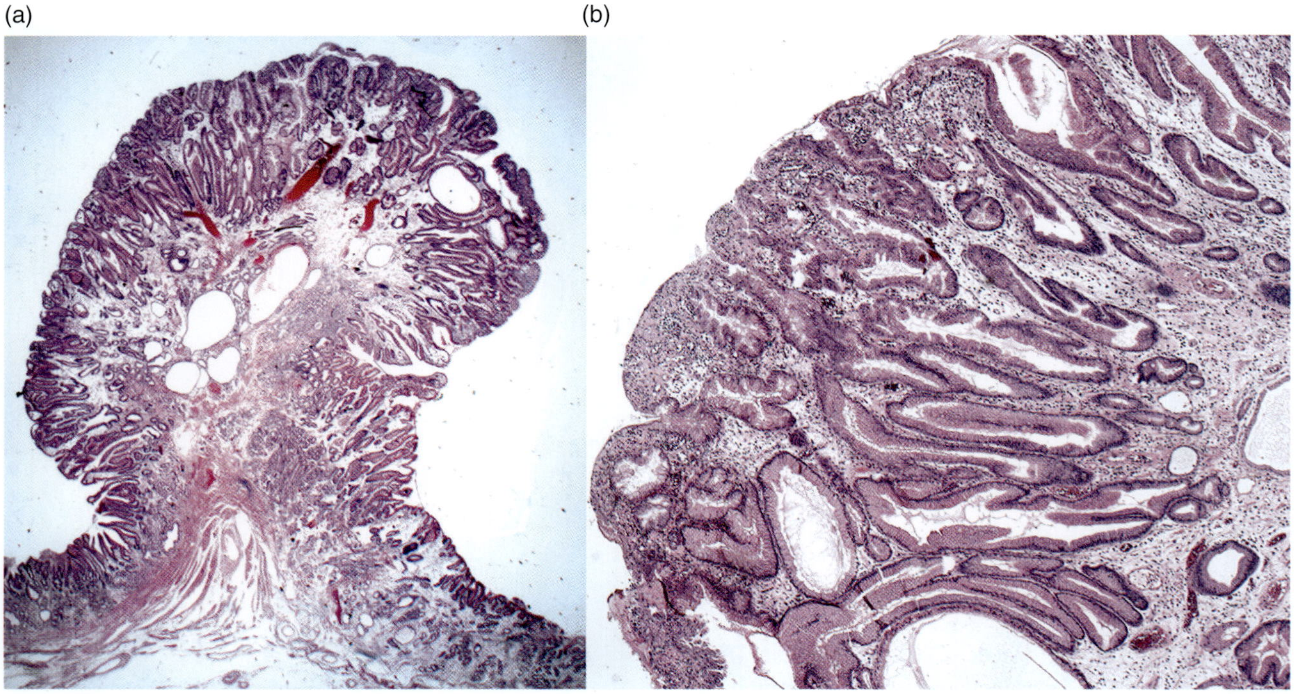

Figure 5.7 Low magnification of a hyperplastic polyp (a), showing gastric foveolar epithelium with intraluminal infolding, irregular branching, and cystic dilatation in higher magnification (b).

(a) (b)

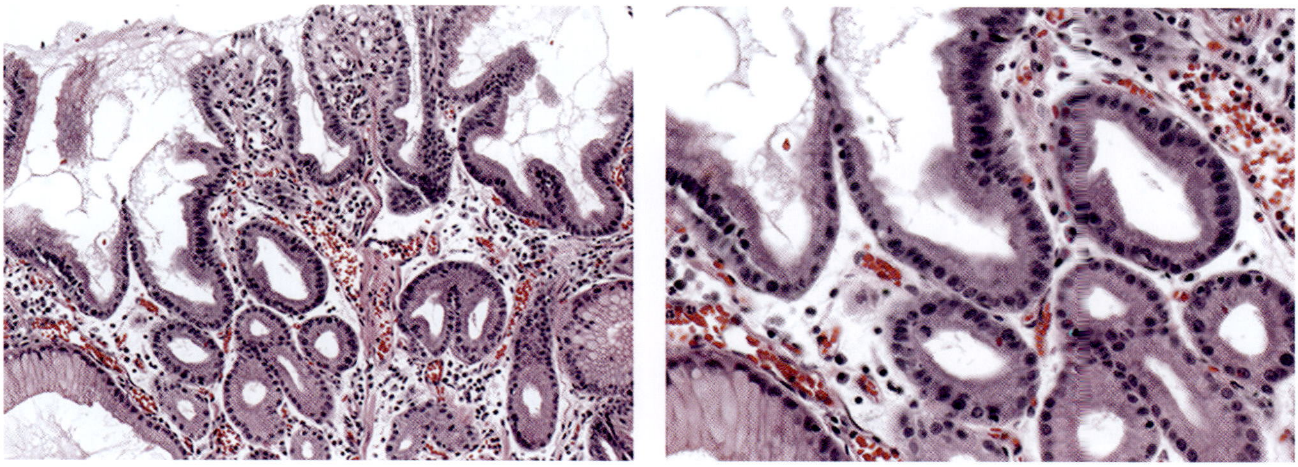

Figure 5.8 Small pyloric type glands beneath the proliferating foveolar epithelium in low (a) and high magnification (b).

(a) (b)

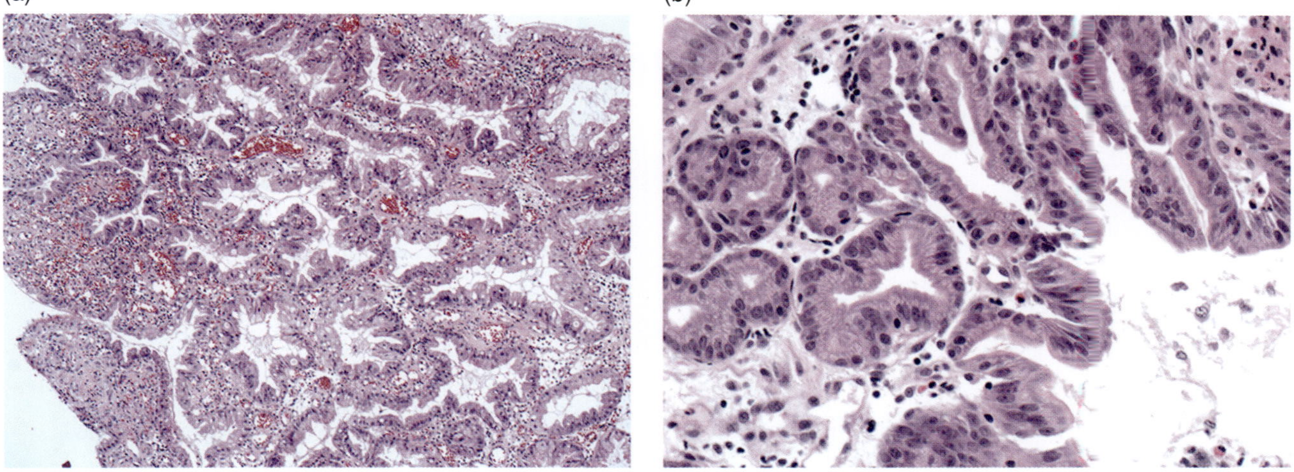

Figure 5.9 Markedly proliferative serrated foveolar epithelium mimicking carcinoma in hyperplastic polyp (a) and regenerative foveolar epithelium mimicking foveolar type dysplasia (b).

Prognosis, Evolution, and Clinical Management

Gastric hyperplastic polyps are the second most common gastric polyps and are generally considered harmless lesions. However, several studies showed that malignant transformations occur in approximately 2–3.3% of gastric hyperplastic polyps. In gastric hyperplastic polyp, malignant changes develop via a hyperplasia–dysplasia–carcinoma sequence (Figure 5.10) and the histology of adenocarcinoma is predominantly well-differentiated gastric adenocarcinoma, and, rarely, signet ring cell or papillary type (Figure 5.11). The risk of malignant transformation is correlated to the size of the polyp, and endoscopic removal of polyps measuring more than 2 cm is recommended. Furthermore, since hyperplastic polyps are associated with mucosal atrophy and intestinal metaplasia, two known risk factors of gastric carcinoma, they should be considered as a surrogate for increased risk of cancer. Notably, associated synchronous or metachronous gastric cancer has been reported in 4–6% of cases.

Thus, *H. pylori* eradication also should be undertaken, if relevant, as well as watchful follow-up.

Variants of Hyperplastic Polyps

Polypoid foveolar hyperplasia: While any mucosal protrusion above the plan of the gastric mucosa may be labeled a polyp by gastroenterologists, the changes may not warrant such a microscopic diagnosis. Polypoid foveolar hyperplasia usually measures 1–2 mm and can be observed at the edges of ulcers or erosions, or in otherwise normal mucosa.

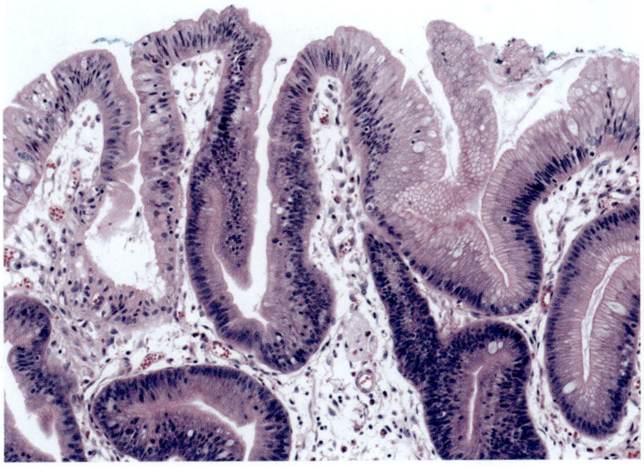

Figure 5.10 Adenomatous low-grade dysplasia found in hyperplastic polyp showing the typical elongated hyperchromatic pencil-shaped nuclei and pseudostratification.

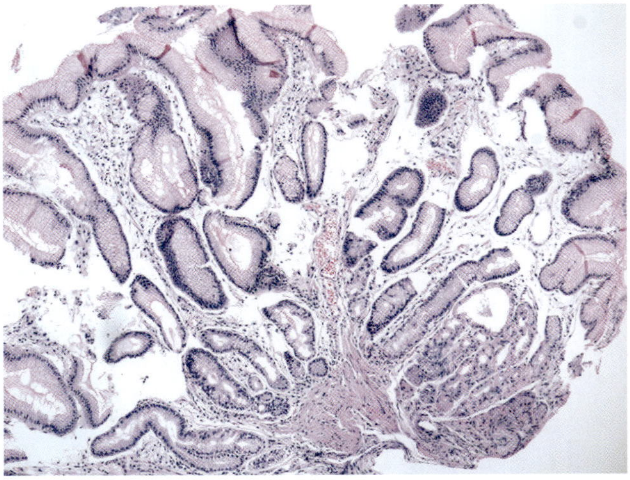

Figure 5.12 A small polypoid foveolar hyperplasia composed solely of proliferating foveolar epithelium and chronic inflammation of the lamina propria without edematous stroma.

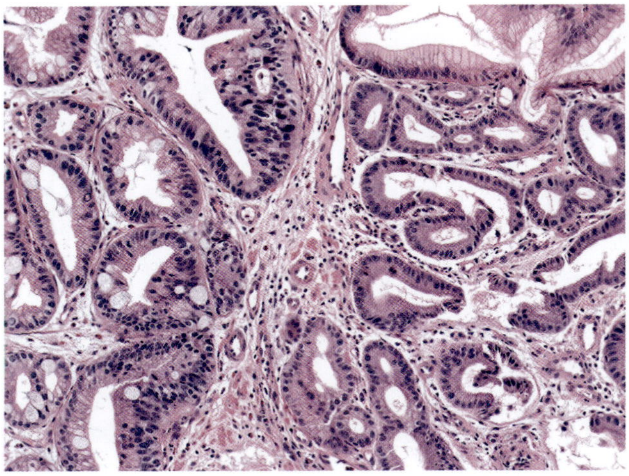

Figure 5.11 Gastric biopsy from polypoid mass showing both hyperplastic polyp and well-differentiated gastric adenocarcinoma on the left.

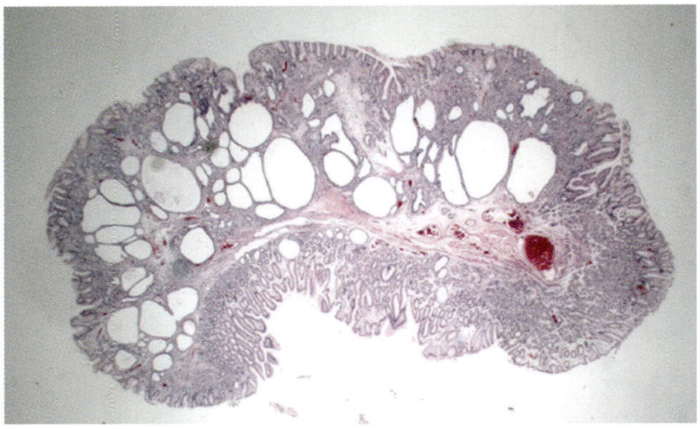

Figure 5.13 Low-power view of gastritis cystica polyposa.

It can be regarded as a precursor lesion to hyperplastic polyps. Microscopic features include simple hyperplasia of the foveolae, but cystic gland changes and distortions are absent. Chronic inflammation of the lamina propria on the periphery is common, but the expanded edematous stroma is missing (Figure 5.12).

Gastritis cystica polyposa/profunda is best defined as a hyperplastic polyp with glandular misplacement in the muscularis mucosa, the submucosa, or the muscularis propria. It is believed to result from trauma-induced entrapment of glands in the gastric wall (frequently seen post-surgery). The term "polyposa" is used when the lesion is mainly intraluminal (Figure 5.13). "Gastritis cystica profunda" is preferred when most of the lesion is intramural. The common location is at the anastomosis of a patient who underwent a partial gastrectomy. The nested organization of the entrapped glandular element, frequently hypertrophic and splaying muscularis mucosae, bland cytology, absent mitotic activity, and lack of desmoplasia are helpful in excluding a neoplasm (Figure 5.14).

Gastric mucosal prolapse polyps have been described recently. These benign polyps display hypertrophic muscle fibers ascending perpendicularly from the muscularis mucosae, and thick-walled blood vessels, while basal glandular elements are noted. These polyps are more commonly sessile than typical hyperplastic polyps. The predominantly antral location, a zone of pronounced peristalsis, and the waxing and waning observed by endoscopists suggest that mucosal prolapse plays a role in the development of these polyps.

Inverted hyperplastic polyps are caused by submucosal glandular proliferation with cystic dilatation and a

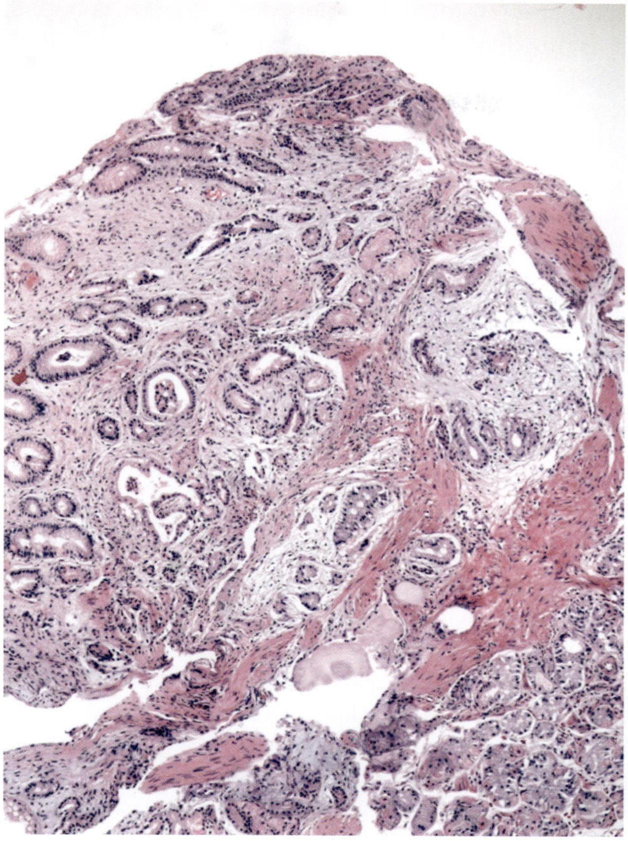

Figure 5.14 Gastric biopsy specimen with bland glands admixed with edematous stroma and hypertrophic muscularis mucosae.

normal-appearing surface mucosa. Some have suggested that they develop after an injury of the muscularis mucosae, resulting in entrapped gastric glands. They may be associated with gastritis cystica profunda and cancer development. Some pathologists call this lesion "herniated gastric mucosa in the submucosa." In cases with carcinomatous transformation (Figure 5.15), mass formation within the cystic spaces mimic submucosal tumor endoscopically.

Hyperplastic polyposis is defined as the presence of 50 or more hyperplastic polyps. A putative association between this rare condition and colorectal cancer has also been suggested.

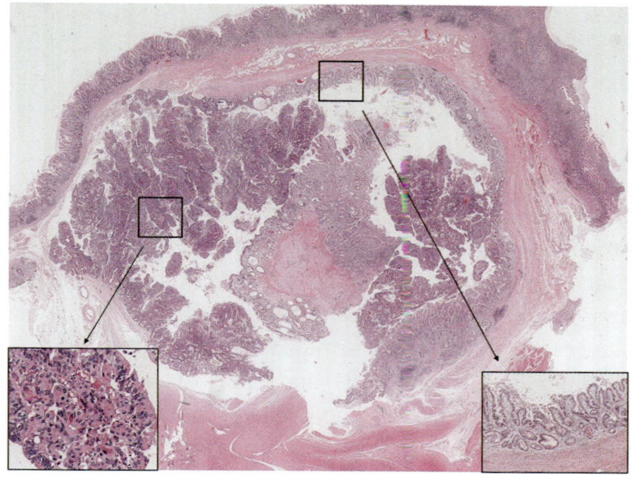

Figure 5.15 Adenocarcinoma observed in the herniated gastric mucosa in the submucosa. Inflamed gastric mucosa (inlet bottom right) and solid areas of adenocarcinoma (inlet bottom left) are present within the cystically dilated spaces surrounded by thickened muscularis mucosae.

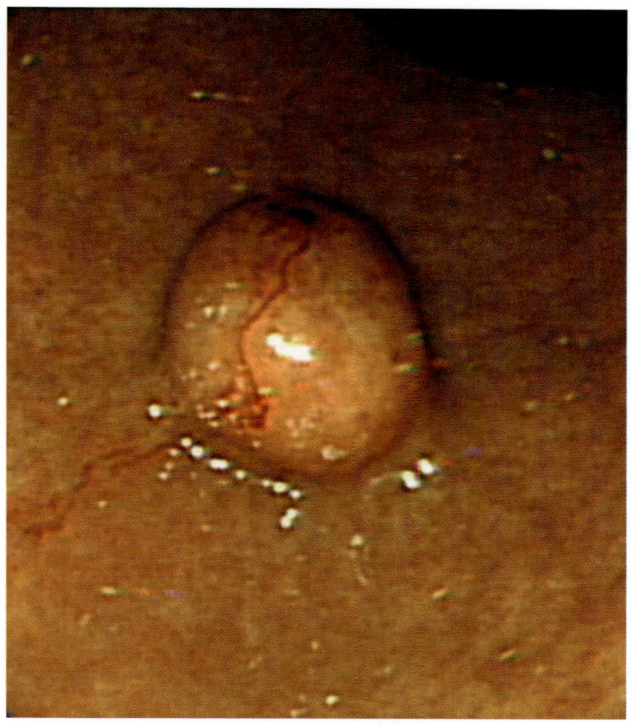

Figure 5.16 Endoscopic view of a pedunculated gastric juvenile polyp.

Gastric Adenoma

Definition and General Features

Adenomas are dysplastic nodules composed of tubular and/or villous structures. Although we favor the term "polypoid dysplasia," we acknowledge that the term "adenoma" remains commonly used in practice.

Clinical Features and Endoscopic Characteristics

Most adenomas are solitary, but multiplicity is noted in 33% of the patients in a Japanese series. These lesions can be sessile or pedunculated (Figure 5.16), and usually measure less than 2 cm. Large adenomas are more frequently composed in part of high-grade dysplastic epithelium. A focus of adenocarcinoma is present in 40–50% of adenomas measuring greater than 2 cm.

Microscopic Features

Gastric adenomas may be architecturally defined as tubular, tubulovillous, or villous. The epithelial lining of gastric adenomas may be of intestinal type (containing goblet cells and/or Paneth cells) or gastric type. Gastric type adenoma can be further subclassified into foveolar type (lined by gastric mucinous foveolar cells) and pyloric gland adenomas. In some cases, it may be impossible to distinguish the epithelial type if there is limited or no mucin production by the neoplastic cells. Gastric adenomas can be graded into two groups: with low-grade dysplasia or with high-grade dysplasia. Those with low-grade dysplasia usually have an indolent clinical course. Alternatively, gastric adenoma with high-grade dysplasia frequently has a cancerous focus, and can rapidly develop into an overt cancer. Thus, the management ought to be individualized based on the degree of dysplasia.

Molecularly, gastric carcinoma arising from adenoma is frequently associated with a mismatch repair deficiency mechanism.

Intestinal Type

An intestinal type epithelium is most common in gastric adenomas, correlating with the intestinalized and atrophic background gastric mucosa. Intestinal type adenomas resemble colonic adenomas and are composed of tubules lined by basophilic columnar cells with hyperchromatic, pencillate nuclei with pseudostratification, and dense eosinophilic cytoplasm. Of practical value, it is important to underscore that the atypical cells extend through the entire thickness of the mucosa, which is different from intestinal metaplasia associated with severe atrophy (Figure 5.17). Goblet and Paneth cells are common. Intestinal type adenomas occur more commonly in the distal stomach compared to gastric type adenomas.

The risk of malignant transformation is directly related to the size, with most carcinoma-associated adenomas measuring >2 cm in diameter. It also may be noted that it may take 10–15 years for a gastric adenoma to transform into carcinoma.

Gastric Foveolar Type

Gastric type adenoma shows cuboidal to columnar foveolar cells with apical mucin caps (Figure 5.18). The cells have pale to clear or sometimes basophilic cytoplasm and hyperchromatic round to oval nuclei. Hyperplasia of the foveolar region with irregular glandular branching and epithelial folding was also frequently noted in this type of adenoma (Figure 5.19). Goblet and Paneth cells are rarely identified. In western populations, they are frequently associated with FAP patients. Most gastric type adenomas were small polyps (<1 cm). Most gastric type adenoma arose in the gastric body and the majority of these patients had little or no inflammatory mucosal pathology in the nonpolypoid gastric mucosa. Foveolar type adenoma usually exhibits low-grade dysplasia and is thought to be associated with a low risk of malignant transformation. In IHC staining, gastric foveolar type epithelium is strongly positive for MUC5AC (Figure 5.18b), but negative for CD10 or MUC2.

(a) (b)

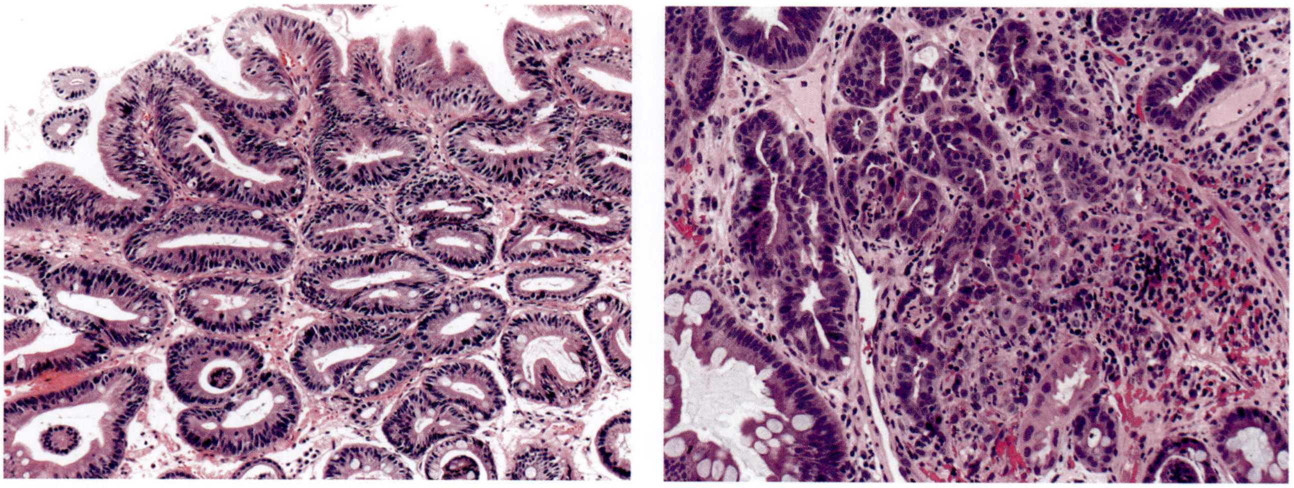

Figure 5.17 Typical microscopic features of intestinal type adenoma with low-grade dysplasia (a) and high-grade dysplasia (b).

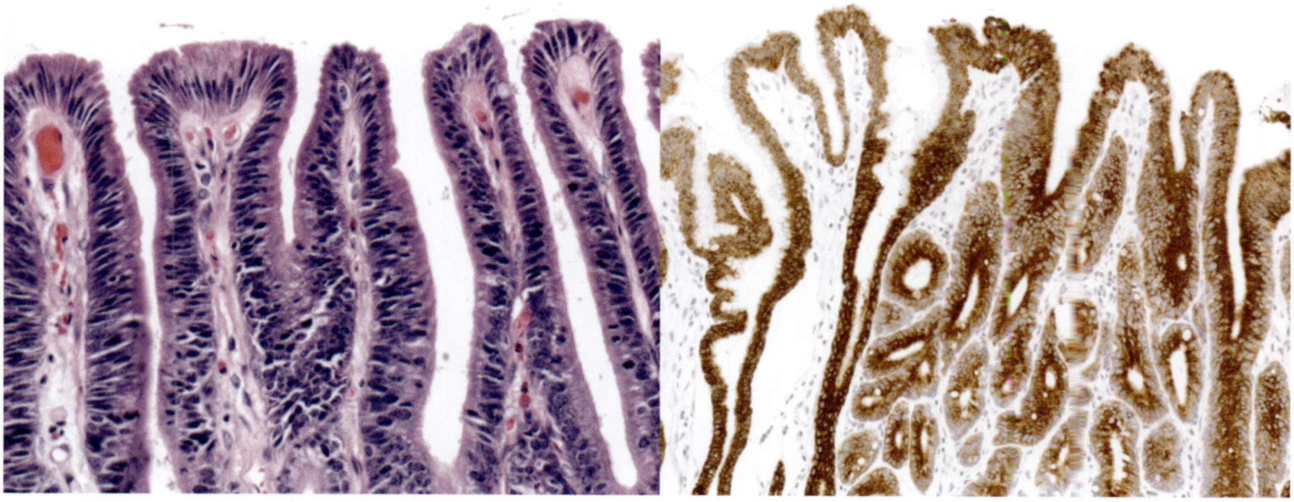

Figure 5.18 Gastric foveolar type adenoma with low-grade dysplasia (left) and immunohistochemistry for MUC5AC positive in adenoma (right). Note the apical mucin caps at the surface.

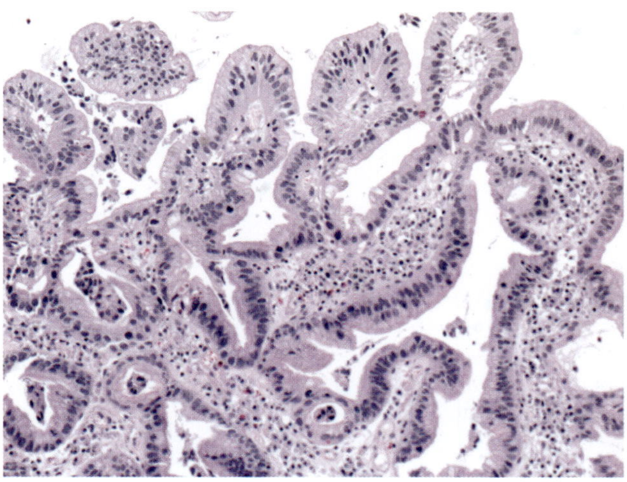

Figure 5.19 Gastric foveolar type adenoma with pale clear cytoplasm and high-grade dysplasia.

Pyloric Gland Type Adenoma

These polyps are composed of closely packed pyloric type glands characteristically lined by cuboidal/columnar cells with round nuclei and pale or eosinophilic cytoplasm (Figure 5.20). Unlike foveolar type adenoma, the cells do not show a well-defined mucin cap, and express both MUC5AC in the surface epithelium and, frequently MUC6 in the glandular component, confirming pyloric gland differentiation. Pyloric gland adenomas have been reported to exhibit high-grade dysplasia and are thought to be associated with a high risk of malignant transformation; 30–39% showed high-grade dysplasia and 12% were associated with adenocarcinoma. Pyloric gland adenoma has been reported in patients with FAP and Lynch syndrome. More than half (64%) of these polyps are located in the fundus.

Pyloric gland adenoma shows frequent TP53 overexpression and chromosomal abnormalities. Activating GNAS mutations are found in 63% and KRAS mutations in 41% of cases. As MLH1 expression loss is rare in sporadic pyloric gland adenomas, simple IHC for MLH1 will help differentiate Lynch syndrome-associated pyloric gland adenoma from sporadic ones.

Prognosis, Evolution, and Clinical Management

The preferred treatment options for gastric adenoma with a biopsy suggestive of low-grade dysplasia is endoscopic resection. For lesions smaller than 1 cm, this is typically done with standard polypectomy. For lesions larger than 1 cm, en bloc resection with endoscopic mucosal resection (EMR) or submucosal dissection (ESD) is preferred due the risk of occult high-grade dysplasia or malignancy. Gastric adenoma with high-grade dysplasia is usually treated by endoscopic resection using various methods including EMR or ESD. According to the eastern series, at least 30% of the endoscopically resected gastric adenomas with high-grade dysplasia have a cancerous focus in the pathologic examination.

Polyposis-Associated Gastric Polyps

The stomach is rarely involved with polyposis syndromes. The hamartomatous polyps observed in juvenile polyposis, Cronkhite–Canada syndrome, and Cowden disease present with overlapping histology as well as typical hyperplastic polyps. Therefore, the diagnosis of a syndromic polyp rests upon receiving the appropriate clinical

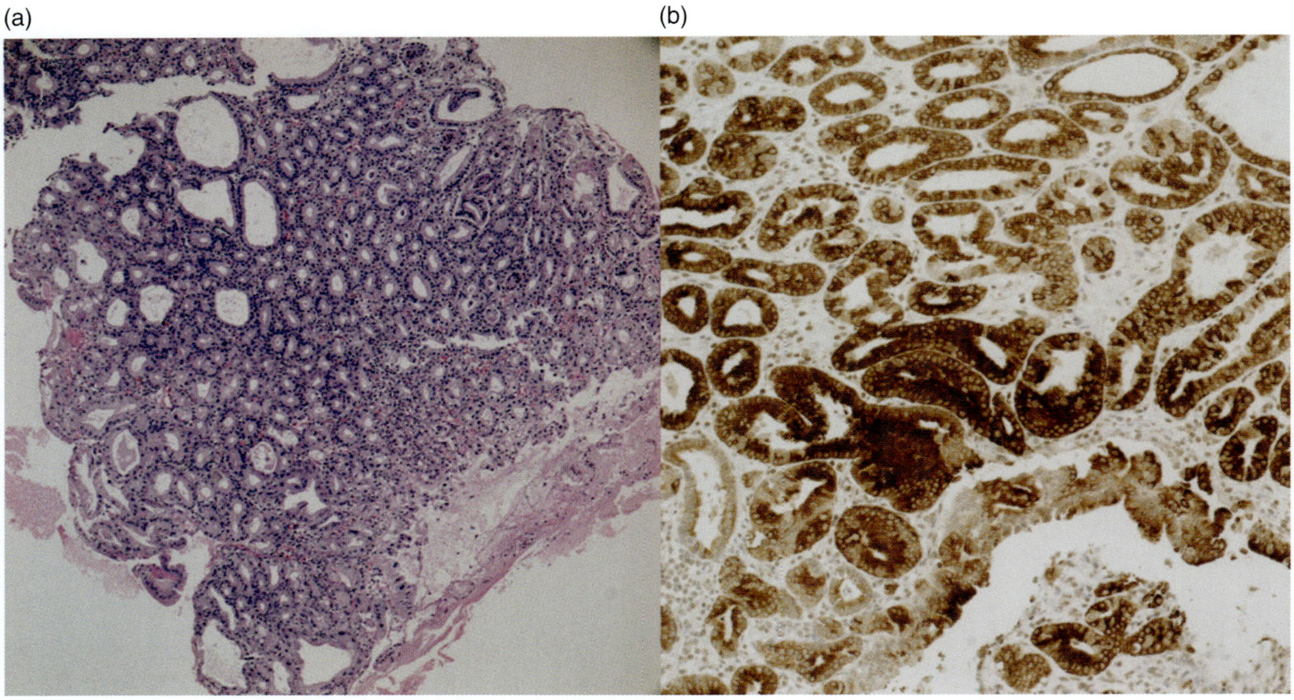

Figure 5.20 Closely packed pyloric type glands lined by cuboidal/columnar cells with round nuclei and pale or eosinophilic cytoplasm (a). MUC6 positivity in proliferated pyloric glands (b).

Table 5.1 Overview of polypoid changes in syndromic settings.

	Juvenile polyposis	Peutz–Jeghers syndrome	Cowden's disease	Cronkhite–Canada syndrome	GAPPS
Inheritance	Autosomal dominant	Autosomal dominant	Autosomal dominant	Non-inherited (sporadic)	Autosomal dominant
Gene	SMAD4 or BMPR1A	STK11/LKB1	PTEN	None	*APC* 1B (GNAS?)
Frequency	Infrequent (15–25%)	25–50%	Common	Common	Common
Location	Antrum > body and fundus	Random	Random	Random	Body and fundus, sparing antrum
Lifetime risk of gastric cancer	15–20%	30%	Rare	About 10%	Unknown

information and knowledge of the endoscopic appearance. Although gastric polyps associated with Peutz–Jeghers syndrome could be diagnosed on the basis of their morphology in the most classic examples, most cases are less developed and may need special evaluation (see Table 5.1). Finally, fundic gland polyps associated with FAP or GAPPS or sporadic fundic gland polyposis are histologically indistinguishable from sporadic and PPI-associated polyps, and only distinguished by their large number (and the clinical history).

Juvenile Polyps

Definition, General Features/Frequency, and Clinical Features

Juvenile polyposis (JP) is an autosomal dominant condition with variable penetrance. Most polyps are noncancerous, but there is an increased risk of cancer of the digestive tract (including the stomach, small intestine, colon, and rectum) in families with JP syndrome. Gastric juvenile polyps are observed in the antrum more frequently than in the body and fundus. They are most often diagnosed in children and young adults.

Clinical Features and Endoscopic Characteristics

Gastric juvenile polyps are rounded and sessile lesions when small, but become pedunculated with a lobulated appearance as they enlarge (Figure 5.21). Diagnostic clinical criteria have been established, including the presence of at least five juvenile polyps in the colon, the presence of juvenile polyps throughout the gut, or the presence of single or multiple juvenile polyps in a patient with an established family history. Rare cases of pyloric obstruction due to large antral polyps are reported. When multiple, they can be associated with iron deficiency anemia and hypoproteinemia.

Microscopic Features

The characteristic features of juvenile polyps include a prominent edematous stroma with mixed inflammatory infiltrate, and cystically dilated glandular and foveolar elements lined with benign epithelium (Figure 5.22). Given the similar histomorphological characteristics, juvenile polyps are difficult to distinguish from hyperplastic polyps based on a pinch biopsy.

Molecular Features

Germline mutations of SMAD4 and BMPR1A, both implicated in the TGFβ-signaling pathway, are the most common molecular abnormalities associated with juvenile polyposis. Each represents 20% of the genetic alterations detected.

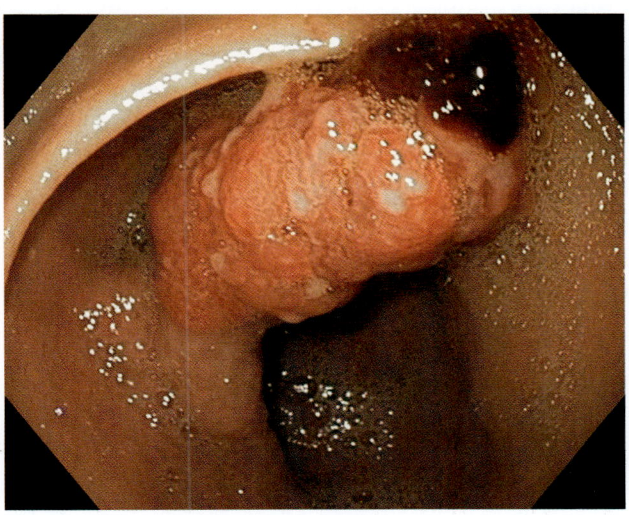

Figure 5.21 Endoscopic appearance of a pedunculated gastric juvenile polyp with a lobulated appearance.

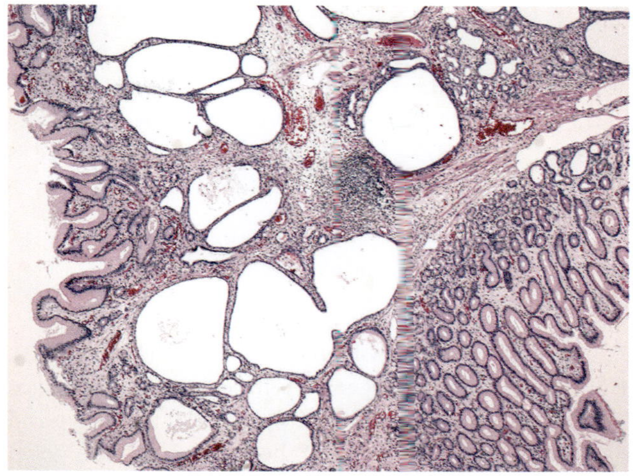

Figure 5.22 Cystically dilated glandular and foveolar elements in juvenile polyp.

Whether germline mutations of SMAD4 are more directly related to the presence of gastric polyps is debated. Mutations in the ENG gene that are also implicated in the TGFβ-signaling pathway have been observed in patients affected in early childhood. Additionally, several cases of juvenile polyps at infancy (diagnosed in the first two years of life and characterized by generalized polyposis) have been associated with germline deletions involving both PTEN and BMPR1A.

Prognosis, Evolution, and Clinical Management

Patients with juvenile polyposis have an increased risk of developing a neoplasm, with as many as 38 and 21% of patients developing colorectal and gastric cancer, respectively. The adenocarcinoma seems to develop following a dysplasia–carcinoma sequence, the risk of cancer increases with the polyps' size, and dysplasia is observed preceding the carcinoma. This increased risk justifies follow-up with screening endoscopy. Most juvenile polyps, even very large ones, can be removed endoscopically with polypectomy and EMR/ESD. In some patients, the polyps may become nearly confluent, in which case, surgical gastrectomy may be necessary.

Peutz–Jeghers Syndrome

Definition, General Features, and Clinical Features

Peutz–Jeghers (P.J) syndrome is an autosomal dominant condition characterized by hamartomatous gastrointestinal polyps, perioral pigmentation, and an increased risk of cancer. Hamartomatous polyps develop all along the gut, but more frequently in the small intestine (90%) than in the colon (78%) or stomach (74%). Only rarely are sporadic Peutz–Jeghers-like polyps detected, and most are diagnosed in a syndromic patient.

In 80% of cases, the syndrome is caused by a germline mutation of the STK11/LKB1 gene, and its prevalence is estimated at about 1/200 000.

Clinical Features and Endoscopic Characteristics

PJ polyps tend to be sessile in the stomach (Figure 5.23). The required clinical diagnostic criteria are (i) the presence of at least two PJ polyps; (ii) the presence of one polyp and classical pigmentation; or (iii) the presence of one polyp along with a family history of PJ polyps.

Microscopic Features

Peutz–Jeghers polyps are characterized by arborizing bundles of smooth muscles emerging from the muscularis mucosae that are covered by cystically distended foveolae (Figure 5.24). The muscular bundles can be thin, and the arborization subtle. Desmin immunoreactivity can be helpful in highlighting the muscular splaying. In practice, when no clinical information is provided, a diagnosis of PJ is uncommonly reached on small or superficial biopsies. Differential diagnoses are broad, but the presence of normal surrounding mucosa can be suggestive of the diagnosis.

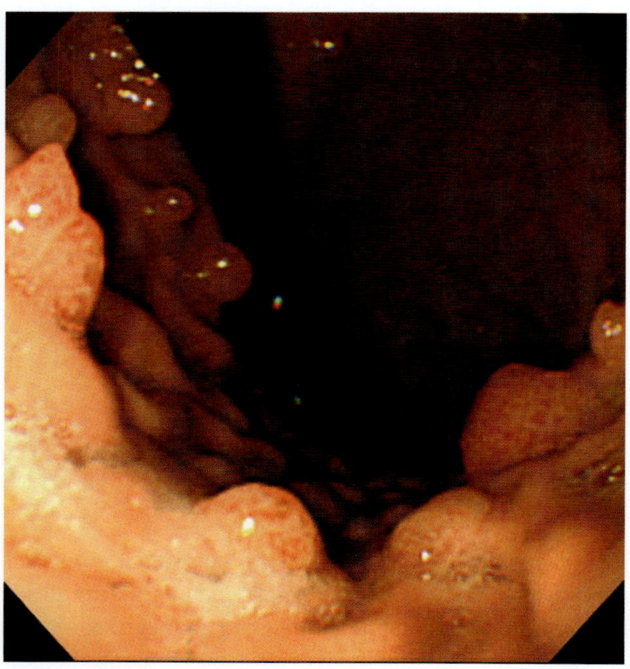

Figure 5.23 Endoscopically many sessile polyps are found in patients with Peutz–Jeghers syndrome.

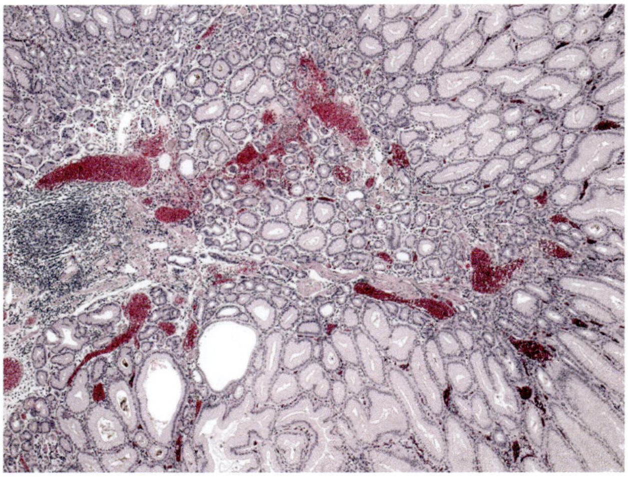

Figure 5.24 Histomorphologically arborizing bundles of smooth muscles emerge from the muscularis mucosae that are covered by cystically distended foveolae.

Molecular Features

STK11/LKB1, which is mutated in Peutz–Jeghers patients, is a serine/threonine kinase involved in cell division, differentiation, and signal transduction. The truncation mutations, which are observed in about 75% of patients, tend to be associated with a higher frequency of gastric involvement and a higher risk of neoplastic transformation than nonsense mutations. There are those who do not have mutations in the STK11 gene. In these cases, the cause of the disorder is unknown.

COX-2 also has been reported to be upregulated in these polyps, leading some authors to recommend the use of COX-2 inhibitors in patients with severe gastric involvement, with a proven reduction in the number of polyps.

Prognosis, Evolution, and Clinical Management

Patients with Peutz–Jeghers syndrome have an increased risk of developing gastrointestinal and extraintestinal malignancies (genitourinary, pancreatic, mammary, and lung). As many as 85% of patients are reported to develop a cancer by the age of 70, and the lifetime risk for gastric cancer is estimated at 30% (Figure 5.25). The risk justifies follow-up for these patients, with surveillance starting as early as the age of eight.

Cowden's Disease

Definition, General Features, Clinical Features, and Endoscopic Characteristics

This rare autosomal dominant condition is caused by germline mutations of the tumor suppressor gene PTEN (phosphatase and tensin homolog). The patients display a

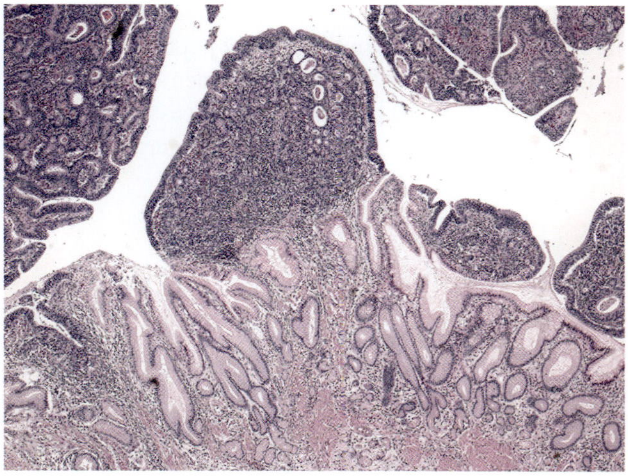

Figure 5.25 Adenocarcinoma developed in patients with hamartomatous polyposis patient. Note the aborizing muscle bundles in the mucosa.

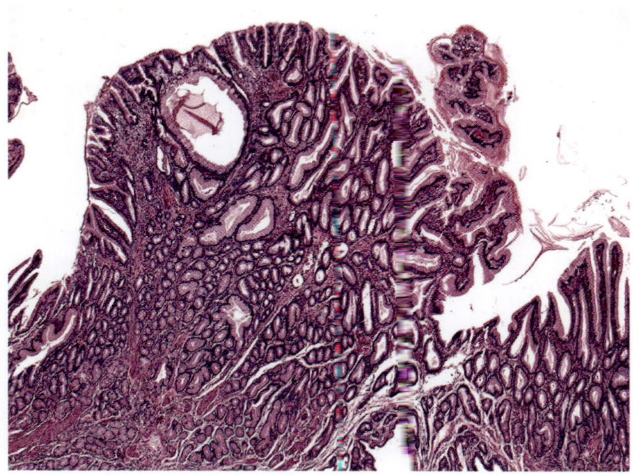

Figure 5.26 Gastric polyp in patient with Cowden's disease with foveolar hyperplasia, cystically dilated glands, and interspersed muscularis mucosae.

wide spectrum of mesodermal, endodermal, and ectodermal alterations with development of multiple hamartomas in various organs. These individuals have an increased risk of breast cancer, but other urogenital, gastrointestinal tract, and thyroid malignancies are reported as well. Gastric cancer is rarely observed. Gastrointestinal polyps are observed in 35–65% of patients.

Microscopic Features

The gastric polyps detected in Cowden's disease bear significant similarities to hyperplastic polyps with foveolar hyperplasia and cystically dilated glands containing papillary infolding. At times, the cysts extend into the submucosa. The stroma may be fibrotic and smooth muscle fibers also may be interspersed among the glands (Figure 5.26). Adenomatous polyps also have occasionally been reported in patients affected by Cowden's disease.

Molecular Features

The diagnosis of PHTS syndrome is made only when a PTEN pathogenic variant is identified. In Cowden's disease, 85% of patients harbor a germline PTEN pathogenic variant.

Prognosis, Evolution, and Clinical Management

There are no clear guidelines. However, in patients with concurrent *H. pylori* infection, eradication of the bacterium has caused the polyps to regress, thus potentially limiting the risk of malignant transformation.

Cronkhite–Canada Syndrome

Definition, General Features, Clinical Features, and Endoscopic Characteristics

Cronkhite–Canada syndrome is a rare non-inherited gastrointestinal polyposis of unknown pathogenesis, although an autoimmune mechanism has been suggested.

Gastric polyps are sessile reddish lesions. This syndrome is diagnosed in the sixth to seventh decades of life, and although examples have been reported worldwide, most cases have been described in Japan. The patients complain of weight loss, malabsorption, diarrhea, and hypoproteinemia. Ectodermal manifestations, primarily changes in skin pigmentation, alopecia, and onychodystrophy, can be observed.

Microscopic Features

The gastric polyps display foveolar hyperplasia with cystic dilated glands, abundant stromal edema, and inflammation (Figure 5.27). A dense eosinophilic infiltrate can be seen in some cases. Cystically dilated glands invaginating in the submucosa can be seen. Cronkhite–Canada syndrome can be difficult to distinguish from other polyposis and hamartomatous syndromes. Of practical value is the recognition that the biopsies of the intervening gastric mucosa are highly inflamed in Cronkhite–Canada syndrome.

Prognosis, Evolution, and Clinical Management

Affected patients generally display a poor prognosis, with mortality associated with gastrointestinal bleeding, sepsis, and congestive heart failure. The risk of cancer remains

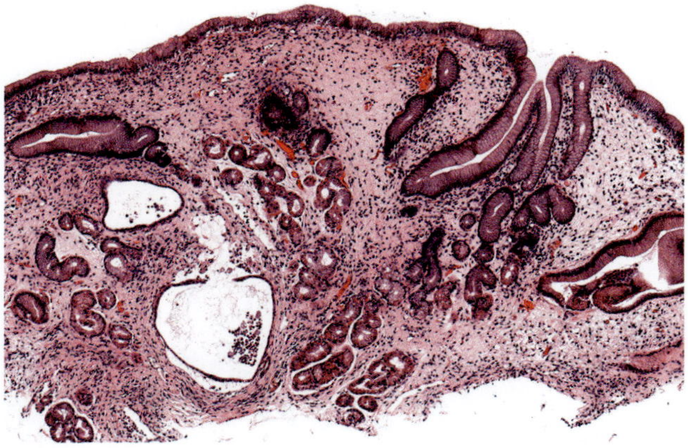

Figure 5.27 Histomorphological appearance of a biopsy from a patient diagnosed with Cronkhite–Canada syndrome showing typical changes like cystic dilation changes of the foveolae and a severe stromal edema.

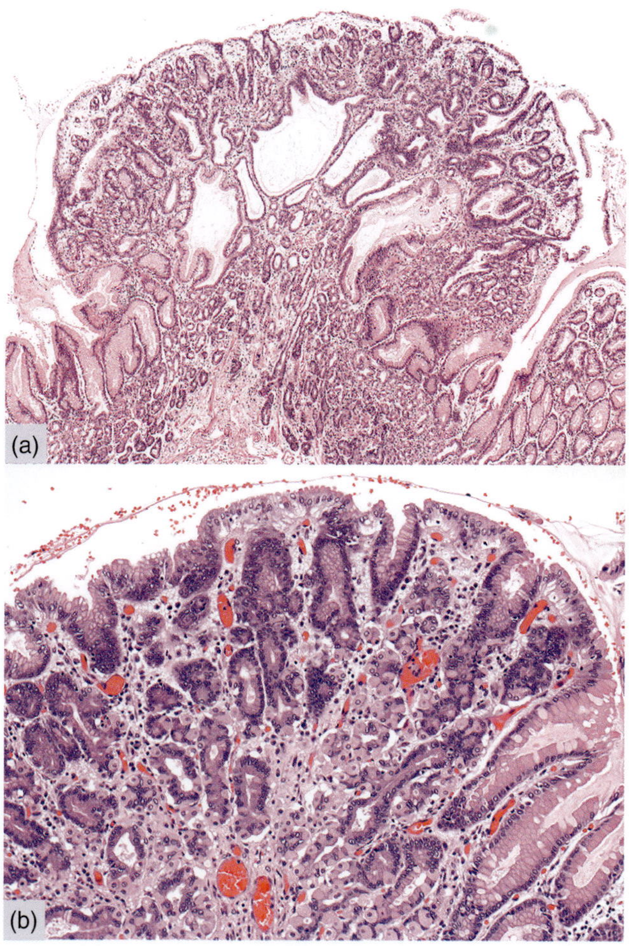

Figure 5.28 A recently described finding in GAPPS are polyps showing hyperproliferative aberrant pits (a) with oxyntic glands reaching up to the mucosal surface (b), whereas this example additionally shows cystic foveolar structures.

controversial, yet colorectal and gastric adenocarcinomas are more frequent than in the general population, with an incidence of approximately 5%. Treatment recommendations are not standardized, but oral corticosteroids remain most commonly prescribed. However, surgery is occasionally proposed.

Gastric Adenocarcinoma and Proximal Polyposis of the Stomach (GAPPS)

GAPPS is a syndromic polyposis, which involves the stomach, especially the fundic and body region.

Definition, General Features, Predisposing Factors

GAPPS is an autosomal dominant syndrome typically showing a severe polyposis of the stomach associated with adenocarcinoma. Only a few studies documented altogether 10 families in the northern and southern hemisphere (Europe, North America, Australia, Asia) fulfilling the criteria of GAPPS. The pathogenesis of this syndrome implicates the *Wnt* pathway.

Clinical Features and Endoscopic Characteristics (Mike)

The age of the patients ranges from 20 to 71 years and women form the largest group. Typically, dyspepsia, epigastric discomfort, or recurrent abdominal pain are reported. Endoscopically, extensive polyposis involving body and fundus are reported, whereas antrum and cardia are not involved. In some cases, sparing of the lesser curve has been reported. The size of the polyps ranges from 1 to 35 mm.

Microscopic Features

The main morphologic findings of GAPPS are fundic gland polyp, characterized by cystic dilatative changes of the foveolar structures. Moreover, some additional findings have been reported including hyperproliferative changes of the pits, characterized by disorganized proliferating oxyntic glands reaching the mucosal surface with infolding of the foveolar epithelium in the pits and foveolae (Figure 5.28). These so-called *hyperproliferative aberrant pits* may represent the early stage of polyp formation.

In addition, flat dysplasia can be present in the intervening mucosa.

One recent study indicates that GAPPS patients may have also a higher risk to develop colonic adenomas compared to the general population

Molecular Features

One study has reported base point mutations of the *APC* gene on chromosome 5q22, affecting promotor 1B. One single study described *APC* mutations in GAPPS while seems to indicate the role of *GNAS* mutation.

Differential Diagnosis

Two differential diagnoses would be possible. One includes the rare event of a gastric hyperplastic polyposis (more than 50 polyps), characterized by hyperplastic polyps. The other differential diagnosis would be upper GI manifestation of FAP, which can be excluded by lower endoscopy with demonstration of multiple colonic adenomas.

Prognosis, Evolution, and Clinical Management

Based on the limited data available and the rarity of the disease, management is evolving. Among the large kindreds reported to date, patients were followed by upper endoscopy beginning around age 10 until polyposis became extensive, at which point patients undergo prophylactic gastrectomy. This typically occurs in the fourth and fifth decade. Colonoscopy in kindreds with GAPP does not suggest a strong association with colon polyps (above what is expected in the general population). Likewise, there is no clear association with duodenal polyps.

Nonepithelial and Malformative Polypoid Lesions

Inflammatory Fibroid Polyps

Definition, General Features, Clinical Features, and Endoscopic Characteristics

Inflammatory fibroid polyps that can be observed throughout the gut are diagnosed predominantly in the stomach (70%) and ileum (20%). Adult men and women are equally affected, and the mean age of patients is 60 years, with rare pediatric cases reported.

The polyps are usually asymptomatic, but larger examples may cause bleeding, anemia, and gastric outlet obstruction. Inflammatory fibroid polyps are broad-based submucosal nodules and either are covered by normal mucosa or show apical depressions (Figure 5.29) or ulcerations. Up to 8% of inflammatory fibroid polyps have been reported near gastric cancer or adenoma despite no evidence of any relationship.

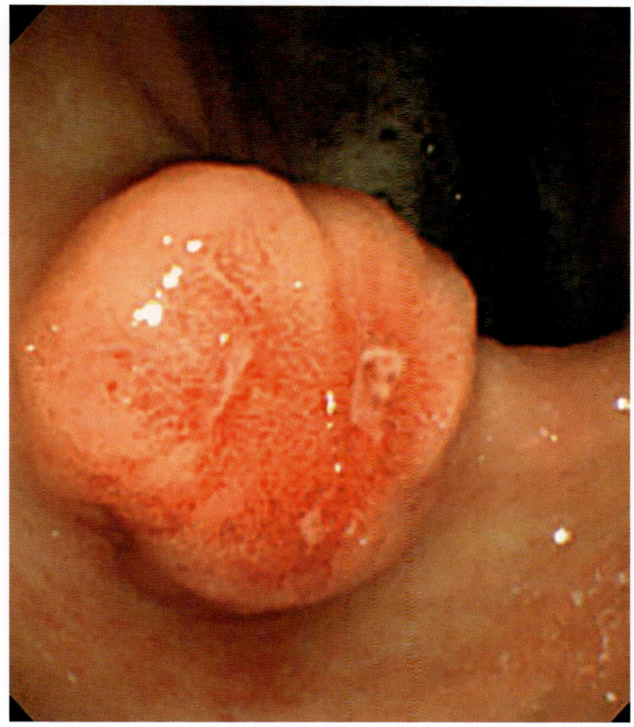

Figure 5.29 Inflammatory fibroid polyp presenting as broad-based submucosal nodule covered by normal mucosa with apical depression.

Gastric polyps are typically located in the antrum, and occur in approximately 3% of gastric biopsies.

Microscopic Features

Inflammatory fibroid polyps result from the proliferation of loose spindle cells arranged in short fascicles or whorled structures (Figure 5.30a). Uncommonly, spindle cells can present a dense eosinophilic cytoplasm, and at times they form an "onion skin" disposition around capillaries. Mitoses are rare. A dense inflammatory infiltrate dominated by eosinophils frequently is intermixed (Figure 5.30b), and loose lymphoid aggregates can form. Giant cells can be detected. Inflammatory fibroid polyps are centered on the submucosa, and overlying mucosa may have branching foveolae that are elongated and distorted. Extension into the muscularis mucosae, muscularis propria, or even the subserosa has been reported.

Practically, the differential diagnoses include gastrointestinal stromal tumor, eosinophilic gastroenteritis, and inflammatory pseudotumor.

(a) (b)

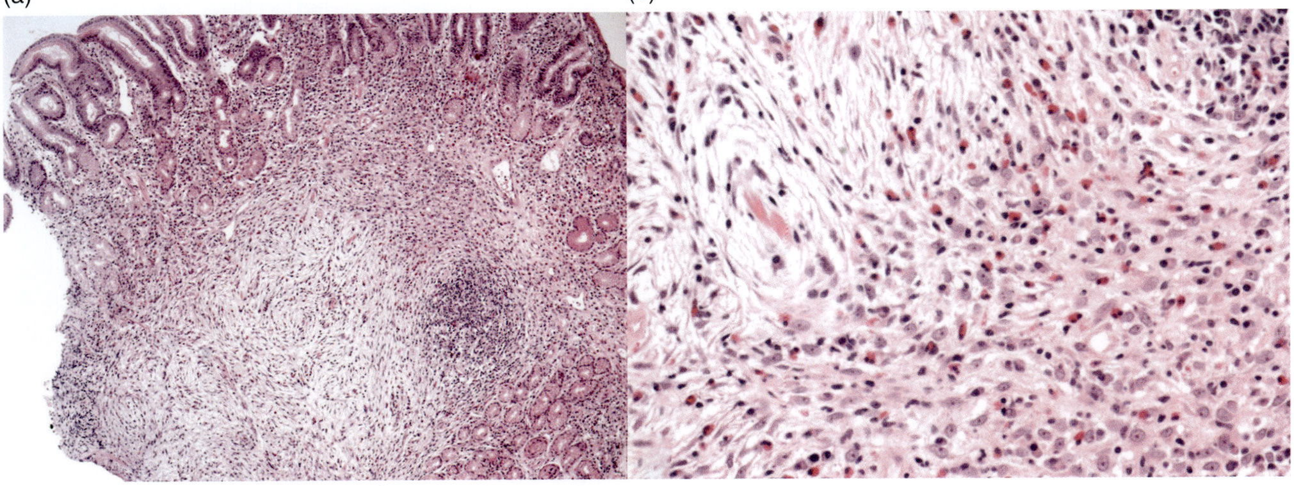

Figure 5.30 Gastric biopsy specimen with proliferation of loose spindle cells arranged in short fascicles or whorled structures (a) and a dense eosinophilic infiltrate intermixed with myofibroblast-like cells (b).

Table 5.2 Immunohistochemical findings in inflammatory fibroid polyps.

Antibody	Positivity
CD34	100%
Fascin	100%
CD35	100% (10% of cells)
Cyclin D1	100%
PDGFRA	90% (diffuse in 94%, focal in 6%)
Calponin	88%
Smooth muscle actin	10–25%
CD117 (KIT), DOG1, S-100 protein	0%
EMA, Keratin, Desmin, bcl2	0%

Immunohistochemical Studies and Molecular Features The immunohistochemical profile is shown in Table 5.2. Immunohistochemically, the spindle cells are positive for CD34, CD35, fascin, and calponin, as well as smooth muscle actin in some cases, but S100 protein, c-kit, desmin, FVIII, and keratin are consistently negative (Figure 5.31). Recent molecular studies have demonstrated that these polyps result from activated mutations of the PDGFRA gene in more than half of the cases, thus suggesting a neoplastic origin.

Lipoma

Definition, General Features, Clinical Features, and Endoscopic Characteristics

Gastric lipomas account for only 2–3% of all benign gastric tumors. They occur more frequently in adults and equally in both sexes.

Abdominal pain and bleeding are the most commonly reported symptoms. Intussusceptions, gastric outlet obstruction, dyspepsia, vomiting, and tachycardia have been reported in association.

Gastric lipomas typically present endoscopically as antral smooth submucosal lesions protruding into the lumen. Mucosal ulcerations or central depressions sometimes are observed. Rare "giant gastric lipomas," which can reach 10 cm, have been described. Rare subserosal lesions have been reported.

Microscopic Features

Gastric lipomas are composed of encapsulated collections of benign adipose tissue, and are composed of mature well-differentiated adipocytes. "Fibrolipoma" composed of both mature adipose tissue and spindle cell-like fibroblasts has been noted. The overlying gastric mucosa can be inflamed and ulcerated, or unremarkable.

The rare liposarcoma will present distinct cytologic atypia.

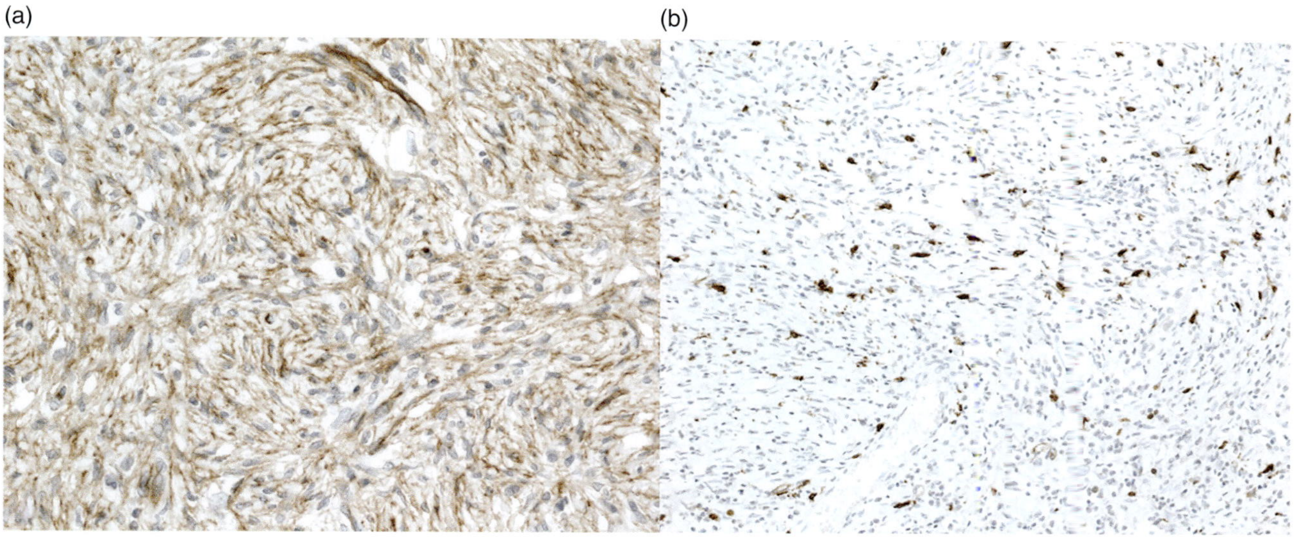

Figure 5.31 Immunohistochemical staining of the inflammatory fibroid polyp (a) positive staining of CD34 in the cytoplasm of spindle tumor cells and (b) negative for c-kit with internal positive control in infiltrating mast cells.

Prognosis, Evolution, and Clinical Management

Lipomas of the gastrointestinal tract are almost universally benign and do not require resection. They can be easily diagnosed by the yellowish appearance on endoscopy and soft "pillow" texture when probed with a biopsy forceps. Endoscopic ultrasound (EUS) is diagnostic when a bright, hyperechoic structure is seen in the submucosa. Biopsy is generally not necessary.

Xanthoma

Definition, General Features, Clinical Features, and Endoscopic Characteristics

Gastric xanthomas are benign accumulations of macrophages with vacuolated sudanophilic cytoplasm. They are not associated with lipid metabolic disorders, but the high percentage of oxidized LDL has led some authors to conclude that these lesions develop secondary to mucosal damage resulting in macrophage chemotactism.

Xanthomas are small (less than 1 cm), rounded, yellowish submucosal lesions seen in 1–7% of endoscopies. They typically are found in the antrum, along the lesser curvature or close to a stoma, or along the greater curvature, in patients who have had gastric surgery. Gastric xanthomas are usually solitary, and it is rare to observe multiple lesions.

Microscopic Features

Xanthomas are composed of benign polygonal histiocytes expanding the lamina propria. The cells have a distinct cell membrane and a small centrally located round or oval nucleus (Figure 5.32). Various lipids (cholesterol, neutral fat, low-density lipoprotein, and oxidized low-density lipoprotein) have been found within these cells. They are commonly located in the upper third of the mucosa. Atypia is absent. Gastric xanthoma can be observed in association with atrophic gastritis, intestinal metaplasia, *H. pylori* gastritis, and gastric carcinoma.

Signet ring cell carcinoma, clear cell variant of carcinoid tumors, and metastatic clear cell renal cell carcinoma are the most common differential diagnoses. Usually, these can be ruled out easily by appropriate immunohistochemical studies. Benign differential diagnoses include Whipple disease and atypical mycobacterial infection. Again, proper use of clinical information and special stains is helpful.

Immunohistochemical Studies

Immunohistochemical positivity for CD68 with negativity for cytokeratins can be used to confirm the histiocytic nature of the cells.

Prognosis, Evolution and Clinical Management

Xanthomas are benign lesions and do not require endoscopic or surgical removal.

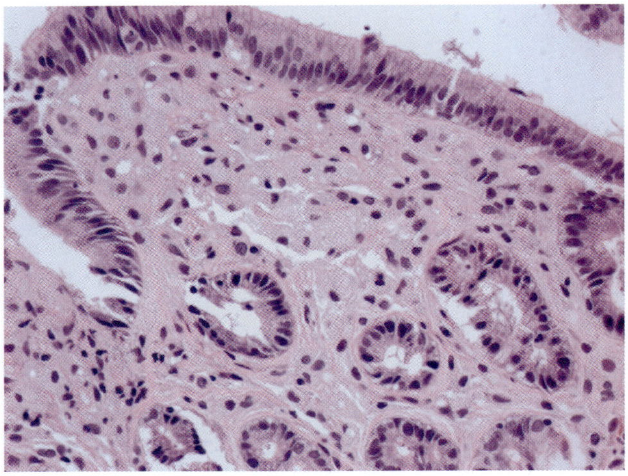

Figure 5.32 Submucosal aggregates of xanthoma cells with a distinct cell membrane, a small centrally located round or oval nucleus and foamy cytoplasm.

Gastric Heterotopic Pancreas

Definition, General Features, Predisposing Factors

This embryologic anomaly is defined by the presence of mature pancreatic tissue within the gastric wall. It represents the second most common pancreatic congenital abnormality after pancreas divisum, likely related to abnormal migration and/or residual rest of pancreatic buds during embryogenesis. It usually develops distally within 5 cm of the pylorus and within the submucosa.

Clinical Features and Endoscopic Characteristics

Most pancreatic heterotopias are asymptomatic but rarely can be associated with abdominal pain, vomiting, gastric outlet obstruction, and even with dysphagia in the rare cases located near the gastroesophageal junction. The typical endoscopic appearance is a small rounded submucosal lesion in the greater curvature side of the antrum, sometimes with central umbilication. In cases with larger lesion with uncommon endoscopic features, differential diagnosis with other types of submucosal tumor can be difficult, so limited surgical resection may be required (Figure 5.33).

Microscopic Features

The appearance is varied and can be classified on the basis of the predominant histologic composition (Figure 5.34). Several different types can be observed synchronously. Some lesions contain all the anatomic components of the pancreatic gland, including ducts, acini, and endocrine islets (type I). Type II consists of pancreatic ducts only. The ducts are commonly dilated and surrounded by smooth muscle bands, and sometimes are reported as "adenomyoma." Type III consists only of acinar tissue, and type IV consists only of islet cells.

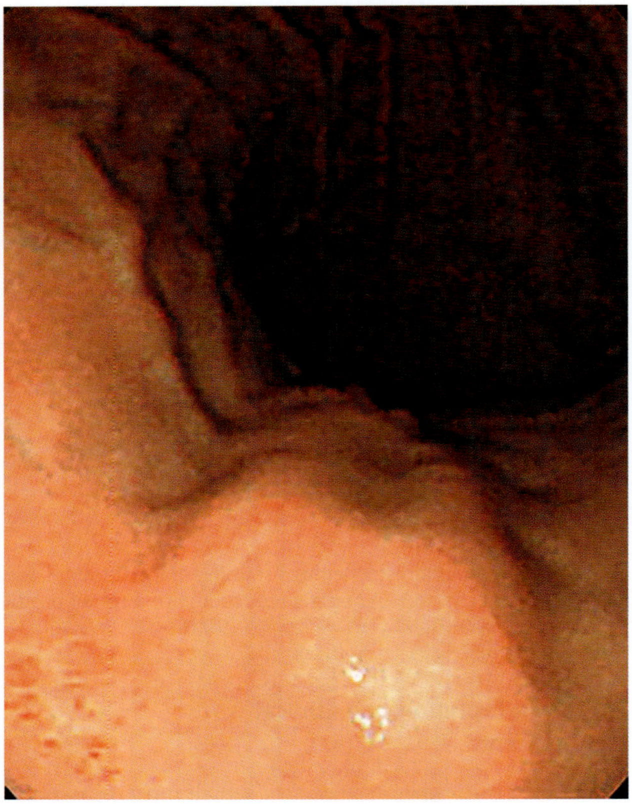

Figure 5.33 Heterotopic pancreas on the posterior wall of the mid-body, an submucosal tumor-like lesion with central depression was seen endoscopically.

Endoscopic pinch biopsies often fail to provide a diagnosis since some of the diagnostic elements are deeply embedded in the gastric wall, but EUS-FNA can be useful in distinguishing ectopic pancreatic tissue from other submucosal lesions such as GIST or leiomyoma, but may not be diagnostically specific.

Prognosis, Evolution, and Clinical Management

Most lesions are identified as subepithelial tumors on endoscopy. Definitive diagnosis usually requires EUS, which shows a hypoechoic (dark) heterogenous structure resembling pancreatic tissue in the submucosal layer. Asyptomatic lesions do not require therapy. In cases of symptomatic lesions, limited resection is the treatment of choice. Successful endoscopic resection has been reported. Various complications have been reported, including acute

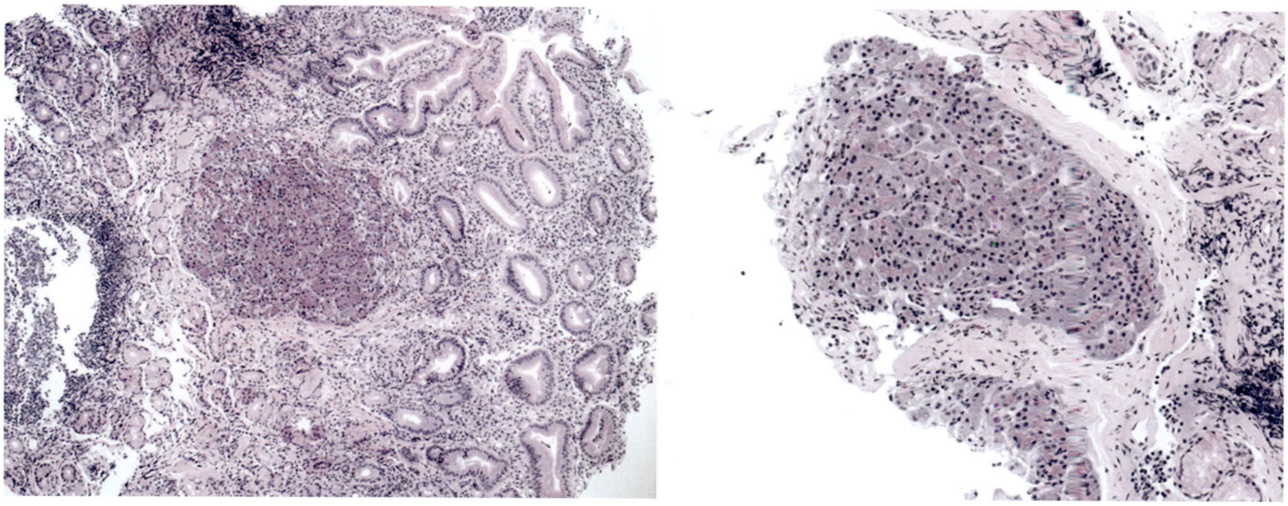

Figure 5.34 In gastric pinch biopsies, observation of pancreatic acini in the gastric, submucosa is pathognomonic for the diagnosis of heterotopia.

pancreatitis, pseudocysts, mucinous cysts, pancreatic intraepithelial neoplasia, and even ductal adenocarcinoma, acinar cell carcinoma, or pancreatic neuroendocrine tumors.

Menetrier's Disease

Definition, General Features, Predisposing Factors

Menetrier's disease is a condition associating diffuse hypertrophic gastropathy, hypochlorhydria, and hypoproteinemia secondary to excessive mucosal protein loss.

It is described not only in adults (often males 40–60 years old), but also pediatric patients. Cytomegalovirus is associated in 70% of children affected. *H. pylori* is revealed in nearly 90% of adult patients, in contrast. Interestingly, a case of Menetrier's disease in an adult with herpes simplex virus infection has been reported.

Clinical Features and Endoscopic Characteristics

Most adult patients show chronic debilitating courses. Conversely, pediatric forms have a self-limited transient course, usually resolving within few months. Vomiting, abdominal pain, and edema are the most common symptoms. Massively thickened irregular "cerebriform" gastric folds with large amounts of viscous mucus and superficial erosions are the characteristic macroscopic features. These changes are seen in the proximal stomach amid edematous mucosa, though localized or diffuse cases have been reported. Localized disease of the gastric antrum, with

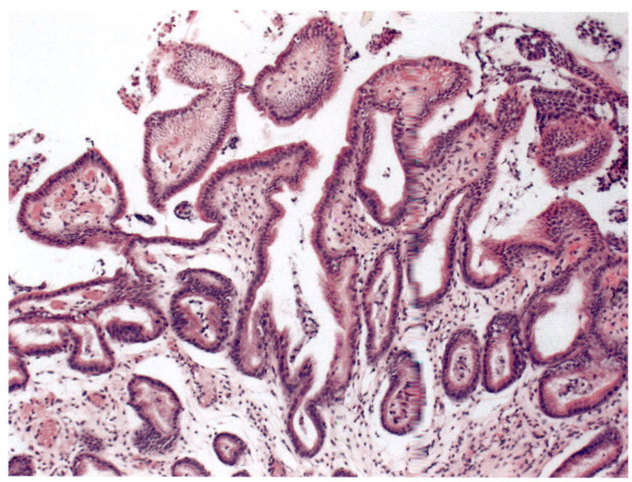

Figure 5.35 Gastric pinch biopsy of a patient with endoscopical appearance of Ménétrier's disease showing typical mucosal changes with foveolar elongation and cystic dilatative changes of the pits.

sparing of the fundus and body, and mainly manifested by polyposis and coexisting with gastritis cystica profunda, has been observed. Examination of conventional pinch biopsies is inadequate to appreciate the massive foveolar hyperplasia, and full-thickness biopsies are recommended if the condition is suspected.

Microscopic Features

Menetrier's disease (Figure 5.35) is characterized by marked elongation and tortuosity of foveolae with cystically dilated pits and marked proliferation of the surface mucus-producing cells. Furthermore, disorganized muscularis mucosae with fascicles of smooth muscles dissecting the lamina propria can be present. Submucosal glandular extension may develop and give rise to a pattern of gastritis cystica profunda. Commonly, atrophy or even loss of glandular parietal and chief cells is observed. Inflammation is uncommon, but marked eosinophilia has been reported. The differential diagnoses include other hypertrophic gastropathies, i.e. Zollinger–Ellison syndrome or hypertrophic gastritis, as well as neoplastic infiltrative processes including gastric lymphoma and diffuse type adenocarcinoma. The diagnosis may be challenging, if only superficial biopsies are provided. However, none of these conditions are associated with such a severe foveolar hyperplasia or profound hypoproteinemia.

Molecular Features

The pathogenesis is unclear, but TGF-α, a ligand for the epidermal growth factor receptor (EGF-R) that causes dose-dependent in vitro proliferation of gastric epithelial cells and dose-dependent reduction of acid secretion, has been implicated.

Prognosis, Evolution, and Clinical Management

If undetected and untreated, the patients will develop profound hypoproteinemia. In addition, iron deficiency anemia can develop secondary to gastric blood loss.

Therapies targeting increased signal of EGF-R have shown some promise, including octreotide (a somatostatin analog) and monoclonal antibodies (e.g. cetuximab) directed against the epidermal growth factor receptor. In case of refractory or complicated cases, massive bleeding, refractory protein loss, or obstructive symptoms, gastrectomy is curative.

Menetrier's disease is reported to carry an increased risk of gastric cancer (a 2–15% lifetime risk), but the exact risk is unknown.

Further Reading

Abraham, S.C., Nobukawa, B., Giardiello, F.M. et al. (2000). Fundic gland polyps in familial adenomatous polyposis: neoplasms with frequent somatic adenomatous polyposis coli gene alterations. *Am. J. Pathol.* 157: 747–754.

Abraham, S.C., Nobukawa, B., Giardiello, F.M. et al. (2001). Sporadic fundic gland polyps: common gastric polyps arising through activating mutations in the beta-catenin gene. *Am. J. Pathol.* 158: 1005–1010.

Abraham, S.C., Park, S.J., Mugartegui, L. et al. (2002). Sporadic fundic gland polyps with epithelial dysplasia: evidence for preferential targeting for mutations in the adenomatous polyposis coli gene. *Am. J. Pathol.* 161: 1735–1742.

Abraham, S.C., Montgomery, E.A., Singh, V.K. et al. (2002). Gastric adenomas: intestinal-type and gastric-type adenomas differ in the risk of adenocarcinoma and presence of background mucosal pathology. *Am. J. Surg. Pathol.* 26: 1276–1285.

Abraham, S.C., Park, S.J., Cruz-Correa, M. et al. (2004). Frequent CpG island methylation in sporadic and syndromic gastric fundic gland polyps. *Am. J. Clin. Pathol.* 122: 740–746.

Alberti, D., Grazioli, L., Orizio, P. et al. (1999). Asymptomatic giant gastric lipoma: what to do? *Am. J. Gastroenterol.* 94: 3634–3637.

Al-Haddad, M., Ward, E.M., Bouras, E.P. et al. (2007). Hyperplastic polyps of the gastric antrum in patients with gastrointestinal blood loss. *Dig. Dis. Sci.* 52: 105–109.

Ally, M.R., Veerappan, G.R., Maydonovitch, C.L. et al. (2009). Chronic proton pump inhibitor therapy associated with increased development of fundic gland polyps. *Dig. Dis. Sci.* 54: 2617–2622.

Alper, M., Akcan, Y., and Belenli, O. (2003). Large pedinculated antral hyperplastic gastric polyp traversed the bulbus causing outlet obstruction and iron deficiency anemia: endoscopic removal. *World J. Gastroenterol.* 9: 633–634.

Amaro, R., Neff, G.W., Karnam, U.S. et al. (2002). Acquired hyperplastic gastric polyps in solid organ transplant patients. *Am. J. Gastroenterol.* 97: 2220–2224.

Anderson, R.D., Patel, R., Hamilton, J.K. et al. (2006). Cronkhite–Canada syndrome presenting as eosinophilic gastroenteritis. *Proc. (Baylor Univ. Med. Cent.)* 19: 209–212.

Antoniou, D., Soutis, M., Stefanaki, K. et al. (2007). Gastric fibrolipoma causing bleeding in a child. *Eur. J. Pediatr. Surg.* 17: 282–284.

Bayerdorffer, E., Ritter, M.M., Hatz, R. et al. (1994). Healing of protein losing hypertrophic gastropathy by eradication of *Helicobacter pylori* – is *Helicobacter pylori* a pathogenic factor in Menetrier's disease? *Gut* 35: 701–704.

Beer, A., Streubel, B., Asari, R. et al. (2017). Gastric adenocarcinoma and proximal polyposis of the stomach (gapps) – a rare recently described gastric polyposis syndrome – report of a case. *Z. Gastroenterol.* 55: 1131–1134.

Bianchi, L.K., Burke, C.A., Bennett, A.E. et al. (2008). Fundic gland polyp dysplasia is common in familial adenomatous polyposis. *Clin. Gastroenterol. Hepatol.* 6: 180–185.

de Boer, W.B., Ee, H., and Kumarasinghe, M.P. (2018). Neoplastic lesions of gastric adenocarcinoma and proximal polyposis syndrome (gapps) are gastric phenotype. *Am. J. Surg. Pathol.* 42: 1–8.

Borch, K., Skarsgard, J., Franzen, L. et al. (2003). Benign gastric polyps: morphological and functional origin. *Dig. Dis. Sci.* 48: 1292–1297.

Brautbar, A., Paz, J., Hadas-Halpern, I. et al. (2005). Menetrier's disease presenting as an acute protein-losing gastroenteropathy in a 27-year-old man with Gaucher disease. *Eur. J. Gastroenterol. Hepatol.* 17: 679–681.

Burdick, J.S., Chung, E., Tanner, G. et al. (2000). Treatment of Menetrier's disease with a monoclonal antibody against the epidermal growth factor receptor. *N. Engl. J. Med.* 343: 1697–1701.

Burkart, A.L., Sheridan, T., Lewin, M. et al. (2007). Do sporadic Peutz–Jeghers polyps exist? Experience of a large teaching hospital. *Am. J. Surg. Pathol.* 31: 1209–1214.

Campos, F.G., Habr-Gama, A., Kiss, D.R. et al. (2006). Cowden syndrome: report of two cases and review of clinical presentation and management of a rare colorectal polyposis. *Curr. Surg.* 63: 15–19.

Carlson, G.J., Nivatvongs, S., and Snover, D.C. (1984). Colorectal polyps in Cowden's disease (multiple hamartoma syndrome). *Am. J. Surg. Pathol.* 8: 763–770.

Carmack, S.W., Genta, R.M., Schuler, C.M. et al. (2009). The current spectrum of gastric polyps: a 1-year national study of over 120,000 patients. *Am. J. Gastroenterol.* 104: 1524–1532.

Carmack, S.W., Genta, R.M., Graham, D.Y. et al. (2009). Management of gastric polyps: a pathology-based guide for gastroenterologists. *Nat. Rev. Gastroenterol. Hepatol.* 6: 331–341.

Chen, Z.M., Scudiere, J.R., Abraham, S.C. et al. (2009). Pyloric gland adenoma: an entity distinct from gastric foveolar type adenoma. *Am. J. Surg. Pathol.* 33: 186–193.

Chongsrisawat, V., Yimyeam, P., Wisedopas, N. et al. (2004). Unusual manifestations of gastric inflammatory fibroid polyp in a child. *World J. Gastroenterol.* 10: 460–462.

Chusid, E.L., Hirsch, R.L., and Colcher, H. (1964). Spectrum of hypertrophic gastropathy; Giant Rugal folds, polyposis, and carcinoma of the stomach – case report and review of the literature. *Arch. Intern. Med.* 114: 621–628.

Cieslak, T.J., Mullett, C.T., Puntel, R.A. et al. (1993). Menetrier's disease associated with cytomegalovirus infection in children: report of two cases and review of the literature. *Pediatr. Infect. Dis. J.* 12: 340–343.

Coffin, C.M. and Dehner, L.P. (1996). What is a juvenile polyp? An analysis based on 21 patients with solitary and multiple polyps. *Arch. Pathol. Lab. Med.* 120: 1032–1038.

Covarrubias, D.J. and Huprich, J.E. (2002). Best cases from the AFIP. Juvenile polyposis of the stomach. Armed Forces Institute of Pathology. *Radiographics* 22: 415–420.

Cronkhite, L.W. Jr. and Canada, W.J. (1955). Generalized gastrointestinal polyposis; an unusual syndrome of polyposis, pigmentation, alopecia and onychotrophia. *N. Engl. J. Med.* 252: 1011–1015.

Daibo, M., Itabashi, M., and Hirota, T. (1987). Malignant transformation of gastric hyperplastic polyps. *Am. J. Gastroenterol.* 82: 1016–1025.

Declich, P., Ambrosiani, L., Bellone, S. et al. (2000). Parietal cell hyperplasia with deep cystic dilations: a lesion closely mimicking fundic gland polyps. *Am. J. Gastroenterol.* 95: 566–568.

Declich, P., Bellone, S., Porcellati, M. et al. (2000). Parietal cell protrusions with fundic gland cysts and fundic gland polyps: are they related or simply similar but distinguishable? *Hum. Pathol.* 31: 1535–1537.

Di Giulio, E., Lahner, E., Micheletti, A. et al. (2005). Occurrence and risk factors for benign epithelial gastric polyps in atrophic body gastritis on diagnosis and follow-up. *Aliment. Pharmacol. Ther.* 21: 567–574.

Dirschmid, K., Walser, J., and Hugel, H. (1984). Pseudomalignant erosion in hyperplastic gastric polyps. *Cancer* 54: 2290–2293.

Dirschmid, K., Platz-Baudin, C., and Stolte, M. (2006). Why is the hyperplastic polyp a marker for the precancerous condition of the gastric mucosa? *Virchows Arch.* 448: 80–84.

Egawa, T., Kubota, T., Otani, Y. et al. (2000). Surgically treated Cronkhite–Canada syndrome associated with gastric cancer. *Gastric Cancer* 3: 156–160.

Evans, J.A., Chandrasekhara, V., Chathadi, K.V. et al. (2015). The role of endoscopy in the management of premalignant and malignant conditions of the stomach. *GIE* 82: 1–8.

Fenoglio-Preiser, C., Noffsinger, A.E., and Stemmermann, G.N. (2008). The nonneoplastic stomach. In: *Gastrointestinal Pathology: An Atlas and Text* (eds. C.M. Fenoglio-Preiser, A.E. Noffsinger and G.N. Stemmermann), 206. Philadelphia: Lippincott Williams & Wilkins.

Friedl, W., Uhlhaas, S., Schulmann, K. et al. (2002). Juvenile polyposis: massive gastric polyposis is more common in MADH4 mutation carriers than in BMPR1A mutation carriers. *Hum. Genet.* 111: 108–111.

Garrean, S., Hering, J., Saied, A. et al. (2008). Gastric adenocarcinoma arising from fundic gland polyps in a patient with familial adenomatous polyposis syndrome. *Am. Surg.* 74: 79–83.

Gencosmanoglu, R., Sen-Oran, E., Kurtkaya-Yapicier, O. et al. (2003). Antral hyperplastic polyp causing intermittent gastric outlet obstruction: case report. *BMC Gastroenterol.* 3: 16.

Genta, R.M., Schuler, C.M., Robiou, C.I. et al. (2009). No association between gastric fundic gland polyps and gastrointestinal neoplasia in a study of over 100,000 patients. *Clin. Gastroenterol. Hepatol.* 7: 849–854.

Giardiello, F.M., Brensinger, J.D., Tersmette, A.C. et al. (2000). Very high risk of cancer in familial Peutz–Jeghers syndrome. *Gastroenterology* 119: 1447–1453.

Gonzalez-Obeso, E., Fujita, H., Deshpande, V. et al. (2011). Gastric "hyperplastic polyps": a heterogenous clinicopathological group including a distinct subset best categorized as mucosal prolypase polyp. *Am. J. Surg. Pathol.* 35 (5): 670–677.

Gravina, A.G., Iacono, A., Alagia, I. et al. (2009). Gastric xanthomatosis associated with gastric intestinal metaplasia in a dyspeptic patient. *Dig. Liver Dis.* 41: 765.

Gursoy, S., Yurci, A., Torun, E. et al. (2005). An uncommon lesion: gastric xanthelasma. *Turk. J. Gastroenterol.* 16: 167–170.

Ha, J.P., Tang, C.N., Cheung, H.Y. et al. (2007). An unusual cause of gastric outlet obstruction. *Gut* 56: 967. 1018.

Hamby, L.S., Lee, E.Y., and Schwartz, R.W. (1995). Parathyroid adenoma and gastric carcinoma as manifestations of Cowden's disease. *Surgery* 118: 115–117.

Hammock, L. and Jorda, M. (2002). Gastric endocrine pancreatic heterotopia. *Arch. Pathol. Lab. Med.* 126: 464–467.

Han, A.R., Sung, C.O., Kim, K.M. et al. (2009). The clinicopathological features of gastric hyperplastic polyps with neoplastic transformations: a suggestion of indication for endoscopic polypectomy. *Gut Liver* 3: 271–275.

Hattori, T. (1985). Morphological range of hyperplastic polyps and carcinomas arising in hyperplastic polyps of the stomach. *J. Clin. Pathol.* 38: 622–630.

Hemmings, C.T. (2007). Menetrier's disease in a patient with ulcerative colitis: a case report and review of the literature. *Pathology* 39: 282–283.

Hirasaki, S., Tanimizu, M., Moriwaki, T. et al. (2005). Acute pancreatitis occurring in gastric aberrant pancreas treated with surgery and proved by histological examination. *Intern. Med.* 44: 1169–1173.

Hirasaki, S., Suzuki, S., Kanzaki, H. et al. (2007). Minute signet ring cell carcinoma occurring in gastric hyperplastic polyp. *World J. Gastroenterol.* 13: 5779–5780.

Hirasaki, S., Matsubara, M., Ikeda, F. et al. (2007). Gastric inflammatory fibroid polyp treated with *Helicobacter pylori* eradication therapy. *Intern. Med.* 46: 855–858.

Hirasaki, S., Kanzaki, H., Fujita, K. et al. (2008). Papillary adenocarcinoma occurring in a gastric hyperplastic polyp observed by magnifying endoscopy and treated with endoscopic mucosal resection. *Intern. Med.* 47: 949–952.

Hizawa, K., Iida, M., Matsumoto, T. et al. (1994). Gastrointestinal manifestations of Cowden's disease. Report of four cases. *J. Clin. Gastroenterol.* 18: 13–18.

Hizawa, K., Fuchigami, T., Iida, M. et al. (1995). Possible neoplastic transformation within gastric hyperplastic polyp. Application of endoscopic polypectomy. *Surg. Endosc.* 9: 714–718.

Howe, J.R., Mitros, F.A., and Summers, R.W. (1998). The risk of gastrointestinal carcinoma in familial juvenile polyposis. *Ann. Surg. Oncol.* 5: 751–756.

Hu, T.L., Hsu, J.T., Chen, H.M. et al. (2002). Diffuse gastric polyposis: report of a case. *J. Formos. Med. Assoc.* 101: 712–714.

Isomoto, H., Furusu, H., Ohnita, K. et al. (2005). Effect of *Helicobacter pylori* eradication on gastric hyperplastic polyposis in Cowden's disease. *World J. Gastroenterol.* 11: 1567–1569.

Iwama, I., Kagimoto, S., Takano, T. et al. Case of pediatric Menetrier disease with cytomegalovirus and *Helicobacter pylori* co-infection. *Pediatr. Int.* 52: e200–e203.

Jalving, M., Koornstra, J.J., Boersma-van Ek, W. et al. (2003). Dysplasia in fundic gland polyps is associated with nuclear beta-catenin expression and relatively high cell turnover rates. *Scand. J. Gastroenterol.* 38: 916–922.

Jalving, M., Koornstra, J.J., Gotz, J.M. et al. (2003). High-grade dysplasia in sporadic fundic gland polyps: a case report and review of the literature. *Eur. J. Gastroenterol. Hepatol.* 15: 1229–1233.

Jalving, M., Koornstra, J.J., Wesseling, J. et al. (2006). Increased risk of fundic gland polyps during long-term proton pump inhibitor therapy. *Aliment. Pharmacol. Ther.* 24: 1341–1348.

Jarvinen, H.J. and Sipponen, P. (1986). Gastroduodenal polyps in familial adenomatous and juvenile polyposis. *Endoscopy* 18: 230–234.

Jass, J.R., Williams, C.B., Bussey, H.J. et al. (1988). Juvenile polyposis – a precancerous condition. *Histopathology* 13: 619–630.

Jeon, S.W. (2010). Endoscopic management of gastric dysplasia: cutting edge technology needs a new paradigm. *World J. Gastrointest. Endosc.* 2: 301–304.

Jeong, Y.S., Park, H., Lee, D.Y. et al. (2004). Gastric xanthomatosis. *Gastrointest. Endosc.* 59: 399–400.

Jewell, K.D., Toweill, D.L., Swanson, P.E. et al. (2008). Gastric hyperplastic polyps in post transplant patients: a clinicopathologic study. *Mod. Pathol.* 21: 1108–1112.

Ji, F., Wang, Z.W., Ning, J.W. et al. (2006). Effect of drug treatment on hyperplastic gastric polyps infected with *Helicobacter pylori*: a randomized, controlled trial. *World J. Gastroenterol.* 12: 1770–1773.

Johnson, G.K., Soergel, K.H., Hensley, G.T. et al. (1972). Cronkite–Canada syndrome: gastrointestinal pathophysiology and morphology. *Gastroenterology* 63: 140–152.

Jun, D.W., Kim, D.H., Kim, S.H. et al. (2007). Menetrier's disease associated with herpes infection: response to treatment with acyclovir. *Gastrointest. Endosc.* 65: 1092–1095.

Kaiserling, E., Heinle, H., Itabe, H. et al. (1996). Lipid islands in human gastric mucosa: morphological and immunohistochemical findings. *Gastroenterology* 110: 369–374.

Kamata, Y., Kurotaki, H., Onodera, T. et al. (1993). An unusual heterotopia of pyloric glands of the stomach with inverted downgrowth. *Acta Pathol. Jpn.* 43: 192–197.

Kantarcioglu, M., Kilciler, G., Turan, I. et al. (2009). Solitary Peutz–Jeghers-type hamartomatous polyp as a cause of recurrent acute pancreatitis. *Endoscopy* 41 (Suppl 2): E117–E118.

Kaufman, A., Storey, D., Lee, C.S. et al. (2007). Mucinous cyst exhibiting severe dysplasia in gastric heterotopic pancreas associated with gastrointestinal stromal tumour. *World J. Gastroenterol.* 13: 5781–5782.

Kawada, M., Seno, H., Wada, M. et al. (2003). Cyclooxygenase-2 expression and angiogenesis in gastric hyperplastic polyp-association with polyp size. *Digestion* 67: 20–24.

Kazantsev, G.B., Schwesinger, W.H., and Heim-Hall, J. (2002). Spontaneous resolution of multiple fundic gland polyps after cessation of treatment with lansoprazole and Nissen fundoplication: a case report. *Gastrointest. Endosc.* 55: 600–602.

Kim, H.S., Woo, D.K., Bae, S.I. et al. (2000). Microsatellite instability in the adenoma–carcinoma sequence of the stomach. *Lab. Investig.* 80: 57–64.

Kono, T., Imai, Y., Ichihara, T. et al. (2007). Adenocarcinoma arising in gastric inverted hyperplastic polyp: a case report and review of the literature. *Pathol. Res. Pract.* 203: 53–56.

Krasinskas, A.M., Abraham, S.C., Metz, D.C. et al. (2003). Oxyntic mucosa pseudopolyps: a presentation of atrophic autoimmune gastritis. *Am. J. Surg. Pathol.* 27: 236–241.

Krasniqi, A.S., Hoxha, F.T., Bicaj, B.X. et al. (2008). Symptomatic subserosal gastric lipoma successfully treated with enucleation. *World J. Gastroenterol.* 14: 5930–5932.

Kurland, J., DuBois, S., Behling, C. et al. (2006). Severe upper-GI bleed caused by gastritis cystica profunda. *Gastrointest. Endosc.* 63: 716–717.

Lagarde, A., Rouleau, E., Ferrari, A. et al. (2010). Germline apc mutation spectrum derived from 863 genomic variations identified through a 15-year medical genetics service to french patients with fap. *J. Med. Genet.* 47: 721–722.

Lai, E.C. and Tompkins, R.K. (1986). Heterotopic pancreas. Review of a 26 year experience. *Am. J. Surg.* 151: 697–700.

Lauwers, G.Y.C.F. and Graham, D.Y. (2010). *Gastric Carcinoma*. Lyon: IARC.

Lauwers, G.Y., Wahl, S.J., Melamed, J. et al. (1993). p53 expression in precancerous gastric lesions: an immunohistochemical study of PAb 1801 monoclonal antibody on adenomatous and hyperplastic gastric polyps. *Am. J. Gastroenterol.* 88: 1916–1919.

Lee, S.E., Kang, S.Y., Cho, J. et al. (2014). Pyloric gland adenoma in lynch syndrome. *Am. J. Surg. Pathol.* 38: 784–792.

Lewin, K.J.A.H. (1996). *Tumors of the Esophagus and Stomach. Atlas of Tumor Pathology*. Washington, DC: Armed Forces Institute of Pathology.

Li, J., Woods, S.L., Healey, S. et al. (2016). Point mutations in exon 1b of apc reveal gastric adenocarcinoma and proximal polyposis of the stomach as a familial adenomatous polyposis variant. *Am. J. Hum. Genet.* 98: 830–842.

Lim, J.K., Jang, Y.J., Jung, M.K. et al. (2010). Menetrier disease manifested by polyposis in the gastric antrum and coexisting with gastritis cystica profunda. *Gastrointest. Endosc.* 72 (5): 1098–1100.

Lin, J., Chen, M., Lei, W. et al. (2009). Eradication of diffuse gastric Peutz–Jeghers polyps by unsedated transnasal snare polypectomy and argon plasma coagulation. *Endoscopy* 41 (Suppl 2): E207–E208.

Lloyd, K.M. 2nd and Dennis, M. (1963). Cowden's disease. A possible new symptom complex with multiple system involvement. *Ann. Intern. Med.* 58: 136–142.

Matsuhashi, N., Nakajima, A., Nomura, S. et al. (2004). Inflammatory fibroid polyps of the stomach and *Helicobacter pylori*. *J. Gastroenterol. Hepatol.* 19: 346–347.

McDuffie, L.A., Sabesan, A., Allgaeuer, M. et al. (2016). Beta-catenin activation in fundic gland polyps, gastric cancer and colonic polyps in families afflicted by 'gastric adenocarcinoma and proximal polyposis of the stomach' (gapps). *J. Clin. Pathol.* 69: 826–833.

Morais, D.J., Yamanaka, A., Zeitune, J.M. et al. (2007). Gastric polyps: a retrospective analysis of 26,000 digestive endoscopies. *Arq. Gastroenterol.* 44: 14–17.

Mori, M., Tamura, S., Enjoji, M. et al. (1988). Concomitant presence of inflammatory fibroid polyp and carcinoma or adenoma in the stomach. *Arch. Pathol. Lab. Med.* 112: 829–832.

Moues, C.M., Steenvoorde, P., Viersma, J.H. et al. (2002). Jejunal intussusception of a gastric lipoma: a review of literature. *Dig. Surg.* 19: 418–420.

Mulholland, K.C., Wallace, W.D., Epanomeritakis, E. et al. (2004). Pseudocyst formation in gastric ectopic pancreas. *JOP* 5: 498–501.

Muller-Lissner, S.A. and Wiebecke, B. (1982). Investigations of hyperplasiogenous gastric polyps by partial reconstruction. *Pathol. Res. Pract.* 174: 368–378.

Murakami, K., Mitomi, H., Yamashita, K. et al. (2001). p53, but not c-Ki-ras, mutation and down-regulation of p21WAF1/CIP1 and cyclin D1 are associated with malignant transformation in gastric hyperplastic polyps. *Am. J. Clin. Pathol.* 115: 224–234.

Muraoka, A., Suehiro, I., Fujii, M. et al. (1998). Type IIa early gastric cancer with proliferation of xanthoma cells. *J. Gastroenterol.* 33: 326–329.

Muto, T. and Ota, K. (1970). Polypogenesis of gastric mucosa. *Gann* 61: 435–442.

Nakajima, A., Matsuhashi, N., Yazaki, Y. et al. (2000). Details of hyperplastic polyps of the stomach shrinking after anti-*Helicobacter pylori* therapy. *J. Gastroenterol.* 35: 372–375.

Nishiyama, Y., Koyama, S., Andoh, A. et al. (2003). Gastric inflammatory fibroid polyp treated with *Helicobacter pylori* eradication therapy. *Intern. Med.* 42: 263–267.

Niv, Y., Delpre, G., Sperber, A.D. et al. (2003). Hyperplastic gastric polyposis, hypergastrinaemia and colorectal neoplasia: a description of four cases. *Eur. J. Gastroenterol. Hepatol.* 15: 1361–1366.

Occena, R.O., Taylor, S.F., Robinson, C.C. et al. (1993). Association of cytomegalovirus with Menetrier's disease in childhood: report of two new cases with a review of literature. *J. Pediatr. Gastroenterol. Nutr.* 17: 217–224.

Ohkusa, T., Miwa, H., Hojo, M. et al. (2003). Endoscopic, histological and serologic findings of gastric hyperplastic polyps after eradication of *Helicobacter pylori*: comparison between responder and non-responder cases. *Digestion* 68: 57–62.

Oncel, M., Remzi, F.H., Church, J.M. et al. (2003). Course and follow-up of solitary Peutz–Jeghers polyps: a case series. *Int. J. Color. Dis.* 18: 33–35.

Ormarsson, O.T., Gudmundsdottir, I., and Marvik, R. (2006). Diagnosis and treatment of gastric heterotopic pancreas. *World J. Surg.* 30: 1682–1689.

Osanai, M., Miyokawa, N., Tamaki, T. et al. (2001). Adenocarcinoma arising in gastric heterotopic pancreas: clinicopathological and immunohistochemical study with genetic analysis of a case. *Pathol. Int.* 51: 549–554.

Ozolek, J.A., Sasatomi, E., Swalsky, P.A. et al. (2004). Inflammatory fibroid polyps of the gastrointestinal tract: clinical, pathologic, and molecular characteristics. *Appl. Immunohistochem. Mol. Morphol.* 12: 59–66.

Paikos, D., Moschos, J., Tzilves, D. et al. (2007). Inflammatory fibroid polyp or Vanek's tumour. *Dig. Surg.* 24: 231–233.

Pantanowitz, L., Antonioli, D.A., Pinkus, G.S. et al. (2004). Inflammatory fibroid polyps of the gastrointestinal tract: evidence for a dendritic cell origin. *Am. J. Surg. Pathol.* 28: 107–114.

Park do, Y. and Lauwers, G.Y. (2008). Gastric polyps: classification and management. *Arch. Pathol. Lab. Med.* 132: 633–640.

Pintiliciuc, O.G., Heresbach, D., de-Lajarte-Thirouard AS et al. (2008). Gastric involvement in juvenile polyposis associated with germline SMAD4 mutations: an entity characterized by a mixed hypertrophic and polypoid gastropathy. *Gastroenterol. Clin. Biol.* 32: 445–450.

Repak, R., Kohoutova, D., Podhola, M. et al. (2016). The first European family with gastric adenocarcinoma and proximal polyposis of the stomach: case report and review of the literature. *Gastrointest. Endosc.* 84: 718–725.

Rodriguez, F.J., Abraham, S.C., Allen, M.S. et al. (2004). Fine-needle aspiration cytology findings from a case of pancreatic heterotopia at the gastroesophageal junction. *Diagn. Cytopathol.* 31: 175–179.

Rothenberg, M., Pai, R., and Stuart, K. (2009). Successful use of octreotide to treat Menetrier's disease: a rare cause of abdominal pain, weight loss, edema, and hypoalbuminemia. *Dig. Dis. Sci.* 54: 1403–1407.

Ryu, D.Y., Kim, G.H., Park do, Y. et al. (2010). Endoscopic removal of gastric ectopic pancreas: an initial experience with endoscopic submucosal dissection. *World J. Gastroenterol.* 16: 4589–4593.

Salloch, H., Reinacher-Schick, A., Schulmann, K. et al. Truncating mutations in Peutz–Jeghers syndrome are associated with more polyps, surgical interventions and cancers. *Int. J. Color. Dis.* 25: 97–107.

Samarasam, I., Roberts-Thomson, J., and Brockwell, D. (2009). Gastric fundic gland polyps: a clinico-pathological study from North West Tasmania. *ANZ J. Surg.* 79: 467–470.

Samet, J.D., Horton, K.M., Fishman, E.K. et al. (2009). Cronkhite–Canada syndrome: gastric involvement diagnosed by MDCT. *Case Rep. Med.* 2009: 148795.

Sanchez, C., Brody, F., Pucci, E. et al. (2007). Laparoscopic total gastrectomy for Menetrier's disease. *J. Laparoendosc. Adv. Surg. Tech. A* 17: 32–35.

Santos Gda, C., Alves, V.A., Wakamatsu, A. et al. (2004). Inflammatory fibroid polyp: an immunohistochemical study. *Arq. Gastroenterol.* 41: 104–107.

Sekine, S., Shibata, T., Yamauchi, Y. et al. (2002). Beta-catenin mutations in sporadic fundic gland polyps. *Virchows Arch.* 440: 381–386.

Sekine, S., Shimoda, T., Nimura, S. et al. (2004). High-grade dysplasia associated with fundic gland polyposis in a familial adenomatous polyposis patient, with special reference to APC mutation profiles. *Mod. Pathol.* 17: 1421–1426.

Shalaby, M., Kochman, M.L., and Lichtenstein, G.R. (2002). Heterotopic pancreas presenting as dysphagia. *Am. J. Gastroenterol.* 97: 1046–1049.

Shand, A.G., Taylor, A.C., Banerjee, M. et al. (2002). Gastric fundic gland polyps in south-East Scotland: absence of adenomatous polyposis coli gene mutations and a strikingly low prevalence of *Helicobacter pylori* infection. *J. Gastroenterol. Hepatol.* 17: 1161–1164.

Shikata, K., Kukita, Y., Matsumoto, T. et al. (2005). Gastric juvenile polyposis associated with germline SMAD4 mutation. *Am. J. Med. Genet. A* 134: 326–329.

Song, D.E., Kwon, Y., Kim, K.R. et al. (2004). Adenocarcinoma arising in gastric heterotopic pancreas: a case report. *J. Korean Med. Sci.* 19: 145–148.

Stolte, M., Sticht, T., Eidt, S. et al. (1994). Frequency, location, and age and sex distribution of various types of gastric polyp. *Endoscopy* 26: 659–665.

Stolte, M., Vieth, M., and Ebert, M.P. (2003). High-grade dysplasia in sporadic fundic gland polyps: clinically relevant or not? *Eur. J. Gastroenterol. Hepatol.* 15: 1153–1156.

Sweet, K., Willis, J., Zhou, X.P. et al. (2005). Molecular classification of patients with unexplained hamartomatous and hyperplastic polyposis. *JAMA* 294: 2465–2473.

Takeuchi, Y., Yoshikawa, M., Tsukamoto, N. et al. (2003). Cronkhite–Canada syndrome with colon cancer, portal thrombosis, high titer of antinuclear antibodies, and membranous glomerulonephritis. *J. Gastroenterol.* 38: 791–795.

Thompson, W.M., Kende, A.I., and Levy, A.D. (2003). Imaging characteristics of gastric lipomas in 16 adult and pediatric patients. *AJR Am. J. Roentgenol.* 181: 981–985.

Tokuhara, D., Okano, Y., Asou, K. et al. (2007). Cytomegalovirus and *Helicobacter pylori* co-infection in a child with Menetrier disease. *Eur. J. Pediatr.* 166: 63–65.

Tomlinson, I.P. and Houlston, R.S. (1997). Peutz–Jeghers syndrome. *J. Med. Genet.* 34: 1007–1011.

Torbenson, M., Lee, J.H., Cruz-Correa, M. et al. (2002). Sporadic fundic gland polyposis: a clinical, histological, and molecular analysis. *Mod. Pathol.* 15: 718–723.

Toubia, N. and Schubert, M.L. (2008). Menetrier's disease. *Curr. Treat Options Gastroenterol.* 11: 103–108.

Udd, L., Katajisto, P., Rossi, D.J. et al. (2004). Suppression of Peutz–Jeghers polyposis by inhibition of cyclooxygenase-2. *Gastroenterology* 127: 1030–1037.

Vasovcak, P., Krepelova, A., Puchmajerova, A. et al. (2007). A novel mutation of PTEN gene in a patient with Cowden syndrome with excessive papillomatosis of the lips, discrete cutaneous lesions, and gastrointestinal polyposis. *Eur. J. Gastroenterol. Hepatol.* 19: 513–517.

Vieth, M. and Stolte, M. (2001). Fundic gland polyps are not induced by proton pump inhibitor therapy. *Am. J. Clin. Pathol.* 116: 716–720.

Vieth, M., Kushima, R., Borchard, F. et al. (2003). Pyloric gland adenoma: a clinico-pathological analysis of 90 cases. *Virchows Arch.* 442: 317–321.

Vinces, F.Y., Ciacci, J., Sperling, D.C. et al. (2005). Gastroduodenal intussusception secondary to a gastric lipoma. *Can. J. Gastroenterol.* 19: 107–108.

Volikos, E., Robinson, J., Aittomaki, K. et al. (2006). LKB1 exonic and whole gene deletions are a common cause of Peutz–Jeghers syndrome. *J. Med. Genet.* 43: e18.

Ward, E.M., Wolfsen, H.C., and Raimondo, M. (2003). Novel endosonographic findings in Cronkhite–Canada syndrome. *Endoscopy* 35: 464.

Watanabe, H., Jass, J.R., and Sobin, L.H. (1990). Histological typing of oesophageal and gastric tumors. In: *Histological Typing of Oesophageal and Gastric Tumors* (eds. H. Watanabe, J.R. Jass and L.H. Sobin), 34–38. Berlin: Springer-Verlag.

Watanabe, T., Kudo, M., Shirane, H. et al. (1999). Cronkhite–Canada syndrome associated with triple gastric cancers: a case report. *Gastrointest. Endosc.* 50: 688–691.

Watanabe, N., Seno, H., Nakajima, T. et al. (2002). Regression of fundic gland polyps following acquisition of *Helicobacter pylori*. *Gut* 51: 742–745.

Weston, B.R., Helper, D.J., and Rex, D.K. (2003). Positive predictive value of endoscopic features deemed typical of gastric fundic gland polyps. *J. Clin. Gastroenterol.* 36: 399–402.

Winkler, A., Hinterleitner, T.A., and Langner, C. (2007). Giant fundic gland polyp mimicking a gastric malignancy. *Endoscopy* 39 (Suppl 1): E34.

Wolfsen, H.C., Carpenter, H.A., and Talley, N.J. (1993). Menetrier's disease: a form of hypertrophic gastropathy or gastritis? *Gastroenterology* 104: 1310–1319.

Wood, M.G., Bates, C., Brown, R.C. et al. (1983). Intramucosal carcinoma of the gastric antrum complicating Menetrier's disease. *J. Clin. Pathol.* 36: 1071–1075.

Wood, L.D., Salaria, S.N., Cruise, M.W. et al. (2014). Upper GI tract lesions in familial adenomatous polyposis (FAP): enrichment of pyloric gland adenomas and other gastric and duodenal neoplasms. *Am. J. Surg. Pathol.* 38: 389–393.

Worthley, D.L., Phillips, K.D., Wayte, N. et al. (2012). Gastric adenocarcinoma and proximal polyposis of the stomach (gapps): a new autosomal dominant syndrome. *Gut* 61: 774–779.

Yamaguchi, K., Ogata, Y., Akagi, Y. et al. (2001). Cronkhite–Canada syndrome associated with advanced rectal cancer treated by a subtotal colectomy: report of a case. *Surg. Today* 31: 521–526.

Yamashita, M., Hirokawa, M., Nakasono, M. et al. (2002). Gastric inverted hyperplastic polyp. Report of four cases and relation to gastritis cystica profunda. *APMIS* 110: 717–723.

Yamashita, K., Saito, M., Itoh, M. et al. (2009). Juvenile polyposis complicated with protein losing gastropathy. *Intern. Med.* 48: 335–338.

Yao, T., Kajiwara, M., Kuroiwa, S. et al. (2002). Malignant transformation of gastric hyperplastic polyps: alteration of phenotypes, proliferative activity, and p53 expression. *Hum. Pathol.* 33: 1016–1022.

Yi, S.Y. (2007). Dyslipidemia and *H. pylori* in gastric xanthomatosis. *World J. Gastroenterol.* 13: 4598–4601.

Zak, Y., Biagini, B., Moore, H. et al. (2006). Submucosal resection of giant gastric lipoma. *J. Surg. Oncol.* 94: 63–67.

6

Gastric Neoplastic Conditions

Precursor Lesions and Early Gastric Cancer

Till S. Clauditz[1] *and Gregory Y. Lauwers*[2]

[1] *Department of Pathology, University-Medical-Center Hamburg-Eppendorf, Hamburg, Germany*
[2] *Moffitt Cancer Center, Tampa, Florida, USA*

Dysplasia in Gastric Mucosa

Definition, General Features, Predisposing Factors

Gastric dysplasia is a condition commonly diagnosed in patients over 60 years of age. The predisposing factors include chronic gastritis, intestinal metaplasia, and atrophic gastritis. It is categorized using two grades (low and high), and it is associated with an increased risk of gastric adenocarcinoma.

Progression of low-grade dysplasia occurs in approximately 25% and is very slow, whereas high-grade lesions are associated with the risk of developing adenocarcinoma in up to 85% of cases.

Currently, modern techniques such as ultrasound, chromoendoscopy, and endoscopic mucosal resection (EMR) can prevent the need for gastrectomy while securing cure.

Clinical Features and Endoscopic Characteristics (MIKE)

Patients with gastric dysplasia rarely present with clinical symptoms. Dysplasia is more common at the lesser curvature and antrum, than in the corpus.

Endoscopically, the mucosa may not always show a distinct lesion (e.g. elevated appearance) and may present only with minimal changes, compared to the normal mucosa. Thus gastric dysplasia is frequently diagnosed on random biopsies. In some cases, the fragile atypical epithelium may result in a lesion mimicking a peptic erosion/ulcer (Figure 6.1a, b).

Flat dysplasia may appear from inconspicuous to elevated mucosa with congestion and nodularity. Depressed lesions with elevated mucosal borders may develop. In all cases, the mucosal irregularity can be highlighted with chromoendoscopy- and/or magnifying-endoscopy as well as narrow-band imaging. Low-grade dysplasia tends to show an elevated profile while high-grade dysplasia is more likely to show a depressed pattern.

Microscopic Features

The typical morphologic features of dysplasia were already mentioned in the polyp section (see Chapter 5). The superficial aspect of the mucosa, foveolar and neck zone of the pits are commonly affected. Full-thickness mucosal involvement and glandular cystic changes can be observed.

Gastric dysplasia is grouped into intestinal (adenomatous) and gastric (foveolar or type II) dysplasia. Low-grade dysplasia characteristically shows limited nuclear hyperchromasia, pleomorphism, and stratification. Furthermore, atypical mitotic figures are rarely seen (Figures 6.2a and 6.3a). Overall, the architecture of the mucosa is generally preserved. On the contrary, high-grade dysplasia shows pleomorphic nuclei with irregular nuclear membrane, chromatin clearing, and prominent nucleoli. Variable degree of architectural disarray is also noted (Figures 6.2b and 6.3b). However, marked glandular crowding, budding, and intraluminal bridges should raise the question of early gastric cancer (Figure 6.4).

Differential Diagnosis

- Acute inflammation can cause reactive atypia with regenerative proliferative changes. It is important to be cautious when diagnosing high-grade dysplasia in the presence of neutrophils in the atypical epithelium. Diffuseness of the atypical changes is usually a pointer

Gastrointestinal Pathology: Correlative Endoscopic and Histologic Assessment, First Edition. Edited by Gregory Y. Lauwers and Michael B. Wallace.

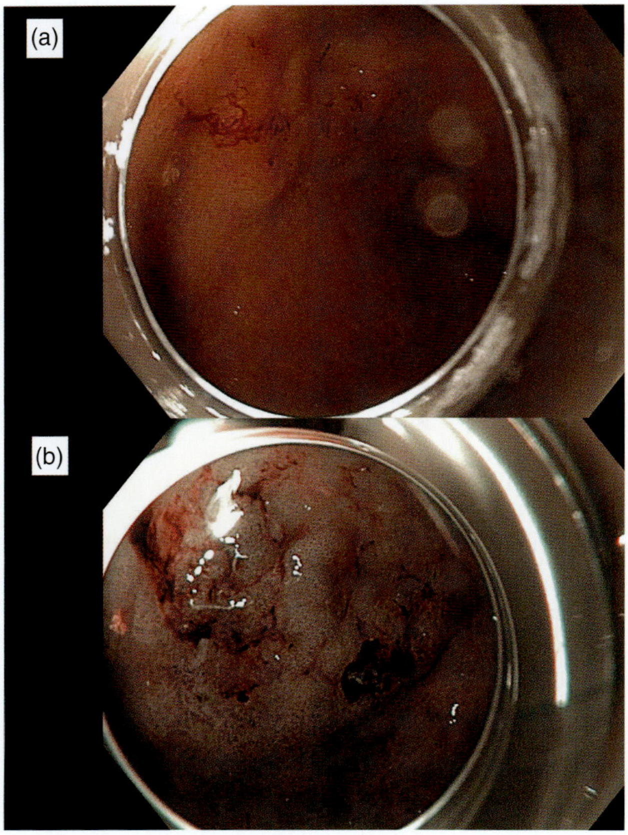

Figure 6.1 Focal gastric neoplasia on lesser curvature of antrum shown in white light (a) and narrow-band imaging (b). The lesion is slightly raised and nodular with increased friability. A following endoscopic submucosal dissection revealed low-grade dysplasia.

for reactive atypia along with seamless transition to the surrounding normal epithelium

- Chemical (reactive) gastritis can cause reactive atypia as well. However, stromal changes such as edema, ectatic superficial capillaries, proliferation, and foveolar hyperplasia with few inflammatory cells can be seen.
- Chemoradiotherapy-related atypia can present severe microscopic changes, but is easily distinguishable by finding atypia in both superficial and deep epithelial components but also in the stroma. Withering microcystic glands and eosinophilic transformation of the cytoplasm may be present as well. Compared to dysplasia, the proliferative activity of reactive atypia is confined to the proliferative zone, i.e. deep foveolae. Furthermore, maturation of the surface epithelium is commonly detected.

In general, some helpful features are the evaluation of the glandular architecture, which is preserved in cases of inflammation or reactive changes. Furthermore, reactive atypia shows round-shaped hyperchromatic nuclei with regular membrane and is located in the center or the base of the cell. The cells are more cuboidal in shape. In the settings of erosion or ulceration, the grading of atypia can be challenging. Findings like fibrin, granulation tissue, and ulcer slough are helpful.

Prognosis, Evolution, and Clinical Management

In case of low-grade dysplasia, progression to invasive carcinoma is slow and occurs in 25% of cases. In cases of the first diagnosis, immediate re-biopsies are recommended to

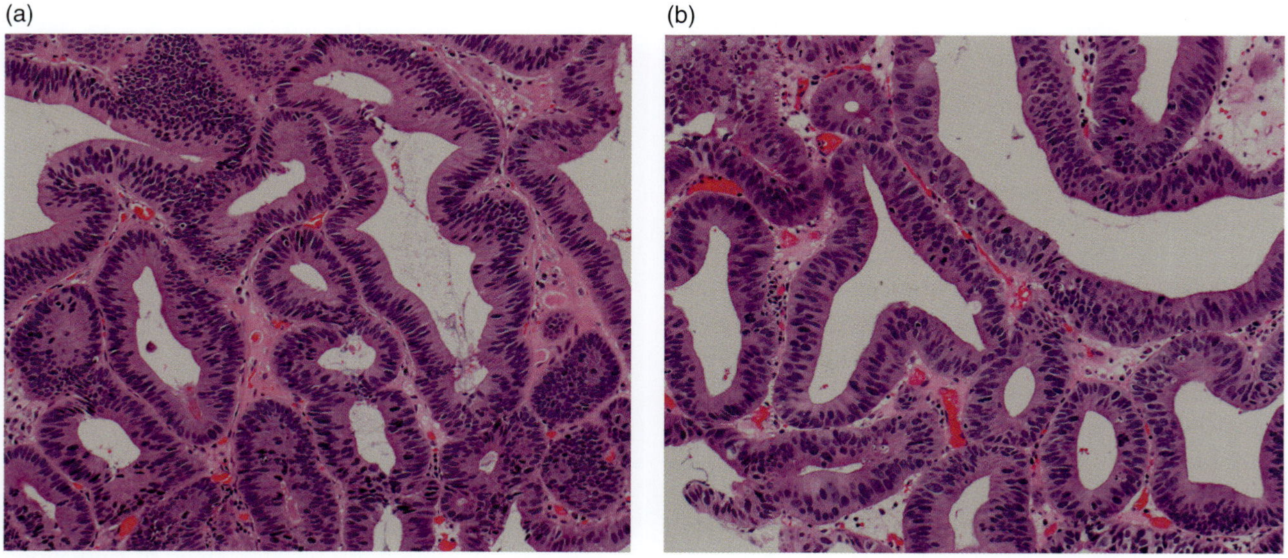

Figure 6.2 Intestinal/adenomatous type dysplasia. (a) Low-grade: It shows limited nuclear hyperchromasia, pleomorphism, and stratification. The architecture is generally preserved. (b) On the contrary, high-grade dysplasia shows pleomorphic nuclei with chromatin clearing, prominent nucleoli as well as architectural disarray.

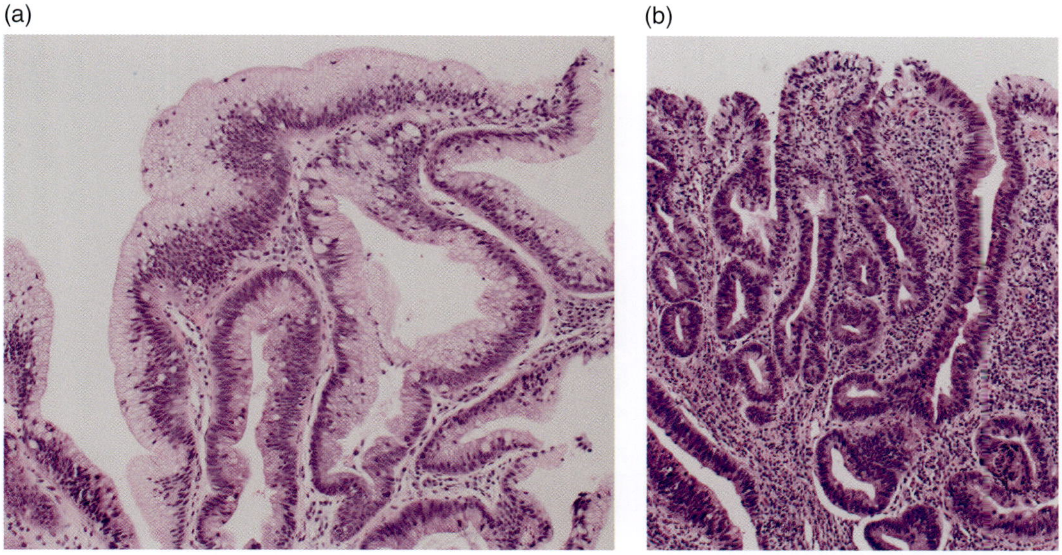

Figure 6.3 Gastric/foveolar/type 2 dysplasia. (a) Low-grade: The lesion displays a papillary architecture and is lined by tall columnar foveolar type cells with low N/C ratio. (b) In high-grade dysplasia, the hyperchromatic nuclei are prominent. The foveolar nature of the epithelium is more challenging but the presence of supranuclear mucin cups is an helpful clue.

exclude carcinoma. This procedure should be followed by biannual endoscopic examinations and annual examination after two negative follow-up biopsies.

With high-grade dysplasia or suspected T1 carcinoma, en bloc endosocpic resection by ESD is warranted. High-resolution, image-enhanced endoscopy (e.g. narrow-band imaging) or equivalent dye-based chromoendoscopy (e.g. indigo carmine) should be used order to precisely localize and estimate depth of invasion. The lesion boundaries should be marked with cautery and followed immediately by ESD (Figure 6.4).

Early Gastric Cancer

Definition, General Features, Predisposing Factors

Adenocarcinomas related to mucosa, lamina muscularis mucosae (pT1a), and submucosa (pT1b) are defined as early gastric cancers and are associated with five-year overall survival of approximately 95%.

Clinical Features and Endoscopic Characteristics

Endoscopically, protruded (type I) early gastric cancer presents as polypoid, nodular, or villous neoplasia. The superficial (type II) early gastric cancer is limited to the plane of the mucosa and only recognized by the presence irregularity/granularity of the mucosal surface. A subclassification system of type IIa (elevated), IIb (flat), and IIc (depressed) has been established. The excavated (type III) early gastric cancer presents as an ulcer. Pure type III cancer is rare (<1%) and appears as a large lesion and shows, contrary to peptic ulcers, rigid, pale, and sloping borders. In practice, most early gastric cancers present mixed lesions. Early gastric cancers are macroscopically classified in three types (protruded, superficial, and depressed). Nodular positivity is low (approximately 7%) in intramucosal cancer (pT1a) and leads to EMR as first-line therapy. Accurate analysis of EMR specimen is of paramount importance to prevent further unnecessary surgical intervention. Deep submucosal and/or lympho-vascular infiltration as well as positive deep margins commonly leads to further surgical treatment.

Microscopic Features

The majority of early gastric cancers are well-differentiated glandular carcinomas.

Type I and IIa more likely to show tubular and papillary architecture represent 52 and 37% of cases, respectively), whereas types IIc and III are more often poorly differentiated (solid or poorly cohesive adenocarcinomas that represent 26 and 14% of cases, respectively) (Figure 6.5).

In type III cancers, the neoplastic elements reach the edge of the ulcer, whereas reactive changes of a chronic peptic ulcer (e.g. scar dense lymphoid infiltrate, endarteritis, fusion of muscularis mucosae and propria) can grossly mimic an invasive adenocarcinoma (Figure 6.5 expand text).

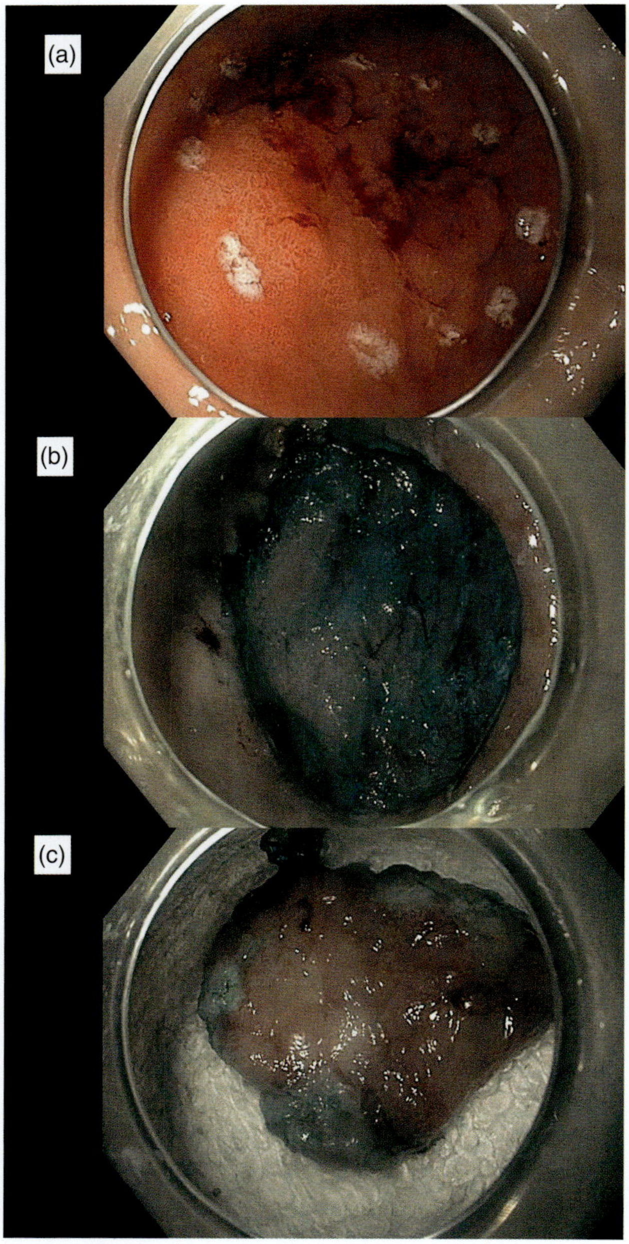

Figure 6.4 When a diagnosis of high-grade dysplasia or T1 carcinoma is made or suspected, en bloc endoscopic resection by ESD is warranted. High-resolution, image-enhanced endoscopy (a) or equivalent dye-based chromoendoscopy (b) used in order to localize precisely the boundaries of the lesion before resection (c).

Prognosis, Evolution, and Clinical Management

Prognostic parameters are depth of invasion, involvement of vessels, or the presence of lymph node metastasis, which is common in cases of submucosal infiltration. Furthermore, approximately 10% patients show second tumor manifestations (synchronous or metachronous). Therefore a precise endoscopic workup before surgical intervention is important.

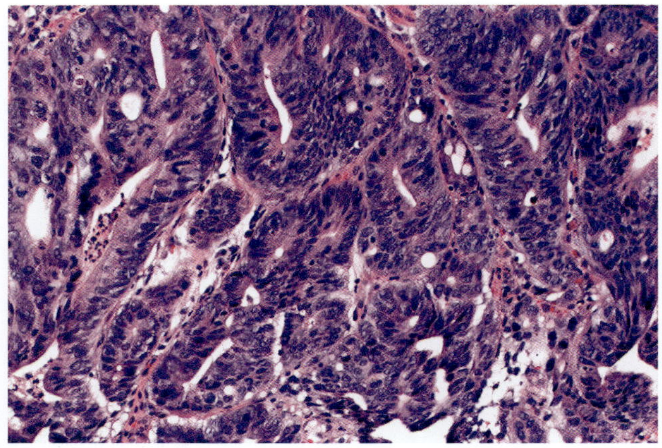

Figure 6.5 Well-differentiated intramucosal adenocarcinoma. This example is differentiated from high-grade dysplasia by the marked glandular crowding and intraluminal bridges.

Adenocarcinoma of the Stomach

Definition, General Features, Predisposing Factors

Adenocarcinoma of the stomach is the most common malignancy and worldwide the third most common malignancy causing death. It affects men more frequently than women. A higher incidence of gastric adenocarcinoma is noted in Japan, Korea, Central America and parts of South America.

Predisposing factors for the development are low socioeconomic status, high intake of salt and dried or pickled foods, and smoking and alcohol consumption. Preventive effect has been reported for Vitamin C, vegetables, carotenoids, and green tea. Although most gastric cancers are sporadic, familial association can be found in approximately 10% of cases. Several germ line mutations have been associated with an increased risk of gastric cancer (see Table 6.1) and are divided into polyp-associated syndromes or hereditary gastric cancer syndromes without polyposis. The most common syndrome is hereditary diffuse gastric cancer (HDGC) associated in most cases with germline mutation of the CDH1 gene locus (E-cadherin).

Several benign conditions such as chronic gastritis (*Helicobacter pylori* associated or autoimmune) with or without intestinal metaplasia, post-surgery (e.g. gastric stump), adenomas, and Ménétrier's disease are known to be associated with development of gastric cancer. In case of chronic *H. pylori* infection, cytotoxin-associated gene (CagA) and vacuolating cytotoxin VacA play a role in the

Table 6.1 An overview of familial syndromes associated with an increased risk of gastric cancer.

Familial syndrome	Inheritance	Affected gene	Risk of gastric cancer
Hereditary diffuse gastric cancer syndrome (HDGC)	Autosomal dominant	CDH1	80%
Hereditary nonpolyposis colon cancer (HNPCC)	Autosomal dominant	MLH1, MSH2, MSH6, PMS2	2–30%
Peutz–Jeghers syndrome	Autosomal dominant	STK11	29%
Juvenile polyposis	Autosomal dominant	SMAD4 BMPR1A	21%
Familial breast cancer	Autosomal dominant	BRCA1 BRCA2	5.5% 2.6%
Li–Fraumeni syndrome	Autosomal dominant	TP53	3.1–4.9%
Familial adenomatous polyposis (FAP)	Autosomal dominant	APC	2.1–4.2%
MYH-associated polyposis	Autosomal recessive	MYH	Very low
Gastric adenocarcinoma and proximal polyposis syndrome (GAPPS)	Autosomal dominant	APC	Unknown

development of gastric cancer. Epstein–Barr virus (EBV) is another infectious agent associated with the development of gastric cancer.

A commonly used classification of gastric adenocarcinoma is the Laurén's classification. It delineates two different tumor types (intestinal and diffuse) with totally different etiology and histopathology. The intestinal type adenocarcinomas are known to be strongly associated with chronic gastritis, intestinal metaplasia as well as geographic differences, which are not reported for diffuse type gastric cancer. Furthermore, intestinal and diffuse type gastric cancers show different dissemination patterns. Intestinal type cancer mainly spreads via the lympho-vascular system while diffuse type cancers are more commonly identified with peritoneal tumor spread.

Clinical Features and Endoscopic Characteristics

Gastric adenocarcinoma mainly arises in antrum and at the lesser curvature, but involvement of the whole stomach is not uncommon. Patients may present several different symptoms ranging from dyspepsia, anorexia, and weight loss to hemorrhage or obstruction. Patients with peptic ulcer-like symptoms frequent the group that is most frequently diagnosed with early gastric cancer.

Endoscopically advanced cancer can present different growth patterns like polypoid, fungating, ulcerated or with the appearance of linitis plastica. Antral and lesser curvature tumors commonly show ulceration, comparable with peptic ulcers. The borders of ulcerative cancer have a more irregularly shaped benign ulcer with elevated rolled edges. In the gastric body polypoid and fungating lesions, sometimes present as ill-defined ulcerated plaque.

Microscopic Features

Adenocarcinomas of the stomach can show several different growth patterns like tubular, acinar, (micro)papillary, and poorly cohesive patterns. Cytologically, the neoplasia can present with gastric or intestinal type differentiation. Parietal, endocrine, chief, and Paneth cells may be detected as well. The WHO classification organizes gastric carcinoma in four different predominant growth patterns (papillary, tubular, mucinous, and poorly cohesive [including signet ring cells]), whereas the papillary as well as tubular subtypes are divided into a three-tier grading system (well, moderately, and poorly differentiated).

Tubular adenocarcinoma predominantly shows neoplastic tubules with irregular branching and anastomosing of the tubules (Figures 6.6 and 6.7). A mucinous component may be detected. The diagnosis of mucinous adenocarcinoma is characterized by the amount extracellular mucin representing more than 50% of the tumor. Therefore, mucinous adenocarcinoma is more likely to be diagnosed on surgical specimen than on biopsies (Figure 6.8).

Papillary adenocarcinoma shows prominent papillae with fibrovascular cores. Furthermore, a micropapillary growth pattern can be recognized, which shows morules like cell clusters occupying lacunar spaces (that should not be misconstrued for lymphatic invasion or stromal retraction). Adenocarcinomas with micropapillary differentiation reveal a more aggressive behavior than standard adenocarcinoma with a high incidence of lymphovascular invasion and nodal metastasis.

Carcinomas of the poorly cohesive type are defined to be composed of isolated cells or small tumor cell clusters. The cytologic features may vary and can resemble lymphocytes, mimic histiocytes, or present with signet ring cells (Figure 6.9). Signet ring cells are defined by intracellular

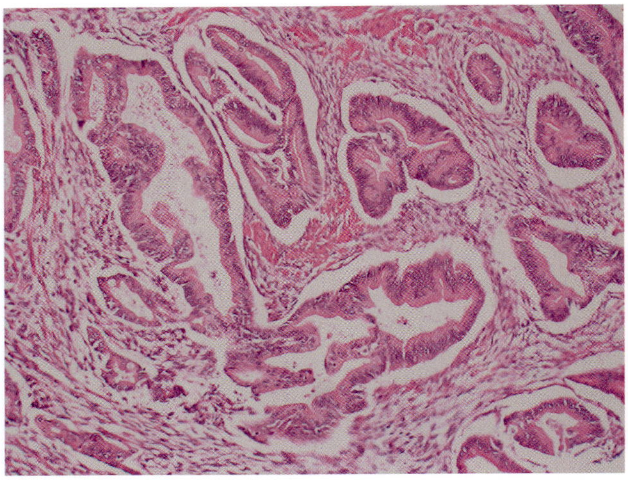

Figure 6.6 Well-differentiated adenocarcinoma of tubular type. The neoplasm is composed of infiltrative well-formed neoplastic glands.

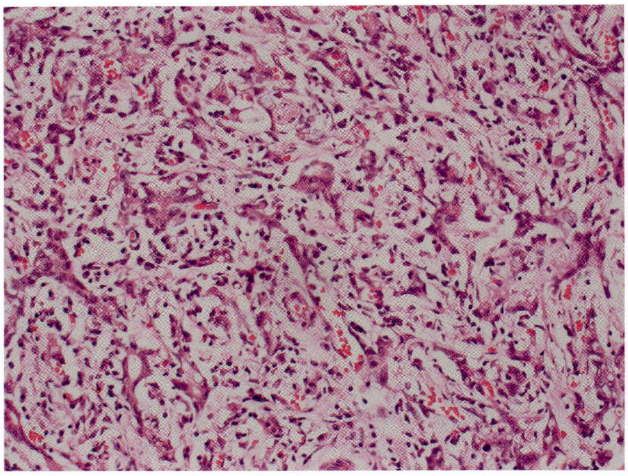

Figure 6.7 Poorly differentiated adenocarcinoma of tubular type. It shows anastomosing poorly formed glandular structures and epithelial cords.

mucin vacuoles, which can be highlighted by Alcian Blue or mucicarmine stains. Comparable to mucinous carcinoma, the cutoff for the diagnosis of a signet ring cell carcinoma is >50% of tumor cells must be present. Additionally, signet ring cell carcinoma can show marked fibrotic stromal changes causing the so-called linitis plastica.

Besides tubular adenocarcinoma with oncocytic differentiation, several other rare histomorphological subtypes were defined according to the WHO classification as shown in Table 6.2.

Despite the updated WHO classification, the Lauren classification remains commonly used in daily practice. It recognizes two types, the intestinal and diffuse type of gastric adenocarcinoma.

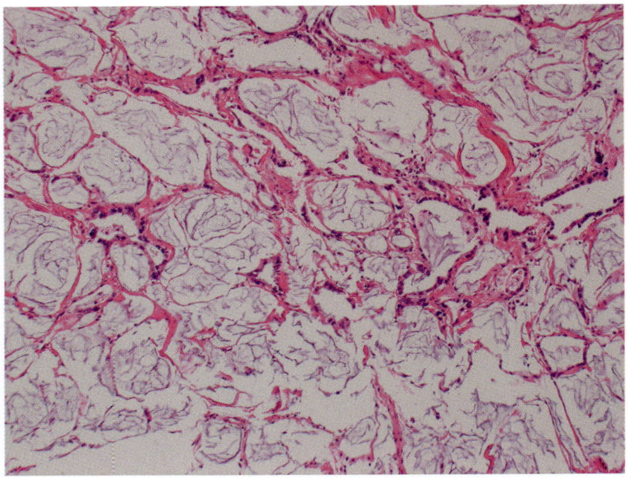

Figure 6.8 Mucinous adenocarcinoma with limited epithelial elements noted at the periphery of the mucinous pools.

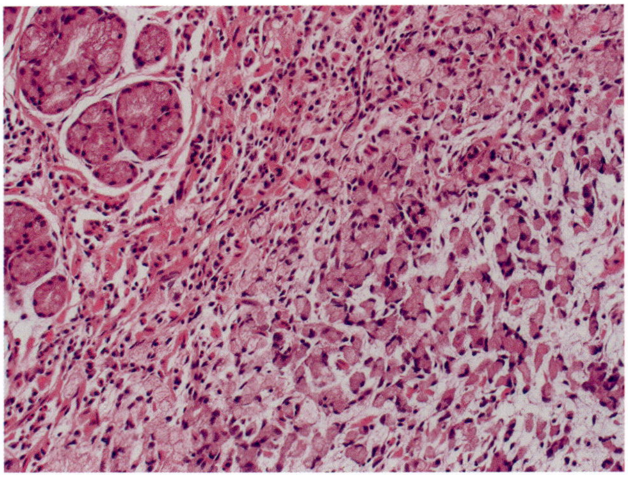

Figure 6.9 Signet ring cell gastric adenocarcinoma composed of individual signet ring tumor cells.

The intestinal type adenocarcinoma is characterized by glandular/tubular structures, which may also present papillary and solid areas. The cytologic component is composed of intestinal type columnar cells and scattered mucin-rich goblet cells. Intestinal type carcinoma shows "pushing" invasive front and the background mucosa classically shows chronic inflammatory changes with or without intestinal metaplasia and dysplasia.

Alternatively, the diffuse type adenocarcinoma shows scattered discohesive or clusters of tumor cells. Glandular differentiation is an uncommon finding. The tumors are poorly demarcated with a ragged infiltrative border with high budding density. The neoplasm is believed to arise from the proliferative foveolar zone located in the gastric pits. Pagetoid spread of tumor cells in gastric foveolae may be observed.

Table 6.2 An overview of rare gastric malignancies with short histological description and other characteristic features.

Subtype	Histology	Special studies	Other
Gastric carcinoma with lymphoid stroma (medullary carcinoma) (Figure 6.10)	Poorly differentiated tubular and/or solid growth; dense lymphoplasmacytic infiltrate; lymphoid follicles and rare giant cells may be present	EBV-positive >80% CD8+ T cells > B cells	Improved survival overexpression/ amplification of PD-L1/L2
Gastric carcinoma with extensive neutrophilic infiltration	Anaplastic tumor with highly pleomorphic discohesive tumor cells embedded in numerous neutrophils	Interleukin-8 production of tumor affects neutrophils	
Adenosquamous	Either the adenocarcinoma or squamous represent at least 25% of the tumor		
Squamous cell carcinoma	Vary from moderately to poorly differentiated with/ without keratinization	Usually late stage diagnosis	Exclusion of metastasis (e.g. esophagus), mapping to exclude adenocarcinoma component
Gastric adenocarcinoma of fundic gland type	Limited to oxyntic mucosa; composed of chief and parietal cells lining anastomosing tubules and glands	MUC6, pepsinogen-I (gastric phenotype), and H+/K+ ATPase positive CD10 and MUC2 negative	Activation Wnt/β-catenin signaling pathway and mutations in GNAS
Hepatoid adenocarcinoma (Figure 6.11)	Large polygonal eosinophilic cells resembling hepatocytes, bile production	Diastase PAS granules present, AFP positive by IHC and serum positive	AFP can also be positive in well-differentiated tubule-papillary carcinoma and yolk sac carcinoma
Carcinoma with rhabdoid features	Diffuse or alveolar growth pattern; poorly cohesive pleomorphic polygonal cells with vesicular nucleus and prominent nucleoli; abundant eosinophilic cytoplasm; paranuclear inclusion	Vimentin, cytokeratin and NSE positive AFP negative	Homogenous neoplasm or mixed with adenocarcinoma; poor prognosis
Carcinosarcoma	Adenocarcinoma in combination with spindle-cell sarcomatoid areas; osteo-, rhabdomyo-, leiomyo-, and/ or chondrosarcomatous differentiation may be present	Mainly located in pyloric region	Rare Poor prognosis
Choriocarcinoma	Composed of malignant syncytiotrophoblast and cytotrophoblast with hemorrhage and otherwise conventional adenocarcinoma	Embryonal carcinoma or yolk sac elements may be present	Rare; disseminated hematogenous and lymphatic metastases are common.

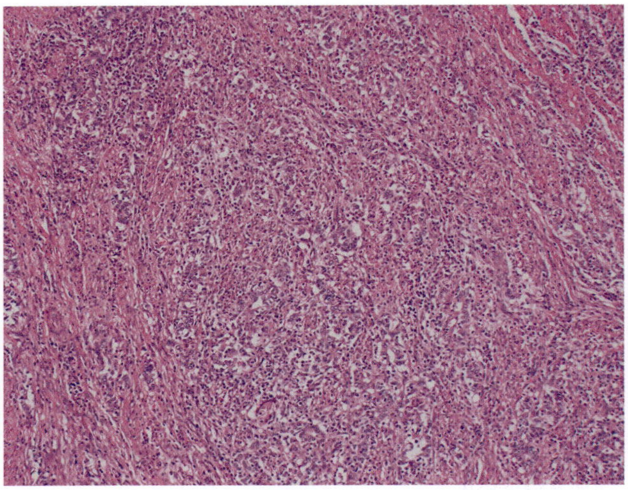

Figure 6.10 EBER-positive gastric adenocarcinoma. Marked lymphocytic infiltrate obscures the epithelial component in this example.

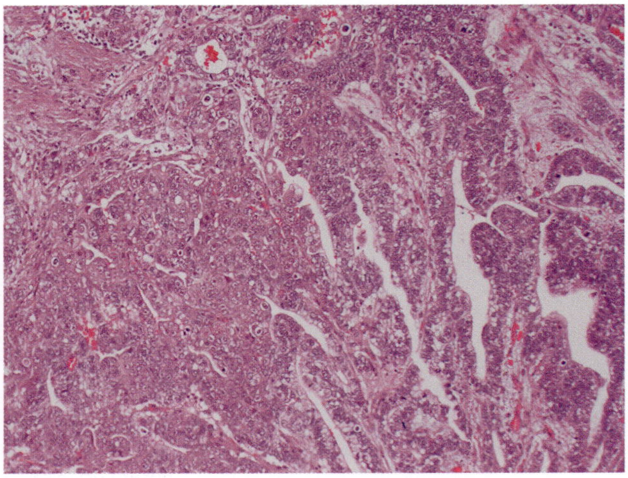

Figure 6.11 AFP-producing gastric adenocarcinoma. Large polygonal eosinophilic cells resembling hepatocytes as well as well-differentiated tubule-papillary component are observed.

Up to 15% of gastric adenocarcinomas are mixed and composed of intestinal and diffuse elements and are categorized as intermediate type.

Immunohistochemical Studies and Molecular Features

In general, gastric adenocarcinomas show a strong and diffuse immunoreactivity for CK7. Moderate to strong nuclear staining for CDX2 may also be present. Papillary adenocarcinoma shows a typical inside-out staining pattern with EMA.

Especially for therapeutic options, HER2 immunohistochemistry is recommended when evaluating gastric adenocarcinomas. A scoring system has been established by Rüschoff et al. with recommendations for surgical and biopsy specimen (see Table 6.3). In case of ambivalent 2+ immunohistochemical staining, additional sliver or fluorescence in situ hybridization is recommended.

Differential Diagnosis

Several benign conditions can cause an overinterpretation on small biopsy fragments. For example, erosive or ulcerative mucosal changes can cause reactive epithelial hyperplasia with regenerative atypia and frequent metastases. Fibrin exudate, reactive fibroblasts, and atypical endothelial cells may also be misleading. Caution is the rule, particularly for patients with long-standing ulcer disease, after radiotherapy or when ulcerated polyps are biopsied.

Table 6.3 Recommendations of HER2 immunohistochemical interpretation.

Score	Surgical specimen-staining pattern	Biopsy specimen-staining pattern	HER2 overexpression assessment
0	No membranous reactivity in <10% of tumor cells	No membranous reactivity in any cell	Negative
1+	Faint/barely perceptible membranous reactivity in ≥10% of tumor cells; cells are reactive only in part of their membrane	Tumor cell cluster with a faint/barely perceptible membranous reactivity irrespective of percentage of tumor cells stained	Negative
2+	Weak to moderate complete, basolateral, or lateral membranous reactivity in ≥10% of tumor cells	Tumor cell cluster with a weak to moderate complete, basolateral, or lateral membranous reactivity irrespective of percentage of tumor cells stained	Equivocal
3+	Strong complete, basolateral, or lateral membranous reactivity in ≥10% of tumor cells	Tumor cell cluster with a strong complete, basolateral, or lateral membranous reactivity irrespective of percentage of tumor cells stained	Positive

Source: From Rüschoff, J., Hanna, W., Bilous, M. et al. (2012). HER2 testing in gastric cancer: a practical approach. *Modern Pathology* 25 (5): 637–650. © 2012 Springer Nature.

Table 6.4 Immunohistochemical panel for mimickers of poorly cohesive gastric adenocarcinoma.

Mimicker	IHC
Muciphages	CD68, CD163
Malignant melanoma	HMB45, SOX10, Melan-A
Lobular breast cancer	CK7, estrogen- and progesterone-receptor, GCDFP
Malignant lymphoma	CD45, CD20, CD3 etc.
GIST	DOG1, CD117

In case of poorly cohesive carcinomas, the neoplastic cells ought to be distinguished from mucin-containing macrophages. Macrophages have vesicular nuclei with one or more small nucleoli, contrary to the neoplastic nuclei that are larger with irregular nuclear membrane, hyperchromasia, and bigger nucleoli.

PAS/D-PAS stains may be positive in both benign and malignant cell types and are not helpful. Immunohistochemistry is more appropriate to distinguish the cell differentiation and to rule out discohesive tumor cells for mimicking macrophages, lymphocytes, or plasma cells.

Other malignancies mimicking poorly cohesive adenocarcinomas can be observed, including malignant melanoma; gastrointestinal stromal tumor (GIST); lymphoma; and lobular carcinoma of the breast, which can easily be distinguished by proper use of an immunohistochemical panels (see Table 6.4). It is important to know that signet ring cell carcinomas are positive for CK20 in up to 65% of the cases and CK7 positivity is found in only 20% of cases. CK7 positive cells are usually CK20 negative. Finally, metastasis of hepatocellular carcinoma can present the same histomorphology and immunohistochemical expression pattern as hepatoid gastric adenocarcinoma. In such cases, a thorough clinical workup is needed to distinguish these entities from each other.

Prognosis, Evolution, and Clinical Management

Gastric adenocarcinoma generally caries a poor prognosis unless detected at early stages. In countries where general screening is performed (Japan, Korea), such early T1a cancers can be treated curatively by endoscopic submucosal resection. Specific strict and expanded criteria have been set by Asian societies, which include differentiated (G1 or 2), superficially invasive (T1a or superficial T1b), negative deep and lateral margins, and absence of lymphovascular invasion. In such cases, lymphatic and vascular metastases are rare. Close coordination between endoscopists and pathologist is critical. Typically endoscopic specimens are mounted on a flat (paraffin) surface with pins to orient the lesion and allow margin assessment.

For more advanced lesions, total gastrectomy is typically warranted, even for palliative purposes in advanced (stage 4) cancers since local complications of unresected tumors, such as obstruction and bleeding, carry very high morbidity.

Neuroendocrine Tumors

Definition, General Features, Predisposing Factors

Neuroendocrine tumors (NETs) of the stomach represent approximately 9% of all diagnosed gastrointestinal NETs and are less than 2% of all gastric malignant neoplasia. They most commonly arise in middle-aged patients. Most NETs are categorized in three types, based on the clinicopathologic features. Most NETs are low-grade neoplasms arising from enterochromaffin-like cells (ECL cell) located in the gastric body oxyntic mucosa. ECL-cell proliferation is usually triggered by hypergastrinemia caused by autoimmune chronic atrophic gastritis (type I), Zollinger–Ellison syndrome/MEN1 (type II), and secondary by achlorhydria (type IV).

Sporadic (type III) NETs that commonly present as large solitary masses are not associated to hypergastrinemia or ECL-cell hyperplasia.

Clinical Features and Endoscopic Characteristics

As noted, most NETs arise as multiple asymptomatic lesions caused by hypergastrinemia. Sporadic cases are less common, are larger, and show a more aggressive behavior. Symptoms caused by atypical hormone secretion of are uncommon.

In general, the gastric primary NETs are small, slowly growing masses with local infiltrative growth pattern. Cases smaller than 1 cm rarely metastasize. Tumor size, involvement of vessels or muscularis mucosae, grade of atypia, and mitotic frequency affect a worse tumor behavior.

Endoscopically, NETs present well-defined nodules or polypoid lesions of the mucosa, whereas larger tumors may present with ulceration. The background mucosa may show atrophic changes in case of type I and prominent folds for type II and IV respectively.

Microscopic Features

NETs can present several growth patterns, i.e. trabecular, nested/nodular, or mixed (Figure 6.12a). They are composed of small uniform cuboidal cells embedded in loose

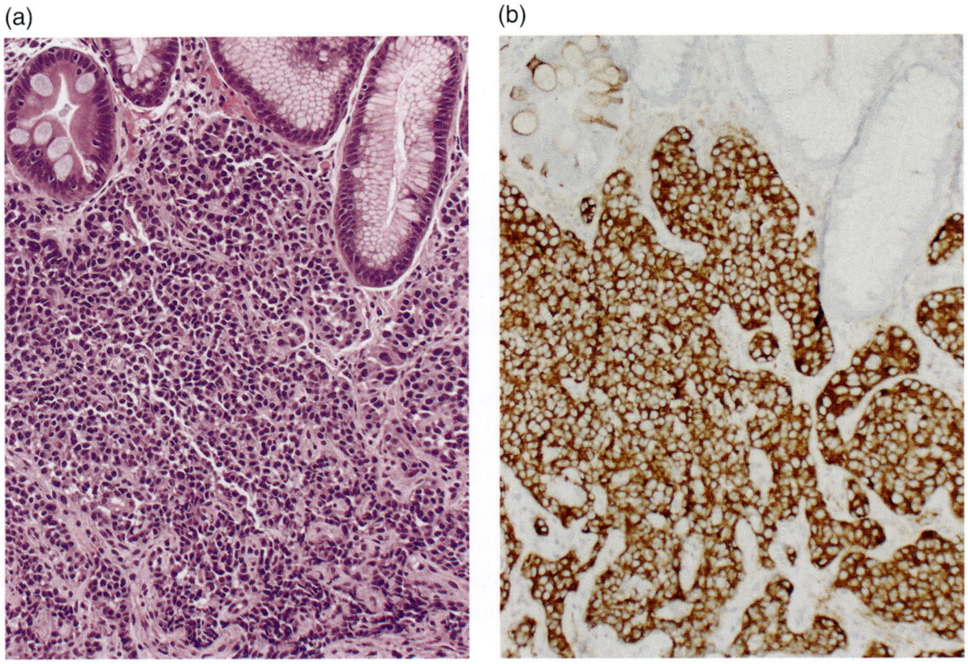

Figure 6.12 Low-grade NET (a) showing a mixed trabecular and nested growth pattern. The cuboidal neoplastic cells are uniform with a light eosinophilic cytoplasm. (b) Synaptophysin immunohistochemical stain confirms the diagnosis.

stroma. Rosettes, tubules, or acinar structures are commonly seen. The cells present with a light eosinophilic cytoplasm with a small round to oval nuclei with dispersed chromatin. Rarely, mitotic figures and nuclear pleomorphism are noted. Retraction artifacts may be present.

ECL cells observed in the background gastric mucosa usually show nodular or linear hyperplasia that may extend into the lamina propria. The diagnosis of adenomatoid ECL-cell hyperplasia is defined by a cluster of five cells. When these micronodules enlarge and fuse, they are defined as dysplastic (with a size up to 0.5 mm). Larger nodules are referred as NETs.

Type I NETs arise in a background of atrophic mucosa with intestinal and/or pyloric pseudo-metaplasia. Type II NETs maybe surrounded by thickened folds with foveolar and oxyntic hyperplasia.

Immunohistochemical Studies and Molecular Features

NETs are consistently positive for synaptophysin and chromogranin A. Hormone stains such as serotonin, gastrin, ghrelin, somatostatin, pancreatic polypeptide, glucagon, calcitonin, and α-human chorionic gonadotropin (α-HCG) may be detected (Figure 6.12b).

Appropriate tumor grading necessitates mitotic count and immunohistochemical staining for Ki67 and counting of at least 500 cells focusing on the hot spot area (see Table 6.5).

Table 6.5 The grading system of NET according to the WHO.

Neuroendocrine tumor grade	Mitoses (per 10 HPFs)[a]	Ki67 proliferation index (%)[b]
1	<2	<3
2	2–20	3–20
3	>20	>20

[a] Mitotic count of at least 50 HPFs; 1 HPF = 2 mm^2.
[b] MIB1 antibody; percentage of 500–2000 counted tumor cells in the areas of highest labeling ("hot spot").

Differential Diagnosis

In practice, glomus tumor, a rare benign mesenchymal neoplasm arising from a glomus body, could be considered. Glomus tumors are small submucosal tumors and are frequently mistaken for the more common gastrointestinal stromal tumors (GISTs) (that could also be considered in the differential diagnosis). Immunohistochemical stains can help guide the diagnosis since the tumor cells are actin and calponin positive but chromogranin, synaptophysin, and CD117 negative.

Prognosis, Evolution, and Clinical Management

Tumor management depends on the NET type. In case of type I and type II NET, patients can be managed conservatively, as endoscopic excision. In cases of multiple tumors of large tumor size, gastrectomy could be considered. Coincidental gastrinoma in cases of type II NET should be removed surgically.

Potentially aggressive sporadic NETs (type III) should be treated with endoscopic excision or partial/total gastrectomy, depending on their size.

NECs are more often diagnosed in advanced tumor disease and are linked with a poor prognosis. The mean survival is reported to be less than one year.

Neuroendocrine Carcinoma

Definition, General Features, and Predisposing Factors

Gastric neuroendocrine carcinomas are malignant tumors composed of cells with neuroendocrine differentiation. They account for less than 2% of gastric neoplasms and are associated with a dismal prognosis. There are two main morphologic variants: small cell and large cell types. They are more common in males. Most affected patients are in the sixth to seventh decade of life.

Clinical Features and Endoscopic Characteristics

NECs usually present as a large and symptomatic neoplasms. Complaints may include epigastric pain, gastrointestinal bleeding, or weight loss. NECs are more frequent in the proximal stomach. Gastric NECs have a mean size of about 5–6.0 cm. In most cases, NECs present as solitary fungating tumor.

Microscopic Features

The majority of NECs show a solid growth pattern composed of solid nests or sheets. Trabecular pattern, scirrhous and tubular growth patterns can also be seen.

The lesions are composed of anaplastic cells that range in shape from round, to polyhedral and spindle with scant cytoplasm. Mitoses and apoptosis are conspicuous.

Large cell NECs represent the most common type. They are defined by the presence of large polygon-shaped cells with abundant cytoplasm with enlarged vesicular nuclei and prominent nucleoli. Rosettes and pseudo-rosettes are common (Figure 6.13). Mucin positivity can be detected in large cell NECs.

Small cell NECs are characterized by high nuclear/cytoplasmic ratio and scant cytoplasm and nuclear molding is common (but rare in large cell variant). However, both histologic variants are usually mixed.

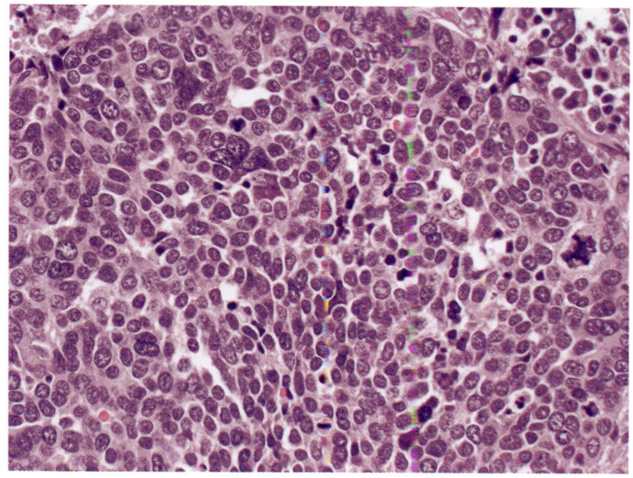

Figure 6.13 Large cell neuroendocrine carcinoma composed of solid sheet of round anaplastic cells. Mitoses and apoptosis are conspicuous.

In most cases, ECL-cell hyperplasia is not detected at the periphery of NEC.

Composite tumors, which are defined as tumors composed of both neuroendocrine and non-neuroendocrine epithelial elements, are common. MANECs are defined as mixed carcinomas in which each element consists of at least 30% of the tumor volume. In most instances, adenocarcinoma component is poorly differentiated.

Immunohistochemical Features

NECs can show immunohistochemical reactivity for chromogranin A, synaptophysin and CD-56. Other peptide hormones, such as serotonin, ghrelin, peptide YY, somatostatin, and gastrin can be demonstrated.

Differential Diagnosis

Poorly differentiated adenocarcinoma, lymphoma, and metastatic malignant melanoma and poorly differentiated squamous cell carcinoma can mimic a NEC. Appropriate use of immunohistochemistry, such as CD45, PAX10, and CK5/6, among others will be useful.

Prognosis, Evolution, and Clinical Management

NEC commonly presents at an advanced stage. Lymphovascular involvement is common in NEC as well as nodal metastases. Early NECS are rare.

Gastrectomy with lymphadenectomy represents the first approach when it can be tolerated by the patient. Platinum-based combination chemotherapy is also commonly used as a first-line treatment for gastric NEC. New combination of irinotecan (anti-angiogenic inhibitor) to cisplatin and amrubicin monotherapy has been proposed.

An exception to this is the type 1 gastric NEC, which occurs in the setting of chronic atrophic gastritis. In this case, the achlorhydric state drives high gastrin production of gastric G-cells, which in turn causes hypertropy of the enterochromaffin cells and low-grade carcinoids. In this setting, there is a very low rate of metastases. Type 1 gastric carcinoids are managed by endoscopic resection of larger (>5–10 mm) lesions and surveillance of smaller lesions.

Nonepithelial Tumors

Gastrointestinal Stroma Tumor (GIST)

Definition, General Features, Predisposing Factors

Gastrointestinal stromal tumors are primary gastric mesenchymal neoplasm, either spindle or epithelioid in appearance and are believed to arise from a precursor of the cells of Cajal. They were believed to be all characterized by ovexpression of tyrosine kinase growth factor receptor KIT (CD117). Over the last few years, additional molecular alterations of several genes have been associated with these neoplasms, including platelet-derived growth factor receptor-α (PDGFRA), BRAF mutation, and SDH.

Clinical Features and Endoscopic Characteristics

The gender distribution of GIST is uniform, whereas affected patients are usually over 30 years of age. GISTs are rare in the pediatric group.

Few patients have inherited predisposing conditions like type 1 neurofibromatosis (showing multiple GIST of the small intestine), or Carney triad (GIST, pulmonary chondroma and/or extra-adrenal paraganglioma) as well as Carney–Stratakis syndrome (GIST + paraganglioma). Few families with KIT or PDGFRA germ line mutations have been reported.

Clinical presentation is broad, ranging from asymptomatic in case of small tumors to hemorrhage or abdominal pain for larger lesions. Infiltrative growth into adjacent organs or structures as well as peritoneal spread may be present. Hematogenous spread may occur and cause distant metastasis. The tumor progression of GIST is related to tumor size, location as well as mitotic count (see Table 6.6).

Table 6.6 Risk stratification of gastric gastrointestinal stromal tumors using tumor size and mitotic activity.

Risk of progression	Tumor characteristics: Size (cm)	Tumor characteristics: Mitotic rate (per 50 HPF[a])	Percentage of patients with progressive disease
Very low	≤2	≤5	0
	>2 to ≤5	≤5	1.9
Low	>5 to ≤10	≤5	3.6
	≤2	≥5	[b]
Intermediate	>10	≤5	10
	>2 to ≤5	>5	16
High	>5 to ≤10	>5	55
	>10	>5	86

[a] High-power field (HPF) of approximately 0.2 mm^2.
[b] Very few cases analyzed to be certain of the clinical outcome.

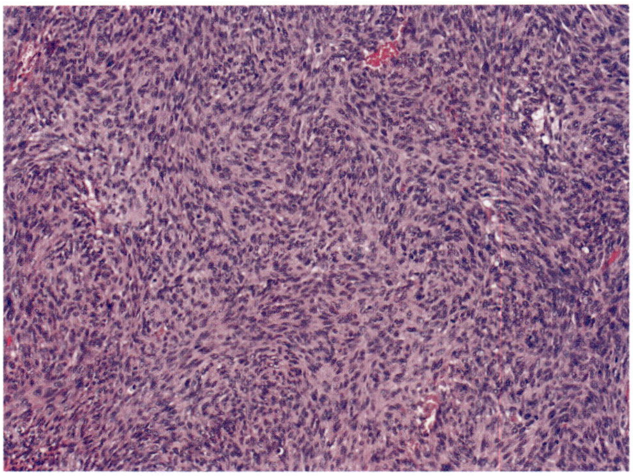

Figure 6.14 GIST, spindle cell variant. The lesion consists of interlacing fascicles of spindle cells. The nuclei have blunt pencil-shaped appearance and are elongated, embedded in a fibrillary eosinophilic cytoplasm.

Microscopic Features

GIST shows a wide morphologic spectrum. Two cell types (spindle and epithelioid) can be seen. Most tumors consist of spindle cells typically forming long interlacing fascicles (Figure 6.14). The nuclei have blunt pencil-shaped appearance and are elongated, embedded in a fibrillary eosinophilic cytoplasm. Paranuclear vacuoles may develop. A sclerosed stroma with or without areas of hyalinization as well as calcification may develop. Myxoid may be detected as well. Multinucleated tumor cells are rarely seen. Several different "subtypes" have been described based on the morphological appearance: sclerosing, palisading, vacuolated, hypercellular, and sarcomatous variants.

Marked cellular pleomorphism is uncommon but may be present in cases of degenerative changes. In rare cases of malignant transformation lipo-, rhabdo-, and chondrosarcomatous components have been described.

The epithelioid GISTs distinctly show round cells with vacuolated clear cytoplasm. The nuclei are round to ovoid in shape. Chromatin structure is finely dispersed with regular small nucleoli. Pleomorphic variant may show large

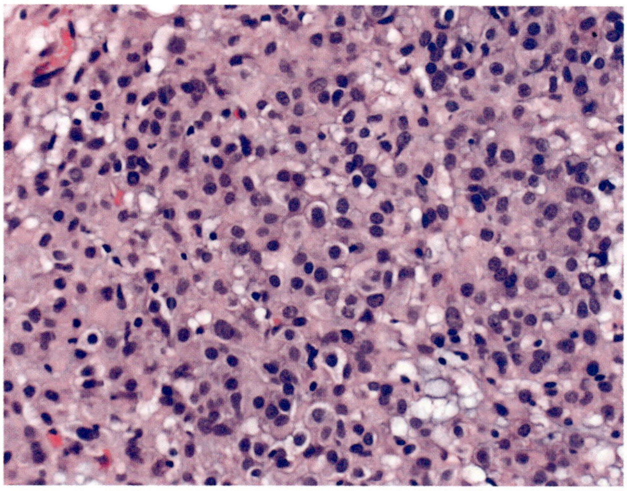

Figure 6.15 GIST, epithelioid variant. The lesion shows distinctly round cells with vacuolated clear cytoplasm. The nuclei are round to ovoid in shape with fine chromatin.

eosinophilic nucleoli. The cells are arranged in sheets or nests with a cohesive growth. Some cases show discohesive growth pattern with signet ring cell-like large tumor cells with abundant eosinophilic cytoplasm and a plasmacytoid appearance. Giant cells can be detected (Figure 6.15).

A system of risk stratification of tumor progression has been proposed by Miettinen et al., which considers parameters like mitotic count and tumor size (see Table 6.6). This system is not reliable on biopsy specimen and should be used only surgical specimen.

Immunohistochemical Studies and Molecular Features

The two most important immunohistochemical stains for the diagnosis of GIST are C-KIT (CD117) and DOG1 ("discovered on GIST 1"). CD117 can be found in more than 90% of cases with a strong and diffuse cytoplasmic and perinuclear dot-like positivity. Weak to moderate expression may also be observed.

DOG1 is a highly sensitive marker for GIST staining tumors with KIT- and PDGFRA-gene mutations. DOG1 successfully stains over 1/3 of CD117 negative cases.

Other markers are less commonly positive like CD34 (>80%), SMA (smooth muscle antigen; 25%), desmin (approx. 5%), and S-100 protein (less than 1%).

CD117 overexpression is caused by exon 11 deletion or mutation of the KIT gene and is commonly found in the spindle cell variant. Platelet-derived growth factor receptor-α (PDGFRA) mutation is found in a smaller group of GIST, commonly showing the epithelioid growth pattern. Immunohistochemically, these tumor phenotypes can also be positive for CD117. CD117 negativity in cases of typical morphology does not exclude GIST. The loss of CD117 as well as CD34 can occur in morphologically mixed or transforming cases. Furthermore, negativity can be observed after imatinib treatment.

Several other genetic alterations may be present in BRAF mutated and SDH-deficient cases. Approximately 30% of GIST show SDHA mutation leading to a negative immunohistochemical stain for SDH. Less common are wild type (WT) GISTs showing V600E BRAF mutations, which present with therapy resistance.

Rare pediatric GISTs present with positive CD117 immunohistochemistry but lack KIT and PDGFRA mutation. Furthermore, they show succinate dehydrogenase B (SDHB) deficiency.

Differential Diagnosis

Several different spindle cells may arise in the stomach and show a histomorphological overlap with GIST.

- Inflammatory fibroid polyp: Usually found in the antrum and mainly located in the submucosa, the diagnosis on punch biopsies can be challenging. Characteristically, the lesion shows small thin-walled vessels surrounded by spindle cells. Multinucleated giant cells with "floret"-like appearance may be present. The background is characterized by an inflammatory infiltrate composed of lymphocytes, plasma cells, and a dominant infiltrate of eosinophils. Inflammatory fibroid polyp should be distinguished from other eosinophil-rich lesions like gastric eosinophilia, hemangioendothelioma, eosinophilic granulomas, inflammatory pseudotumor, or parasite infection. The spindle cell component is positive for CD34, fascin, and calponin immunohistochemistry. CD117 and DOG1 are negative. Molecular analysis can show PDGFRA gene mutation.
- Schwannoma: Characteristically, the lesion is surrounded by a cuff of lymphocytes. The spindle cells are arranged in bundles embedded in a fibrous stroma. Nuclear atypia may be present, but mitotic rate is low. Typical findings like Antoni A and B growth pattern, vascular hyalinization, and verocay bodies are rarely seen. Ancient schwannomas can show severe degenerative changes and can sometimes hardly be distinguished from degenerative GIST (e.g. after treatment). Immunohistochemical studies reveal positivity for S-100 and GFAP (glial fibrillary acidic protein). CD 34 can be positive, whereas CD117, DOG1, and smooth muscle markers are negative.
- Leiomyoma rarely occurs in the stomach but shows a comparable growth pattern like already described for the esophagus (see Chapter 3). They show a strong expression of desmin, myosin, or SMA. CD117 and DOG1 are negative.

Several other entities like melanoma, epithelioid hemangioendothelioma, Kaposi sarcoma, epithelioid angiosarcoma,

Table 6.7 Few examples of soft tissue tumors with possible histomorphological overlapping.

Benign	Malignant
Rhabdomyoma	Rhabdomyosarcoma
Lipoma, angiolipoma	Liposarcoma
Granular cell tumor	Paraganglioma
Ganglioneuroma	Ganglioneuroblastoma
	Clear cell sarcoma

or glomus tumor enter differential diagnosis of GIST to distinguish these entities. Immunohistochemical stains are helpful. It is important to mention that Melan-A may be positive in epithelioid GIST, whereas melanoma markers like HMB45, S100, and SOX10 are negative.

Several other soft tissue neoplasia (see Table 6.7) can show overlapping features with GIST.

Prognosis, Evolution, and Clinical Management

GISTs are relatively common findings during routine upper endoscopy. Removal by endoscopic resection or surgery is generally recommended although small (<1–2 cm), low-risk lesions can be monitored by surveillance endoscopic ultrasound. Endoscopic ultrasound allows core biopsy and risk stratification by assessment of mitosis rate and Ki-67 staining, as well as confirmatory immunohistochemistry stains.

Endoscopic resection is effective for small endophytic tumors using endoscopic submucosal dissection (ESD) or submucosal tunnel endoscopic resection (STER) methods. For exophytic tumors, surgical resection or combined endoscopic/surgical resection is advised.

Further Reading

Abraham, S.C., Carney, J.A., Ooi, A. et al. (2005). Achlorhydria, parietal cell hyperplasia, and multiple gastric carcinoids: a new disorder. *Am. J. Surg. Pathol.* 29: 969–975.

Agaimy, A., Bihl, M.P., Tornillo, L. et al. (2010). Calcifying fibrous tumor of the stomach: clinicopathologic and molecular study of seven cases with literature review and reappraisal of histogenesis. *Am. J. Surg. Pathol.* 34: 271–278.

Amy, C., Lazure, T., Sales, J.P. et al. (2001). Gastric epithelioid angiosarcoma, a biopsy diagnostic pitfall. *Ann. Pathol.* 21: 439–441.

Ban, S. (2011). Early and advanced gastric carcinomas. In: *Advances in Surgical Pathology. Gastric Cancer* (eds. D. Tan and G. Lauwers). Philadelphia: Lippincott Williams & Wilkins.

Billings, S.D., Meisner, L.F., Cummings, O.W. et al. (2000). Synovial sarcoma of the upper digestive tract. *Mod. Pathol.* 13: 68–76.

Borch, K., Ahren, B., Ahlman, H. et al. (2005). Gastric carcinoids: biologic behavior and prognosis after differentiated treatment in relation to type. *Ann. Surg.* 242: 64–73.

Bosman, F.T., Carneiro, F., Hruban, R.H. et al. (2010). *World Health Organization Classification of Tumours. Classification of Tumours of the Digestive System*. Lyon: IARC Press.

Bosman, F.T., Carneiro, F., Hruban, R.H., and Theise, N.D. (eds.) (2010). *WHO Classification of the Digestive System*. Lyon: International Agency for Research on Cancer (IARC) Press.

Brien, T.P., Farraye, F.A., and Odze, R.D. (2001). Gastric dysplasia-like epithelial atypia associated with chemoradiotherapy for esophageal cancer: a clinicopathologic and immunohistochemical study of 15 cases. *Mod. Pathol.* 14: 389–396.

Campbell, F. and Lauwers, G.Y. (2013). Tumors of the esophagus and stomach. In: *Diagnostic Histopathology of Tumors*, 4e (ed. C.D. Fletcher), 378–433. Philadelphia: Elsevier/Saunders.

Capella, C., Frigerio, B., Cornaggia, M. et al. (1984). Gastric parietal cell carcinoma – a newly recognized entity: light microscopic and ultrastructural features. *Histopathology* 8: 813–824.

Capella, C., Heitz, P., Hofler, H. et al. (1995). Revised classification of neuroendocrine tumours of the lung, pancreas and gut. *Virchows Arch.* 425: 547–560.

Charlton, A., Blair, V., Shaw, D. et al. (2004). Hereditary diffuse gastric cancer: predominance of multiple foci of signet-ring cell carcinoma in distal stomach and transitional zone. *Gut* 53: 814–820.

Cheng, N., Hui, D.Y., Liu, Y. et al. (2015). Is gastric lymphoepithelioma-like carcinoma a special subtype of EBV-associated gastric carcinoma? New insight based on clinicopathological features and EBV genome polymorphisms. *Gastric Cancer* 18: 246–255.

Chompret, A., Kannengiesser, C., and Barrois, M. (2004). PDGFRA germline mutation in a family with multiple cases of gastrointestinal stromal tumor. *Gastroenterology* 126: 318–321.

Debiec-Rychter, M., Wasag, B., Stul, M. et al. (2004). Gastrointestinal stromal tumors (GISTs) negative for KIT (CD117 antigen) immunoreactivity. *J. Pathol.* 202: 430–438.

Delbecque, K., Legrand, M., Boniver, J. et al. (2004). Calcifying fibrous tumour of the gastric wall. *Histopathology* 44: 399–400.

Dixon, M.F., O'Connor, H.J., Axon, A.T. et al. (1986). Reflux gastritis: a distinct histopathologic entity? *J. Clin. Pathol.* 39: 524–530.

Doyle, L.A. and Hornick, J.L. Gastrointestinal stromal tumours: from KIT to succinate dehydrogenase. *Histopathology* 64: 53–67.

Fay, D.E. and Nisbeth, H. (1990). Massive gastrointestinal hemorrhage in an immunosuppressed man due to gastric Kaposi's sarcoma. *Am. J. Gastroenterol.* 85: 607–609.

Ferlay J, Soerjomataram I, Ervik M, et al. *GLOBOCAN 2012 v1.0, Cancer Incidence and Mortality Worldwide: IARC CancerBase No. 11 [Internet]*. Lyon: International Agency for Research on Cancer; 2013. http://globocan.iarc.fr. (accessed November 2017)

Fletcher, C.D.M., Berman, J.J., Corless, C. et al. (2002). Diagnosis of gastrointestinal stromal tumors: a consensus approach. *Hum. Pathol.* 33: 459–465.

Fox, K.R., Moussa, S.M., Mitre, R.J. et al. (1990). Clinical and pathologic features of primary gastric rhabdomyosarcoma. *Cancer* 66: 772–778.

Fuller, C.E. and Williams, G.T. (1991). Gastrointestinal manifestations of type I neurofibromatosis (von Recklinghausen's disease). *Histopathology* 19: 1–11.

Gill, A.J., Chou, A., Vilain, R. et al. (2010). Immunohistochemistry for SDHB divides gastrointestinal stromal tumors into 2 distinct types. *Am. J. Surg. Pathol.* 34: 636–644.

Guler, M., Daniels, J.A., Abraham, S.C. et al. (2008). Expression of melanoma antigens in epithelioid gastrointestinal stromal tumors. A potential diagnostic pitfall. *Arch. Pathol. Lab. Med.* 132: 1302–1306.

Heinrich, M.C., Corless, C.L., Demetri, G.D. et al. (2003). Kinase mutations and imatinib response in patients with metastatic gastrointestinal stromal tumor. *J. Clin. Oncol.* 21: 4342–4349.

Heinrich, M.C., Corless, C.L., Duensing, A. et al. (2003). PDGFRA activating mutations in gastrointestinal stromal tumors. *Science* 299: 708–710.

Hidaka, Y., Mitomi, H., Saito, T. et al. (2013). Alteration in the Wnt/β-catenin signaling pathway in gastric neoplasias of fundic gland (chief cell predominant) type. *Hum. Pathol.* 44: 2438–2448.

Hou, Y., Tan, Y., Xu, J. et al. (2006). Schwannoma of the digestive tract: a clinicopathologic, immunohistochemical and ultrastructural study of 33 cases. *Histopathology* 48: 536–545.

Ishida, M., Sekine, S., Fukagawa, T. et al. (2013). Neuroendocrine carcinoma of the stomach: morphologic and immunohistochemical characteristics and prognosis. *Am. J. Surg. Pathol.* 37: 949–959.

Jiang, S.X., Mikami, T., Umezawa, A. et al. (2006). Gastric large cell neuroendocrine carcinomas: a distinct clinicopathologic entity. *Am. J. Surg. Pathol.* 30: 945–953.

Johnston, J. and Helwig, E.B. (1981). Granular cell tumors of the gastrointestinal tract and perianal region. A study of 74 cases. *Dig. Dis. Sci.* 26: 807–816.

Kang, S.H., Kim, K.H., Seo, S.H. et al. (2014). Neuroendocrine carcinoma of the stomach: a case report. *World J. Gastrointest. Surg.* 6: 77–79.

Kobayashi, A., Hasebe, T., Endo, Y. et al. (2005). Primary gastric choriocarcinoma: two case reports and a pooled analysis of 53 cases. *Gastric Cancer* 8: 178–185.

Kodama, Y., Inokuchi, K., Soejima, K. et al. (1983). Growth patterns and prognosis in early gastric carcinoma: superficially spreading and penetrating growth types. *Cancer* 51: 320–326.

La Rosa, S., Inzani, F., Vanoli, A. et al. (2011). Histopathologic characterization and improved prognostic evaluation of 209 gastric neuroendocrine neoplasms. *Hum. Pathol.* 42: 1373–1384.

Lasota, J., Dansonka-Mieszkowska, A., Sobin, L.H. et al. (2004). A great majority of GISTs with PDGFRA mutations represent gastric tumors of low or no malignant potential. *Lab. Investig.* 84: 874–883.

Laurén, P. (1965). The two histologic main types of gastric carcinoma: diffuse and so-called intestinal-type carcinoma. *Acta Pathol. Microbiol. Scand.* 64: 31–49.

Lauwers, G.Y. and Riddell, R.H. (1999). Gastric epithelial dysplasia. *Gut* 45: 784–790.

Lauwers, G.Y., Ban, S., Mino, M. et al. (2004). Endoscopic mucosal resection for gastric epithelial neoplasms: a study of 39 cases with emphasis on the evaluation of specimens and recommendations for optimal pathologic analysis. *Mod. Pathol.* 17: 2–8.

Lazure, T., Ferlicot, S., and Gauthier, F. (2002). Gastric inflammatory myofibroblastic tumors in children: an unpredictable course. *J. Pediatr. Gastroenterol. Nutr.* 34: 319–322.

Lee, K.C., Ng, W.F., and Chan, J.K.C. (1988). Epithelioid haemangioendothelioma presenting as a gastric polyp. *Histopathology* 12: 335–337.

Lee, W.A., Lee, M.K., and Jeen, Y.M. (2004). Solitary fibrous tumor arising in gastric serosa. *Pathol. Int.* 54: 436–439.

Liegl, B., Hornick, J.L., and Corless, C.L. (2009). Monoclonal antibody DOG1.1 shows higher sensitivity than KIT in the diagnosis of gastrointestinal stromal tumors, including unusual subtypes. *Am. J. Surg. Pathol.* 33: 437–446.

Lim, H., Park, Y.S., Lee, J.H. et al. (2015). Features of gastric carcinoma with lymphoid stroma associated with Epstein–Barr virus. *Clin. Gastroenterol. Hepatol.* 13: 1738–1744.

Liu, X., Cheng, Y., Sheng, W. et al. (2010). Analysis of clinicopathologic features and prognostic factors in hepatoid adenocarcinoma of stomach. *Am. J. Surg. Pathol.* 34: 1465–1471.

Lustbader, I. and Sherman, A. (1987). Primary gastrointestinal Kaposi's sarcoma in a patient with acquired immune deficiency syndrome. *Am. J. Gastroenterol.* 82: 894–895.

Matsubara, Y., Ando, T., Hosakawa, A. et al. (2018). Neuroendocrine carcinoma of the stomach: a response to combination chemotherapy consisting of ramucirumab plus paclitaxel. *Intern. Med.* 57: 671–675.

Matsui, K., Jin, X.M., Kitagawa, M., and Miwa, A. (1998). Clinicopathologic features of neuroendocrine carcinomas of the stomach: appraisal of small celland large cell variants. *Arch. Pathol. Lab. Med.* 122: 1010–1017.

McGregor, D.H., Kerley, S.W., and McGregor, M.S. (1993). Gastric angiolipoma with chronic hemorrhage and severe anemia. *Am J Med Sci* 305: 229–235.

Medeiros, F., Corless, C.L., Duensing, A. et al. (2004). KIT-negative gastrointestinal stromal tumors. *Am. J. Surg. Pathol.* 28: 889–894.

Miettinen, M. and Lasota, J. (2001). Gastrointestinal stromal tumors—definition, clinical, histological, immunohistochemical, and molecular genetic features and differential diagnosis. *Virchows Arch.* 438: 1–12.

Miettinen, M., Paal, E., Lasota, J. et al. (2002). Gastrointestinal glomus tumors: a clinicopathologic, immunohistochemical, and molecular genetic study of 32 cases. *Am. J. Surg. Pathol.* 26: 301–311.

Miettinen, M., Lasota, J., and Sobin, L.H. (2005). Gastrointestinal stromal tumors of the stomach in children and young adults: a clinicopathologic, immunohistochemical, and molecular genetic study of 44 cases with long-term follow-up and review of the literature. *Am. J. Surg. Pathol.* 29: 1373–1381.

Miettinen, M., Sobin, L.H., and Lasota, J. (2005). Gastrointestinal stromal tumors of the stomach: a clinicopathologic, immunohistochemical, and molecular genetic study of 1765 cases with long-term follow-up. *Am. J. Surg. Pathol.* 29: 52–68.

Miettinen, M., Wang, Z.F., and Lasota, J. (2009). DOG1 antibody in the differential diagnosis of gastrointestinal stromal tumors. A study of 1840 cases. *Am. J. Surg. Pathol.* 33: 1401–1408.

Miettinen, M., Dow, N., Lasota, J. et al. (2009). A distinctive novel epitheliomesenchymal biphasic tumor of the stomach in young adults ("gastroblastoma"): a series of 3 cases. *Am. J. Surg. Pathol.* 33: 1370–1377.

Miettinen, M., Makhlouf, H.R., and Sobin, L.H. (2009). Plexiform fibromyxoma: a distinctive benign gastric antral neoplasm not to be confused with a myxoid GIST. *Am. J. Surg. Pathol.* 33: 1624–1632.

Minamoto, T., Mai, M., Watanabe, K. et al. (1990). Medullary carcinoma with lymphocytic infiltration of the stomach. *Cancer* 66: 945–952.

Mori, M., Iwashita, A., and Enjoji, M. (1986). Adenosquamous carcinoma of the stomach: a clinicopathologic analysis of 28 cases. *Cancer* 57: 333–339.

Nomura, R., Saito, T., Mitomi, H. et al. (2014). GNAS mutation as an alternative mechanism of activation of the Wnt/β-catenin signaling pathway in gastric adenocarcinoma of the fundic gland type. *Hum. Pathol.* 45: 2488–2496.

Okita, N.T., Kato, K., Takahari, D. et al. (2011). Neuroendocrine tumors of the stomach: chemotherapy with cisplatin plus irinotecan is effective for gastric poorly-differentiated neuroendocrine carcinoma. *Gastric Cancer* 14: 161–165.

Ono, H., Yao, K., Fujishiro, M. et al. (2016). Guidelines for endoscopic submucosal dissection and endoscopic mucosal resection for early gastric cancer. *Dig. Endosc.* 28 (1): 3–15.

Ooi, A., Nakanishi, I., Itoh, T. et al. (1991). Predominant Paneth cell differentiation in an intestinal type gastric cancer. *Pathol. Res. Pract.* 187: 220–225.

Ooi, A., Ota, M., Katsuda, S. et al. (1995). An unusual case of multiple gastric carcinoids associated with diffuse endocrine cell hyperplasia and parietal cell hypertrophy. *Endocr. Pathol.* 3: 229–237.

Pantanowitz, L., Antonioli, D.A., Pinkus, G.S. et al. (2004). Inflammatory fibroid polyps of the gastrointestinal tract: evidence for a dendritic cell origin. *Am. J. Surg. Pathol.* 28: 107–114.

Park, D.Y., Srivastava, A., Kim, G.H. et al. (2008). Adenomatous and foveolar gastric dysplasia: distinct patterns of mucin expression and background intestinal metaplasia. *Am. J. Surg. Pathol.* 32: 524–533.

Pasini, B., McWhinney, S.R., Bei, T. et al. (2008). Clinical and molecular genetics of patients with the Carney–Stratakis syndrome and germline mutations of the genes coding for the succinate dehydrogenase subunits SDHB, SDHC, and SDHD. *Eur. J. Hum. Genet.* 16: 79–88.

Pauwels, P., Debiec-Rychter, M., Sciot, R. et al. (2002). Clear cell sarcoma of the stomach. *Histopathology* 41: 526–530.

Pauwels, P., Debiec-Rychter, M., Stul, M. et al. (2005). Changing phenotype of gastrointestinal stromal tumours under imatinib mesylate treatment: a potential diagnostic pitfall. *Histopathology* 47: 41–47.

Rege, T.A., Wagner, A.J., Corless, C.L. et al. (2011). Pediatric-type gastrointestinal stromal tumors in adults: distinctive histology predicts genotype and clinical behavior. *Am. J. Surg. Pathol.* 35: 495–504.

Ribeiro, M.J., Alonso, T., Gajate, P. et al. (2018). Huge recurrent gastric neuroendocrine tumor: a second-line chemotherapeutic dilemma. *Autops. Case Rep.* 8: e2018005.

Rindi, G. and Solcia, E. (2012). Neuroendocrine tumors and non neoplastic neudocrine cell changes. In: *Advances in*

Surgical Pathology: Gastric Cancer (eds. D. Tan and G.Y. Lauwers), 94–104. Wolters Kluwer Health Adis (ESP).

Rogers, W.M., Dobo, E., Norton, J.A. et al. (2008). Risk-reducing total gastrectomy for germline mutations in E-cadherin (CDHI): pathologic findings with clinical implications. *Am. J. Surg. Pathol.* 32: 799–809.

Roh, J.H., Srivastava, A., Lauwers, G.Y. et al. (2010). Micropapillary carcinoma of stomach. A clinicopathologic and immunohistochemical study of 11 cases. *Am. J. Surg. Pathol.* 34: 1139–1146.

Rüschoff, J., Hanna, W., Bilous, M. et al. (2012). HER2 testing in gastric cancer: a practical approach. *Mod. Pathol.* 25 (5): 637–650.

Saito, R., Abe, H., Kunita, A. et al. (2017). Overexpression and gene amplification of PD-L1 in cancer cells and PD-L1$^+$ immune cells in Epstein–Barr virus-associated gastric cancer: the prognostic implications. *Mod. Pathol.* 30: 427–439.

Schildhaus, H.U., Cavlar, T., Binot, E. et al. (2008). Inflammatory fibroid polyps harbour mutations in the platelet-derived growth factor receptor alpha (PDGFRA) gene. *J. Pathol.* 216: 176–182.

Schlemper, R.J., Riddell, R.H., Kato, Y. et al. (2000). The Vienna classification of gastrointestinal epithelial neoplasia. *Gut* 47: 251–255.

Schmid, C., Beham, A., Steindorfer, P. et al. (1990). Non functional malignant paraganglioma of the stomach. *Virchows Arch. A* 417: 261–266.

Setia, N., Clark, J.W., Duda, D.G. et al. (2015). Familial gastric cancers. *Oncologist* 20: 1365–1377.

Shia, J., Tang, L.H., Weiser, M.R. et al. (2008). Is nonsmall cell type high-grade neuroendocrine carcinoma of the tubular gastrointestinal tract a distinct disease entity? *Am. J. Surg. Pathol.* 32: 719–731.

Shin, D.H., Lee, J.H., and Kang, H.J. (2010). Novel epitheliomesenchymal biphasic stomach tumour (gastroblastoma) in a 9-year-old: morphological, ultrastructural and immunohistochemical findings. *J. Clin. Pathol.* 63: 270–274.

Shokouh-Amiri, M.H., Hansen, C.P., and Moesgaard, F. (1986). Liposarcoma of the stomach: a case report. *Acta Chir. Scand.* 152: 389–391.

Solcia, E. (2010). *Neuroendocrine Neoplasms of the Stomach. WHO Classification of Tumours of the Digestive System*, 64–68. Lyon: IARC Press.

Solcia, E., Capella, C., Fiocca, R. et al. (1990). Gastric argyrophil carcinoidosis in patients with Zollinger–Ellison syndrome due to type 1 multiple endocrine neoplasia. *Am. J. Surg. Pathol.* 14: 503–513.

Solcia, E., Fiocca, R., Villani, L. et al. (1995). Hyperplastic, dysplastic and neoplastic enterochromaffin-like cell proliferations of the gastric mucosa: classification and histogenesis. *Am. J. Surg. Pathol.* 19 (Suppl 1): S1–S7.

Son, H.J., Song, S.Y., Kim, S. et al. (2005). Characteristics of submucosal gastric carcinoma with lymph node metastatic disease. *Histopathology* 46: 158–165.

Su, J.S., Chen, Y.T., Wang, R.C. et al. (2013). Clinicopathological characteristics in the differential diagnosis of hepatoid adenocarcinoma: a literature review. *World J. Gastroenterol.* 19: 321–327.

Takubo, K., Honma, N., Sawabe, M. et al. (2002). Oncocytic adenocarcinoma of the stomach: parietal cell carcinoma. *Am. J. Surg. Pathol.* 26: 458–465.

Taxy, J.B. and Battifora, H. (1988). Angiosarcoma of the gastrointestinal tract. A report of three cases. *Cancer* 62: 210–216.

Tohda, G., Osawa, T., Asada, Y. et al. (2016). Gastric adenocarcinoma of fundic gland type: endoscopic and clinicopathological features. *World J. Gastrointest. Endosc.* 8: 244–251.

Ueyama, H., Yao, T., Nakashima, Y. et al. (2010). Gastric adenocarcinoma of fundic gland type (chief cell predominant type): proposal for a new entity. *Am. J. Surg. Pathol.* 34: 609–619.

Verweij, J., Casali, P.G., Zalcberg, J. et al. (2004). Progression-free survival in gastrointestinal stromal tumours with high-dose imatinib: randomised trial. *Lancet* 364: 1127–1134.

Volpe, C.M., Hameer, H.R., Masetti, P. et al. (1995). Squamous cell carcinoma of the stomach. *Am. Surg.* 61: 1076–1078.

Wang, W.Y., Li, J.N., and Li, G.D. (2010). Plexiform angiomyxoid myofibroblastic tumour of the gastric fundus: successful diagnosis and treatment by endoscopy. *J. Clin. Pathol.* 63: 569–570.

Xie, J.W., Sun, Y.Q., Feng, C.Y. et al. (2016). Evaluation of clinicopathological factors related to the prognosis of gastric neuroendocrine carcinoma. *Eur. J. Surg. Oncol.* 42: 1464–1470.

Zhang, Q., Ming, J., Zhang, S. et al. (2015). Micropapillary component in gastric adenocarcinoma: an aggressive variant associated with poor prognosis. *Gastric Cancer* 18: 93–99.

Gastric Neoplastic Conditions

Lymphoid Lesions of the Stomach

Mounir Trimeche and Laurence de Leval

Centre Hospitalier Universitaire Vaudois, University Institute of Pathology, Lausanne, Switzerland

Extranodal Marginal Zone Lymphoma of Mucosa-Associated Lymphoid Tissue (MALT Lymphoma)

Definition, General Features, and Predisposing Factors

Extranodal mucosa-associated lymphoid tissue (MALT) lymphoma is a low-grade lymphoma of small B cells that arise from the marginal zone surrounding lymphoid follicles. This neoplasm comprises 7–8% of all B-cell lymphomas and occurs in a wide range of extranodal sites, most commonly in the stomach. Gastric MALT lymphoma accounts for nearly half of primary gastric lymphomas (Table 6.8), and occurs predominantly in male individuals over 50 years, but can also affect younger patients. Acquired MALT in the stomach, caused by *Helicobacter pylori*-induced gastritis, provides the seed bed for MALT lymphoma development.

Table 6.8 Main histological types of primary gastric lymphomas.

B-cell lymphomas
Marginal zone B-cell lymphoma of MALT type
Diffuse large B-cell lymphoma
With MALT component
Without MALT component
Mantle cell lymphoma (malignant lymphomatous polyposis)
Burkitt lymphoma
Miscellaneous rare types
T/NK-cell lymphomas
HTLV1-associated adult T-cell lymphoma/leukemia
Peripheral T-cell lymphoma, not otherwise specified
Enteropathy associated T-cell lymphoma
Anaplastic large cell lymphoma
Immunodeficiency-related lymphoproliferative disorders
HIV-associated lymphoproliferations
Post-transplant lymphoproliferative disorders
Congenital immunodeficiency lymphoproliferative diseases

MALT, mucosa-associated lymphoid tissue; NK, natural killer; HTLV1, human T-lymphotropic virus-1; HIV, human immunodeficiency virus.

Clinical Features and Endoscopic Characteristics

Symptoms are nonspecific including abdominal pain, dyspepsia, bloating, and heartburn. Bleeding, vomiting, and weight loss are reported in less than 1/3 of cases while systemic symptoms are uncommon. The antrum is most commonly involved, but multifocal involvement is frequent. Various macroscopic appearances can be observed: ulcerative lesions, mucosal granularity, and rugal fold thickening and/or diffusely infiltrative lesions. Occasionally, MALT lymphomas may form localized polypoid tumors. However, in some cases, the mucosa may appear macroscopically normal or with slight petechiae only. Deep infiltration, mass formation, and ulceration are less frequent than in high-grade lymphomas.

Microscopic Features

The cardinal morphological features of MALT lymphoma are:

- diffuse and/or nodular dense infiltrate of neoplastic lymphoid B cells cytologically resembling marginal zone B cells and showing a marginal zone distribution,
- lympho-epithelial lesions (LELs),
- reactive lymphoid follicles with germinal centers.

Typically, the neoplastic cells are small lymphoid cells with irregular nuclei and scant cytoplasm resembling centrocytes (centrocyte-like cells). In other instance, they resemble small lymphocytes with round nuclei or show features of medium-sized monocytoid cells, with abundant pale cytoplasm, well-defined cell membranes, and round to oval, smoothly contoured nuclei (Figure 6.16). The proportion of cells with these features varies. In some tumors, there is a relatively monotonous population, while others comprise a mixture of cell types. The neoplastic infiltrate also usually contains scattered large cells resembling centroblasts or immunoblasts.

Plasmacytic differentiation, present in about 30% of cases, tends to be more prominent in the upper portion of the mucosa (Figure 6.17). The neoplastic plasma cells may appear as normal mature plasma cells, may have crystalline inclusions in the cytoplasm, or may possess nuclei with Dutcher bodies (Figure 6.17b). In some cases, intracytoplasmic immunoglobulin may be so abundant that the nucleus is pushed to one side and the cells resemble the signet ring cells of diffuse type adenocarcinoma.

LELs are an important and characteristic feature of gastric MALT lymphoma. They are defined as the unequivocal invasion of individual crypts by aggregates of three or more neoplastic cells, eventually leading to degenerative changes or destruction and disintegration of the crypt epithelium. The LELs are usually easily found but, occasionally, they

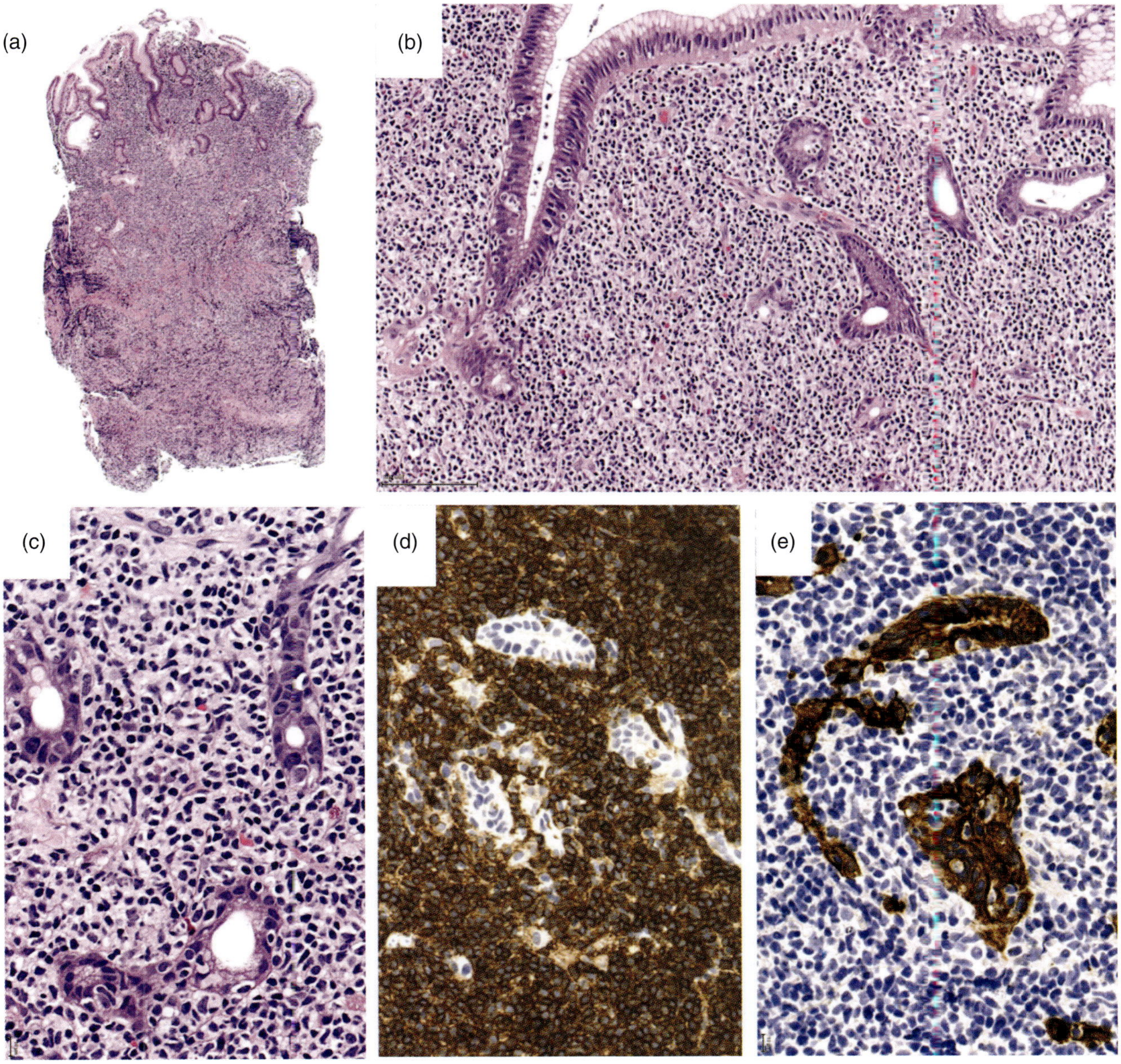

Figure 6.16 Microscopic aspect of gastric MALT lymphoma. (a) Low magnification of the endoscopic biopsy showing a diffuse lymphoid infiltrate involving the mucosa and submucosa with disruption of the muscularis mucosa. (b, c) The monotonous lymphoid infiltrate obliterates the crypts and the glands, and comprises small- to medium-sized lymphoid cells with moderately abundant clear cytoplasm and scattered large cells. The gastric crypts and glands are infiltrated and disrupted by small aggregates of lymphoid cells forming typical lymphoepithelial lesions, better highlighted by immunostainings for (d) CD20 and (e) cytokeratins (immunoperoxidase).

are scarce and require a careful search that may be aided by immunohistochemical tools, especially cytokeratin immunohistochemistry, which highlights the associated epithelial destruction (Figure 6.16c–e). Although LELs are highly suggestive of MALT lymphoma, they are not specific for a diagnosis of malignancy and may be seen in non-MALT lymphomas.

An important component of MALT lymphomas are reactive lymphoid follicles, around which the neoplastic cells tend to be distributed. The neoplastic MALT lymphoid cells may invade the reactive germinal centers, producing follicular colonization. Eventually, the lymphoma may completely overrun and destroy the lymphoid follicles, creating a nodular pattern, which may sometimes be mistaken and resemble follicular lymphoma (FL). Within the germinal centers, the neoplastic cells may undergo marked plasma cell differentiation or show transformation to large cell morphology.

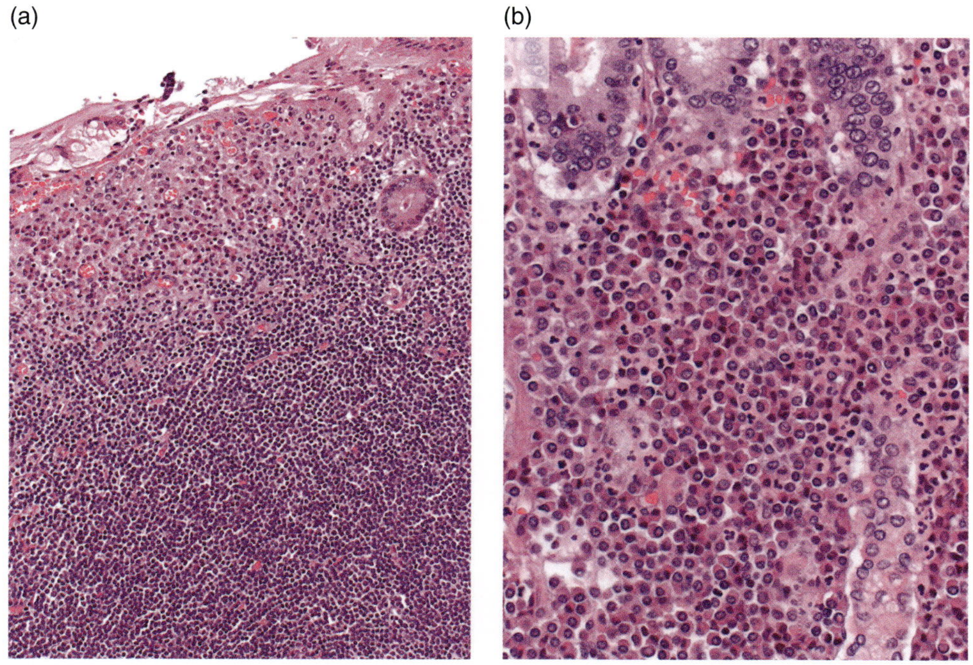

Figure 6.17 Gastric MALT lymphoma with plasma cell differentiation. (a) The neoplastic cells with plasma cell differentiation preferentially distribute in the upper mucosa and (b) frequently contain nuclear inclusions (Dutcher bodies).

Gastric MALT lymphoma is usually multifocal and microscopic tumor foci may be seen throughout the gastric mucosa at a distance from the main tumor mass.

Regional lymph node involvement may be subtle, as the lymphoma cells initially localize to the marginal zones without architectural distortion. Further involvement is characterized by spread to the interfollicular areas or producing follicular colonization.

Immunohistochemical and Molecular Features

The neoplastic cells express B-cell markers (CD20, CD19, CD79a, and PAX5) and BCL2. They are negative for CD5 with few exceptions. MALT lymphoma cells do not express CD10, BCL6, CD23, or cyclin D1. About half of cases show aberrant co-expression of CD43. Except in areas with marked plasma cellular differentiation, the lymphoma cells are also frequently positive for the recently characterized marginal zone B cell-associated IRTA-1 (immunoglobulin superfamily receptor translocation-associated-1) antigen (Figure 6.18).

The neoplastic cells usually express IgM and are generally negative for IgD. Occasional cases are positive for IgA or IgG. Monotypic immunoglobulin with light chain restriction is expressed at the membrane and, to a lesser extent, in the cytoplasm, according to the degree of plasmacytic differentiation.

CD21 and CD23 are useful for highlighting follicular dendritic cells. Whereas reactive germinal centers are typically associated with tight, dense follicular dendritic cell meshwork, neoplastic follicular colonization may be associated with large expanded irregular aggregates of follicular dendritic cells.

Cytokeratin immunohistochemistry is also useful for demonstrating the epithelial destruction associated with LELs. Nonneoplastic reactive T cells, highlighted by CD3 and CD5, are usually found in substantial numbers.

Immunoglobulin heavy and light chains are rearranged and show somatic hypermutation of their variable regions, consistent with derivation from a post-germinal center memory B cell.

A number of genetic alterations are specifically associated with MALT lymphomas and are detectable in routinely processed endoscopic biopsies by FISH or reverse-transcriptase PCR assays. The most frequently detected translocations in primary gastric lymphomas are the t(11;18)(q21;q21)/*API2-MALT1* and the t(1;14)(p22;q32)/*BCL10-IGH*, present respectively in up to 25 and 5% of cases. The t(11;18) translocation is more frequent in CagA positive strains of *H. pylori* and is predictive of low response to *H. pylori* eradication.

Differential Diagnosis

Reactive Lymphoid Hyperplasia

The most common challenge in the diagnosis of gastric MALT lymphoma is differentiating it from *H. pylori*-associated gastritis that may have prominent marginal zones

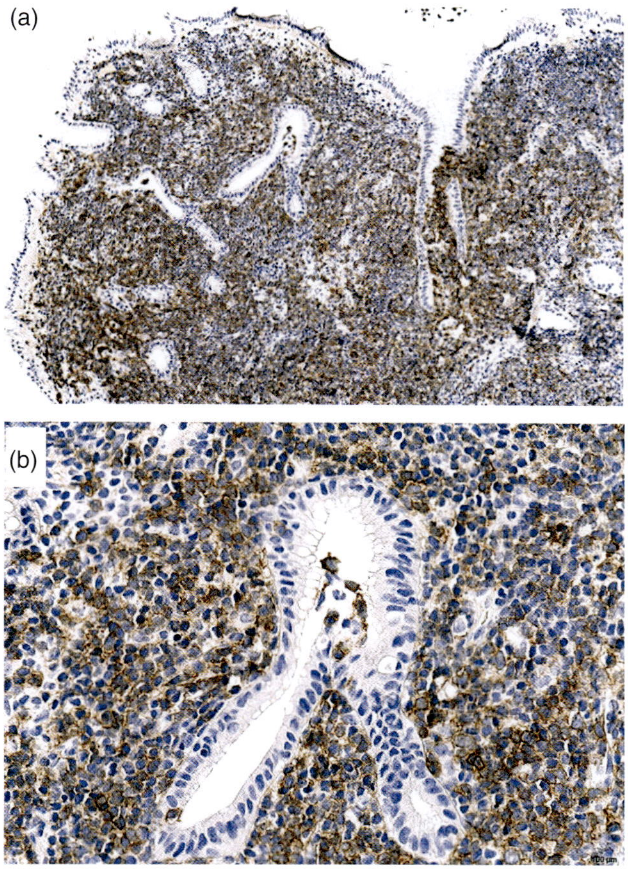

Figure 6.18 IRTA1 expression in gastric MALT lymphoma. Positive staining in a large proportion of tumor cells, particularly near the epithelial structures, and in tumor cells forming lymphoepithelial lesions (immunoperoxidase).

Table 6.9 Wotherspoon scoring system for gastric lymphoid infiltrates.

Score	Diagnosis	Histological features
0	Normal	Scattered plasma cells in lamina propria, no lymphoid follicles
1	Chronic active gastritis	Small clusters of lymphocytes in lamina propria, no lymphoid follicles, no lympho-epithelial lesions
2	Chronic active gastritis with florid lymphoid follicle formation	Prominent lymphoid follicles with a surrounding mantle zone and plasma cells, no lympho-epithelial lesions
3	Suspicious lymphoid infiltrate, probably reactive	Lymphoid follicles surrounded by small lymphocytes that infiltrate diffusely in lamina propria and occasionally into the epithelium
4	Suspicious lymphoid infiltrate, probably lymphoma	Lymphoid follicles surrounded by marginal zone cells that infiltrate diffusely in lamina propria and into the epithelium in small groups
5	MALT lymphoma	Presence of dense diffuse infiltrate of marginal zone cells in lamina propria with prominent lympho-epithelial lesions

Source: From Wotherspoon, A., Doglioni, C., Diss, T. et al. (1993). Regression of primary low grade B-cell gastric lymphoma of mucosa-associated lymphoid tissue type after eradication of *Helicobacter pylori*. *Lancet* 342: 575-577. © 1993 Elsevier.

with some marginal zone cells infiltrating the juxtaposed glands, creating small LELs adjacent to the lymphoid follicles.

In favor of lymphoma are the presence of an expansile, destructive infiltrate with loss of normal architecture, the cytological features of the infiltrating cells (with the appearance of marginal zone cells rather than small lymphocytes), the presence of Dutcher bodies, infiltration of the muscularis mucosae and well-formed LELs. However, many biopsies lack some of these features. The histologic scoring system of Wotherspoon is useful to assess the likelihood of gastric lymphoid infiltrates being reactive versus malignant (Table 6.9). Immunohistochemical analyses are helpful by revealing monotypic immunoglobulin expression and/or co-expression of CD43. B-cell clonality analysis by PCR-based methods helps resolve difficult cases.

Other Small B-Cell Lymphomas

MALT lymphoma must be distinguished from other small B-cell lymphomas that may involve the stomach, including mantle cell lymphoma (most frequently encountered), small lymphocytic lymphoma/chronic lymphocytic leukemia (CLL), and FL (both rarely seen in gastric biopsies). The differential diagnosis with other small B-cell lymphomas relies upon a combination of morphological, immunophenotypical, and molecular features (Table 6.10).

- Mantle cell lymphoma may display histopathological features similar to those of MALT lymphoma, including the presence of occasional LELs. Distinctive immunophenotypic features include positivity for CD5, cyclin D1 and SOX11, and IgD.
- Small lymphocytic lymphoma/CLL involving the gastric mucosa may be confused with MALT lymphoma but the cytological features are different, as CLL comprises small lymphocytes with round nuclei and occasional prolymphocytes. Additional distinguishing features include the absence of reactive follicles, usual lack of prominent LEL and the immunophenotypic features of CLL (CD5+, CD23+, IgD+).
- FL is rarely encountered in the stomach and most cases represent secondary involvement of the stomach in the

Table 6.10 Differential diagnosis of small B-cell lymphomas involving the stomach.

	MALT lymphoma	Mantle cell lymphoma	Small lymphocytic lymphoma	Follicular lymphoma
Neoplastic cell morphology	Centrocytes like or monocytoid lymphoid cells ± plasma cell differentiation	Monotonous small/ medium-size cells	Small lymphoid cells	Centrocytes and centroblasts (grade 1–2, or 3)
Architecture and microenvironment	Lymphoepithelial lesions, reactive and colonialized follicles Abundant T-cells	Mantle, nodular or diffuse pattern of growth Follicles usually absent	Proliferating centers No lymphoid follicles	Neoplastic follicles
Immunophenotype	CD5−/+, CD10−, CD43−/+, BCL6−, IRTA1+. Monotypic plasma cells (30%)	CD5+, cyclin D1+, SOX11+, CD23−, CD43+, BCL2+, BCL6−, CD10−	CD5+, CD23+, CD43+, BCL2+, BCL6−, CD10−, LEF1+	CD5−, BCL2+, BCL6+, CD10+
Genetics	t(11;18)(q21;q21)/*API2-MALT1* t(1;14)(p22;q32)/*BCL10-IGH*	t(11;14) (q13;q32)/*CCND1-IGH*	Deletions of 13q14.3 11q12-q23, 17p13 Trisomy 12	(14;18) (q32;q21)/*IGH-BCL2*
Clinical features	Indolent, responding to antibiotic therapy	Usually aggressive	Indolent	Indolent

context of systemic disease. The presence of follicular structures in association with follicular dendritic cells and a mixed cytological composition comprising small lymphoid cells with scattered larger cells are common to both FL and MALT lymphoma, but FL is usually CD10+, BCL2+, and BCL6+.

Transformation to Diffuse Large B-Cell Lymphoma (DLBCL)

Transformation of MALT lymphoma to DLBCL is diagnosed when sheets or confluent clusters of large transformed cells are found outside follicles in a background of MALT lymphoma. Clusters filling one high-power microscopic field or more are needed to consider large cell transformation. Conversely, diffusely scattered large cells, representing 5–10% or even up to 20% of the total population, are not associated with a worse prognosis, as long as they do not form clusters.

Before considering large cell transformation, the possibility that the large cells represent residual reactive germinal center cells or large neoplastic cells confined to colonized follicles must be excluded. Immunohistochemical stains for follicular dendritic cell meshwork (CD21, CD23) may be helpful to delineate the underlying architecture.

Plasma Cell Neoplasia

The stomach is an uncommon site for extramedullary plasmacytomas or dissemination of multiple myeloma. However, MALT lymphoma with extensive plasma cell differentiation may suggest the alternative diagnosis of a plasma cell neoplasm. In favor of lymphoma are the presence of a component of B lymphocytes, the presence of Dutcher bodies, LELs and reactive lymphoid follicles, and expression of IgM by the neoplastic cells (although some MALT lymphomas express other heavy chains, but conversely plasma cell neoplasms are infrequently IgM+).

Poorly Preserved High-Grade Lymphoma

In small biopsies with crush artifact harboring DLBCL or Burkitt lymphoma, there may be distortion leading to the impression of a small cell tumor. The presence of apoptotic debris, necrosis, and/or numerous mitotic figures should raise the suspicion of a high-grade malignancy. Staining with Ki67 is helpful for identifying highly proliferative tumors. Clinical information, such as the endoscopic appearance of the tumor and/or its apparent growth rate, can also provide evidence for the correct diagnosis.

Prognosis, Evolution, and Clinical Management

MALT lymphomas are characterized by a distinctive indolent clinical course, with an overall survival rate of approximately 90% at five years.

The treatment method of MALT lymphoma is determined according to the clinical stage and *H. pylori* infection status. Eradication of *H. pylori* is recommended regardless the clinical stage. Most patients with histological residual disease after successful *H. pylori* eradication will have a favorable course without additional treatment but lifelong surveillance is mandatory to detect late relapses (5–20%) and metachronous gastric cancer.

Translocation t(11;18)-positive cases and perigastric lymphadenopathy are the main negative predictors of response to *H. pylori* eradication. In advanced clinical stages, residual disease after *H. pylori* eradication, or *H. pylori*-negative cases, radiotherapy and/or chemotherapy can be administered subsequently. Rituximab, a chimeric antibody directed against CD20, has shown efficacy in MALT lymphoma and its combination with chlorambucil was successfully tested for the treatment of patients with t(11;18)-positive gastric MALT lymphomas.

Post-treatment Evaluation of Gastric MALT Lymphoma

Follow-up for gastric MALT lymphoma includes serial gastroscopy with histological assessment of multiple biopsies from all parts of the stomach.

A good histological response to treatment is characterized by regression of the diffuse lymphoid infiltrate and LELs with frequent persistence of small basal aggregates of lymphocytes and an "empty' lamina propria composed of loose connective tissue with scattered plasma cells and glandular loss.

In order to standardize the pathological evaluation of follow-up gastric biopsies, the Groupe d'Etude des Lymphomes de l'Adulte (GELA) has proposed a grading system based on histological features, independent of immunohistochemical or molecular studies. The morphological features are classified into four categories: complete histological remission, probable minimal residual disease, responding residual disease, and no change (Figure 6.19). The category of "probable minimal residual disease" is of uncertain significance, as half of these cases are associated with a clonal *IGH* gene rearrangement by PCR but it is not an indication for further treatment and, since it is not associated with active disease, it can be considered as a state of remission.

Most patients who achieve complete remission and "probable minimal residual disease" remain in remission

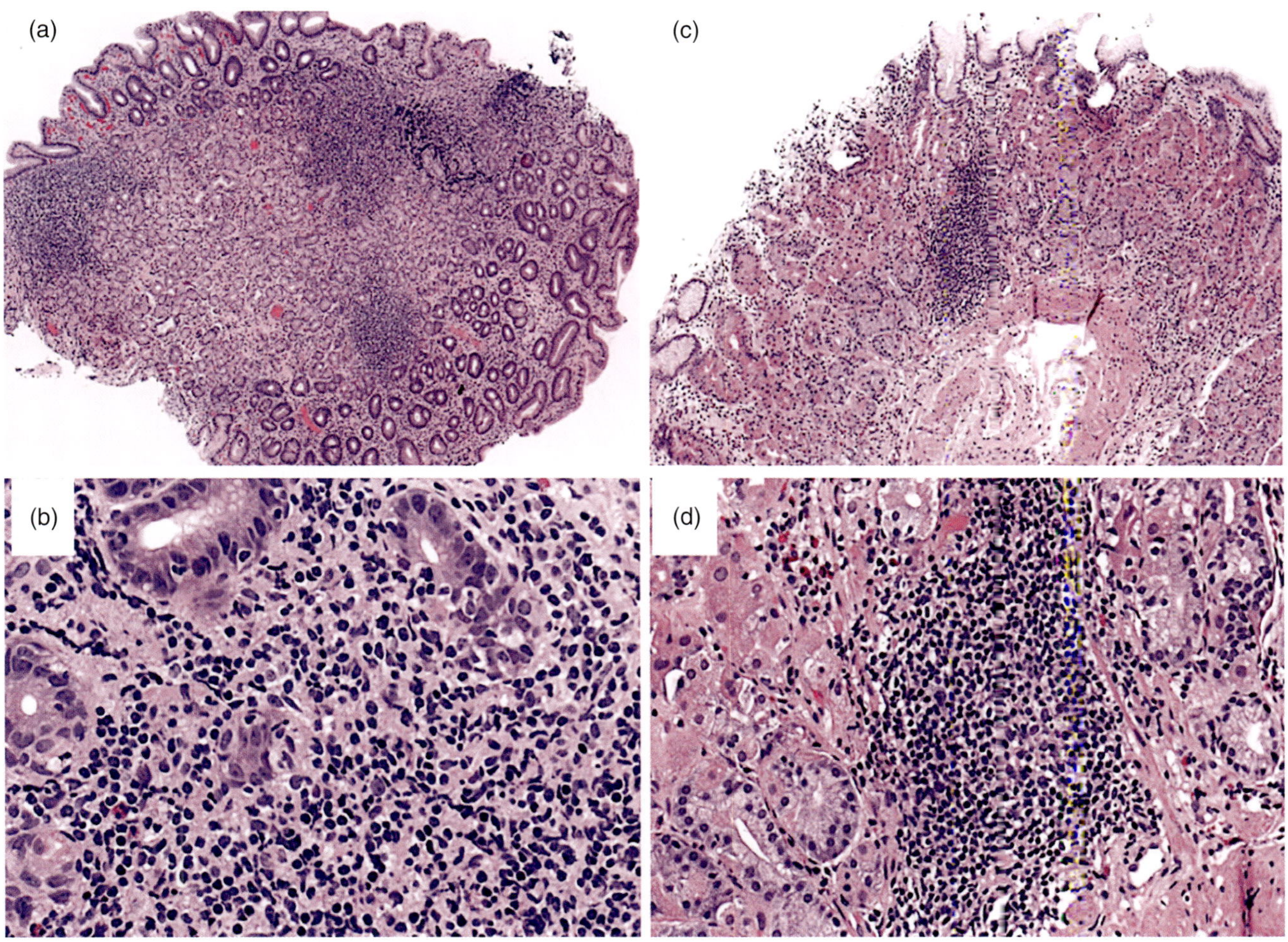

Figure 6.19 Control gastric biopsies after antibiotic therapy for *H. pylori*-associated MALT lymphoma. (a, b) Responding residual disease (rRD): dense, diffuse, and nodular, lymphoid infiltrate in the lamina propria with focal lymphoepithelial lesions and stromal fibrosis. (c, d) Probable minimal residual disease (pMRD): small limited lymphoid infiltrate in the deep mucosa without lymphoepithelial lesions.

but relapse occurs in about 20% of cases, whether or not in association with *H. pylori* reinfection. Relapses may occur several years after initial remission and can be focal. In *H. pylori*-positive relapses, antibiotic therapy usually results in a further remission.

Long-term endoscopic follow-up of gastric MALT lymphoma patients is also recommended to detect preneoplastic or neoplastic changes of the gastric epithelium, as gastric MALT lymphoma shows an association and an increased risk of transformation of the gastric epithelium.

The use of PCR-based tests for assessing B-cell clonality in the follow-up gastric biopsies after antibiotic therapy for gastric MALT lymphoma is not recommend in routine diagnostic practice.

Gastric Diffuse Large B-Cell Lymphoma (DLBCL)

Definition, General Features, and Predisposing Factors

Diffuse large B-cell lymphoma (DLBCL) is a neoplasm of large B cells featuring a diffuse growth pattern. Primary gastric DLBCL is very close to gastric MALT lymphoma in terms of prevalence and represents one of the two most common lymphoid malignancies of the stomach. It occurs in patients between 50 and 60 years old and shows a slight male predominance.

Gastric DLBCL may arise de novo or from transformation of other types of small B-cell lymphomas. The role of *H. pylori* infection in gastric DLBCL is controversial but the bacterium is detected in about 1/3 of the cases, especially in patients with concomitant gastric MALT lymphoma. Additional risk factors include Epstein–Barr virus (EBV) especially in immunocompromised and elderly patients.

Clinical Features and Endoscopic Characteristics

The clinical presentation of gastric DLBCL is nonspecific. The most common symptom is epigastric pain or dyspepsia but patients can present with anorexia, nausea or vomiting, weight loss, bleeding, and perforation.

DLBCL is usually associated with a solitary large mass that is likely to show ulceration (Figure 6.20), but occasionally, more diffuse infiltration with an intact mucosa is seen. A polypoid pattern may also be encountered. The antrum is the most common site but any part of the stomach may be involved. Local lymph node involvement is common.

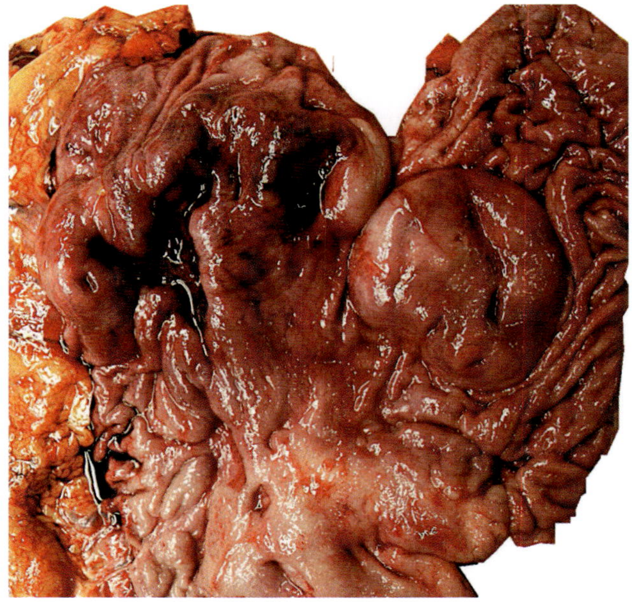

Figure 6.20 Primary gastric diffuse large B-cell lymphoma presenting as a voluminous ulcerated polypoid mass.

Microscopic Features

DLBCL is characterized by the presence of compact aggregates of large atypical lymphoid cells infiltrating the lamina propria and submucosa, with nuclei at least twice the size of a small lymphocyte, usually larger than those of macrophages (Figure 6.21). Several morphologic variants are recognized. In most cases, the predominant cells resemble either centroblasts or immunoblasts, or there is often a mixture of both. Occasional cases comprise large, bizarre, or even multinucleated cells. The large cells infiltrate in sheets between the glands, which ultimately atrophy and disappear, but invasion of individual glands and formation of LELs are uncommon.

When DLBCL is seen in association with MALT lymphoma, the extent of the secondary high-grade component varies. Some cases are comprised of small foci of cohesive sheets of large transformed cells, while others are characterized by a predominance of large cell lymphoma with only minor residual foci of small cell lymphoma that may be difficult to identify.

Immunohistochemical and Molecular Features

Similar to other DLBCLs, the tumor cells express CD20 and other pan-B-cell antigens (CD19, CD22, CD79a, PAX5) with surface and/or cytoplasmic immunoglobulin, usually IgM, and show a high proliferation rate (Ki67 > 50%).

A variable number of CD3+ reactive T cells are scattered throughout the tumor. Residual follicular dendritic cell

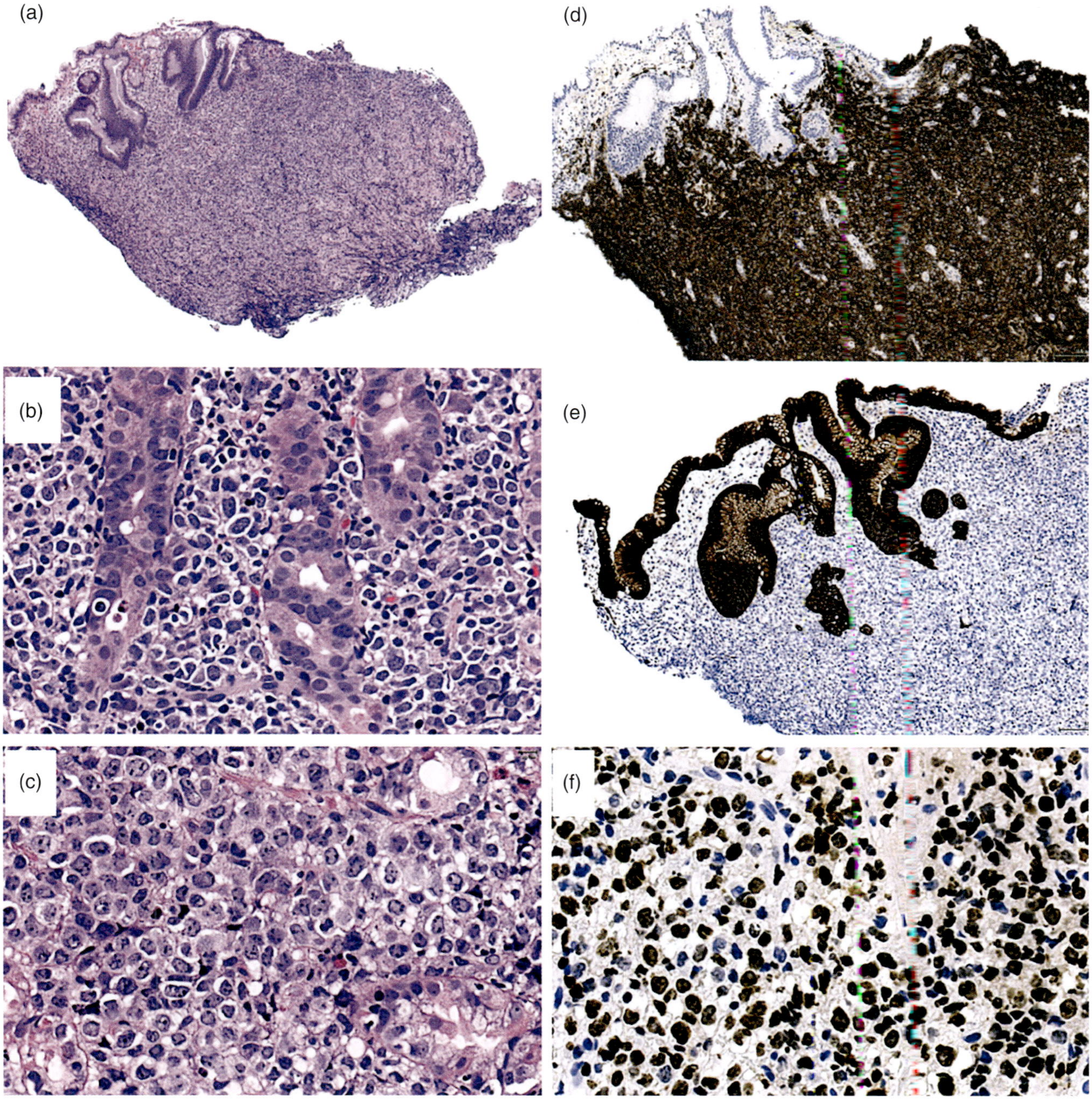

Figure 6.21 Diffuse large B-cell lymphoma of the stomach. (a) Low-power view of an endoscopic biopsy showing a dense and diffuse lymphoid infiltrate involving the mucosa and infiltrating the muscularis mucosa. (b, c) Large lymphoid cells infiltrate the lamina propria between epithelial structures and scattered cells infiltrate the epithelium without evidence of clear lymphoepithelial lesions. (d) The neoplastic cells are strongly positive for CD20. (e) Cytokeratin stain highlights the crypts and residual glands in the lamina propria. (f) High proliferation rate shown by a nuclear Ki67 staining in most cells.

meshworks highlighted by CD21 or CD23, if present, may suggest transformation from MALT lymphoma.

When DLBCL coexists with a low-grade component, both components show the same light chain restriction and identical immunoglobulin gene rearrangements. DLBCLs arising from MALT lymphoma are frequently negative for BCL2 and CD10 but, in contrast to MALT lymphoma, frequently express BCL6. Conversely, de novo gastric DLBCL may express CD10 and/or BCL2. However, there are no reliable immunophenotypic features distinguishing gastric lymphomas arising de novo from those transformed from MALT lymphomas.

Gastric DLBCL may be subclassified into molecular subgroups, similar to DLBCL arising in lymph node or elsewhere. The "germinal center B-cell like" (GCB) and "non-GCB" categories can be defined by immunohistochemistry for expression of CD10, BCL6, and MUM1, according to Hans' algorithm, but the clinical usefulness of this stratification remains controversial.

Compared to nodal DLBCL, *BCL2* gene rearrangements are rare in primary gastric DLBCL. In contrast, rearrangements of *BCL6* can be detected in up to 1/2 of primary gastric DLBCL cases and were found predictive of complete remission and better survival. *MYC* rearrangements can also be detected in nearly 10% of cases, and are associated with clinically aggressive behavior. MALT-specific translocations such as t(11;18) are rarely present in gastric DLBCL. EBV can be demonstrated by EBER in situ hybridization in rare cases, especially in elderly patients.

Differential Diagnosis

DLBCL must be distinguished from:

- MALT lymphoma with increased number of large cells (discussed previously, in the Section "Extranodal Marginal Zone Lymphoma of Mucosa-Associated Lymphoid Tissue (MALT Lymphoma)").
- Burkitt lymphoma (see Section "Burkitt Lymphoma").
- Other high-grade B-cell neoplasms (Table 6.11) including high-grade B-cell lymphoma (HGBCL) not otherwise specified (NOS) and HGBCLs with combined *MYC* and *BCL2* and/or *BCL6* translocations, referred to as "double-hit" or "triple hit" lymphomas (Figure 6.22).
- Poorly differentiated carcinoma, especially in poorly preserved biopsy specimens and in rare cases where the malignant lymphoid cells have the appearance of signet ring cells but this differential diagnosis is easily resolved by histochemical and immunohistochemical analyses.

Prognosis, Evolution, and Clinical Management

DLBCLs usually present at a more advanced stage than MALT lymphomas and their prognosis is worse with a five-year survival rate of 60–70%. There are conflicting reports as to whether the presence of an associated low-grade component influences the outcome of primary gastric DLBCL.

The treatment of gastric DLBCL is based on a combination of chemotherapy and Rituximab, supplemented by antibiotics in *H. pylori*-positive cases. The role of radiotherapy consolidation is debated but it has been associated with a lower recurrence rate in some series. Surgery is used only for patients with major complications such as severe bleeding, perforation, or obstruction.

Mantle Cell Lymphoma

Definition, General Features, and Predisposing Factors

Mantle cell lymphoma is a distinctive small B-cell lymphoma entity with a relatively aggressive course, affecting middle-aged to older adults with a male predominance. Patients usually present widespread disease at initial diagnostic, often with involvement of the gastrointestinal tract. However, primary isolated gastric mantle cell lymphoma is rare.

Clinical Features and Endoscopic Characteristics

Mantle cell lymphoma often manifests with abdominal pain, weight loss, diarrhea, and rectal bleeding. As a primary gastrointestinal disease, mantle cell lymphoma may present as numerous polypoid lesions, so-called multiple lymphomatous polyposis. Any portion of the gastrointestinal tract may be involved, especially the ileo-caecal region. Gastric involvement is noted in 50% of cases, as large cerebroid folds and in some cases as a mass. In addition, microscopic involvement of the gastrointestinal tract without endoscopic lesions is extremely frequent in patients with systemic mantle cell lymphoma (80% of cases).

Microscopic Features

Mantle cell lymphoma is composed of a diffuse or vaguely nodular monotonous infiltrate of uniform small- to medium-sized lymphoid cells with irregular nuclei and scant cytoplasm (Figure 6.23). Scattered epithelioid histiocytes may be dispersed among the neoplastic cells. The infiltrate may surround small residual involuted germinal centers. The neoplastic cells tend to displace and obliterate glandular structures and LELs can been seen, but are not a typical feature.

A spectrum of morphological variants is recognized, in particular the blastoid variant with cells resembling lymphoblasts with high mitotic activity, and the pleomorphic variant in which the lymphomatous cells display more variable size with prominent nuclei potentially mimicking DLBCL.

Immunohistochemical and Molecular Features

The neoplastic cells are usually positive for pan-B lymphocyte markers, such as CD19, CD20, CD79a, and PAX5, and typically show strong expression of surface IgM and IgD, with lambda light chain more frequently than kappa. They often also express CD5, CD43, BCL2, but lack CD23, CD10, and BCL6.

Table 6.11 Differential diagnosis of high-grade mature B-cell lymphomas involving the stomach.

	Burkitt lymphoma	DLBCL-NOS	HGBCL, double-/triple hit	HGBCL-NOS
Epidemiology	Adolescents or adults, male predominance, HIV, immunodeficiency	Any age, more common in older adults	Adults	Adults
Morphology	Diffuse growth with "starry-sky" pattern Uniform, medium-sized cells Mitotic and apoptotic figures	Diffuse growth Large cells: centroblasts and/or immunoblasts and/or anaplastic cells	Diffuse growth +/− "starry-sky" pattern Intermediate between DLBCL and Burkitt lymphoma OR blastoid OR large cell morphology	Diffuse growth +/− "starry-sky" pattern Intermediate between DLBCL and Burkitt lymphoma OR blastoid
Immunophenotype	CD20+, CD79a+, CD10+, BCL6+, MUM1−, BCL2−, MYC+, Ki67 = 100%	CD20+, CD79a+, CD10−/+, BCL6+/−, MUM1+/−, BCL2+/−, MYC−/+, Ki67 < 90%	CD20+, CD79a+, CD10+/−, BCL6+/−, MUM1+/−, BCL2 variable, MYC+, Ki67 > 90%, TdT−	CD20+, CD79a+, CD10+/−, BCL6+/−, MUM1+/−, BCL2 variable, MYC−/+, Ki67 > 90%, TdT−
Genetics	*MYC* rearrangement constant, *TCF3* or *ID3* mutations in 70% of cases	*BCL6, MYC* (or *BCL2*) rearrangement in a subset of cases (no double hit)	*MYC* and *BCL2*, and/or *BCL6* rearrangements (double/triple hit)	*MYC, BCL2*, or *BCL6* rearrangement in a subset of cases (no double hit)
EBV status	Subset of cases EBV+	Rare cases EBV+ (EBV+ DLBCL, NOS)	EBV-negative	EBV-negative

DLBCL, diffuse large B-cell lymphoma; HGBCL, high-grade B-cell lymphoma; EBV, Epstein–Barr virus; NOS, not otherwise specified.

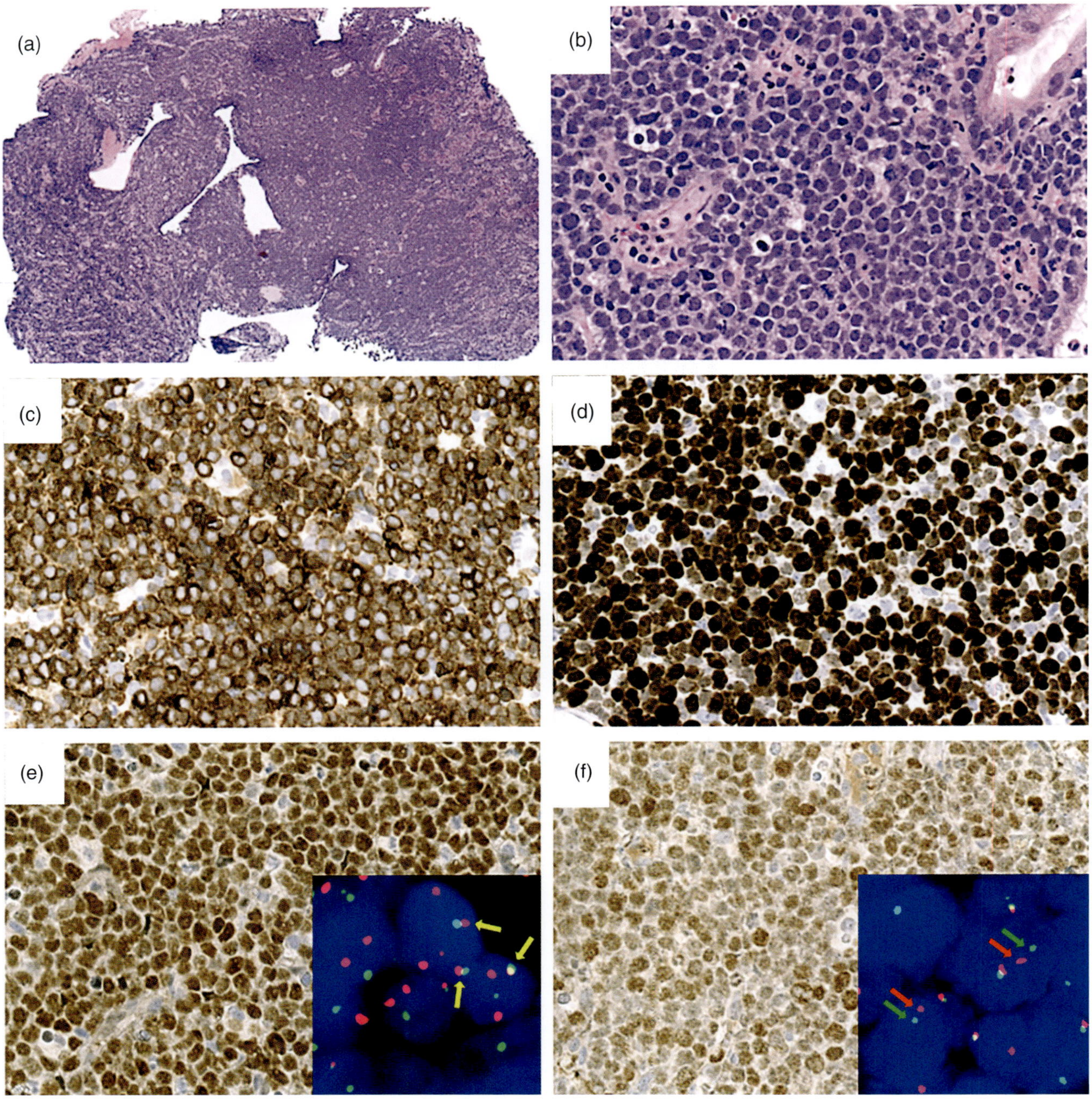

Figure 6.22 Primary gastric "double-hit" high-grade B-cell lymphoma with *MYC* and *BCL6* rearrangements showing intermediate features between diffuse large B-cell lymphoma and Burkitt lymphoma, in a 42-year-old HIV-positive woman. (a) The tumor cells densely infiltrate the mucosa with a focally prominent "starry-sky" pattern. (b) The tumor is composed of medium-sized and occasional larger lymphoid cells, suggestive of Burkitt lymphoma but with slightly more pleomorphism including blastic cells with moderately prominent nucleoli. (c) The neoplastic cells are CD79a-positive with (d) a Ki67 proliferation rate nearly 100%, and are EBV-negative by in situ hybridization (not shown). (e) Strong nuclear expression of MYC in the majority of the nuclei with *MYC-IGH* gene rearrangement by fluorescence in situ hybridization (FISH) (fusion probe with fusion signals indicate by yellow arrow). (f) Moderate nuclear expression of BCL6 in almost all the malignant cells with *BCL6* gene rearrangement by FISH (break-apart probe with signals indicated by red and green arrows).

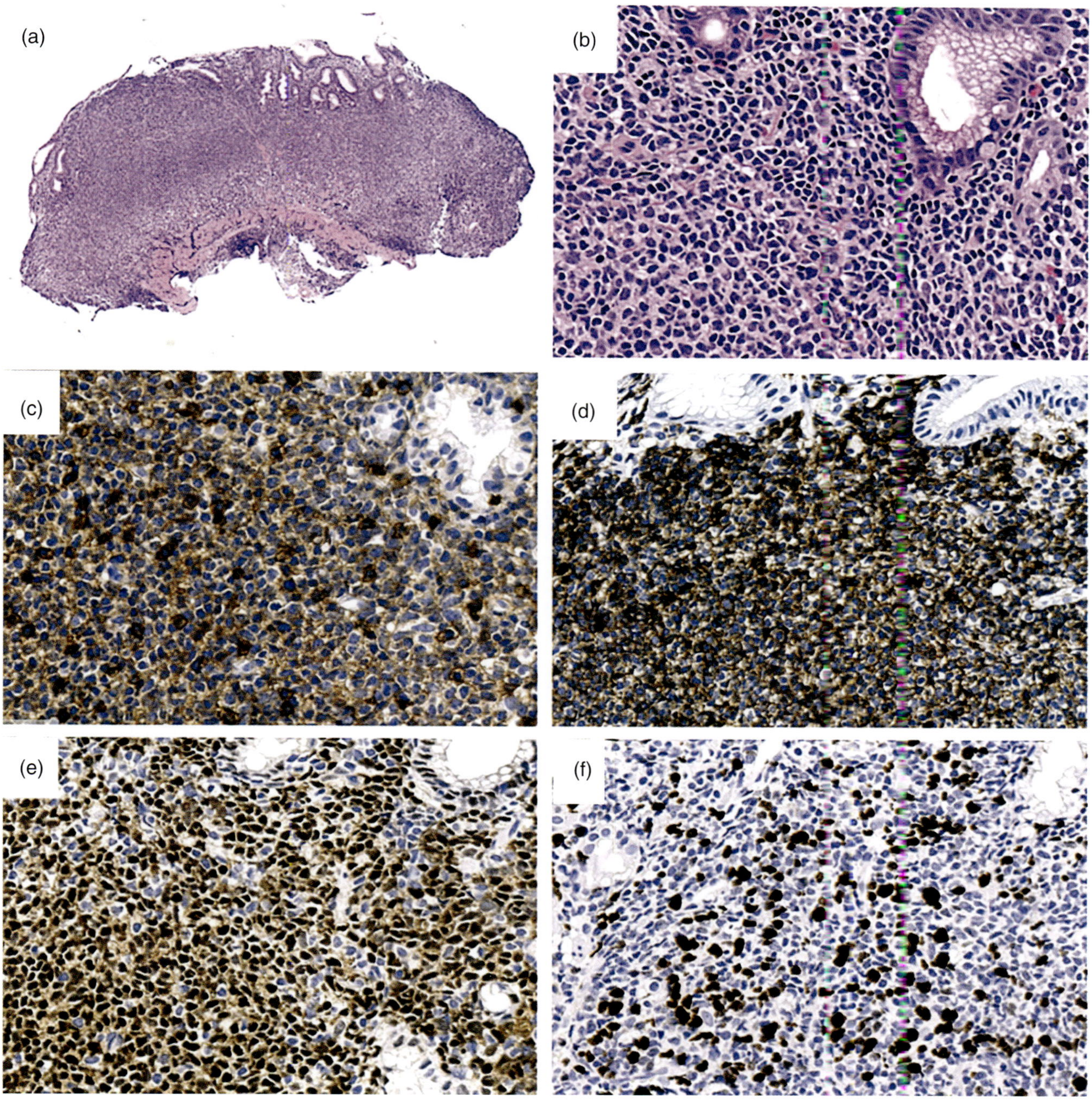

Figure 6.23 Mantle cell lymphoma diagnosed on gastric biopsies in a 80-year-old man. (a) Low-power view showing a diffuse and dense vaguely nodular lymphoid infiltrate obliterating the mucosa and the submucosa. (b) The lymphoid infiltrate is composed of monotonous small- to medium-sized lymphoid cells with irregular nuclei and scant cytoplasm. The neoplastic cells are positive for CD20 (not shown) and (c) CD5, with (d) co-expression of CD43, (e) strong nuclear expression of cyclin D1 and (f) a Ki67 labeling index of about 30%.

Cyclin D1 is overexpressed as a consequence of the t(11;14)(q13;q32) translocation involving the *CCND1* and *IGH* genes (Figure 6.23e). Rare cases of mantle cell lymphoma are cyclin D1-negative by immunohistochemistry and do not harbor *CCND1* rearrangement, and often show alternative rearrangement of *CCND2* but such cases should be diagnosed with extreme caution. SOX11 expression is a characteristic feature of mantle cell lymphoma distinctive from other small B-cell lymphoma and useful to identify cyclin D1-negative cases.

Differential Diagnosis

The differential diagnosis of mantle cell lymphoma is mainly with other small B-cell lymphomas for the common form (see Table 6.10). In contrast, the blastoid and the pleomorphic variants of mantle cell lymphoma can be very similar in appearance to DLBCL and myeloid or precursor lymphoid neoplasm.

Prognosis, Evolution, and Clinical Management

Mantle cell lymphoma is a relatively aggressive disease compared to other small B-cell lymphomas, with a median survival of three to five years.

The proliferation index evaluated by Ki67 immunohistochemistry is an important prognostic biomarker that should be reported.

Burkitt Lymphoma

Definition, General Features, and Predisposing Factors

Burkitt lymphoma is a highly aggressive neoplasm composed of mature B cells with very high proliferative activity, preferentially affecting children and young adults. Three clinical variants are recognized: endemic, sporadic, and immune deficiency-associated.

Burkitt lymphoma has a predilection for extranodal sites, including gastrointestinal tract, especially the ileo-caecal region, and may also occur in the stomach.

Clinical Features and Endoscopic Characteristics

The tumors are often bulky, sometimes with ulceration, and are usually located in the gastric body or antrum.

Microscopic Features

The tumor is composed of a diffuse infiltrate of uniform, medium-sized lymphoid cells containing round nuclei with granular chromatin and multiple nucleoli and a rim of basophilic cytoplasm. Mitotic figures are usually numerous, with abundant apoptotic activity and scattered macrophages containing apoptotic cellular debris imparting a "starry-sky" appearance (Figure 6.24). A subset of cases shows plasmacytoid differentiation.

Immunohistochemical and Molecular Features

The neoplastic cells are CD20+, IgM+, CD10+, BCL2−, and BCL6+, with a proliferation fraction approaching 100%. The tumor cells are positive for the EBV in the majority of endemic cases and in a subset of the other clinical variants.

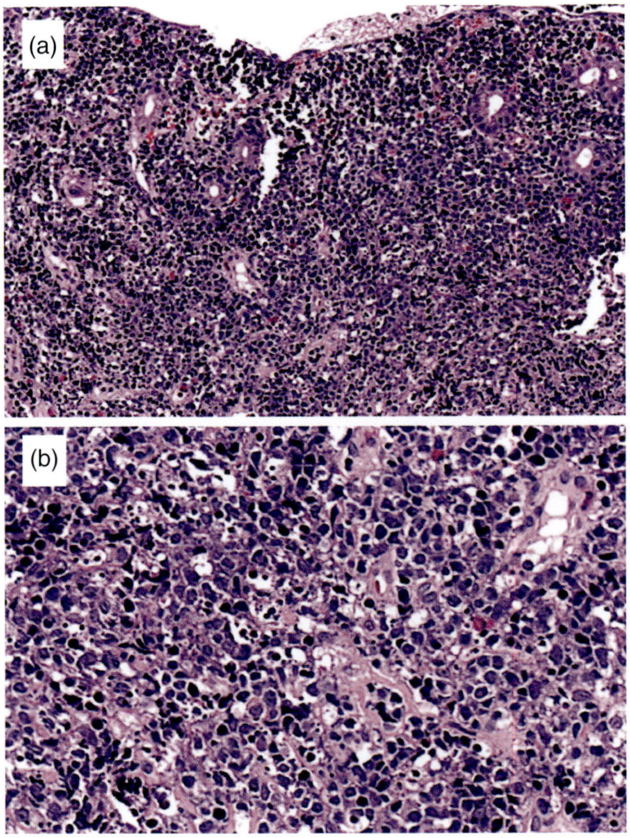

Figure 6.24 Primary gastric sporadic Burkitt lymphoma, EBV-negative, in a 34-year-old HIV-negative man. (a, b) A dense monotonous infiltrate of medium-sized lymphoid cells with scant cytoplasm, numerous mitoses and apoptotic bodies and a starry-sky appearance obscures the mucosa. A *MYC* rearrangement was demonstrated by FISH (not shown).

The hallmark molecular abnormality is a translocation of the *MYC* gene to *IGH*, *IGK* or *IGL*, most frequently t(8;14)(q24;q32).

Differential Diagnosis

Burkitt lymphoma must be distinguished from other high-grade lymphomas especially DLBCLs, and HGBCLs, NOS, or with *MYC* and *BCL2* and/or *BCL6* translocations (Table 6.12). Burkitt lymphoma must also be distinguished from lymphoblastic lymphoma due to the overlapping cytological features and the common presence of a starry-sky pattern, but immature lymphoid neoplasms uncommonly involve the stomach.

Prognosis, Evolution, and Clinical Management

A better outcome has been reported for patients with gastric Burkitt lymphoma compared to non-gastric Burkitt lymphoma, especially when the disease was localized to the stomach.

A complete remission after eradication of *H. pylori* in gastric Burkitt lymphoma has been reported, suggesting a role for the bacterium in its pathogenesis and the importance of seeking and eradicating the bacterium in combination with conventional chemotherapy.

Peripheral T-Cell Lymphomas

Definition, General Features, and Predisposing Factors

Peripheral T-cell lymphomas (PTCLs) are overall rare and primary gastric presentation is exceptional. Notably there is some geographic variation, especially with respect to specific histological types. Lymphomas associated with human T-lymphotropic virus-1 (HTLV1) may represent the primary manifestation of adult T-cell leukemia/lymphoma (ATLL).

Primary gastric T-cell lymphomas without HTLV1 infection mostly fall into the category of peripheral T-cell lymphoma, NOS. Some of them are positive for EBV or occur in association with *H. pylori* infection. Gastric involvement with enteropathy-associated T-cell lymphoma (EATL) can also be seen, especially in northern Europe where coeliac disease is prevalent. Anaplastic large cell lymph can also arise in the stomach, but such presentation is extremely rare. Extranodal NK/T-cell lymphoma (ENKTCL), nasal type, may also involve the stomach (Figure 6.25).

Clinical Features and Endoscopic Characteristics

Gastric T-cell lymphomas are often present as ulcerated masses in the middle or upper corpus or are more widely distributed.

Microscopic Features

- T-cell lymphomas HTLV1+: The cytomorphology ranges from monomorphic to polymorphic and may comprise medium-sized cells with round or irregular nuclei and medium- to large-sized cells or cells with anaplastic morphology.
- EATL: It is composed of pleomorphic medium- to-large cells with high mitotic rates and polymorphic inflammatory infiltrate rich in histiocytes and eosinophils.
- PTCL-NOS: The majority display large cell morphology or, less commonly, comprise a population of small- to medium-sized cells. Tumors composed of smaller cells may show clear cell features and epitheliotropism, potentially mimicking the LELs of MALT B-cell lymphoma. The neoplastic infiltrates may show a pronounced eosinophilia that may partially obscure the neoplastic cells.
- ENKTCL: The cytomorphological features are heterogeneous from case to case and the lymphoma cells range from monomorphic small- and medium-sized to polymorphic large cells. An angiocentric and angiodestructive infiltration pattern reported as a characteristic but inconstant feature is responsible for ischemic necrosis, leading to mucosal ulceration or perforation.

Immunohistochemical and Molecular Features

HTLV1-associated T-cell lymphomas are usually CD4+, CD7−, and CD8−; strongly express CD25; and are positive for FOXP3.

Most PTCL-NOS show a helper-inducer phenotype (CD4+, CD8−), whereas some cases show a suppressor-cytotoxic phenotype (CD4−, CD8−/+, TIA1+, granzyme B+). Expression of CD30 by the tumor cells is frequently detected in cases with large cell morphology. A subset of the latter with the immunophenotype of intraepithelial lymphocytes may express CD103 and/or show enteropathy-like features and may represent gastric localizations of the EATL, which are typically CD3+, CD5−, CD4−, CD8−, CD56−, CD30+, CD103+, TCR$\alpha\beta$−. Few cases present typical features of anaplastic large cell lymphoma and cases positive for ALK are extremely rare.

The usual immunophenotype for ENKTCL derived from natural killer (NK) cells, which harbor polyclonal *TCR* genes, is CD2+, cCD3+, CD5−, CD4−, CD8−, CD56+, with co-expression of TIA-1, perforin, and/or granzyme B, indicative of an activated cytotoxic phenotype. ENKTCL is by definition associated with EBV.

Prognosis, Evolution, and Clinical Management

The outcome of patients with primary gastric peripheral T-cell lymphoma is in general poorer compared with gastric B-cell lymphomas. However the prognosis of patients with gastric anaplastic large lymphoma and peripheral T-cell lymphoma, NOS, is better than that of patients with intestinal EATLs.

Indolent T/NK-Cell Lymphoproliferations of the Gastrointestinal Tract

In addition to the "usual" forms of aggressive T- and NK-cell neoplasms, more indolent lymphoproliferations derived from T/NK cells may affect the gastrointestinal tract. These are important to recognize because they can easily be mistaken for "high-grade" lymphomas.

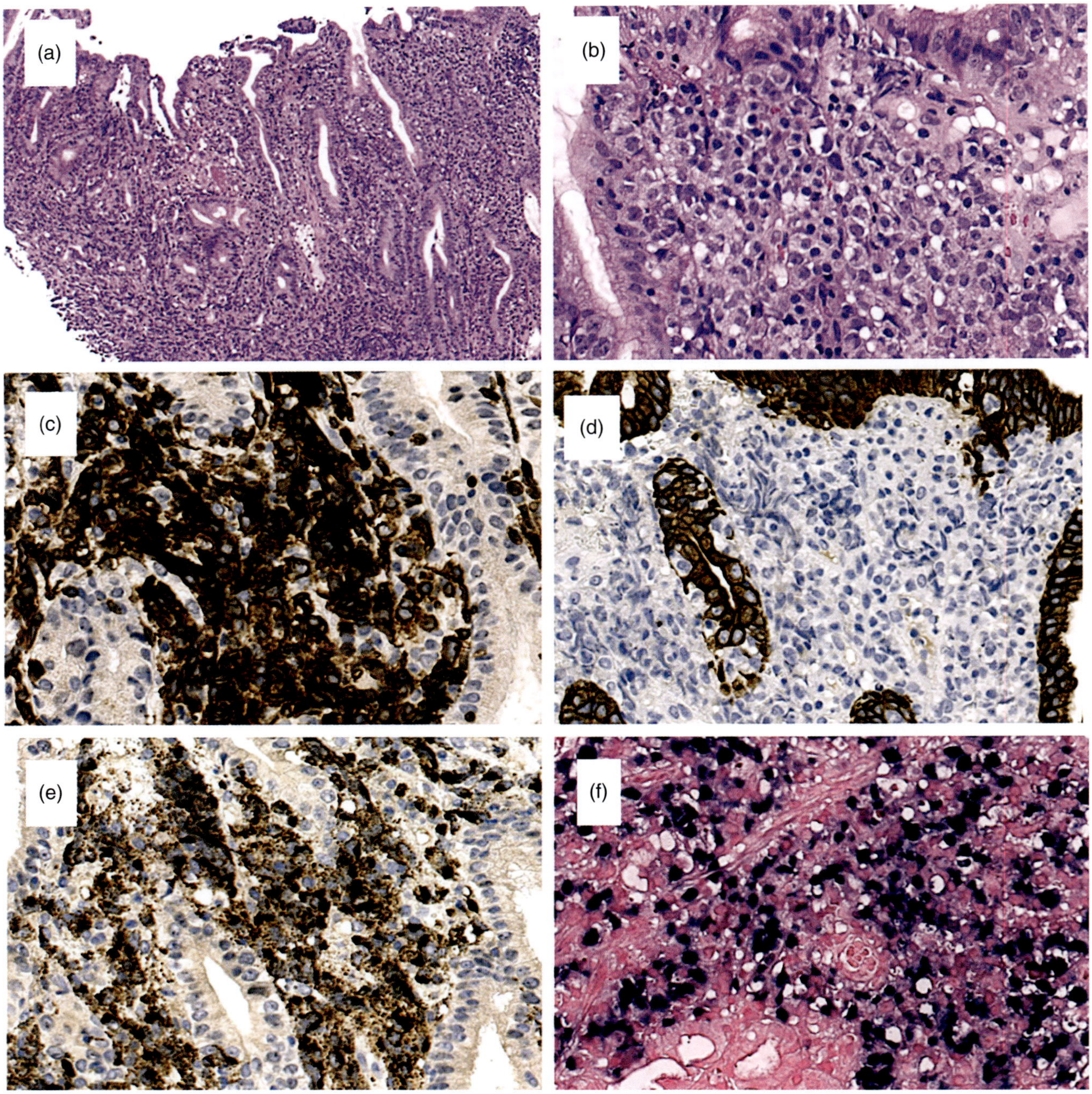

Figure 6.25 Gastric involvement by an extranodal NK/T-cell lymphoma nasal-type in a 37-year-old man with an advanced clinical stage at presentation. (a) A diffuse lymphoid infiltrate is seen in the gastric mucosa, (b) composed of medium- to large-sized lymphoid cells with irregular nuclei and scant cytoplasm admixed with some eosinophils. (c) The atypical lymphoid cells are positive for CD3, (d) infiltrate the crypts and glands as shown by cytokeratin stain, (e) express cytotoxic granules-associated granzyme-B, and (f) are positive for Epstein–Barr virus (EBERs in situ hybridization).

Indolent T-Cell Lymphoproliferative Disorders of the Gastrointestinal Tract

Rare primary clonal T-cell proliferations of the gastrointestinal tract with an indolent clinical behavior were recently recognized and introduced as a provisional entity in the newly revised World Health Organization (WHO) classification. These occur more commonly in middle-aged individuals with chronic diarrhea, weight loss, abdominal pain, and/or rectal bleeding. Endoscopic findings include mucosal erythema, erosions, or small ulcerations and in some instances small polyps, without mass lesions. Patients usually had multiple lesions along the gastrointestinal tract, and rare cases have evidence of distant disease.

Mucosal biopsies reveal a dense infiltrate of small, monotonous lymphoid cells in the lamina propria without destruction of the epithelial structures and, in some cases, an extension to the submucosa. The lymphoid cells express CD3 and can be CD4+, CD8+ or CD4− CD8−. They often lack expression of CD5 or CD7, and they do not express CD56, CD30, FOXP3, or PD1. Ki67 is generally low (<10%) and EBV is typically absent.

NK-Cell Gastropathy/Enteropathy

This very rare disorder derived from NK cells, with a benign clinical course and features distinct from NK-cell lymphoma, has been variably reported as "lymphomatoid gastropathy" or "NK-cell enteropathy." Most cases occur in middle-aged to older individuals who were either asymptomatic or presented with middle gastrointestinal symptoms. The lesions are either localized or in multiple sites and may appear as small polyps or nodules or erosions/ulcers, with edema.

The biopsy shows an atypical lymphoid infiltrate composed of medium- to large-sized cells with abundant clear or slightly eosinophilic cytoplasm, diffusely infiltrating the lamina propria, with occasional epitheliotropism and glandular destruction but absence of angiocentricity and angiodestruction. The atypical cells have a NK-cell immunophenotype (CD3+, CD4−, CD5−, CD7+, CD8−, CD56+), with an activated cytotoxic profile (TIA1, granzym B, perforin), a moderate Ki67 proliferation index (10–30%), and a negative EBV status.

Gastric Lymphomas in Abnormal Immune States

Lymphomas in human immunodeficiency virus (HIV)-positive individuals often involve the gastrointestinal tract. However, the stomach is involved relatively infrequently compared to the colon, rectum, and small intestine. Most cases are HGBCLs, classified as DLBCL or Burkitt lymphoma and show an association with EBV infection more commonly than those occurring in the HIV-negative population.

Post-transplant lymphoproliferative disorders (PTLD) may also occur in the stomach. They are classified as early lesions, polymorphic PTLDs, monomorphic PTLDs, and classical Hodgkin lymphoma-type. The polymorphic and monomorphic PTLDs of B-cell lineage are most frequently encountered in the gastrointestinal tract. A few cases of EBV-negative gastric MALT lymphomas have also been reported in allograft recipients.

Further Reading

Andriani, A., Zullo, A., Di Raimondo, F. et al. (2006). Clinical and endoscopic presentation of primary gastric lymphoma: a multicentre study. *Aliment. Pharmacol. Ther.* 23: 721–726.

Auer, I.A., Gascoyne, R.D., Connors, J.M. et al. (1997). t(11;18)(q21;q21) is the most common translocation in MALT lymphomas. *Ann. Oncol.* 8: 979–985.

Bacon, C.M., Du, M.Q., and Dogan, A. (2007). Mucosa-associated lymphoid tissue (MALT) lymphoma: a practical guide for pathologists. *J. Clin. Pathol.* 60: 361–372.

Banerjee, D., Walton, J.C., Jory, T.A. et al. (1990). Primary gastric T-cell lymphoma of suppressor-cytotoxic (CD8+) phenotype: discordant expression of T-cell receptor subunit beta F1, CD7and CD3 antigens. *Hum. Pathol.* 21: 872–874.

Baumgaertner, I., Copie-Bergman, C., Levy, M. et al. (2009). Complete remission of gastric Burkitt's lymphoma after eradication of *Helicobacter pylori*. *World J. Gastroenterol.* 15: 5746–5750.

Beck, P.L., Gill, M.J., and Sutherland, L.R. (1996). HIV-associated non-Hodgkin's lymphoma of the gastrointestinal tract. *Am. J. Gastroenterol.* 91: 2377–2381.

Castro, F.A., Jansen, L., Krilaviciute, A. et al. (2015). Survival of patients with gastric lymphoma in Germany and in the United States. *J. Gastroenterol. Hepatol.* 30: 1485–1491.

Cogliatti, S., Schmid, U., Schumacher, U. et al. (1991). Primary B-cell gastric lymphoma: a clinicopathological study of 145 patients. *Gastroenterology* 101: 1159–1170.

Copie-Bergman, C., Gaulard, P., Lavergne-Slove, A. et al. (2003). Proposal for a new histological grading system for post-treatment evaluation of gastric MALT lymphoma. *Gut* 52: 1656.

Falini, B., Agostinelli, C., Bigerna, B. et al. (2012). IRTA1 is selectively expressed in nodal and extranodal marginal zone lymphomas. *Histopathology* 61: 930–941.

Ferreri, A.J. and Montalban, C. (2007). Primary diffuse large B-cell lymphoma of the stomach. *Crit. Rev. Oncol. Hematol.* 63: 65–71.

Ferreri, A.J., Freschi, M., Dell'Oro, S. et al. (2001). Prognostic significance of the histopathologic recognition of low- and high grade components in stage I–II B-cell gastric lymphomas. *Am. J. Surg. Pathol.* 25: 95–102.

Hans, C.P., Weisenburger, D.D., Greiner, T.C. et al. (2004). Confirmation of the molecular classification of diffuse large B-cell lymphoma by immunohistochemistry using a tissue microarray. *Blood* 103: 275–282.

Hasserjian, R.P., Ott, G., Elenitoba-Johnson, K.S. et al. (2009). Commentary on the WHO classification of tumours of lymphoid tissues (2008): "gray zone" lymphomas overlapping with Burkitt lymphoma or classical Hodgkin lymphoma. *J. Hematop.* 2: 77–81.

He, M., Chen, K., Li, S. et al. (2016). Clinical significance of "double-hit" and "double-protein" expression in primary gastric B-cell lymphomas. *J. Cancer* 7: 1215–1225.

Holanda, D., Zhao, M.Y., Rapoport, A.P. et al. (2008). Primary gastric T cell lymphoma mimicking marginal zone B cell lymphoma of mucosa-associated lymphoid tissue. *J. Hematop.* 1: 29–35.

Hsi, E.D., Singleton, T.P., Swinnen, L. et al. (2000). Mucosa-associated lymphoid tissue-type lymphomas occurring in post-transplantation patients. *Am. J. Surg. Pathol.* 24: 100–106.

Isaacson, P.G. and Du, M.Q. (2004). MALT lymphoma: from morphology to molecules. *Nat. Rev. Cancer* 4: 644–653.

Isaacson, P., Wotherspoon, A., Diss, T., and Pan, L. (1991). Follicular colonization in B-cell lymphoma of mucosa-associated lymphoid tissue. *Am. J. Surg. Pathol.* 15: 819–828.

Isaacson, P., Chott, A., Nakamura, S. et al. (2008). Extranodal marginal zone lymphoma of mucosa-associated lymphoid tissue (MALT lymphoma). In: *WHO Classification of Tumours of Haematopoietic and Lymphoid Tissues* (eds. S. Swerdlow, E. Campo, N. Harris, et al.), 214–217. Lyon: International Agency for Research on Cancer.

Iwamizu-Watanabe, S., Yamashita, Y., Yatabe, Y. et al. (2004). Frequent expression of CD30 antigen in the primary gastric non-B, non-Hodgkin lymphomas. *Pathol. Int.* 54: 503–509.

de Jong, D.J.B., van Heerde, P., and Hart, A. (1997). Histological grading in gastric lymphoma: pretreatment criteria and clinical relevance. *Gastroenterology* 112: 1466–1474.

de Jong, D., Boot, H., and Taal, B. (2000). Histological grading with clinical relevance in gastric mucosa-associated lymphoid tissue (MALT) lymphoma. *Recent Results Cancer Res.* 156: 27–32.

Kawamoto, K., Nakamura, S., Iwashita, A. et al. (2009). Clinicopathological characteristics of primary gastric T-cell lymphoma. *Histopathology* 55: 641–653.

Leoncini, L., Raphael, M., Stein, H. et al. (2008). Burkitt lymphoma. In: *WHO Classification of Tumours of Haematopoietic and Lymphoid Tissues* (eds. S. Swerdlow, E. Campo, N. Harris, et al.), 262–266. Lyon: International Agency for Research on Cancer.

de Leval, L. and Hasserjian, R.P. (2009). Diffuse large B-cell lymphomas and Burkitt lymphoma. *Hematol. Oncol. Clin. North Am.* 23: 791–827.

Levy, M., Copie-Bergman, C., Gameiro, C. et al. (2005). Prognostic value of translocation t(11;18) in tumoural response of low grade gastric lymphoma of mucosa-associated lymphoid tissue type to oral chemotherapy. *J. Clin. Oncol.* 23: 5061–5066.

Levy, M., Copie-Bergman, C., Molinier-Frenkel, V. et al. (2010). Treatment of t(11;18)-positive gastric mucosa-associated lymphoid tissue lymphoma with rituximab and chlorambucil: clinical, histological and molecular follow-up. *Leuk. Lymphoma* 51: 284–290.

Liang, R., Chan, W.P., Kwong, Y.L. et al. (1997). High incidence of BCL-6 gene rearrangement in diffuse large B-cell lymphoma of primary gastric origin. *Cancer Genet. Cytogenet.* 97: 114–118.

Liu, H., Ruskon-Fourmestraux, A., Lavergne-Slove, A. et al. (2001). Resistance of t(11;18) positive gastric mucosa-associated lymphoid tissue lymphoma to Helicobacter pylori eradication therapy. *Lancet* 357: 39–40.

Maeshima, A.M., Taniguchi, H., Toyoda, K. et al. (2016). Linicopathological features of histological transformation from extranodal marginal zone B-cell lymphoma of mucosa-associated lymphoid tissue to diffuse large B-cell lymphoma: an analysis of 467 patients. *Br. J. Haematol.* 174: 923–931.

Matnani, R., Ganapathi, K.A., Lewis, S.K. et al. (2017). Indolent T- and NK-cell lymphoproliferative disorders of the gastrointestinal tract: a review and update. *Hematol. Oncol.* 35 (1): 3–16.

Ohshima, K., Jaffe, E., and Kikuchi, M. (2008). Adult T-cell leukaemia/lymphoma. In: *WHO Classification of Tumours of Haematopoietic and Lymphoid Tissues* (eds. S. Swerdlow, E. Campo, N. Harris, et al.), 281–284. Lyon: International Agency on Cancer Research.

O'Malley, D.P., Goldstein, N.S., and Banks, P.M. (2014). The recognition and classification of lymphoproliferative disorders of the gut. *Hum. Pathol.* 45: 899–916.

Omonishi, K., Yoshino, T., Sakuma, I. et al. (1998). BCL-6 protein is identified in high grade but not low grade mucosa-associated lymphoid tissue lymphomas of the stomach. *Mod. Pathol.* 11: 181–185.

Park, Y.H., Kim, W.S., Kang, H.J. et al. (2006). Gastric Burkitt lymphoma is a distinct subtype that has superior outcomes to other types of Burkitt lymphoma/leukemia. *Ann. Hematol.* 85: 285–290.

Perry, A.M., Warnke, R.A., Hu, Q. et al. (2013). Indolent T-cell lymphoproliferative disease of the gastrointestinal tract. *Blood* 122: 3599–3606.

Qin, Y., Greiner, A., Trunk, M.J. et al. (1995). Somatic hypermutation in low grade mucosa-associated lymphoid tissue-type B-cell lymphoma. *Blood* 86: 3528–3534.

Raderer, M., Streubel, B., Woehrer, S. et al. (2005). High relapse rate in patients with MALT lymphoma warrants lifelong follow-up. *Clin. Cancer Res.* 11: 3349–3352.

Ruskone-Fourmestraux, A. and Audouin, J. (2010). Primary gastrointestinal tract mantle cell lymphoma as multiple lymphomatous polyposis. *Best Pract. Res. Clin. Gastroenterol.* 24: 35–42.

Ruskone-Fourmestraux, A., Delmer, A., Lavergne, A. et al. (1997). Multiple lymphomatous polyposis of the gastrointestinal tract: prospective clinicopathologic study of 31 cases. Groupe D'etude des Lymphomes Digestifs. *Gastroenterology* 112: 7–16.

Salaverria, I., Royo, C., Carvajal-Cuenca, A. et al. (2013). CCND2 rearrangements are the most frequent genetic events in cyclin D1(-) mantle cell lymphoma. *Blood* 121: 1394–1402.

Swerdlow, S., Campo, E., Seto, M., and Müller-Hermelink, H. (2008). Mantle cell lymphoma. In: *WHO Classification of Tumours of Haematopoietic and Lymphoid Tissues* (eds. S. Swerlow, E. Campo, N. Harris, et al.), 229–232. Lyon: International Agency for Research on Cancer.

Swerdlow, S., Webber, S., Chadburn, A., and Ferry, J. (2008). Post-transplant lymphoproliferative disorders. In: *WHO Classification of Tumours of Haematopoietic and Lymphoid Tissues* (eds. S. Swerdlow, E. Campo, N. Harris, et al.), 343–349. Lyon: International Agency on Cancer Research.

Swerdlow, S.H., Campo, E., Pileri, S.A. et al. (2016). The 2016 revision of the World Health Organization classification of lymphoid neoplasms. *Blood* 127: 2375–2390.

Takeshita, M., Iwashita, A., Kurihara, K. et al. (2000). Histologic and immunohistologic findings and prognosis of 40 cases of gastric large B-cell lymphoma. *Am. J. Surg. Pathol.* 24: 1641–1649.

Wotherspoon, A.C., Pan, L.X., Diss, T.C., and Isaacson, P.G. (1992). Cytogenetic study of B-cell lymphoma of mucosa-associated lymphoid tissue. *Cancer Genet. Cytogenet.* 58: 35–38.

Wotherspoon, A., Doglioni, C., Diss, T. et al. (1993). Regression of primary low grade B-cell gastric lymphoma of mucosa-associated lymphoid tissue type after eradication of Helicobacter pylori. *Lancet* 342: 575–577.

Ye, H., Liu, H., Attygalle, A. et al. (2003). Variable frequencies of t(11;18)(q21;q21) in MALT lymphomas of different sites: significant association with CagA strains of *H. pylori* in gastric MALT lymphoma. *Blood* 102: 1012–1018.

Yokoi, T., Nakamura, T., Kasugai, K. et al. (1999). Primary low grade gastric mucosa-associated lymphoid tissue (MALT) lymphoma with polypoid appearance. Polypoid gastric MALT lymphoma: a clinicopathologic study of eight cases. *Pathol. Int.* 49: 702–709.

Zamboni, G., Franzin, G., Scarpa, A. et al. (1996). Carcinoma-like signet-ring cells in gastric mucosa-associated lymphoid tissue (MALT) lymphoma. *Am. J. Surg. Pathol.* 20: 588–598.

Zucca, E., Copie-Bergman, C., Ricardi, U. et al. (2013). Gastric marginal zone lymphoma of MALT type: ESMO Clinical Practice Guidelines for diagnosis, treatment and follow-up. *Ann. Oncol.* 24: 144–148.

7

Inflammatory and Miscellaneous Conditions of the Small Intestine

Ian Brown[1] *and Michael B. Wallace*[2]

[1] *Envoi Specialist Pathologists, Brisbane, Australia*
[2] *Mayo Clinic, Jacksonville, Florida, USA*

Inflammatory Conditions

Intraepithelial Lymphocytosis with Normal Villous Architecture (Lymphocytic Duodenosis)

Definition, Frequency, Predisposing Factors

This inflammatory pattern is defined by an increase in intraepithelial T lymphocytes with preservation of the villous architecture. It is noted in 1.3–2.2% of proximal small intestinal biopsies, and has been associated with multiple etiologies (see Table 7.1).

Clinical Features/Endoscopic Characteristics

Lymphocytic duodenosis can be difficult to distinguish from celiac disease. Patients typically present with symptoms of diarrhea and irritable bowel syndrome. Patients with lymphocytic duodenitis can be distinguished based on the absence of autoantibodies characteristic of celiac disease, as well as the absence of extraintestinal manifestations such as thyroiditis, dermatitis herpetiformis, and IgA deficiency. Although less frequent than celiac disease, some LD patients have typically HLA types (DQ2, DQ8) raising suspicion that there may be overlap between the two diseases.

Microscopic Features

Characteristically, the villous length is preserved (villous-to-crypt ratio of at least 3 : 1). Mild crypt hyperplasia may be evident in some cases. The primary abnormality is an increase in intraepithelial T lymphocytes. The normal range was originally regarded as less than 40 intraepithelial lymphocytes (IELs)/100 epithelial cells (EC) (based on jejunal biopsies); more recent studies evaluating duodenal biopsies have concluded that the upper limit of normal is 25 IEL/100EC with 25–29 IEL/100EC regarded as a borderline abnormality and ≥30 IEL/100EC definitely abnormal. In practice, a count of IELs in a span of 20 enterocytes at the tip of five randomly chosen villi is the best way to document subtle abnormality. An average IEL density of ≥6/20 EC has been demonstrated to separate celiac disease-related cases from normal controls. Various degrees of chronic inflammation in the lamina propria may also be seen (Figure 7.1a, b).

Differential Diagnosis

A variety of stimuli potentially can cause this inflammatory pattern. Most can also be associated with villous blunting if the reaction is severe and/or prolonged. Gluten sensitivity is responsible in 9–40% of cases, and characteristically displays villous tip predominance of the IEL infiltrate with reduction in IEL density from villous tip to base, (i.e. "decrescendo sign"). Although not a specific feature, its absence is good histological evidence against celiac disease.

Suggestions for Reporting

A diagnosis of lymphocytic duodenitis pattern should be accompanied by a comment highlighting the nonspecific nature of the finding.

Example Report

"The duodenal mucosa has normal villous architecture and a preserved villous to crypt ratio. There is an increase of intraepithelial lymphocytes in the surface villous epithelium."

Gastrointestinal Pathology: Correlative Endoscopic and Histologic Assessment, First Edition. Edited by Gregory Y. Lauwers and Michael B. Wallace.

Table 7.1 Intraepithelial lymphocytosis with normal villous architecture – causes/associations.

Common:
- Gluten sensitivity—including dermatitis herpetiformis, first-degree relatives of celiac patients, celiac patients on GFD
- Infection—viral enteritis, Helicobacter pylori infection, Giardia, Cryptosporidia, tropical sprue
- Drugs—NSAIDs, others
- Autoimmune disease—Rheumatoid arthritis, systemic lupus erythematosus, Hashimoto thyroiditis, Graves' disease, psoriasis, ankylosing spondylitis, type 1 diabetes, scleroderma
- Idiopathic (a subset meets clinical criteria for irritable bowel syndrome)

Uncommon:
- Non-gluten food hypersensitivity—cereals, cow's milk, soy products, fish, rice, chicken
- Autoimmune enteropathy
- Immunodeficiency disorders—IgA deficiency, chronic variable immunodeficiency
- Inflammatory bowel disease
- Lymphocytic and collagenous colitis
- Morbid obesity
- Bacterial overgrowth
- Secondary to local GIT inflammation

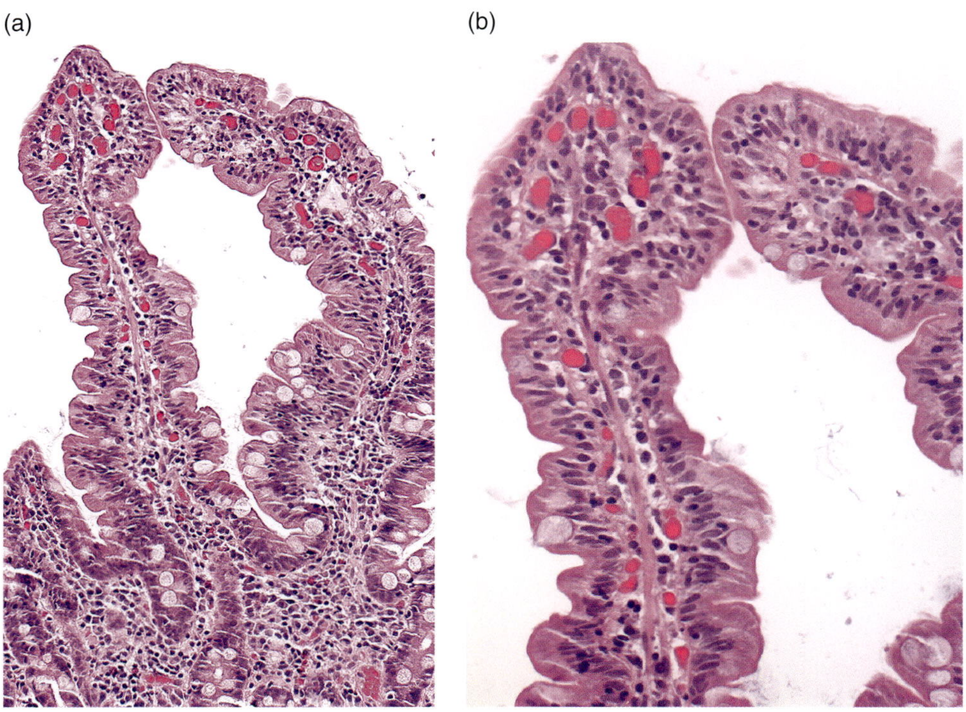

Figure 7.1 (a) Duodenal intraepithelial lymphocytosis with normal villous architecture. (b) High-power view of duodenal intraepithelial lymphocytosis. The lymphocytes are readily identified as basophilic round nuclei at the base of the epithelium.

Comment: This pattern of intraepithelial lymphocytosis with normal villous architecture is not specific. It is estimated that approximately 10% of cases represent an early form of celiac disease. Other causes include recent viral infection, concurrent autoimmune disease, and nonsteroidal anti-inflammatory (NSAID) effect.

Treatment/Prognosis/Evolution

Treatment for lymphocytic duodenitis should be aimed at specific etiologies, generally applying the least invasive/intrusive therapy first. Avoidance of NSAID medications, treatment of *Helicobacter pylori* or parasitic infection, and if no response, a gluten-free diet have been the most effective therapies.

Microvillus Inclusion Disease

Definition, General Features (Frequency), and Predisposing Factors

This rare autosomal recessive disorder presents in the neonatal period with severe intractable diarrhea, and is due to a defect in assembly and differentiation of the brush border. A mutation that impairs the globular tail domain (GTD) component of the apo-MyoVa-GTD (class V myosin) structure that is important in apical membrane recycling is responsible. It occurs in infants of all ethnic groups. An inherited predisposition is supported by familial clustering.

Clinical Features/Endoscopic Characteristics

Microvillus Inclusion Disease (MID) typically presents in infancy with severe secretory diarrhea with volume depletion and metabolic acidosis. A less severe form may present at several months of age. Treatment is largely supportive with total parenteral nutrition. The endoscopic appearance is typically normal or with mild erythema of the mucosa with subtle villous atrophy ("scalloping").

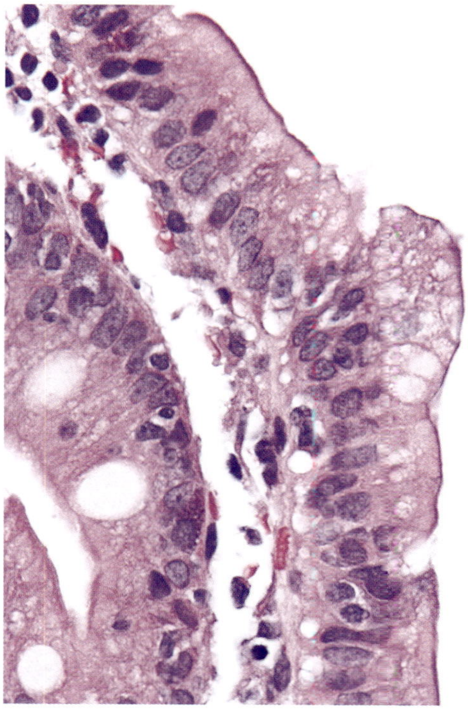

Figure 7.2 Microvillous inclusion disease with vacuolization of surface epithelium.

Microscopic Features

The mucosa displays diffuse villous shortening with little or no crypt hyperplasia (i.e. crypt hypoplastic atrophy) and normal or even decreased mucosal inflammatory cells. Enterocytes have a "bubbly" cytoplasmic appearance with a lack of luminal brush border that may resemble gastric metaplasia (Figure 7.2).

Ancillary Investigations

The primary defect in brush border assembly results in cytoplasmic displacement of the surface microvilli. These are well demonstrated as PAS-positive inclusions in the supranuclear cytoplasm of the enterocytes that also stain strongly for carcinoembryonic antigen and alkaline phosphatase and display cytoplasmic rather than cell membrane immunostaining for CD10. Electron microscopy demonstrates vesicles lined by microvilli that are structurally unremarkable (Figure 7.3—Courtesy of Dr. E. Montgomery).

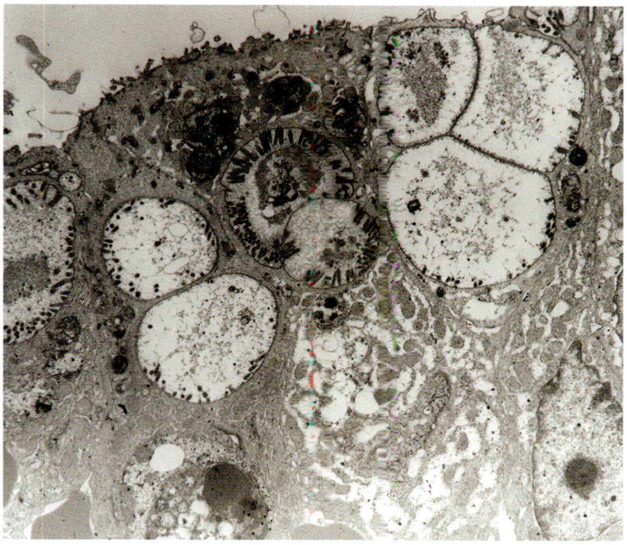

Figure 7.3 Electron microscopic image characteristic of the microvillous inclusion disease. *Source:* Courtesy of Dr. E. Montgomery.

Treatment/Prognosis/Evolution

Treatment is largely supportive with total parenteral nutrition. The prognosis is very poor with a high fatality by three years of age. Those who have later onset may have a better prognosis but typically suffer from severe mental and physical growth retardation. Small bowel transplantation, with or without concomitant liver transplantation has been applied although the prognosis is not clearly improved compared with nutritional support alone. In one large cohort, there was 63% long-term survival with supportive care versus 77% with small bowel transplantation.

Intestinal Epithelial Dysplasia (Tufting Enteropathy)

Definition, General Features, and Predisposing Factors

This autosomal recessive disorder usually presents in infancy with severe intractable diarrhea. A genetic abnormality of the EpCAM gene on chromosome 2p21 is responsible. The disorder results from a basement membrane disturbance with abnormal cell–matrix and cell–cell interaction.

Intestinal epithelial dysplasia (IED) is a congenital disease of the small bowel that presents in infancy with severe diarrhea and intestinal failure. The prevalence is approximately 1/50 000–100 000 births in western countries.

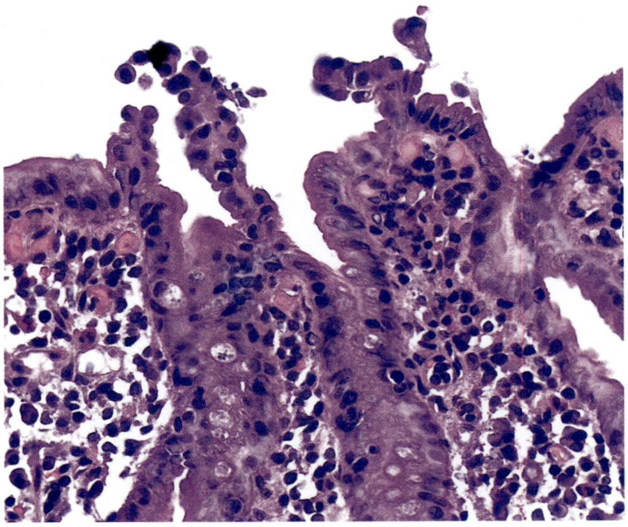

Figure 7.4 Histologic evidence of a tufting enetropathy.

Predisposing Factors

An autosomal recessive inheritance is supported by familial clustering and a higher incidence of disease in areas of high consanguinity.

Clinical Features

Infants typically present with severe intractable diarrhea at birth. Some cases have associated dysmorphic facial features, nonspecific punctuated keratitis, choanal atresia, esophageal atresia, and imperforate anus.

Microscopic Features

The characteristic feature is widespread enterocyte cell tufts of the small intestine and to some extent large intestinal epithelium. The tufts represent cells detached from the basement membrane. Within the tufts, cells exhibit apical rounding, which induces a teardrop shape. The associated loss of mucosal integrity allows antigens access to the lamina propria inducing an immunological reaction with villous blunting, crypt hyperplasia, and normal or increased inflammatory cells in the lamina propria. There is no increase in intraepithelial lymphocytes (Figure 7.4).

Immunohistochemical features

Absence of staining for the mutated gene product EpCAM/MOC31 antibody by immunohistochemistry helps confirm the diagnosis.

Differential Diagnosis

Conditions associated with villous atrophy could be considered, particularly those presenting early in infancy.

Treatment/Prognosis/Evolution

Most affected patients require total parenteral nutrition. More recently, intestinal transplantation has been effective and should generally be considered before severe complications develop.

Acrodermatitis Enteropathica

Definition, General Features (Frequency), and Predisposing Factors

This rare autosomal recessive disorder results from deficiency of a zinc-specific transporter protein. The resultant inability to absorb zinc produces a syndrome of diarrhea, dermatitis, alopecia, and mental deficiency. The condition is inherited in an autosomal recessive fashion due to a mutation in the solute carrier family (SLC) 39 gene (at 8q24.3), with consequent deficiency of a zinc-specific transporter protein resulting in the zinc deficiency that produces the clinical disorder.

Clinical Features

Acrodermatitis enteropathica (AE) patients typically develop skin manifestations of erythema and vesiculobullous dermatitis as well as alopecia, diarrhea, and delayed growth and sexual maturation.

Microscopic Features

The small intestine can be normal or show variable villous blunting with crypt hyperplasia and inflammation in the lamina propria. Intraepithelial lymphocytes are not increased. Ultrastructural studies show distinctive lysosomal inclusions in Paneth cells.

Treatment/Prognosis/Evolution

Patients response to oral zinc replacement of 3 mg/kg/day elemental zinc or 13.2 mg/kg/day of zinc sulfate.

Infections

Giardiasis

Definition, General Features, and Predisposing Factors

This protozoan infection by *Giardia lamblia* is acquired via a fecal-oral route or by exposure to contaminated water. The infection is more commonly encountered in children and immunocompromised patients, and with travel to underdeveloped countries. Secondary bacterial overgrowth may contribute to pathological findings.

Clinical Features/Endoscopic Characteristics

Only about half of infected individuals have symptoms, which typically include diarrhea, malaise, foul smelling greasy stools, nausea, and vomiting. There is wide variability in the severity, which is related to the virulence of the organism, microbial burden, and host immunity (see Hopkins et al.'s "Acute giardiasis: an improved clinical case definition for epidemiologic studies.") Upper endoscopy is usually normal or with nonspecific features of inflammation and atrophy. Diagnosis should be made on stool sampling.

Microscopic Features

In most cases, the mucosa is normal and Giardia are appreciated in the intervillous space as kite-shaped or sickle-shaped, depending on whether they appear end on or side on in the sections (Figure 7.5). The characteristic trophozoites contain two ovoid nuclei. When present, mucosal injury is characterized by mild chronic inflammation, usually with increased eosinophils. Mild villous blunting, crypt hyperplasia, and intraepithelial lymphocytosis can occur. Sparse or absent plasma cells may indicate a predisposing primary immunodeficiency disease, e.g. Chronic Variable Immunodeficiency (CVID) or IgA immunodeficiency.

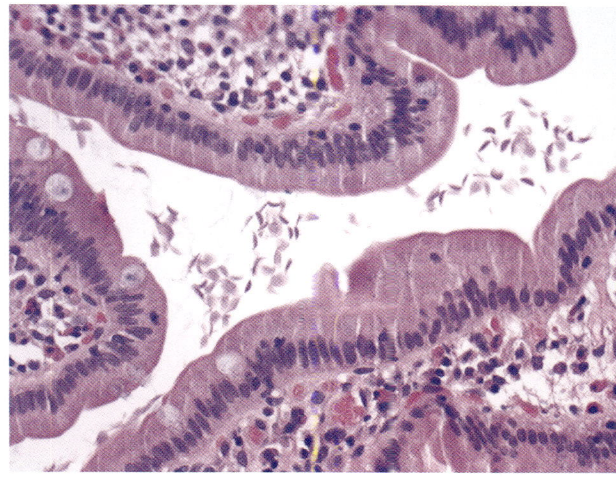

Figure 7.5 Duodenal giardiasis. Note the variable shapes of the organisms in the intervillous space.

Differential Diagnosis

It includes normal small intestine with epithelial denudation. Care needs to be taken in assessment of the cellular morphology.

Treatment/Prognosis/Evolution

Symptomatic patients should be treated with antibiotics. Asymptomatic carriers usually do not require therapy except in cases where the carrier may have direct/close exposure to immunocomprised, pregnant individuals, or day care facilities. Multiple antibiotics are effective, most commonly metronidazole for five days. Many patients have secondary lactose intolerance; so, milk should be avoided for approximately one month.

Cryptosporidiosis

Definition, General Features, and Predisposing Factors

This coccidian protozoan infection is caused by *Cryptosporidium parvum*. The transmission is by the fecal-oral route or via ingestion of contaminated water. The infection is more common in immunocompromised patients.

Clinical Features/Endoscopic Characteristics

In immunocompetent individuals, cryptosporidia usually manifests as mild diarrhea but can rarely be severe with biliary involvement. Particularly in AIDS patients with CD4 counts <100 cells/μl, diarrhea is severe along with associated cholangitis, hepatitis, pancreatitis, and respiratory symptoms.

Microscopic Features

Organisms are appreciable as 2–5 μm round basophilic bead-like structures on the luminal surface (both villous and gland) of the epithelial cells. The organisms can be highlighted on Giemsa or Gram stains and are located both within the apical cytoplasm of the epithelial cells and free within the lumen. A mixed inflammatory cell infiltrate and variable villous blunting are usually seen (Figure 7.6).

Differential Diagnosis

Other coccidian infections ought to be ruled out. These include: *Cyclospora*, which are larger organisms located in the cytoplasm but lacking the apical predisposition of cryptosporidia; microsporidia, which are much smaller intracytoplasmic organisms without the apical cytoplasmic location of cryptosporidia; and *Isospora* (see below).

Treatment/Prognosis/Evolution

Treatment is aimed at both the primary infection and, if present, the underlying immunocompromised state. In immunocompetent patients, therapy is often unnecessary as most individuals recover spontaneously within several weeks. If symptoms do not improve, treatment with nitazoxanide is preferred. In immunocompromised patients, typically HIV, the most effective treatment is aimed at HIV itself with antiretrovirals and supportive care for diarrhea. In a large randomized controlled trial, nitazoxanide was effective for patients with CD4 counts >50 cells/μl but not those with lower CD4.

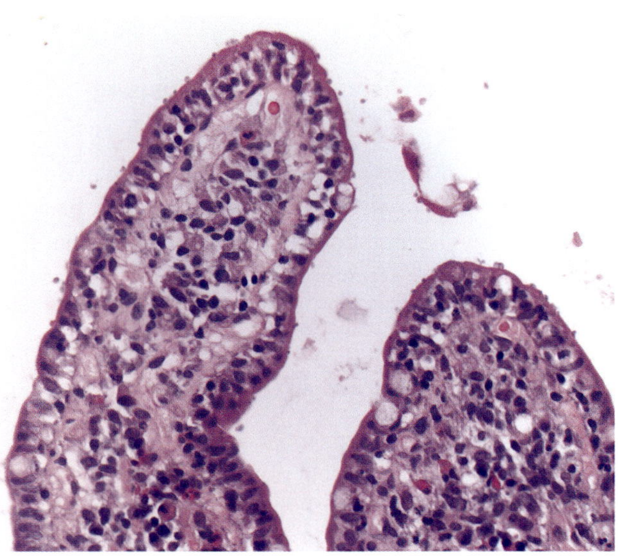

Figure 7.6 Cryptosporidiosis with secondary lymphocytosis. Observe the organisms adherent to the intestinal brush border.

Isospora

Definition

This protozoan coccidial infection produces diarrhea and, in some cases, malabsorption.

Clinical Features/Endoscopic Characteristics

Cystoisospora belli (formerly Isospora belli) causes a mild, self-limited diarrhea in immunocompetent individuals but may cause severe diarrhea/wasting in immunocompromised patients.

Microscopic Features

A characteristic feature is the development of villous blunting with compensatory crypt hyperplasia. An associated mixed inflammatory cell infiltrate is present, sometimes with prominent eosinophilia. Epithelial cells appear disorganized, and contain characteristic peri- or subnuclear inclusions, which may be banana-shaped or rounded with prominent nucleus depending on the stage in the parasite life cycle. Giemsa or silver-based stains can better highlight the organisms.

Treatment/Prognosis/Evolution

Treatment of immunocompetent patients is supportive with oral rehydration. In immunocompromised patients, and others with severe symptoms, antibiotics such as trimethoprim/sulfamethoxazole are effective.

Microsporidiosis

Definition and Predisposing Factors

This infection by a protozoan coccidial parasite is most commonly encountered in immunosuppressed patients. The organisms are within the cytoplasm of the epithelial cells of the gastrointestinal tract (GIT).

Clinical Features/Endoscopic Characteristics

Clinical features are similar to cryptosporidium although additional non-gastrointestinal manifestations such as ocular and cerebral infections may occur as well as myositis.

Microscopic Features

Biopsies often show no abnormality. Minor villous change is encountered in some infections. The organisms are identified in supranuclear vacuoles, and consist of spore and plasmodial forms. Silver stains best highlight the organisms.

Spread

The infection can disseminate widely (e.g. *E. intestinalis*).

Treatment/Prognosis/Evolution

Treatment with albendazole is recommended for both immunocompetent and compromised patients although the course is typically longer (two to four weeks) in immunocompromised patients or those with disseminated infection.

Strongyloidiasis

Definition, General Features, and Predisposing Factors

Infection by the nematode parasite *Strongyloides stercoralis* is endemic in tropical regions and immigrants from these areas. Immunocompromised patients are at particular risk for multisystem disease.

Clinical Features/Endoscopic Characteristics

Most carriers are asymptomatic but gastrointestinal (duodenitis, diarrhea, nausea, vomiting), skin (dermatitis), and pulmonary symptoms can occur. Hyperinfection syndrome due to autoinfection with high parasite load can cause disseminated infection of almost any solid organ and septic shock.

Microscopic Features

In immunocompetent patients there is a marked lamina propria eosinophil infiltrate often accompanied by neutrophils surrounding the invasive parasites. Adult worms, larvae, and eggs may be found in the crypts. In immunocompromised patients or in the setting of mild disease, there may be minimal inflammation (Figure 7.7).

Differential Diagnosis

Eosinophilic enteritis ought to be ruled out, and identification of the parasite is key to the diagnosis.

Treatment/Prognosis/Evolution

Treatment of uncomplicated infection is typically with ivermectin in two doses of 200 mcg/kg/day over two days.

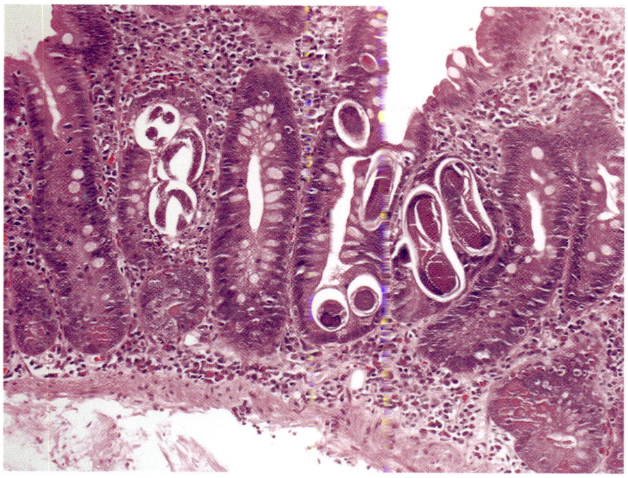

Figure 7.7 Example of strongyloides in the duodenal crypts.

Mycobacterial Infection—*Mycobacterium avium* Intracellulare Complex (MAIC) and *Mycobacterium tuberculosis*

Definition and Predisposing Factors

Infection by typical and atypical forms of acid fast mycobacterial infection is most commonly acquired in the setting of compromised immunity. *Mycobacterium tuberculosis* almost always occurs with active pulmonary disease.

Clinical Features/Endoscopic Characteristics

The Clinical features of Mycobacteria avium intracellulare and Mycobacterium tuberculosis vary widely but primarily manifest as pulmonary disease. The GIT is involved as part of disseminated infection, most commonly in immunocompromised patients, and may present as nausea, anorexia, hepatosplenomegaly, diarrhea, or abdominal pain.

Microscopic Features

Mycobacterium avium intracellulare (MAI)-associated intestinal disease is characterized by an infiltrate of histiocytes in the intestinal lamina propria. Villi are distended and secondarily blunted. Other inflammation is uncommon. Poorly formed granulomata may be seen. Acid fast stains and PAS stain will highlight numerous organisms within the cytoplasm of the histiocytes (lesser numbers if immunocompetent) (Figure 7.8a–c).

M. tuberculosis is characterized by well-formed granulomata, sometimes with caseous necrosis, a mixed

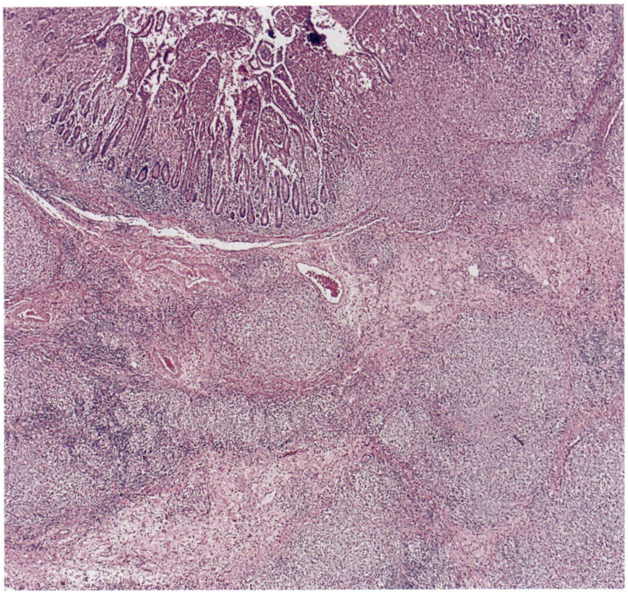

Figure 7.8 Low-power view of MAI-associated enteritis with diffuse histiocytic infiltrate of the lamina propria and poorly formed granulomata. Acid fast stain did highlight numerous organisms within the cytoplasm of the histiocytes.

inflammatory cell infiltrate, and mucosal ulceration. Architectural distortion, fibrosis, and dystrophic calcification are seen in older lesions.

Molecular Features

Polymerase chain reaction (PCR) techniques are available.

Differential Diagnosis

Common conditions to be distinguished from MAIC are Whipple's disease, fungal infection, and other histiocyte-rich disorders. Conditions sharing morphologic features with *M. tuberculosis* are Crohn's disease and yersiniosis (see text).

Treatment/Prognosis/Evolution

A detailed discussion of treatment of MAIC and MTb is beyond the scope of this book. Readers are referred to in-depth excellent resources on this topic.

Whipple's Disease

Definition

Infection by the bacterium *Tropheryma whipplei* gives rise to multiorgan disease. When severe, small intestine involvement may produce malabsorption.

Microscopic Features

The main feature is infiltration of the lamina propria by histiocytes with foamy cytoplasm. Granuloma formation occasionally may be seen. Aside from a variable neutrophil infiltrate, inflammation is inconspicuous. Villi are often blunted, and there may be prominent cytoplasmic vacuolation of enterocytes. Organisms within the histiocytes are strongly PAS positive (Figure 7.9a–c).

Molecular Features

PCR specific for *T. whipplei* is available and can be performed on paraffin shavings from the tissue block.

Differential Diagnosis

Various conditions can mimic Whipple's disease, including MAIC, fungal infections such as *Cryptococcus* and histoplasmosis, normal muciphages, and macroglobulinemia.

Spread

The disease frequently involves other organs and the disease manifestations are protean.

Treatment/Prognosis/Evolution

Treatment of Whipple's disease is based on the organ involved. For generalized infection including gastrointestinal involvement, ceftriaxone 2 g IV daily or penicillin G two million units daily for two weeks followed by trimethoprim/sulfamethoxazole suppression for one year is recommended. For central nervous system (CNS) and endocarditis, treatment is typically four weeks.

Yersiniosis

Definition and General Features

Gram negative coccoid bacteria affect the small and large intestine. The most common human infections are by *Yersinia enterocolitica* and *Yersinia pseudotuberculosis* species. Infection is acquired from contaminated water, dairy, and meat products.

Clinical Features/Endoscopic Characteristics

Yersinia can present with both an acute gastroenteritis as well as delayed postinfectious sequelae. Acute yersiniosis

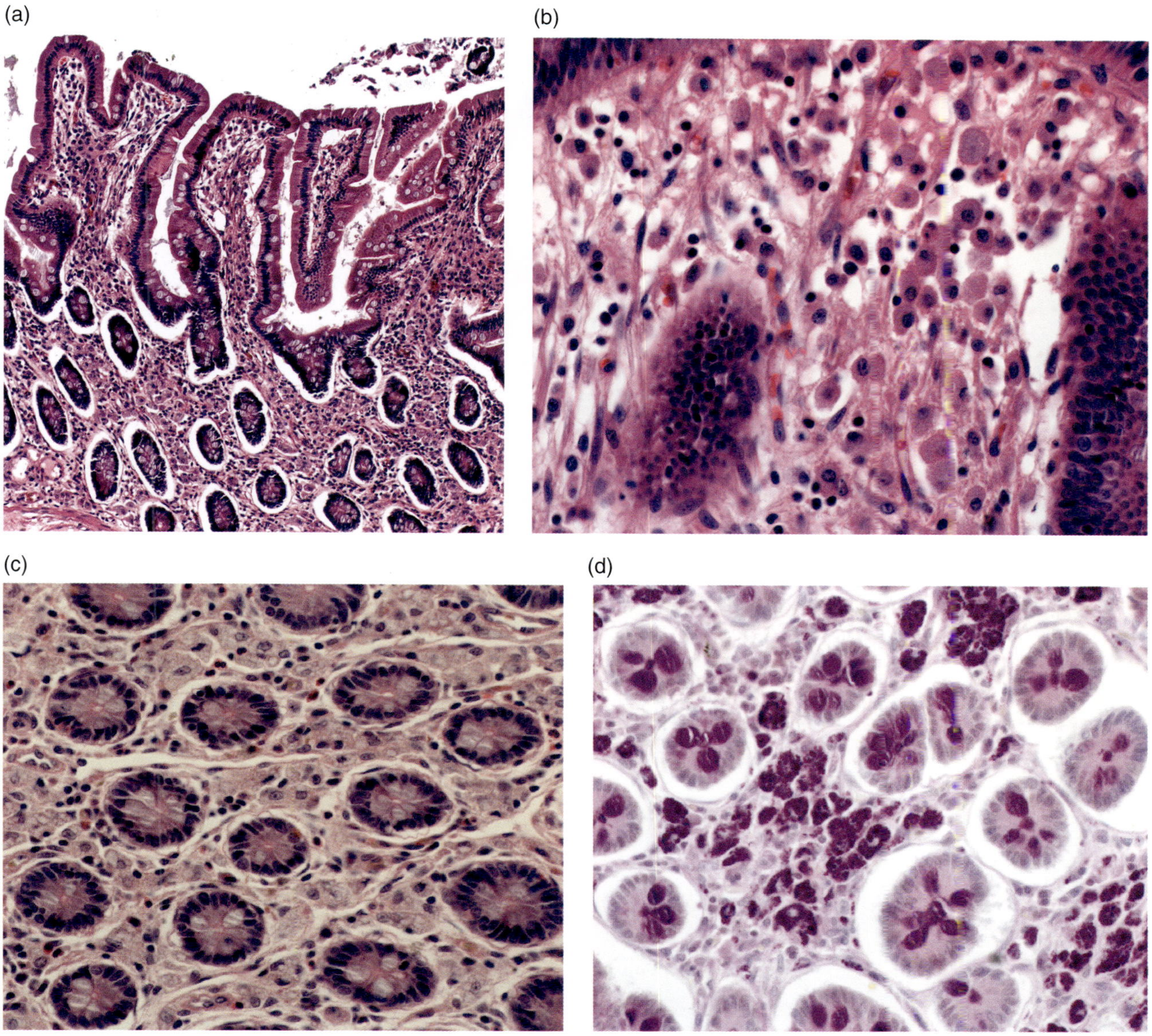

Figure 7.9 (a–c) Example of Whipple's disease, characterized by infiltration of the lamina propria by histiocytes with foamy cytoplasm. Organisms within the histiocytes are strongly PAS positive (d).

involves nonspecific symptoms of fever, diarrhea, abdominal pain, nausea, and vomiting. A specific manifestation is acute pseudoappendicitis with right lower quadrant pain, and at surgery inflammation of the appendix, terminal ileum, and adjacent lymphadenitis.

Microscopic Features

The ileum, right colon, and appendix are typically affected. The characteristic findings are large geographic granulomata with central microabscess formation. These are often centered on reactive Peyer's patches. Ulceration is common. Usually, very few organisms are found on Gram stain.

Molecular Testing

PCR performed on paraffin shavings from the tissue block are useful in confirming infection.

Differential Diagnosis

Crohn's disease; other bacterial infections associated with ileitis, particularly Salmonella, and Campylobacter; and mycobacterial infection are to be excluded.

Treatment/Prognosis/Evolution

Antimicrobial therapy is unproven in Yersinia enterocolitis. In most cases, supportive care is appropriate. In

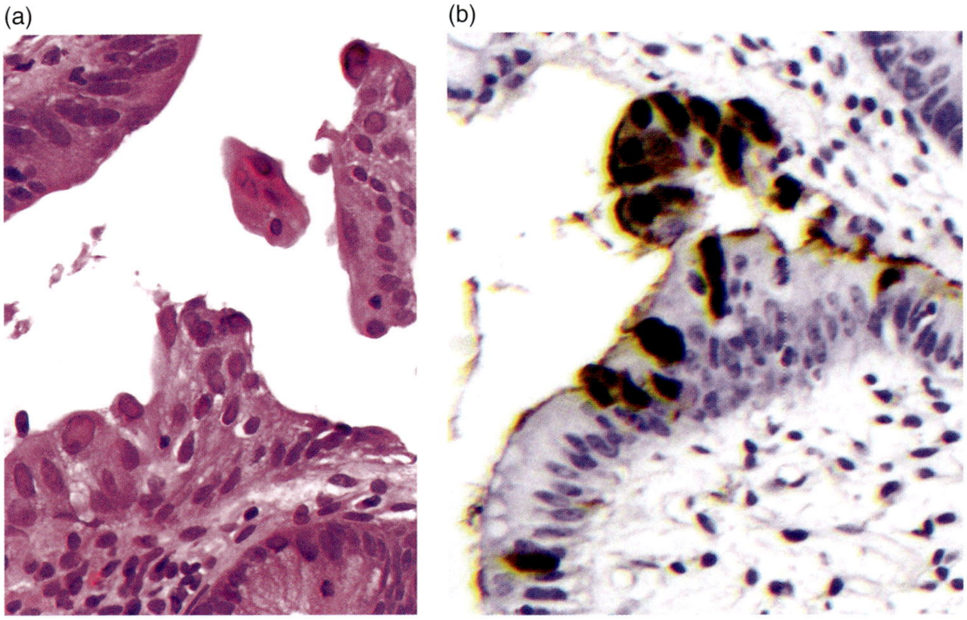

Figure 7.10 (a) Adenovirus infection with typical eosinophilic intranuclear inclusions which can be highlighted by (b) immunohistochemistry.

severe cases, or immunocompromised patients, fluoroquinolone or trimethoprim/sulfamethoxazole may be used.

Adenovirus

Definition

This systemic viral infection only occasionally involves the GIT.

Clinical Features/Endoscopic Characteristics

Adenovirus may cause gastrointestinal symptoms such as acute diarrhea, particularly the subgroup F adenovirus types 40 and 41. Fatal hepatitis has been reported in pediatric liver transplant patients.

Microscopic Features

Two types of intranuclear changes seen on light microscopy are (i) eosinophilic nuclear inclusion bodies and (ii) "smudge cells," in which the nucleus is slightly enlarged, homogeneous, and basophilic (Figure 7.10a, b).

Treatment/Prognosis/Evolution

Treatment is not required for uncomplicated cases. In immunocompromised patients, antivirals should be used, most commonly cidofovir.

Cytomegalovirus

Definition, General Features, and Predisposing Factors

In this systemic viral infection by Herpesviridae, gastrointestinal involvement is usually the result of immunosuppression and reactivation of latent disease. Primary infection is uncommon.

Clinical Features/Endoscopic Characteristics

Cytomegalovirus (CMV) causes a wide spectrum of symptoms. The most common gastrointestinal symptoms occur in immunocompromised patients and include diarrhea, fever, abdominal pain, and bleeding. Given the nonspecific nature of the symptoms, a low threshold is needed to confirm disease, typically by endoscopy with biopsy of suspicious regions. The endoscopic features are typically ulcerations, which may be very large.

Microscopic Features

Characteristic viral inclusions are found, typically in the endothelial, epithelial, or stromal cells. These can be confirmed by immunohistochemistry. Inflammation or ulceration may develop (Figure 7.11).

Treatment/Prognosis/Evolution

Treatment of symptomatic patients, particularly immunocompromised patients is recommended. Multiple antivirals such as ganciclovir have been effective.

Human Immunodeficiency Virus

Definition

Infection with the human immunodeficiency virus can affect the small bowel.

Clinical Features/Endoscopic Characteristics

HIV causes a wide variety of gastrointestinal symptoms. A full discussion is beyond the scope of this book. However, acute GI manifestations include nausea, diarrhea, anorexia, and weight loss. Chronic symptoms are typically related to opportunistic infections, which are discussed elsewhere in this text.

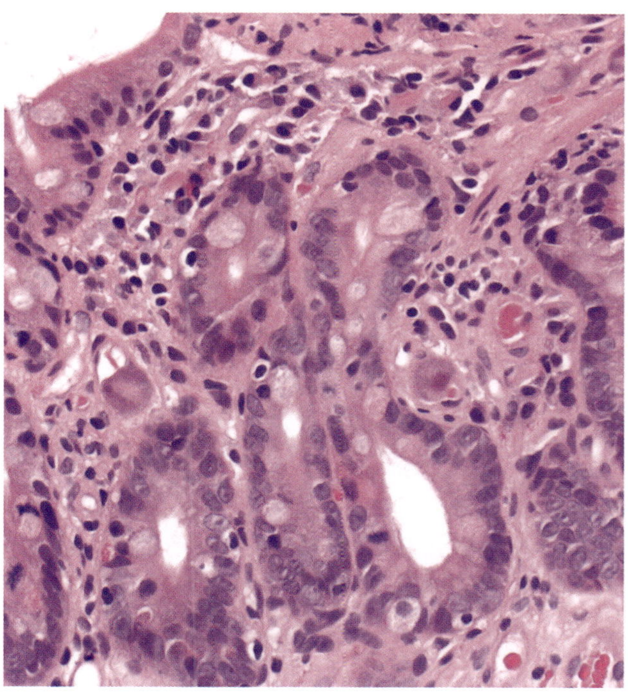

Figure 7.11 CMV duodenitis with classic CMV inclusions in endothelial cell carousels.

Microscopic Features

HIV targets and depletes CD4-positive T cells. In the intestine, mucosal biopsies exhibit a lamina propria depleted of lymphocytes, and normal lymphoid follicles may show fibrosis. In the setting of highly active antiretroviral therapy, commensal infections are uncommon.

Treatment/Prognosis/Evolution

Treatment of HIV is complex and beyond the scope of this this text. For most individuals, highly active anti-retroviral therapy (HAART) with multiple agents has revolutionized the treatment and prognosis of HIV to the point that most cases can now be managed effectively.

Celiac Disease

Definition, General Features (Frequency), and Predisposing Factors

This malabsorptive condition results from inflammation and epithelial injury induced by an immunological response to gluten, a large peptide protein found in the *Triticum* grain family (i.e. wheat, barley, and rye).

This autoimmune condition develops in response to the ingestion of gliadins, which are amino acids rich in proline and glutamine that contain abundant sulfhydryl groups. These sulfhydryl groups are the enzymatic target of tissue transglutaminase (TTG), a process referred to as deamidation. Deamidated gliadin binds to HLA-specific receptors on antigen presenting cells inducing both cell-mediated and humoral immune response. Carriage of HLADQ2 or HLADQ8 haplotype is a genetic prerequisite. Mucosal injury, for example by viral infection, appears to be an important precipitating step by allowing the initial access of gluten (and the responsible antigens, i.e. gliadins) to the immune effector cells in the mucosa.

Clinical Features/Endoscopic Characteristics

Celiac disease presents in both classical (diarrhea, weight loss, malabsorption, anemia, dermatitis herpetiformis) and atypical (bloating, nonspecific malaise, minor laboratory

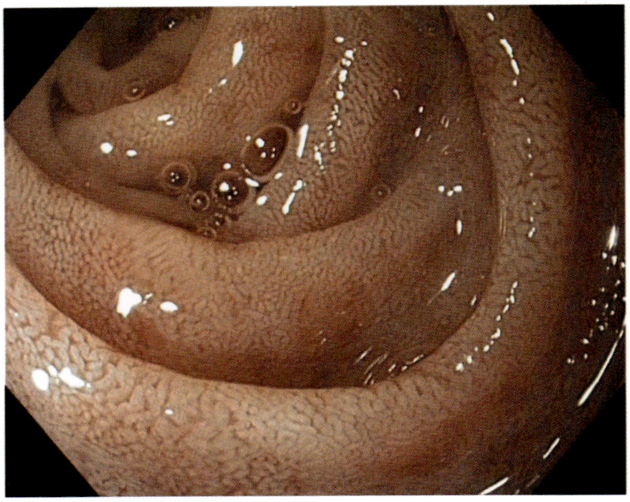

Figure 7.12 Endoscopic celiac disease with scalloping of the duodenal folds.

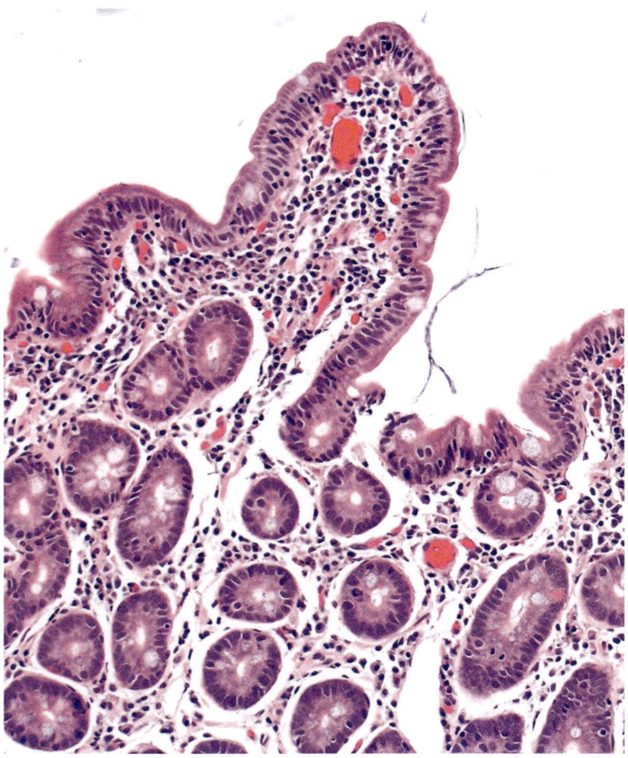

Figure 7.13 Example of celiac disease, Marsh grade 1 with the characteristic intraepithelial lymphocytosis, minimal expansion of the lamina propria.

abnormalities) forms. The increasing use of endoscopic biopsy of the duodenum, and serological testing for autoantibodies has raised awareness and changed the understanding of the epidemiology, recognizing this as a common disease. Population studies suggest a prevalence of 1 in 184 adults although only 1 in 8 cases were clinically diagnosed. Endoscopic features are typically only present in more advanced disease and should not be relied upon to exclude disease. Features include "scalloping" and gross blunting of the villi (Figure 7.12).

Microscopic Features

The earliest histological change is increased intraepithelial CD3/CD8-positive T lymphocytes (>30/high power field (HPF)) that trigger enterocyte loss by apoptotic cell death (Figure 7.13). Initially enterocyte loss is compensated by crypt epithelial proliferation with crypt hyperplasia; however, continuous injury produces villous blunting and eventually flat mucosa. Concomitant lamina propria inflammation rich in plasma cells and lymphocytes occurs. Plasma cells are responsible for the production of the antibodies that are serological markers of celiac disease (i.e. TTG). In some cases, eosinophils may be conspicuous, and occasionally, neutrophils are found in the lamina propria, surface, or crypt epithelium. Injured enterocytes may fail to package and process absorbed lipid adequately, leading to cytoplasmic vacuolation ("lipid hang up sign"). Minimal thickening of the subepithelial collagen layer not exceeding 5 μm, sometimes accompanied by epithelial denudation, is encountered in 36–60% of biopsies. This should not be interpreted as representing collagenous sprue. As the villi shorten, goblet cells may become less readily identified, particularly at the surface. Gastric metaplasia may be observed in up to 2/3 of biopsies but is never as prominent as in peptic duodenitis.

The extent of villous and crypt architectural abnormality has been used in establishing the morphological Marsh classification (see Table 7.2). In practice, type 1 and type 3 patterns are most commonly encountered; type 2 pattern is infrequent and almost never a uniform finding. Problems exist in the distinction between type 1 and type 2 lesions and in the subclassification of type 3 lesions. To address this, Corazza and Villanacci have proposed a simplified, more

Table 7.2 Modified Marsh classification scheme.

	0	1	2	3a	3b	3c
IEL	<30	≥30	≥30	≥30	≥30	≥30
Crypts	Normal	Normal	Hypertrophic	Hypertrophic	Hypertrophic	Hypertrophic
Villi	Normal	Normal	Normal	Atrophy +	Atrophy ++	Absent

Table 7.3 Villanicci–Corazza classification scheme.

Type A	Infiltrative, non-atrophic; incorporating type 1 and 2
Type B1	Atrophic with shortened but still detectable villi, incorporating types 3a and b
Type B2	Complete atrophy without detectable villi, corresponding to type 3c

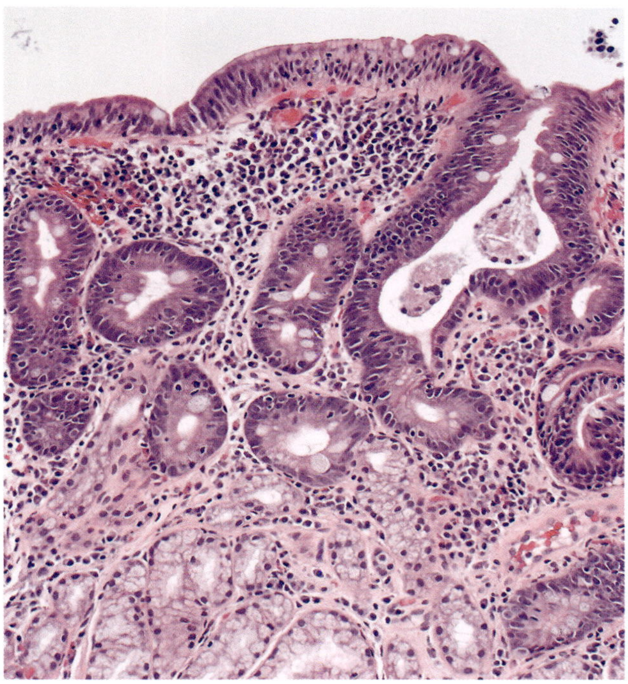

Figure 7.14 Marsh grade 3a of celiac disease with definite villous blunting.

reproducible grading system (Table 7.3). The major problem for both classifications is the variability in the degree of injury between biopsy fragments and even within individual biopsy fragments that occurs in up to 50% of biopsies. Rarely, the histological changes may be restricted to the duodenal bulb. This makes the designation of a single pattern type impossible in most cases. At least three biopsies taken throughout the duodenum is recommended to avoid underdiagnosis related to sampling error (Figure 7.14a, b).

Differential Diagnosis

It is useful to view the differential diagnosis in terms of conditions causing intraepithelial lymphocytosis without villous blunting (lymphocytic duodenosis; Marsh type 1/2 mimics) see (Table 7.1) and conditions displaying intraepithelial lymphocytosis with villous blunting or flat mucosa (Marsh type 3 pattern) (Table 7.4). Serology, HLADQ status, and histological response to gluten-free diet remain the mainstays in separating celiac disease from its histological mimics.

Table 7.4 Intraepithelial lymphocytosis with villous blunting/flat mucosa—cause/associations

Celiac disease (majority of cases)
Non-gluten food hypersensitivity (e.g. cereals, cow's milk, soy products, fish, rice, and chicken)
Infection, e.g. viral/bacterial enteritis, tropical sprue
Bacterial overgrowth
Autoimmune enteropathy
Immunodeficiency disorders, e.g. IgA deficiency, CVID
Drugs (e.g. NSAIDs, olmesartan, methotrexate)
Inflammatory bowel disease
Collagenous sprue
Idiopathic

Treatment/Prognosis/Evolution

Treatment is a strict gluten-free diet, which is curative in >95% of individuals. The challenge is in compliance with the diet due to both advertent and inadvertent exposure to gluten. True nonresponders (i.e., refractory celiac disease) are subclassified as type 1 (with normal intraepithelial lymphocytes) and type 2, which have monoclonal T-cells with a high risk of developing enteropathy associated T-cell lymphoma.

Autoimmune Enteropathy

Definition, General Features, and Predisposing Factors

This malabsorption enteropathy results from mucosal injury induced by autoantibodies to mucosal epithelial cells, principally to the enterocytes, but sometimes Paneth cells and goblet cells. Most cases present in childhood; however, adult cases are increasingly recognized. The pathogenesis involves the development of autoantibodies that target epithelial intestinal cells. The precipitant for autoantibody development is unknown. A subset of autoimmune enteropathy cases occur in patients with Immune dysregulation, polyendocrinopathy, enteropathy, X-linked (IPEX) syndrome, an X-linked recessive disorder usually presenting in infancy. IPEX is characterized by immunodysregulation, polyendocrinopathy, and enteropathy in the affected males. It results from mutations in the FOXP3 gene that cause deficiency of CD25+, CD4+ regulatory T cells with consequent loss of self-tolerance and development of autoantibodies targeting self-antigens such as gut enterocytes. A loss of self-tolerance may also underlie other cases of autoimmune enteropathy. A 75 kDa antigen, encoded on chromosome 19p13 and involved in gut epithelial cell tight junction regulation appears to be important. Its dysfunction could allow antigens into the lamina propria, initiating an inflammatory reaction.

Clinical Features/Endoscopic Characteristics

Autoimmune enteropathy (AIE) is a rare disease, which typically presents in children with severe refractory diarrhea in the setting of autoantibodies and often with other associated autoimmune disorders. The endoscopic appearance is similar to celiac sprue. By definition they are refractory to a gluten-free diet.

Microscopic Features

Three main patterns are recognized, and a fourth pattern consists of features of two or more of these:

1) Active chronic duodenitis (IBD-like) pattern with villous blunting, expansion of the lamina propria by mixed but predominantly mononuclear inflammation, and neutrophilic cryptitis (with or without crypt abscesses). Increased apoptosis of crypt epithelium may not be noted. Crypt architectural disturbance is common, and pseudopyloric gland metaplasia may be seen.
2) Celiac disease-like pattern with villous blunting and increased intraepithelial lymphocytes (>25 IELs/100 enterocytes). Crypt epithelial apoptosis is typically inconspicuous. In contrast to celiac disease the $\gamma\sigma$ T-cell receptor (TCR) density is not increased.
3) Graft versus host disease-like pattern characterized by increased apoptosis with or without crypt dropout, and minimal inflammation (Figure 7.15).

In cases associated with anti-goblet cell or anti-Paneth cell antibodies, loss of the corresponding cell type occurs.

Molecular Features

Circulating antibodies to enterocytes are most commonly found. Occasionally the antibodies are against goblet cells and/or Paneth cells. These are not specific to autoimmune enteropathy as they can develop in other chronic inflammatory gut disorders, such as inflammatory bowel disease. Indirect immunofluorescence can confirm the diagnosis.

Differential Diagnosis

Usually, the clinical context helps guide the diagnosis.

1) Celiac disease should be considered particularly in cases displaying intraepithelial lymphocytosis. The presence of basal crypt apoptosis or the absence/reduced density of one mucosal cell type are important pointers to AIE. Celiac serology (elevated TTG) is negative and HLADQ2/8 haplotype is often not detected.
2) Graft versus host disease (GVHD): The clinical history normally suggests this possibility.

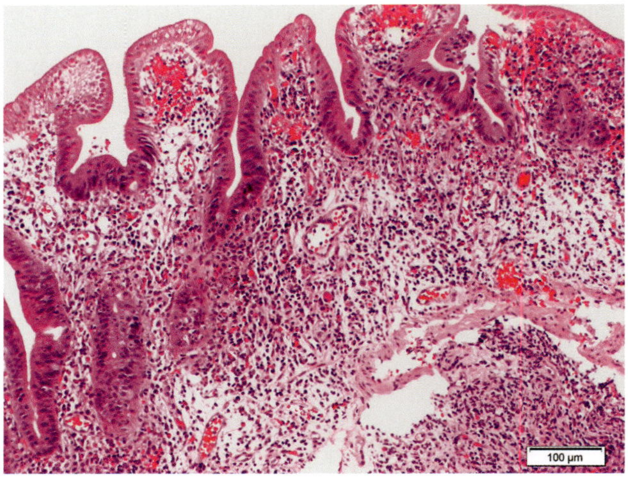

Figure 7.15 Low-power view of autoimmune enteropathy characterized by blunting of villi and expansion of lamina propria by mixed inflammatory cells and glandular apoptosis in a pattern similar to GVHD.

3) CVID: One histological manifestation of CVID has features of autoimmune enteropathy. However, the clinical setting is important in reaching the proper conclusion.
4) Drugs: Immunomodulatory drugs such as mycophenolate and ipilimumab can induce an enteropathy with epithelial apoptosis and architectural disturbance. Olmesartan can also produce mucosal damage that may mimic autoimmune enteropathy both clinically and histologically. In all cases, review of clinical history and treatment are helpful.
5) Crohn's disease: In some cases, the marked inflammation, architectural abnormality, and sometimes diffuse GIT involvement of AIE can suggest Crohn's disease. Crypt apoptosis and absence of ulceration and granuloma formation point to AIE.

Treatment/Prognosis/Evolution

The largest experience reported with AIE is from Mayo clinic with 15 adult patients. Immunosuppressive therapy was used in 93% of patients and 60% responded within two months of treatment.

Tropical Sprue

Definition, General Features, and Predisposing Factors

Tropical sprue (enteropathy) is an acquired chronic inflammatory disorder of the intestinal mucosa. A persistent infection is favored to be the cause; hence, the disease is sometimes referred to as "post-infective tropical malabsorption."

Residence in, or visitation to, tropical areas (30° North or South of the equator), in particular India, much of South East Asia, Puerto Rico, parts of the Caribbean, northern South America, and West Africa, which are the areas of high prevalence. It is postulated that acquisition of enterotoxigenic coliforms injures the enterocytes and crypt cells and induces the inflammatory process. Particular HLA haplotypes may confer higher risk.

Clinical Features/Endoscopic Characteristics

Tropical sprue presents similar to other small bowel malabsorptive diseases with diarrhea, weight loss, and nutritional deficiencies. Individuals must be exposed to tropical regions for typically one month or more to contract the disease. Endoscopic features are similar to celiac sprue.

Microscopic Features

The histological features closely resemble celiac disease with villous blunting, inflammation of the lamina propria, and intraepithelial lymphocytosis. The lymphocytic infiltrate may be marked and involves both crypts and surface epithelium. Villous blunting is typically incomplete. The changes involve the entire small intestine, and in contradictinction to celiac disease, the ileum is often more severely affected than the duodenum. Eosinophils are prominent in many cases and may provide a subtle histological diagnostic clue (Figure 7.16).

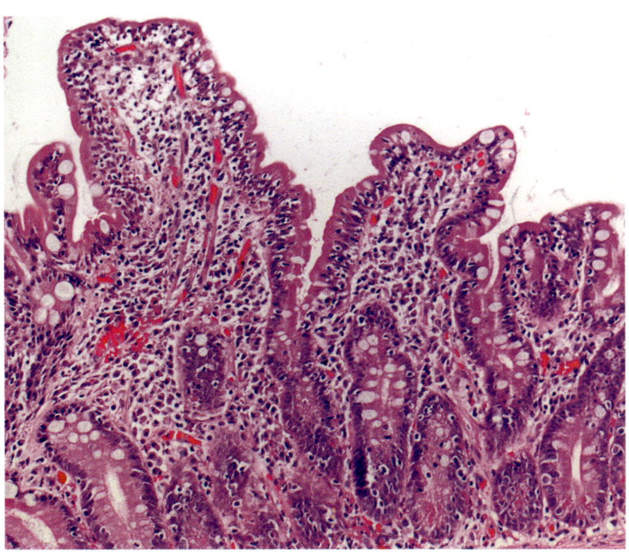

Figure 7.16 Example of a tropical sprue with intraepithelial lymphocytosis and minimal expansion of lamina propria.

Differential Diagnosis

1) Distinguishing celiac disease is usually a primary step: A history of travel to a tropical region, negative celiac serology, and absence of a response to gluten free diet are discriminating features. Involvement of the ileum and a uniform IEL density from crypt to villous tip are morphologic clues suggesting tropical sprue rather than celiac disease.
2) Bacterial overgrowth may share a similar pathogenesis with tropical sprue; however, the clinical setting allows distinction. Neutrophils in the surface epithelium favor bacterial overgrowth, as they are rarely seen in tropical sprue.
3) Infective enteritis (see conditions discussed above).

Treatment/Prognosis/Evolution

Most cases require antimicrobial therapy, typically with tetracycline 250 mg PO four times daily plus folic acid for three to six weeks. One in five patients may relapse, usually those living persistently in the tropics.

Small Intestinal Bacterial Overgrowth

Definition, General Features, and Predisposing Factors

This condition results from colonization of the small intestine by aerobic Gram negative bacteria or anaerobic bacteria derived from the colon or, less commonly, the oropharynx. It is characterized by >10 colony forming units (cfu)/ml of bacteria in small intestinal aspirates. It may cause malabsorption or diarrhea.

Predisposing factors include surgical blind loop, adhesions, fistulae, scleroderma, chronic renal failure, resections involving the ileocecal valve, chronic pancreatitis, reduced gastric acid secretion and intestinal dysmotility, or occasionally large or multiple small bowel diverticula.

Clinical Features/Endoscopic Characteristics

Small intestinal bacterial overgrowth (SIBO) presents similar to other malabsorptive conditions. There are usually no visible endoscopic abnormalities except in severe cases where it may present with ulceration. A diagnosis can be confirmed by endoscopic aspiration of intestinal fluid for quantitative bacterial culture or breath test.

Microscopic Features

The mucosa may appear histologically normal or can show villous blunting accompanied by crypt hyperplasia and inflammation that typically have a patchy distribution. An increase in intraepithelial lymphocytes and a mild lamina propria neutrophil infiltrate are often present. Neutrophils seen in the surface epithelium are a helpful indicator of SIBO.

Differential Diagnosis

Celiac disease and tropical sprue are the most common conditions to rule out.

Treatment/Prognosis/Evolution

Treatment is aimed at the underlying condition if reversible, dietary change, and antimicrobial therapy. Surgical bypass can rarely be reversed but should be considered when feasible. Removal of antimotility drugs (narcotics, anticholinergics) and avoidance of acid suppression may also help by allowing natural acidification and sterilization of the stomach contents. Dietary therapy consisting of high fat, low carbohydrate, and low fiber may help. In cases where these fail, use of antimicrobial, particularly non-absorbed agents such as rifaximin, is helpful.

Chronic Variable Immunodeficiency (CVID)

Definition, General Features, and Predisposing Factors

Under this heading is a heterogeneous group of disorders characterized by a defect in B-cell maturation resulting in hypogammaglobulinemia. Usually sporadic, up to 20% of patients exhibit an autosomal dominant inheritance. Mutations of TACI (transmembrane activator and calcium-modulator and cyclophilin ligand [CAML] interactor) encoded by TNFRSF13B on the short arm of chromosome 17 are found in 5–10% of cases. This impedes immunoglobulin formation and/or plasma cell maturation.

Clinical Features/Endoscopic Characteristics

20–60% of patients have gastrointestinal manifestations, typically diarrhea, weight loss, and evidence of malabsorption.

Microscopic Features

The biopsies are characterized by an increase in lymphocytes in the lamina propria with lymphoid nodule formation. Plasma cells are absent or markedly reduced, although some lymphocytes may have plasmacytoid features. Lymphoid nodules are composed of T cells rather than B cells. A sprue-like pattern of villous blunting or flat mucosa with intraepithelial lymphocytosis may occur. Apoptosis of the crypt epithelium is common, and may be predominant. A histiocyte infiltrate may occur in the lamina propria. True granulomata may also develop. Giardia and other parasitic infections may be present as a result of the immune defect.

Differential Diagnosis

CVID can mimic several conditions, including

1) Celiac disease: Lymphoid nodules, crypt apoptosis, and the relative or absolute absence of plasma cells in the lamina propria are the major features suggestive of CVID when a biopsy displays villous blunting and inflammation.
2) GVHD: A clinical history of hematopoietic cell transplant or other transplant will suggest this diagnosis.
3) Autoimmune enteropathy: The relative absence of plasma cells and presence of lymphoid follicles will suggest CVID.
4) Crohn's disease: CVID with granuloma is often initially misdiagnosed as Crohn's disease. The clinical setting is critical in guiding the diagnosis. Crypt apoptosis and reduced plasma cell infiltration are important clues.
5) Whipple's disease: Important to consider when a prominent histiocytic infiltrate is detected. PAS-positive bacilli will be found in the cytoplasm of the histiocytes in Whipple's disease.
6) Only males are affected with X-linked agammaglobulinemia. Patients with CVID present at an older age.

Treatment/Prognosis/Evolution

Treatment is largely based on replacement of immune globulin, treatment of specific infectious complications, prophylaxis for lung infections in patients with ongoing lung disease despite adequate immune globulin, and occasionally glucocorticoid therapy for patients with autoimmune or inflammatory disorders. A detailed summary of treatment options is described by Cunningham-Rundles.

Selective IgA Deficiency

Definition, General Features, and Predisposing Factors

Immunoglobulin A (IgA) deficiency is the most common primary immunodeficiency. The diagnosis requires detection of a decreased serum level of IgA in the presence of normal levels of other immunoglobulin isotypes. This condition is 10–15 times more likely in celiac disease patients than in the general population.

Clinical Features/Endoscopic Characteristics

Patients with IgA deficiency are prone to gastrointestinal infections, particularly *G. lamblia*, as well as inflammatory bowel disease including both ulcerative colitis and Crohn's disease. Endoscopic features are similar to non-IgA inflammatory bowel disease.

Microscopic Features

The features are similar to CVID with nodular lymphoid hyperplasia, sprue-like, and/or GVHD-like patterns and occasional infection by giardia. IgA-secreting plasma cells are absent but IgM-producing plasma cells are not affected, so the total plasma cell number may not always be appreciably reduced. Since associated celiac disease is common, there may be morphologic features of this disease, and separation from pure IgA deficiency-related changes is often challenging.

Differential Diagnosis

The same differential diagnosis as CVID can be entertained (see above). Exclusion of celiac disease may require IgG-based serology, HLADQ haplotype testing, and/or a trial of gluten-free diet.

Treatment/Prognosis/Evolution

Treatment is primarily indicated for those with sinopulmonary manifestations and included antimicrobial therapy for active infections, vaccination, and chronic prophylactic antibiotics for recurrent infections, and immune globulin in those that do not respond to these measures.

Graft Versus Host Disease

Definition, General Features (Frequency), and Predisposing Factors

GVHD develops in transplant graft recipients when immunocompetent donor cells induce an immunological reaction against alloantigens of the native cells of the host. GVHD is most commonly seen following bone marrow transplantation or in solid organ transplantation.

Clinical Features/Endoscopic Characteristics

GVHD can affect the entire GIT and liver. The most common manifestation is diarrhea, as well as upper GI symptoms of anorexia, vomiting. Endoscopic findings are often normal but may appear as nonspecific inflammation with erythema, granularity, or ulceration of any part of the GI tract. Endoscopic biopsy should be performed even of normal appearing mucosa with the highest yield from rectal mucosa, being positive in more than 85% of cases.

Microscopic Features

Crypt apoptosis with various degrees of epithelial cell loss is the key finding. Often the lamina propria appears depleted of inflammatory cells as a result of bone marrow transplantation. A mild neutrophil infiltrate may be seen. Occasionally, lymphocytes may infiltrate the epithelium near areas of active apoptosis. The severity of changes may be graded according to the Lerner system (Table 7.5).

Differential Diagnosis

This includes diseases with crypt loss and those characterized by crypt apoptosis. Attention to the clinical setting is most important.

1) Conditions with crypt loss include ischemic injury, chemotherapy effect, and radiotherapy effect.
2) Ailments to consider on the basis of increased apoptosis include immunodeficiency disorders (CVID, selective IgA), autoimmune enteropathy, thymoma-associated enteritis, AIDS-related enteropathy, and iatrogenic damage (e.g. chemotherapy, ipilimumab, mycophenolate).

Treatment/Prognosis/Evolution

Treatment is based on the severity and extent of organ involvement. Mild, grade-1 disease affecting the skin may be treated with topical corticosteroids. More severe diseases, including GVHD of the GIT, are typically treated with systemic corticosteroids. In a large series of 469 patients with acute GVHD, 41% had a durable initial response. Of those that did not respond initially, 70% developed chronic GVHD.

Table 7.5 Grading of GVHD.

Grade	Pathology
Grade 1	Isolated apoptotic epithelial cells, without crypt loss
Grade 2	Loss of isolated crypts, without loss of contiguous crypts
Grade 3	Loss of two or more contiguous crypts
Grade 4	Extensive crypt loss with mucosal denudation.

Collagenous Sprue

Definition, General Features (Frequency), and Predisposing Factors

This disorder is characterized by deposition of collagen in the immediate subepithelial zone of the proximal small intestine. Up to 50% of cases occur in the setting of celiac disease. Olmesartan and NSAIDs account for some cases. An association with autoimmune disease is also reported.

Clinical Features/Endoscopic Characteristics

Collagenous sprue is a rare condition, which presents in a similar manner to celiac sprue but may have a more refractory course and often overlaps with celiac sprue and collagenous involvement of the colon. Endoscopic features are similar to celiac sprue.

Microscopic Features

The characteristic feature is deposition of collagen to a thickness >10 μm in the subepithelial zone. The lower border of this deposition is irregular with capillary entrapment and dilatation. Villous blunting is typical and an increased chronic inflammatory cells and eosinophils are usually seen in the lamina propria. Intraepithelial lymphocytosis is present in the celiac disease-related cases (Figure 7.17).

Molecular Features

An abnormal intraepithelial lymphocyte population may be identified, particularly in a setting of type 2 refractory celiac disease (RCD). Loss of reaction for CD8 in the majority of intraepithelial T cells is an indicator of a neoplastic T-cell population. Clonal TCR gene rearrangement and abnormal findings on flow cytometry are confirmatory.

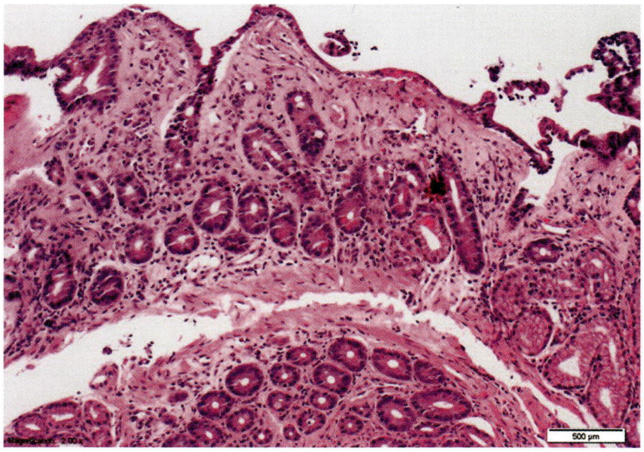

Figure 7.17 Collagenous sprue with obvious expansion of the lamina propria by dense collagen band.

Differential Diagnosis

The stromal scarring of radiation-induced enteropathy can mimic collagenous sprue.

Treatment/Prognosis/Evolution

Small case series describe responses to gluten-free diet, often combined with glucocorticoids.

Refractory Celiac Disease (RCD)

Definition, General Features, and Predisposing Factors

Proven celiac disease that either does not show improvement despite 12 months of a strict gluten-free diet, or requires further intervention because of severe or deteriorating clinical symptoms.

Clinical Features/Endoscopic Characteristics

Clinical and endoscopic features are the same as celiac disease apart from the nonresponse to gluten-free diet. Patient should be thoroughly investigated and questioned regarding occult gluten ingestion. A subgroup however may develop enteropathy-associated T-cell lymphoma, which includes ulcerative jejunitis. This condition is particularly aggressive and nearly half are fatal.

Microscopic Features

Histologically, despite therapeutic intervention, there is a persisting enteropathy with minimal or no improvement in villous architecture, intraepithelial lymphocytosis, or lamina propria inflammation from the initial biopsies. Morphologic features infrequently encountered include subepithelial collagen deposition, a basal pattern of lymphoid infiltration, crypt atrophy, and a reduction in Paneth cell numbers.

Molecular Features

- RCD is divided on the basis of IEL immunophenotype into type 1 (with normal immunophenotype) and type 2 (with aberrant IEL immunophenotype). Type 2 is associated with a risk for development of overt enteropathy-associated T-cell lymphoma (EATL). Distinction relies on the immunophenotyping of the intraepithelial T cells,

Table 7.6 Differentiating features of celiac disease and refractory celiac disease type 1 and 2.

	TCR rearrangement	CD3/CD8 immunohistochemistry	Flow cytometry
Celiac disease	Polyclonal	Preserved	No loss of surface T cell markers
RCD 1	Polyclonal (usually)	Preserved	No loss of surface T cell markers
RCD 2	Monoclonal	CD8 lost in >50% of CD3 positive IEL	Loss of surface CD3, CD7, and CD8 in >20% of IEL

flow cytometric analysis of unfixed biopsy tissue, and PCR TCR clonality studies (Table 7.6).

- In type 1 RCD the IEL phenotype is identical to usual celiac disease with expression of surface CD3, CD7, CD8, CD103, and TCRβ on flow cytometry. Expression of CD8 is identified in the majority of the CD3-positive IEL. TCR gene rearrangement should be polyclonal, although, a dominant clone can occasionally produce a false monoclonal result.
- Type 2 RCD is characterized by loss of multiple surface T-cell markers including CD3, CD7, and CD8 on flow cytometry. CD103 is expressed as is cytoplasmic CD3 (due to preservation of the immunoreactive epsilon component), which is demonstrable by immunohistochemistry. Loss of multiple surface markers (CD3, CD7, and CD8) in >20% of IEL determined by flow cytometric analysis and immunohistochemical loss of CD8 in >50% of IEL is abnormal and indicative of RCD2. Monoclonal TCR is consistently identified.

Differential Diagnosis

Once noncompliance with a strict gluten-free diet is excluded, then the major conditions to consider are collagenous sprue, autoimmune enteropathy, tropical sprue, immunodeficiency disorders such as CVID, and Crohn's disease (see respective sections).

Treatment/Prognosis/Evolution

In type 1 RCD, treatment is typically glucocorticoids alone, which are tapered over several months to the lowest dose needed to maintain remission. In type 2 RCD, glucocorticoids tapers are usually combined with chronic immunomodulators such as azathioprine or 6-mercaptopurine.

Crohn's Disease

Definition, General Features, and Predisposing Factors

Crohn's disease is a chronic inflammatory bowel disease characterized by discontinuous, transmural inflammation variously associated with granuloma formation, sinus/fistula formation, and fibrosis related stenosis (see chapter on colonic manifestations).

Clinical Features/Endoscopic Characteristics

Crohn's disease may present with a wide variety of clinical manifestations but are generally divided into inflammatory enterocolitis, fistulizing disease, and fibrostenotic disease. Any aspect of the GI tract can be involved. Common symptoms include diarrhea, bleeding, fistulization (entero-entero, entero-cutaneous, entero-vesical, entero-vaginal, etc.), abscess, and malabsorption. Upper GI manifestations such as oral, esophageal, and gastroduodenal ulceration are less common. Ulceration of the colon is typical in "skip" patterns with varying degrees of inflammation from mild erythema and granularity, to deep serpiginous ulcers (Figure 7.18).

Microscopic Features

The terminal ileum is the most commonly affected site, and the biopsies are characterized by patchy variable intensity active chronic inflammation with architectural disturbance and pseudopyloric gland metaplasia. Ulceration and granuloma formation may be identified. The proximal

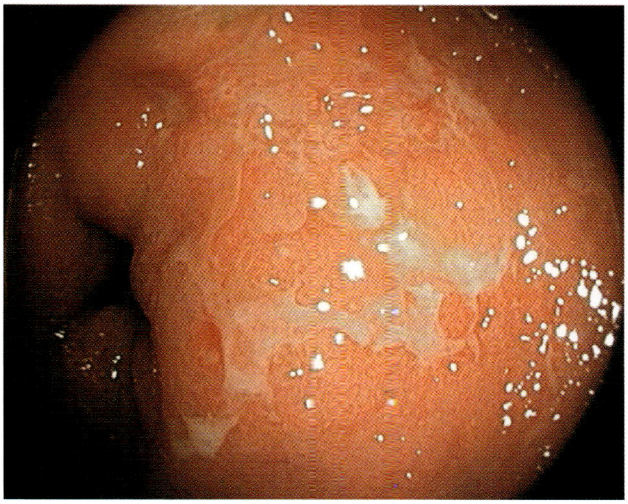

Figure 7.18 Example of Crohn's ileitis with deep serpiginous ulceration, erythema, and granular appearance of the mucosa.

(a) (b)

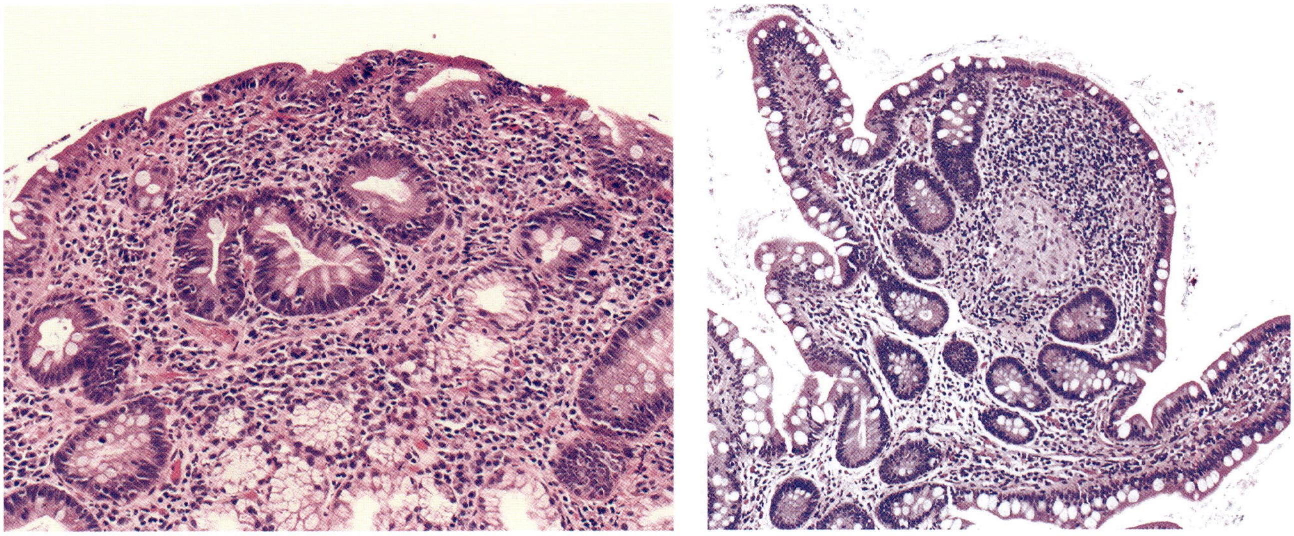

Figure 7.19 Microscopic evidence of active Crohn's ileitis (a) and granuloma (b).

small intestine is involved in up to 1/3 of the occasions that ileocolonic involvement is encountered. Discontinuous active chronic inflammation of variable severity is seen. There is often ulceration. Granuloma formation is occasionally present (Figure 7.19a, b).

Differential Diagnosis

The differential diagnosis is wide, including iatrogenic injury. NSAID enteropathy is to be considered, yet it is devoid of granulomata and generally has less chronic inflammation. Eosinophils may be frequent, although not numerous enough to suggest eosinophilic enteritis.

- Infection, in particular Yersinia and Mycobacterium infection, ought to be considered.
- Chronic granulomatous disease: The mucosal ulceration and inflammation with granuloma formation closely resemble Crohn's disease. The finding of histiocytes with dark brown cytoplasmic contents is a clue to chronic granulomatous disease. A history of recurrent infections is helpful.
- CVID enteropathy, particularly with granuloma, is to be excluded, as well.
- Finally, diffuse pattern of duodenal inflammation may occur, albeit rarely, with ulcerative colitis. This is particularly the case in a setting of diffuse pancolitis in young patients.

Treatment/Prognosis/Evolution

Therapy of Crohn's is increasing complex and based on the clinical manifestations. Multiple immunosuppressive and immunomodulatory drugs are available. Two general approaches are used: step-up therapy typically beginning with aminosalicylates, followed by glucocorticoids, immunomodulators, and biologics; and step-down therapy, which begins with the more potent biologics to achieve remission then progresses to lower potency treatment to maintain remission. Treatment of each specific manifestation is beyond the scope of this chapter but interested readers are referred to several excellent references.

Food Protein-Induced Enteropathy

Definition, General Features, and Predisposing Factors

This condition is a (non IgE) cell-mediated hypersensitivity in response to ingested proteins and polypeptides most commonly found in cow's milk, soy protein, oats, peanuts, egg, fish, rice, or chicken.

Clinical Features/Endoscopic Characteristics

Food protein-induced enterocolitis syndrome typically presents in infants with vomiting, diarrhea, loss of weight, and failure to thrive. It may have an acute or chronic form depending on whether there is infrequent or chronic ingestion of the food allergen. Other atopic diseases are seen in approximately 1/3 of infants.

Microscopic Features

Variable villous blunting and an increase in intraepithelial lymphocytes are characteristic. A flat mucosa typically is not found. Lymphonodular hyperplasia of the duodenal bulb is nearly universal. Eosinophil infiltration is usually present, and may be numerous enough to warrant a designation of eosinophilic enteritis. Neutrophils are frequently identified in the lamina propria and sometimes the crypt epithelium.

Differential Diagnosis

Celiac disease is the main differential diagnosis. Villus blunting is seldom severe in food allergy enteropathy. Instead, lymphonodular hyperplasia, and the often prominent eosinophils are additional distinguishing features.

Treatment/Prognosis/Evolution

Return to normal mucosal morphology and rapid clinical improvement follow withdrawal of the offending antigen. In infants, return to breastfeeding is preferred. If not possible, a hypoallergenic, non-cow's milk formula is recommended.

Eosinophilic Enteritis

Definition and General Features

This condition is a symptomatic eosinophil-rich inflammatory disorder either limited to the small intestine or involving the small intestine as part of more extensive gastrointestinal disease. Disorders associated with eosinophilic enteritis are myriad (Table 7.7).

Clinical Features/Endoscopic Characteristics

Eosinophilic enteritis is most commonly part of the spectrum of diffuse eosinophilic gastroenteritis. Manifestations are often classified based on the layer of intestinal involvement including mucosal, muscle layer, or subserosal disease. Approximately, 80% of patients have concurrent elevations in serum eosinophils. Endoscopic features are nonspecific including erythema, thickened folds, and erosions.

Table 7.7 Causes of eosinophilic infiltration in small bowel.

- Idiopathic[a]
- Parasitic infection[a], e.g. Strongyloides, hookworms
- Allergy[a]: food—cow's milk, soy protein
- Drugs: NSAIDs, gold, L-tryptophan, carbamazepine, methotrexate, tacrolimus, azathioprine, rifampicin, clozapine, enalapril, mycophenolate
- Crohn's disease (quiescent)
- Connective tissue disorders
- Vasculitis: Churg–Strauss syndrome, occasionally polyarteritis nodosa (PAN), and others
- Neoplasia: Lymphoma, Langerhans cell histiocytosis, Systemic Mastocytosis, myeloid neoplasms
- Inflammatory fibroid polyp
- Solid organ and bone marrow transplantation
- Hypereosinophilic syndrome

[a] Most common.

Microscopic Features

The normal mean enteric eosinophil count is <10/HPF with peak eosinophil counts in pediatric duodenum and ileum being 26/HPF and 28/HPF respectively. In eosinophilic enteritis, mucosal involvement is characterized by diffuse eosinophil infiltrate >20–30/HPF accompanied by villous blunting of variable degree, eosinophil infiltration of epithelium, eosinophilic crypt abscess formation, and infiltration of muscularis mucosae. Mucosal edema may be prominent in some case.

Report

Where no specific cause is known or found, the pathologist should report mucosal eosinophilia as a reaction pattern with multiple possible etiologies. When a potential cause is microscopically evident, it should be stated in the report specifically. Otherwise, a comment to the effect that "mucosal eosinophilia is not specific. Common causes include allergic reaction to food or drugs and parasitic infection" is useful.

Treatment/Prognosis/Evolution

If tolerated, the most effective therapy is avoidance of the food antigen. Since there is no established method to confirm a specific food antigen, empiric elimination diets of the six most common food antigens (soy, wheat, egg, milk, peanut/tree nuts, fish/shellfish) is recommended. A prospective clinical trial consists of six-food elimination diet or elemental diet in the treatment of adults with eosinophilic gastroenteritis. At least six weeks are usually needed to achieve remission and noncompliance is common. Patient symptoms and peripheral eosinophil counts serve as markers of response. For patient who cannot comply with or does not respond to elimination diets, glucocorticoids, cromolyn, ketotifen, or anti-leukotriene agents (montelukast) may be effective.

Histiocytic/Granulomatous Enteritis

Definition

Conditions leading to the collection of histiocytes or well-developed granulomata in the small intestine fall into this category (see Table 7.8).

Table 7.8 Common causes of histiocytic and granulomatous infiltration.

Histiocytes	Xanthoma, malakoplakia, Whipple's, MAIC, lipid storage disorders
Granulomata	Foreign body granuloma, sarcoidosis, Crohn's disease, pneumatosis, CVID, chronic granulomatous disease, *M. tuberculosis*

Microscopic Features

See specific sections.

Necrotizing Enterocolitis (NEC)

Definition, General Features, and Predisposing Factors

This idiopathic ischemic disorder is characterized by hemorrhagic necrosis of the small intestine and proximal colon. It develops most commonly in premature infants ("neonatal NEC"). Predisposing conditions include prematurity, as well as Paneth cell deficiency, luminal bacteria, and commencement of enteral feeding.

Clinical Features/Endoscopic Characteristics

NEC is a common emergency of infants, occurring in 4–11.5% of underweight births with increasing frequency among the lowest birth weight infants. Symptoms typically present at three to four weeks of life, beginning with nonspecific lethargy, poor feeding with progression to more severe symptoms of vomiting, diarrhea, gastrointestinal obstruction, and sepsis. Endoscopy should generally be avoided as it may induce perforation and characteristic findings are seen on radiographic studies including pneumatosis intestinalis.

Microscopic Features

Focal or diffuse coagulative necrosis of the intestinal mucosa or deeper layers of the intestinal wall is noted, associated with hemorrhage. Inflammation is minimal. Pneumatosis intestinalis may develop. Healing may produce fibrosis.

Differential Diagnosis

Conditions to exclude are ischemia (see below); Crohn's disease in small intestine (at the healing stage); and tropical necrotizing colitis. The former condition affects all age groups. "Pigbel" in Papua New Guinea is due to undercooked pork allowing *C. perfringens* infection.

Treatment/Prognosis/Evolution

Treatment is based on severity of disease. For stage 1 (mild) and stage 2 (moderate) disease, supportive care including total parenteral nutrition, antibiotics, and radiographic monitoring, is used. For stage 3 (severe) disease manifesting as pneumatosis intestinalis with significant systemic features (sepsis, disseminated intravascular coagulation (DIC), perforation, metabolic acidosis), surgical exploration is warranted with resection of the affected region of bowel.

Intestinal Ischemia (Syn. Ischemic Enteritis)

Definition and Predisposing Factors

This pattern of injury results from an inadequate supply of nutrients to the cellular and supporting elements. This is typically the result of inadequate blood supply. The causes are myriad (see Table 7.9).

Microscopic Features

These encompass a broad spectrum, depending on the severity. The earliest change is epithelial cell apoptosis followed by crypt atrophy and villous blunting. Edema and red cell extravasation are prominent if venous obstruction is the cause. Later, hyalinization of the lamina propria may develop. Inflammation is generally limited, but focal acute inflammation may develop, particularly when the blood supply is restored. The muscularis mucosa may be atrophic or disappear.

Radiation Enteritis

Definition, General Features, and Predisposing Factors

This is the injury to the small intestine secondary to pelvic or abdominal radiation.

Clinical Features/Endoscopic Characteristics

Patients typically present with diarrhea, bleeding, or obstruction. Endoscopic features range from erythema with telangiectasia or stenosis.

Table 7.9 Etiologies of ischemic disease.

Vascular obstruction
1) External compression
• Adhesions
• Volvulus
• Incarceration in hernia sac
• Iatrogenic, e.g. surgical ligation
2) Vessel wall abnormality
• Atherosclerosis
• Vasculitis: PAN, Churg–Strauss (EGPA), Takayasu's, Wegener's granulomatosis, (GPA) connective tissue disorder related. Behcet's
• Radiotherapy-related intimal hyperplasia
• Amyloidosis
• Arterial dissection
• Scleroderma
• Fibromuscular hyperplasia
• Hemolytic uremic syndrome (HUS)/thrombotic thrombocytopenic purpura (TTP)/thrombotic microangiopathies
3) Vascular Lumen
• Thrombosis
• Hypercoagulable state (e.g. embolus)
• Thromboembolus
• Cholesterol emboli
• Tumor emboli
• Foreign body
Intestinal hypoperfusion
• Hypovolemia
• Cardiac failure
• Excessive exercise
Drugs
• Digoxin
• Cocaine
• NSAIDs
• Pseudoephedrine
• Vasopressor agents
• OCP (oral contraceptive pill)/estrogenic compounds
Luminal obstruction with backpressure
• Tumors
• Hirschsprung's disease
Infection, e.g. CMV
Miscellaneous, e.g. necrotizing enterocolitis

Microscopic Features

The alterations occur throughout the entire wall and can be acute or chronic. Acute mucosal changes range from edema to frank ulceration or necrosis. Villous blunting and a mild increase in chronic inflammation can be seen. Acute inflammation, crypt apoptosis, and crypt loss occur with more severe injury. Atypical appearing stellate cells ("radiation" fibroblasts) may be seen in the granulation tissue of an ulcer. Chronic damage is characterized by crypt architectural irregularity with pyloric gland metaplasia and fibrosis in the lamina propria.

Differential Diagnosis

Depending on severity, conditions to rule out include Crohn's disease, vasculitis, and NSAID injury.

Treatment/Prognosis/Evolution

Treatments include dietary (low residue), antidiarrheal agents (e.g. loperamide), antibiotics if small intestinal bacterial overgrowth is present, and hyperbaric oxygen, which is particularly effective for ulcerative/severe inflammatory disease. Surgery is to be avoided except in cases of severe, refractory stasis.

Peptic Duodenitis

Definition, General Features, and Predisposing Factors

This injury to the proximal small intestinal mucosa is induced by abnormal gastric acid exposure. There is a well-established association with gastric Helicobacter pylori infection leading to increased acid secretion. Excessive gastric acid exposure induced by a gastrin-producing tumor (Zollinger–Ellison syndrome) is another established etiology. Iatrogenic influences may potentiate the injurious effect of gastric acid (e.g. NSAIDs), but also tobacco, chronic renal disease, and alcohol.

Clinical Features/Endoscopic Characteristics

Erosions and ulceration of the duodenum are very common in patients infected with *H. pylori* or those taking chronic NSAID medication. Symptoms include dyspepsia, bleeding, or rarely perforation. Endoscopy is commonly used, particularly in patients with "red flag" symptoms such as elderly onset, bleeding, or vomiting. The endoscopic appearance is one of ulceration with loss of mucosal integrity and white ulcers of varying depth (Figure 7.20).

Microscopic Features

Characteristic features include a variable degree of villous blunting, gastric foveolar metaplasia, and acute and chronic inflammation in the lamina propria. Erosion and

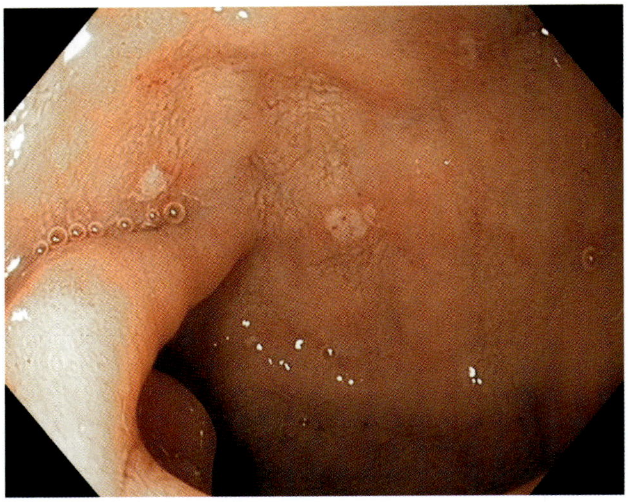

Figure 7.20 NSAIDs enteropathy with superficial erosion and multifocal white patches of epithelial denudation (center and left of image).

ulceration develop when injury is severe. Helicobacter pylori may colonize the metaplastic gastric epithelium. Reactive cytological changes occur in inflamed epithelium, but they are insufficient to evoke a diagnosis of dysplasia. Brunner gland hyperplasia is common and is typified by a nodular proliferation of glands that extends into the mucosa. Typically, the changes are most marked in the duodenal bulb region.

Differential Diagnosis

The astute pathologist should eliminate:

1) A peptic duodenitis-like pattern of celiac disease characterized by a prominent neutrophil infiltrate. The associated features, such as intraepithelial lymphocytosis, villous blunting, and inflammation beyond the duodenal bulb secure the diagnosis.
2) NSAID enteropathy. A relevant clinical history is crucial. Involvement beyond the duodenal bulb, a conspicuous eosinophil infiltrate, and subtle ischemic injury features such as lamina propria hyalinization and crypt atrophy are supportive of NSAID injury.
3) Crohn's disease. Inflammation is often variable in intensity. Ulceration and granuloma formation may be present.

Treatment/Prognosis/Evolution

Treatment is twofold. Endoscopic therapy of acute bleeding duodenitis includes injection of adrenaline, cautery of bleeding or visible large vessels, or mechanical closure with clip devices. Following acute therapy, treatment is aimed at acid suppression and at underlying causes including eradication of *H. pylori* when present and avoidance of NSAIDs.

NSAID Enteropathy

Definition, General Features (Frequency), and Predisposing Factors

This injury to the small intestine is mediated by microvascular alterations associated with NSAID ingestion. It may affect the mucosa and/or submucosa and lead to mucosal inflammation, erosion, or diaphragm-like strictures.

Clinical Features/Endoscopic Characteristics

NSAID enteropathy overlaps with peptic duodenitis as discussed above (Figure 7.20).

Microscopic Features

Various degrees of villous blunting (even sometimes flat mucosa) are usual. Acute and chronic inflammation is mild, but conspicuous eosinophils are sometimes found. Erosion and gastric metaplasia of antral or pseudopyloric gland type can occur with chronic damage. Prominent lipid-induced cytoplasmic vacuolization in the surface epithelium can be seen as well as ischemic features. The epithelium may acquire a serrated pattern as well. Abnormal crypt architecture develops with chronic use.

Differential Diagnosis

Conditions to exclude are:

1) Peptic duodenitis (see above).
2) Crohn's disease, particularly in ileum in the setting of long-term NSAID use. Clinical history is relevant. The finding of granulomata and a fissuring rather than a broad-based pattern of ulceration favor Crohn's disease, along with prominent lymphangiectasia and marked active chronic inflammation.
3) Vasculitis/Behcet's (see below)
4) Infection (see below).

Treatment/Prognosis/Evolution

Treatment is the same as for peptic duodenitis associated with NSAID use as discussed above.

Isolated Ileitis/Erosion

Definition, General Features (Frequency), and Predisposing Factors

This term represents inflammation and/or ulceration limited to the distal terminal ileum and detected by ileoscopy. Various etiologies can be at play (see table): (i) Crohn's disease limited to the ileum; (ii) infection—Yersinia, *M. tuberculosis*, Campylobacter, Salmonella; rarely viral e.g. CMV and fungal e.g. Histoplasma; (iii) medications—NSAID use, calcium channel blockers (Nicorandil), others; (iv) spondyloarthropathy—ankylosing and non-ankylosing type; (v) idiopathic disease.

Clinical Features/Endoscopic Characteristics

Clinical features are discussed within the specific sections for each etiology.

Microscopic Features

The main feature is acute inflammation with cryptitis and crypt abscess formation. There may be associated superficial erosion, although this may only be identified on multiple levels. The latter may overlie reactive lymphoid tissue (aphthous type erosion). Eosinophils are usually present and may be numerous. Lymphocytes and plasma cells are increased, particularly if erosion is present. Features of chronicity may be encountered, including crypt branching and shortening, villus blunting, basal plasmacytosis, and pseudopyloric gland metaplasia.

Differential Diagnosis

Common conditions to rule out include backwash ileitis in ulcerative colitis and vasculitis, particularly Behcet's disease.

Treatment/Prognosis/Evolution

Treatment is discussed within the specific section for each etiology.

Behcet's Disease

Definition, General Features (Frequency), and Predisposing Factors

This condition of unknown etiology is a multisystem vasculitic disorder involving both small and large vessels. Infection and genetic predisposition have been proposed as predisposing factors. There is an increased prevalence in countries along the Silk Road, with the highest incidence in Turkey. HLA B51 has been associated.

Clinical Features/Endoscopic Characteristics

Behcet's disease involves the GIT as part of a diffuse mucocutaneous spectrum. The most common sites of involvement are terminal ilium, and proximal colon. Symptoms include nausea, abdominal pain, and diarrhea. At endoscopy, ulcerations may be seen but there are no specific features, which distinguish these from other ulcerating conditions so biopsy and clinical exclusion of other entities such as Crohn's and NSAID are critical.

Microscopic Features

The disease may manifest throughout the gut, with the ileocecal region being most commonly affected. Mucosal involvement varies from nonspecific focal active inflammation to extensive and deep mucosal ulceration. An aphthous pattern of erosion is commonly encountered. Endoscopic biopsies are unlikely to show the vasculitis, which is present in the submucosa especially in the veins or deeper in the intestinal wall.

Differential Diagnosis

The differential diagnosis is broad, including Crohn's disease, Henoch–Schonlein purpura, and enterocolic lymphocytic phlebitis.

Treatment/Prognosis/Evolution

Treatment of gastrointestinal manifestations is typically recommended when ulceration of significant symptoms are present. Treatment options include glucocorticoids often combined with azathioprine for one to two months followed by tapering of the glucocorticoids. Other therapies include anti-TNF agents and aminosalicylates similar to therapy for Crohn's disease.

Cryptogenic Multifocal Ulcerating and Stenosing Enteritis (CMUSE)

Definition, General Features (Frequency), and Predisposing Factors

This uncommon disorder is characterized by multifocal ulceration and stenosis of the small intestine. The etiology is uncertain. Associations with complement 2 deficiency and polyarteritis nodosa have been reported.

Clinical Features/Endoscopic Characteristics

CMUSE is a rare entity with features of recurrent small bowel obstruction and diffuse enteral ulceration. Endoscopic features are nonspecific other than multifocal shallow ulcers.

Microscopic Features

Ulceration involving mucosa or superficial submucosa is always found in the segment of intestinal stenosis. A mild mixed inflammatory infiltrate with some eosinophils is seen. There is no abnormality in the intestine away from the ulcers.

Differential Diagnosis

Ischemia, Crohn's disease, iatrogenic injury (e.g. NSAIDs, potassium, chemotherapy), and ulcerating jejunoileitis can all mimic this rare disorder.

Treatment/Prognosis/Evolution

Treatment of CMUSE is typically with glucocorticoids. In cases of stenosis, small case series report response to endoscopic balloon dilation.

Miscellaneous Disorders

Pigment Disorders

Various endogenous or exogenous pigmented material can be detected within the small intestine.

Clinical Features/Endoscopic Characteristics

Pigmented changes of the small bowel are rare. Ferrous pigments are most common with typical appearance of "peppery speckles" in the mucosa.

Microscopic Features

- Iron: Deposition may occur in hereditary hemochromatosis or as result of multiple blood transfusions or administration of oral or parenteral iron. In hemochromatosis and secondary causes of iron overload, the iron deposition can be within the lamina propria and within the epithelium of both the mucosa and Brunner glands. Oral iron tablets may be associated with mucosal erosion, and brown crystalline iron is often seen in the surface exudate.
- Carbon: Carbon can be found to a variable extent within the ileal Peyer's patches of city dwellers.
- Pseudomelanosis: This is a deposition of brown pigment, usually within the villous stroma. The pigment contains variable amounts of iron, ceroid, sulfur, and melanin. A Perls stain will highlight the iron. Alternatively, true melanosis can be associated with metastatic melanoma in the local area.
- "Brown bowel" syndrome: This disorder develops secondary to deficiency in vitamin E, which is essential for stabilizing mitochondrial membranes. Vitamin E deficiency may lead to primary or secondary fat malabsorption. A secondary smooth muscle "mitochondrial myopathy" results in cytoplasmic lipofuscin deposition within the cytoplasm of cells of the muscularis mucosa, muscularis propria, and vascular media or within histiocytes throughout the GIT. Cell atrophy develops with extensive deposition.

Special Studies

Perls stain will be helpful for the diagnosis of pseudomelanosis and hemosiderin. Conversely, Fontana Masson stain will be helpful for lipofuscin. Electron microscopy and chemical microanalysis may be required in some cases.

Treatment/Prognosis/Evolution

These conditions typically require no treatment.

Deposition Disorders

Waldenstrom Macroglobulinemia

Definition, General Features (Frequency), and Predisposing Factors

This clinicopathologic disorder is characterized by the production and tissue deposition of IgM paraprotein that is produced by the neoplastic cells of a lymphoplasmacytic lymphoma.

Clinical Features/Endoscopic Characteristics

Clinical manifestations are nonspecific with dyspepsia, diarrhea, or early satiety. Endoscopic features are also nonspecific and include erythema and thickened gastrointestinal folds.

Microscopic Features

The IgM paraprotein deposition is evidenced by brightly eosinophilic, homogenous, and strongly PAS+ material. Initially noted within the villous lymphatics and between the epithelial cells, it eventually fills the lamina propria (Figure 7.21). Villous blunting and lymphangiectasia develop, with foamy histiocytes frequently found within the dilated lymphatics. Occasionally the neoplastic plasmacytoid cells may infiltrate the lamina propria. Secondary infection, in particular giardiasis, may result because of loss of normal immunoglobulin function.

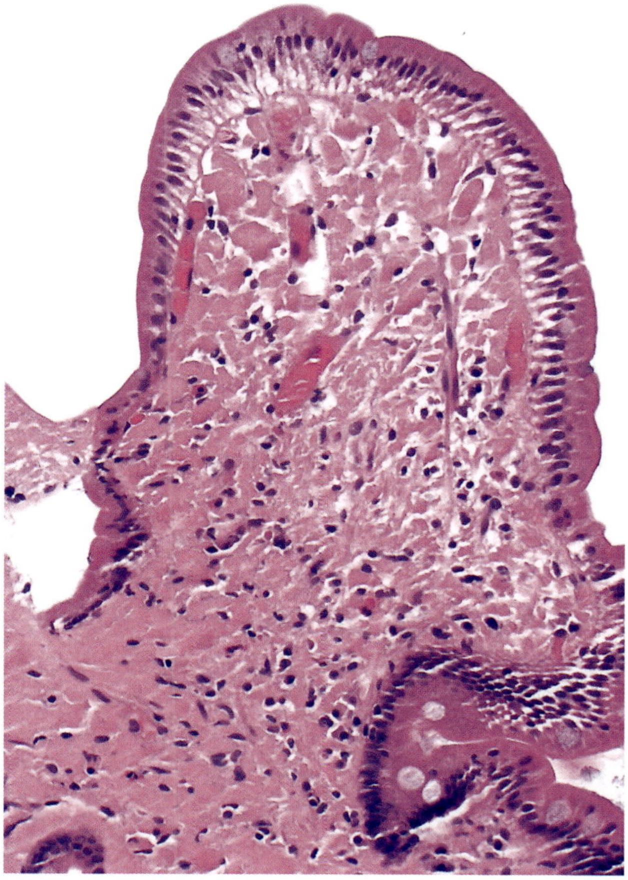

Figure 7.21 Example of the Waldenstrom disease with expansion of the lamina propria by eosinophilic paraprotein deposition.

Differential Diagnosis

Conditions that could confuse the unwary observer include amyloidosis, intestinal lymphangiectasia, and Whipple's disease.

Treatment/Prognosis/Evolution

Treatment is aimed at the underlying disorder and is beyond the scope of this text. Symptomatic patients are typically treated with chemotherapy such as rituximab. The addition of rituximab to front-line therapy with cyclophosphamide, doxorubicin hydrochloride (hydroxydaunorubicin), vincristine sulfate (Oncovin), and prednisone (CHOP) (R-CHOP) results in a higher response rate and longer time to treatment failure in patients with lymphoplasmacytic lymphoma: results of a randomized trial of the German Low-Grade Lymphoma Study Group (GLSG).

Amyloidosis

Definition, General Features (Frequency), and Predisposing Factors

This generic term encompasses the accumulation and tissue deposition of various proteins with distinctive structural arrangement (β pleated sheet) and staining properties (green birefringence with Congo red). Three main clinical categories are recognized—AA, AL, and hereditary. Classification is also based on the type of amyloid protein.

Clinical Features/Endoscopic Characteristics

Patients with amyloid have a wide variety of gastrointestinal features including hepatosplenomegaly, poor intestinal motility (gastroparesis/constipation), and malabsorption. Biopsy is often obtained from subcutaneous fat, although rectal biopsy at endoscopy has good sensitivity but may be prone to bleeding.

Microscopic Features

Amyloidosis is characterized by homogeneous, amorphous, and light eosinophilic staining extracellular deposits on H&E sections. Typically there is deposition in the wall of submucosal vessels and around nerves (initially in familial amyloid polyneuropathy) and within the muscle of the muscularis mucosae and propria. This may coalesce into a uniform deposition replacing much of the normal lamina propria and submucosa. A globular pattern of deposition is occasionally encountered. Secondary changes due to vascular involvement may be seen and include ischemic ulceration and hemorrhage due to vessel wall weakness. Perforation may occur (Figure 7.22a, b).

Special Studies

Standard confirmation is by way of Congo red staining with apple green birefringence on polarization. Immunohistochemistry for amyloid P component is confirmatory but is often faint. Ultrastructurally, randomly oriented fibrils measuring 7–10 nm in diameter are observed.

Typing of amyloid

This requires a multidisciplinary approach, including clinical evaluation combined with immunohistochemical studies (of low specificity and sensitivity) and, variously, biochemical tests, genetic studies, and functional imaging (Table 7.10).

Differential Diagnosis

The two conditions to rule out are hyaline fibrosis and light chain deposition.

Treatment/Prognosis/Evolution

Treatment is aimed at the underlying disorder and details are beyond the scope of this text. In general, treatment is aimed at the primary etiology such as the chronic inflammatory, infectious, or neoplastic disorder.

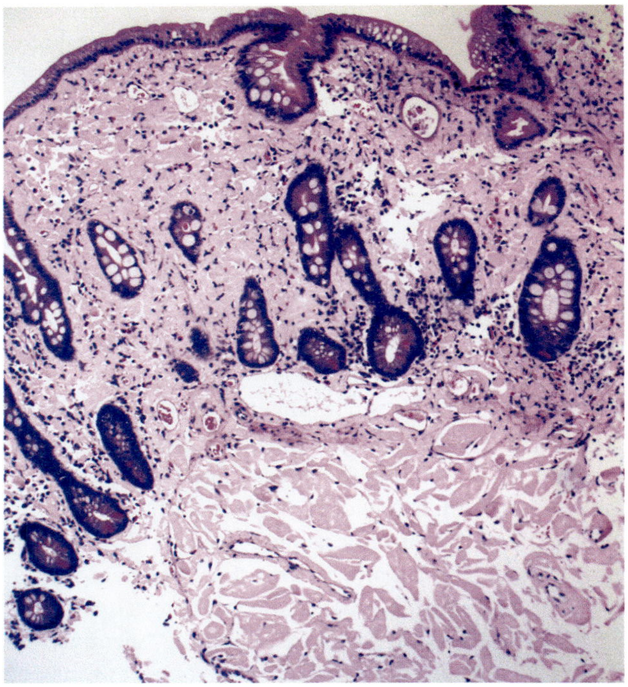

Figure 7.22 Amyloid deposition resulting in the expansion of the lamina propria and blunting the villi. Confirmation can be easily established by Congo Red stain.

Table 7.10 Major types of amyloid affecting the small intestine.

Type of amyloid	Precursor protein	Clinical setting
AA	Serum amyloid A protein	Chronic inflammatory conditions Familial Mediterranean fever
AL	Monoclonal immunoglobulin light chain	Plasma cell neoplasia, B-cell lymphoma
ATTR	Transthyretin	Familial amyloidotic polyneuropathy
Alys	Lysozyme	Autosomal dominant systemic amyloidosis with prominent visceral deposition
AApoA1	Apolipoprotein A1	Autosomal dominant systemic amyloidosis with prominent visceral deposition
Aβ2M	β_2-microglobulin	Renal dialysis associated

Abetalipoproteinemia

Definition, General Features (Frequency), and Predisposing Factors

This rare autosomal recessive disorder is due to mutations in the gene encoding for microsomal triglyceride transfer protein. The subsequent absence of plasma apo B-containing lipoproteins compromise absorption of fat and fat soluble vitamins.

Clinical Features/Endoscopic Characteristics

Patients with this disorder typically develop steatorrhea with typically onset within the first five to seven years of life. Endoscopy may show "white" villous tips do to lipid retention.

Microscopic Features

Marked foamy vacuolization of the cytoplasm of enterocytes covering the upper 2/3 of the villi is characteristic, resulting from the retention of absorbed lipid that cannot be transported to the bloodstream. The villous architecture remains normal, and there is no associated inflammation.

Differential Diagnosis

Failure to fast prior to endoscopic biopsy may yield similar histology. "Lipid hang-up" due to enteropathy is another mimic.

Treatment/Prognosis/Evolution

Treatment is focused on high-dose fat soluble vitamins, particularly vitamin E, which prevents neuropathy and retinopathy.

Further Reading

Abraham, S.C., Yardley, J.H., and Wu, T.T. (1999). Erosive injury to the upper gastrointestinal tract in patients receiving iron medication. *Am. J. Surg. Pathol.* 23: 1241–1247.

Akram, S., Murray, J.A., Pardi, D.S. et al. (2007). Adult autoimmune enteropathy: Mayo Clinic Rochester experience. *Clin. Gastroenterol. Hepatol.* 5: 1282.

Al-Daraji, W.I., Zelger, B., Zelger, B., and Hussein, M.R. (2010). Microvillous inclusion disease: a clinicopathologic study of 17 cases from the UK. *Ultrastruct. Pathol.* 34 (6): 327–332.

Al-Toma, A., Verbeek, W.H., Hadithi, M. et al. (2007). *Gut* 56 (10): 1373.

Al-Toma, A., Verbeek, W.H., and Mulder, C.J. (2007). Update on the management of refractory coeliac disease. *J. Gastrointestin. Liver Dis.* 16: 57.

Ament, M.E. and Rubin, C.E. (1972). Soy protein—another cause of the flat intestinal lesion. *Gastroenterology* 62: 227.

Antonioli, D. (2003). Celiac disease: a Progress report. *Mod. Pathol.* 16 (4): 342–346.

Aslanian, H., Chander, B., Robert, M. et al. (2012). Prospective evaluation of acute graft-versus-host disease. *Dig. Dis. Sci.* 57 (3): 720–725.

Aziz, I., Evans, K.E., Hopper, A.D. et al. (2010). A prospective study into the aetiology of lymphocytic duodenosis. *Aliment. Pharmacol. Ther.* 32: 1392–1397.

Batheja, M.J., Leighton, J., Azueta, A., and Heigh, R. (2010). The face of tropical sprue in 2010. *Case Rep. Gastroenterol.* 4 (2): 168–172.

Bell, S.W., Kerner, J.A. Jr., and Sibley, R.K. (1991). Microvillous inclusion disease. The importance of electron microscopy for diagnosis. *Am. J. Surg. Pathol.* 15: 1157.

Biagi, F., Luinetti, O., Campanella, J. et al. (2004). Intraepithelial lymphocytes in the villous tip: do they indicate potential coeliac disease? *J. Clin. Pathol.* 57: 835.

Bohane, T.D., Cutz, E., Hamilton, J.R., and Gall, D.G. (1977). Acrodermatitis enteropathica, zinc, and the Paneth cell. A case report with family studies. *Gastroenterology* 73: 587.

Bonamico, M., Thanasi, E., Mariani, P. et al. (2008). Duodenal bulb biopsies in celiac disease: a multicenter study. *J. Pediatr. Gastroenterol. Nutr.* 47: 618.

Brandt, L.J., Davidoff, A., Bernstein, L.H. et al. (1981). Small-intestine involvement in Waldenstrom's macroglobulinemia. Case report and review of the literature. *Dig. Dis. Sci.* 26: 174.

Brenchley, J.M., Schacker, T.W., Ruff, L.E. et al. (2004). CD4+ T cell depletion during all stages of HIV disease occurs predominantly in the gastrointestinal tract. *J. Exp. Med.* 200 (6): 749–759.

Brown, I.S., Bettington, A., Bettington, M., and Rosty, C. (2014). Tropical Sprue – revisiting an under recognised condition. *Am. J. Surg. Pathol.* 38 (5): 666–672.

Brown, I., Mino-Kenudson, M., Deshpande, V., and Lauwers, G.Y. (2006). Intraepithelial lymphocytosis in architecturally preserved proximal small intestinal mucosa – an increasing diagnostic problem with a wide differential diagnosis. *Arch. Pathol. Lab. Med.* 130 (7): 1020–1025.

Brown, I., Smith, J., and Rosty, C. (2012). Gastrointestinal pathology in celiac disease: a case series of 150 consecutive newly diagnosed patients. *Am. J. Clin. Pathol.* 138 (1): 42–49.

Buske, C., Hoster, E., Dreyling, M. et al. (2009). German low-grade lymphoma study group. *Leukemia* 23 (1): 153.

Caselli, M., Gaudio, M., Chiamenti, C.M. et al. (1998). Histologic findings and helicobacter pylori in duodenal biopsies. *J. Clin. Gastroenterol.* 26 (1): 74–80.

Castigli, E., Wilson, S.A., Garibyan, L. et al. (2005). TACI is mutant in common variable immunodeficiency and IgA deficiency. *Nat. Genet.* 37: 829–834.

Catassi, C., Fabiani, E., Rätsch, I.M. et al. (1996). The coeliac iceberg in Italy. A multicentre antigliadin antibodies screening for coeliac disease in school-age subjects. *Acta Paediatr. Suppl.* 412: 29–35.

Cellier, C., Delabesse, E., Helmer, C. et al. (2000). Refractory sprue, coeliac disease, and enteropathy-associated T-cell lymphoma. French Coeliac Disease Study Group. *Lancet* 356 (9225): 203–208.

Chang, F., Mahadeva, U., and Deere, H. (2005). Pathological and clinical significance of increased intraepithelial lymphocytes (IELs) in small bowel mucosa. *APMIS* 113: 385.

Chin, D.P., Hopewell, P.C., Yajko, D.M. et al. (1994). Mycobacterium avium complex in the respiratory or gastrointestinal tract and the risk of M. avium complex bacteremia in patients with human immunodeficiency virus infection. *J. Infect. Dis.* 169 (2): 289–295.

Conte, D., Velio, P., Brunelli, L. et al. (1987). Stainable iron in gastric and duodenal mucosa of primary hemochromatosis patients and alcoholics. *Am. J. Gastroenterol.* 82: 237–240.

Corazza, G.R. and Villanacci, V. (2005). Coeliac disease. *J. Clin. Pathol.* 58: 573.

Courville, E.L., Siegel, C.A., Vay, T. et al. (2009). Isolated asymptomatic ileitis does not progress to overt Crohn disease on long-term follow-up despite features of chronicity in ileal biopsies. *Am. J. Surg. Pathol.* 33 (9): 1341–1347.

Cover, T.L. et al. (1989). Yersinia enterocolitica. *N. Engl. J. Med.* 321 (1): 16.

Cunningham-Rundles, J., Zhou, Z., Mankarious, S., and Courter, S. (1993). Long-term use of IgA-depleted

intravenous immunoglobulin in immunodeficient subjects with anti-IgA antibodies. *Clin. Immunol.* 13 (4): 272–278.
Cunningham-Rundles, C. (2010). How I treat common variable immune deficiency. *Blood* 116 (1): 7–15.
Cutz, E., Rhoads, J.M., Drumm, B. et al. (1989). Micro inclusion disease: an inherited defect of brush border assembly and differentiation. *N. Engl. J. Med.* 320: 646.
Cutz, E., Sherman, P.M., and Davidson, G.P. (1997). Enteropathies associated with protracted diarrhea of infancy: clinicopathological features, cellular and molecular mechanisms. *Pediatr. Pathol. Lab. Med.* 17: 335.
Daniels, J.A., Lederman, H.M., Maitra, A., and Montgomery, E.A. (2007). Gastrointestinal tract pathology in patients with common variable immunodeficiency (CVID): a clinicopathologic study and review. *Am. J. Surg. Pathol.* 31 (12): 1800–1812.
Daum, S., Cellier, C., and Mulder, C.J. (2005). Refractory coeliac disease. *Best Pract. Res. Clin. Gastroenterol.* 19: 413.
De Petris, G. and López, J.I. (2008). Histopathology of diaphragm disease of the small intestine. *Am. J. Clin. Pathol.* 130: 518–525.
DeBrosse, C.W., Case, J.W., Putnam, P.E. et al. (2006). Quantity and distribution of eosinophils in the gastrointestinal tract of children. *Pediatr. Dev. Pathol.* 9 (3): 210–218.
Di Sabatino, A., Miceli, E., Dhaliwal, W. et al. (2008). Distribution, proliferation, and function of Paneth cells in uncomplicated and complicated adult celiac disease. *Am. J. Clin. Pathol.* 130: 34.
Dignass, A. et al. (2010). The second European evidence-based consensus on the diagnosis and management of Crohn's disease: current management. *J. Crohns Colitis* 4: 28.
Ebert, E.C. (2009). Gastrointestinal manifestations of Behçet's disease. *Dig. Dis. Sci.* 54 (2): 201–207.
Ebert, E.C. and Nagar, M. (2008). Gastrointestinal manifestations of amyloidosis. *Am. J. Gastroenterol.* 103 (3): 776–787.
Eddleston, M., Peacock, S., Juniper, M., and Warrell, D.A. (1997). Severe cytomegalovirus infection in immunocompetent patients. *Clin. Infect. Dis.* 24 (1): 52–56.
Farthing, M.J. (1996). Giardiasis. *Gastroenterol. Clin. N. Am.* 25: 493.
Feldmeier, J.J. and Hampson, N.B. (2002). A systematic review of the literature reporting the application of hyperbaric oxygen prevention and treatment of delayed radiation injuries: an evidence based approach. *Undersea Hyperb. Med.* 29 (1): 4.
Feurle, G.E. and Marth, T. (1994). An evaluation of antimicrobial treatment for Whipple's Disease. Tetracycline versus trimethoprim-sulfamethoxazole. *Dig. Dis. Sci.* 39 (8): 1642–1648.
Foster, C.S. (1979). The brown bowel syndrome: a possible smooth muscle mitochondrial myopathy. *Histopathology* 3: 1.
Freeman, H.J. (2009). Multifocal stenosing ulceration of the small intestine. *World J. Gastroenterol.* 15 (39): 4883–4885.
Freeman, H.J. (2010). Update on collagenous sprue. *World J. Gastroenterol.* 16 (3): 296–298.
Gad, A., Willén, R., Carlén, B. et al. (1995). Duodenal involvement in Waldenström's macroglobulinemia. *J. Clin. Gastroenterol.* 20 (2): 174–176.
Galland, R.B. and Spencer, J. (1986). Surgical management of radiation enteritis. *Surgery* 99 (2): 133.
Goka, B.Q., Rolston, D.D., Mathan, V.I., and Farthing, M.J. (1990). The relative merits of faecal and duodenal juice microscopy in the diagnosis of giardiasis. *Trans. R. Soc. Trop. Med. Hyg.* 84 (1): 66–67.
Goldstein, N.S. (2006). Isolated ileal erosions in patients with mildly altered bowel habits. A follow-up study of 28 patients. *Am. J. Clin. Pathol.* 125: 838–846.
Goldstein, N.S. and Underhill, J. (2001). Morphologic features suggestive of gluten sensitivity in architecturally normal duodenal biopsy specimens. *Am. J. Clin. Pathol.* 116: 63–71.
Gonsalves, N., Doerfler, B., Yang, G., and Hirano, I. (2009). S1861 A prospective clinical trial of six food elimination diet or elemental diet in the treatment of adults with eosinophilic gastroenteritis. *Gastroenterology* 136 https://doi.org/10.1016/S0016-5085(09)61276-2.
Gould, M., Zarrin-Khameh, N., and Sellin, J. (2013). Small bowel amyloidosis. *Curr. Gastroenterol. Rep.* 15: 350.
Goulet, O.J., Brousse, N., Canioni, D. et al. (1998). Syndrome of intractable diarrhoea with persistent villous atrophy in early childhood: a clinicopathological survey of 47 cases. *J. Pediatr. Gastroenterol. Nutr.* 26: 151.
Goulet, O. et al. (2007). Intestinal epithelial dysplasia (tufting enteropathy). *Orphanet J. Rare Dis.* 2: 20.
Greenwood, N. (1976). The jejunal mucosa in two cases of a-beta-lipoproteinemia. *Am. J. Gastroenterol.* 65: 160.
Groisman, G.M., Amar, M., and Livne, E. (2002). CD10: a valuable tool for the light microscopic diagnosis of microvillous inclusion disease (familial microvillous atrophy). *Am. J. Surg. Pathol.* 26: 902.
Groisman, G., Ben-Izhak, O., Schwersenz, A. et al. (1993). The value of polyclonal carcinoembryonic antigen immunostaining in the diagnosis of micro inclusion disease. *Hum. Pathol.* 24: 1232.
Gross, T. et al. (1986). AIDS and multiple system involvement with cryptosporidium. *Am. J. Gastroenterol.* 81: 456–458.
Haboubi, N.Y., Lee, G.S., and Montgomery, R.D. (1991). Duodenal mucosal morphometry of elderly patients with small intestinal bacterial overgrowth: response to antibiotic treatment. *Age Ageing* 20: 29.

Haghighi, P. and Wolf, P.L. (1997). Tropical sprue and subclinical enteropathy: a vision for the nineties. *Crit. Rev. Clin. Lab. Sci.* 34: 313.

Harris, M., Burton, I.E., and Scarffe, J.H. (1983). Macroglobulinaemia and intestinal lymphangiectasia: a rare association. *J. Clin. Pathol.* 36 (1): 30–36.

Hayat, M., Cairns, A., Dixon, M.F., and O'Mahony, S. (2002). Quantitation of intraepithelial lymphocytes in human duodenum: what is normal? *J. Clin. Pathol.* 55: 393.

Hemmer, P.R., Topazian, M.D., Gertz, M.A., and Abraham, S.C. (2007). Globular amyloid deposits isolated to the small bowel: a rare association with AL amyloidosis. *Am. J. Surg. Pathol.* 31: 141–145.

Hings, I.M., Severson, R., Filipovich, A.H. et al. (1994). Treatment of moderate and severe acute GVHD after allogeneic bone marrow transplantation. *Transplantation* 58 (4): 437–442.

Horbar, J.D., Badger, G.J., Carpenter, J.H. et al. (2002). Trends in mortality and morbidity for very low birth weight infants, 1991–1999. *Pediatrics* 110 (1 Pt 1): 143.

Horn, T., Svendsen, L.B., and Nielsen, R. (1990). Brown-bowel syndrome. Review of the literature and presentation of cases. *Scand. J. Gastroenterol.* 25: 66.

Ho-Yen, C., Chang, F., van der Walt, J. et al. (2009). Recent advances in refractory coeliac disease: a review. *Histopathology* 54: 783.

Isaacs, P.E., Sladen, G.E., and Filipe, I. (1987). Mefenamic acid Enteropathy. *J. Clin. Pathol.* 40 (10): 1221–1227.

Joo, M., Shim, S.H., Chang, S.H. et al. (2009). Nodular lymphoid hyperplasia and histologic changes mimicking celiac disease, collagenous sprue, and lymphocytic colitis in a patient with selective IgA deficiency. *Pathol. Res. Pract.* 205 (12): 876–880.

Kakar, S., Mehra, V. et al. (2003). Significance of intraepithelial lymphocytosis in small bowel biopsy samples with normal mucosal architecture. *Am. J. Gastroenterol.* 98/9: 2027–2033.

Kaye, P., Abdulla, K., Wood, J. et al. (2008). Iron-induced mucosal pathology of the upper gastrointestinal tract: a common finding in patients on oral iron therapy. *Histopathology* 53 (3): 311–317.

Keiser, P.B. and Nutman, T.B. (2004). Strongyloides stercoralis in the immunocompromised population. *Clin. Microbiol. Rev.* 17 (1): 208–217.

Kesuaai, I., Kuitonen, P., Savilahti, E., and Sippenen, P. (1984). Mast cells and eosinophils in the jejunal mucosa of patients with intestinal cows' milk allergy and coeliac disease of childhood. *J. Pediatr. Gastroenterol. Nutr.* 3: 368.

Khulusi, S., Badve, S., Patel, P. et al. (1996). Pathogenesis of gastric metaplasia of the human duodenum: role of helicobacter pylori, gastric acid, and ulceration. *Gastroenterology* 110 (2): 452–458.

Kobayashi, Y., Suzuki, H., Konno, T. et al. (1983). Ultrastructural alterations of Paneth cells in infants associated with gastrointestinal symptoms. *Tohoku J. Exp. Med.* 139: 225.

Kokkonen, J., Holm, K., Karttunen, T.J., and Mäki, M. (2000). Children with untreated food allergy express a relative increment in the density of duodenal gammadelta+ T cells. *Scand. J. Gastroenterol.* 35: 1137.

Kuitunen, P., Kosnai, I., and Savilahti, E. (1982). Morphometric study of the jejunal mucosa in various childhood enteropathies with special reference to intraepithelial lymphocytes. *J. Pediatr. Gastroenterol. Nutr.* 1: 525.

Kyle, R.A. and Bayrd, E.D. (1975). Amyloidosis: review of 236 cases. *Medicine* 54 (4): 271.

Lappinga, P.J., Abraham, S.C., Murray, J.A. et al. (2010). Small intestinal bacterial overgrowth: histopathologic features and clinical correlates in an underrecognized entity. *Arch. Pathol. Lab. Med.* 134: 264–270.

Leder, K. et al. (1998). Microsporidial disease in HIV-infected patients: a report of 42 patients and review of the literature. *Scand. J. Infect. Dis.* 30: 331.

Lucendo, A.J. and Arias, A. (2012). Eosinophilic gastroenteritis: an update. *Expert Rev. Gastroenterol. Hepatol.* 6 (5): 591–601.

Maguire, A.A., Greenson, J.K., Lauwers, G.Y. et al. (2009). Collagenous Sprue: a clinicopathologic study of 12 cases. *Am. J. Surg. Pathol.* 33: 1440.

Mahadeva, S., Wyatt, J.I. et al. (2002). Is a raised intraepithelial lymphocyte count with normal duodenal villous architecture clinically relevant? *J. Clin. Pathol.* 55: 424–428.

Malamut, G., Verkarre, V., Suarez, F. et al. (2010). The enteropathy associated with common variable immunodeficiency: the delineated frontiers with celiac disease. *Am. J. Gastroenterol.* 105 (10): 2262–2275.

Martin, P.J., Rizzo, J.D., Wingard, J.R. et al. (2012). *Biol. Blood Marrow Transplant.* 18 (8): 1150–1163.

Maverakis, E., Fung, M.A., Lynch, P.J. et al. (2007). Acrodermatitis enteropathica and an overview of zinc metabolism. *J. Am. Acad. Dermatol.* 56 (1): 116–124.

Mino-Kenudson, M., Brown, I., and Lauwers, G.Y. (2005). Histopathological diagnosis of gluten-sensitive enteropathy. *Curr. Diagn. Pathol.* 11 (4): 274–283.

Molina, J.M. et al. (1998). Albendazole for treatment and prophylaxis of microsporidiosis due to Encephalitozoon intestinalis in patients with AIDS: a randomized double-blind controlled trial. *J. Infect. Dis.* 177 (5): 1373.

Montalto, M., D'Onofrio, F., Santoro, L. et al. (2009). Autoimmune enteropathy in children and adults. *Scand. J. Gastroenterol.* 44: 1029.

Moran, C.J., Kolman, O.K., Russell, G.J. et al. (2012). Neutrophilic infiltration in gluten-sensitive enteropathy is neither uncommon nor insignificant: assessment of duodenal biopsies from 267 pediatric and adult patients. *Am. J. Surg. Pathol.* 36 (9): 1339–1345.

Nath, S.K. (2005). Tropical sprue. *Curr. Gastroenterol. Rep.* 7 (5): 343–349.

Neldner, K.H. et al. (1975). Zinc therapy of acrodermatitis enteropathica. *N. Engl. J. Med.* 292: 879–882.

Neu, J. and Walker, W.A. (2011). Necrotising enterocolitis. *N. Engl. J. Med.* 364: 255–264.

Nightingale, S.D., Byrd, L.T., Southern, P.M. et al. (1992). Incidence of Mycobacterium avium-intracellulare complex bacteremia in human immunodeficiency virus-positive patients. *J. Infect. Dis.* 165 (6): 1082–1085.

Nowak-Wegrzyn, A. and Muraro, A. (2009). Food protein-induced enterocolitis syndrome. *Curr. Opin. Allergy Clin. Immunol.* 9 (4): 371.

Oberhuber, G., Granditsch, G., and Vogelsang, H. (1999). The histopathology of coeliac disease: time for a standardized report scheme for pathologists. *Eur. J. Gastroenterol. Hepatol.* 11: 1185.

Oberhuber, G., Kastner, N., and Stolte, M. (1997). Giardiasis: a histologic analysis of 567 cases. *Scand. J. Gastroenterol.* 32: 48–51.

O'Donnell, S., Crotty, P.L., O'Sullivan, M. et al. (2013). Isolated active ileitis: is it a mild subtype of Crohn's disease? *Inflamm. Bowel Dis.* 19 (9): 1815–1822.

Owens, S.R. and Greenson, J.K. (2007). The pathology of malabsorption: current concepts. *Histopathology* 50 (1): 64–82.

Paerregaard, A. (2009). What does the IBD patient Hide in the upper gastrointestinal tract? *Inflamm. Bowel Dis.* 15 (7): 1101–1104.

Patey-Mariaud de Serre, N., Canioni, D., Ganousse, S. et al. (2009). Digestive histopathological presentation of IPEX syndrome. *Mod. Pathol.* 22: 95.

Patey-Mariaud De Serre, N., Cellier, C. et al. (2000). Distinction between coeliac disease and refractory sprue: a simple immunohistochemical method. *Histopathology* 37: 70.

Perlemuter, G., Chaussade, S., Soubrane, O. et al. (1996). Multifocal stenosing ulcerations of the small intestine revealing vasculitis associated with C2 deficiency. *Gastroenterology* 110: 1628–1632.

Pons, V., Rolland, C., Nauze, M. et al. (2011). A severe form of abetalipoproteinemia caused by new splicing mutations of microsomal triglyceride transfer protein (MTTP). *Hum. Mutat.* 32: 751–759. https://doi.org/10.1002/humu.21494.

Ramakrishna, B.S., Venkataraman, S., and Mukhopadhya, A. (2006). Tropical malabsorption. *Postgrad. Med. J.* 82 (974): 779–787.

Rana, S.V. and Bhardwaj, S.B. (2008). Small intestinal bacterial overgrowth. *Scand. J. Gastroenterol.* 43: 1030–1037.

Ranganathan, S., Schmitt, L.A., and Sindhi, R. (2014). Tufting enteropathy revisited: the utility of MOC31 (EpCAM) immunohistochemistry in diagnosis. *Am. J. Surg. Pathol.* 38 (2): 265–272.

Ravelli, A., Bolognini, S., Gambarotti, M., and Villanacci, V. (2005). Variability of histologic lesions in relation to biopsy site in gluten-sensitive enteropathy. *Am. J. Gastroenterol.* 100: 177.

Rex, D.K. and Jersild, R.A. Jr. (1988). Further characterization of the pigment in pseudomelanosis duodeni in three patients. *Gastroenterology* 95 (1): 177–182.

Riordan, S.M., McIver, C.J., Wakefield, D. et al. (2001). Small intestinal mucosal immunity and morphometry in luminal overgrowth of indigenous gut flora. *Am. J. Gastroenterol.* 96: 494.

Robert, M.E. (2005). Gluten sensitive enteropathy and other causes of small intestinal lymphocytosis. *Semin. Diagn. Pathol.* 22 (4): 284–294.

Robert, M.E., Ament, M.E., and Weinstein, W.M. (2000). The histologic spectrum and clinical outcome of refractory and unclassified sprue. *Am. J. Surg. Pathol.* 24: 676.

Rolny, P., Sigurjonsdottir, H.A., Remotti, H. et al. (1999). Role of immunosuppressive therapy in refractory sprue-like disease. *Am. J. Gastroenterol.* 94: 219.

Rosinach, M. et al. (2012a). Approximately one in four LD patients has *H. pylori* infection. *Dig. Liver Dis.* 44 (8): 643–648.

Rosinach, M. et al. (2012b). Lymphocytic duodenosis: aetiology and long-term response to specific treatment. *Dig. Liver Dis.* 44 (8): 643–648.

Rossignol, J.F., Hidalgo, H., Feregrino, M. et al. (1998). A double-'blind' placebo-controlled study of nitazoxanide in the treatment of cryptosporidial diarrhoea in AIDS patients in Mexico. *Trans. R. Soc. Trop. Med. Hyg.* 92 (6): 663–666.

Rossignol, J.F. et al. (2001). Treatment of diarrhea caused by *Cryptosporidium parvum*: a prospective randomized, double-blind, placebo-controlled study of Nitazoxanide. *Trans. R. Soc. Trop. Med. Hyg.* 184 (1): 103–106.

Rubio-Tapia, A. and Murray, J.A. (2010). Classification and management of refractory coeliac disease. *Gut* 59 (4): 547–557.

Ruemmele, F.M., Schmitz, J., and Goulet, O. (2006). Microvillous inclusion disease (microvillous atrophy). *Orphanet J. Rare Dis.* 1: 22.

Sanchez, T.H., Brooks, J.T., Sullivan, P.S. et al. (2005). Bacterial diarrhea in persons with HIV infection, United States, 1992–2002. *Clin. Infect. Dis.* 41: 1621–1627.

Satsangi, J., Silverberg, M.S., Vermeire, S., and Colombel, J.F. (2006). The Montreal classification of inflammatory bowel disease: controversies, consensus, and implications. *Gut* 55 (6): 749–753.

Sattianayagam, P.T., Hawkins, P.N., and Gillmore, J.D. (2009). Systemic amyloidosis and the gastrointestinal tract. *Nat. Rev. Gastroenterol. Hepatol.* 6: 608–617.

Schmitt, S., Küry, S., Giraud, M. et al. (2009). An update on mutations of the SLC39A4 gene in acrodermatitis enteropathica. *Hum. Mutat.* 30: 926.

Segarra-Newnham, M. (2007). For hyperinfection syndrome, there is no generally agreed upon regimen although a prolonged course of ivermectin and reduction of any immunosuppressive drugs is most common. *Ann. Pharmacother.* 41 (12): 1992.

Shepherd, N.A., Crocker, P.R., Smith, A.P., and Levison, D.A. (1987). Exogenous pigment in Peyer's patches. *Hum. Pathol.* 18 (1): 50–54.

Shmidt, E., Smyrk, T.C., Faubion, W.A., and Oxentenko, A.S. (2013). Duodenal intraepithelial lymphocytosis with normal villous architecture in pediatric patients: Mayo Clinic experience, 2000–2009. *J. Pediatr. Gastroenterol. Nutr.* 56 (1): 51–55.

Shorter, J., Thompson, M.D., Mooney, D.P., and Modlin, J.F. (1998). Surgical aspects of an outbreak of Yersinia enterocolitis. *Pediatr. Surg. Int.* 13 (1): 2–5.

Siberry, G.K., Abzug, M.J., and Nachman, S. (2013). Panel on Prevention and Treatment of Opportunistic Infections in HIV-Exposed and HIV-Infected Children. Executive summary: 2013 update of the guidelines for the prevention and treatment of opportunistic infections in HIV-exposed and HIV-infected children. *Pediatr Infect Dis J* 32 (12): 1303–1307.

Singh, V.V. and Toskes, P.P. (2004). Small bowel bacterial overgrowth: presentation, diagnosis, and treatment. *Curr. Treat. Options Gastroenterol.* 7 (1): 19–28.

Sivagnanam, M., Mueller, J.L., Lee, H. et al. (2008). Identification of EpCAM as the gene for congenital tufting enteropathy. *Gastroenterology* 135 (2): 429–437.

Snover, D.C. (1990). Graft-versus-host disease of the gastrointestinal tract. *Am. J. Surg. Pathol.* 14 (Suppl 1): 101–108.

South, M.A., Dolen, J., Beach, D.K., and Mirkovic, R.R. (1982). Fatal adenovirus hepatic necrosis in severe combined immune deficiency. *Pediatr. Infect. Dis.* 1 (6): 416–419.

Swanson, V.L. and Thomassen, R.W. (1965). Pathology of the jejunal mucosa in tropical sprue. *Am. J. Pathol.* 46: 511–551.

Symeonidis, N., Jakubowski, A., Pierre-Louis, S. et al. (2007). Invasive adenoviral infections in T-cell-depleted allogeneic hematopoietic stem cell transplantation: high mortality in the era of cidofovir. *Transpl. Infect. Dis.* 9 (2): 108–113.

Talley, N.J., Shorter, R.G., Phillips, S.F., and Zinsmeister, A.R. (1990). Eosinophilic gastroenteritis: a clinicopathological study of patients with disease of the mucosa, muscle layer, and subserosal tissues. *Gut* 31 (1): 54.

Tankel, H.I., Clark, D.H., and Lee, F.D. (1965). Radiation enteritis with malabsorption. *Gut* 6: 560–569.

Ugur, H. et al. (2011). *J. Pediatr. Gastroenterol. Nutr.* 52 (4): 460–465.

Urbanski, S.J., Arsenault, A.L., Green, F.H., and Haber, G. (1989). Pigment resembling atmospheric dust in Peyer's patches. *Mod. Pathol.* 2 (3): 222–226.

Variend, S., Placzec, M., Raafat, F., and Walker-Smith, J.A. (1984). Small intestinal mucosal fat in childhood enteropathies. *J. Clin. Pathol.* 37: 373.

Verress, B., Franzen, L., Bodin, L., and Borch, K. (2004). Duodenal intraepithelial lymphocyte-count revisited. *Scand. J. Gastroenterol.* 4: 138.

Vitoria, J.C., Camerero, C., Sojo, A. et al. (1982). Enteropathy related to fish, rice, and chicken. *Arch. Dis. Child.* 57: 44.

Walker, M.M. (2003). What is tropical sprue? *J. Gastroenterol. Hepatol.* 18: 887.

Ward, E.M., Woodward, T.A., Mazlumzadeh, M., and Calamia, K. (2003). Gastrointestinal disease in Behçet's disease. *Adv. Exp. Med. Biol.* 528: 459.

Washington, K. and Jagasia, M. (2009). Pathology of graft-versus-host disease in the gastrointestinal tract. *Hum. Pathol.* 40 (7): 909–917.

Washington, K., Stenzel, T.T., Buckley, R.H., and Gottfried, M.R. (1996). Gastrointestinal pathology in patients with common variable immunodeficiency and X-linked agammaglobulinemia. *Am. J. Surg. Pathol.* 20 (10): 1240–1252.

Weir, D.C., Glickman, J.N., Roiff, T. et al. (2010). Variability of histopathological changes in childhood celiac disease. *Am. J. Gastroenterol.* 105 (1): 207–212.

West, B. (1988). Pseudomelanosis duodeni. *J. Clin. Gastroenterol.* 10 (2): 127–129.

Wheby, M.S., Swanson, V.L., and Bayless, T.M. (1971). Comparison of ileal and jejunal biopsies in tropical sprue. *Am. J. Clin. Nutr.* 24: 117–123.

Wyatt, J.I., Rathbone, B.J., Sobala, G.M. et al. (1990). Gastric epithelium in the duodenum: its association with helicobacter pylori and inflammation. *J. Clin. Pathol.* 43 (12): 981–986.

Yantiss, R.K. and Odze, R.D. (2009). Optimal approach to obtaining mucosal biopsies for assessment of inflammatory disorders of the gastrointestinal tract. *Am. J. Gastroenterol.* 104: 774.

Yu, V.Y., Tudehope, D.I., and Gill, G.J. (1977). Neonatal necrotizing enterocolitis: 1. Clinical aspects. *Med. J. Aust.* 1 (19): 685.

Zaha, S., Hirata, T., Kinjo, F. et al. (2002). Efficacy of ivermectin for chronic strongyloidiasis: two single doses given 2 weeks apart. *J. Infect. Chemother.* 8 (1): 94–98.

Zamel, R., Khan, R., Pollex, R.L., and Hegele, R.A. (2008). Abetalipoproteinemia: two case reports and literature review. *Orphanet J. Rare Dis.* 3: 19.

Zanini, B. et al. (2014). Clinical expression of lymphocytic duodenosis in "mild enteropathy" celiac disease and in functional gastrointestinal syndromes. *Scand. J. Gastroenterol.* 49 (7): 794–800.

8

Polyps of the Small Intestine

Ian Brown[1] and Michael B. Wallace[2]

[1] *Envoi Specialist Pathologists, Brisbane, Australia*
[2] *Mayo Clinic, Jacksonville, Florida, USA*

Many neoplasms of the small intestine present as polyps, and these are discussed in Chapter 9. This chapter deals only with non-neoplastic lesions and conditions presenting as polypoid lesions.

Heterotopia

Gastric Heterotopia

Definition and Predisposing Factors

Gastric heterotopia is the presence of oxyntic mucosa commonly detected in the duodenal bulb. A genetic basis remains unproven. *Helicobacter pylori* infection plays no role, in contrast to its etiologic role in foveolar gastric metaplasia.

Clinical Features/Endoscopic Characteristics

Gastric heterotopia of the duodenum is a common endoscopic finding. It typically develops when proximal duodenal mucosa is exposed to gastric acid and may be more common in hyper-secretory condition. The endoscopic appearance is of nodular mucosa, typically in the proximal duodenal bulb (Figure 8.1). The nodules may have surface pit patterns that resemble gastric mucosa. The main issue is distinguishing these from neoplastic duodenal polyps. This is best done by the location (proximal bulb versus more distal location for neoplasia) and surface pit patterns.

Microscopic Features

Gastric heterotopia is characterized by well-organized and demarcated gastric body type glands within the intestinal mucosa (Figure 8.2). It varies from a few glands to extensive replacement of native mucosa. Mild inflammation is common, and *H. pylori* can be found in case of concomitant gastric infection. Secondary changes of ulceration (usually with *H. pylori* infection), glandular cystic dilatation resembling cystic fundic gland polyp (in patients taking proton pump inhibitor medication), foveolar hyperplasia, and gastric hyperplastic type polyp are occasionally encountered. There is no risk for dysplasia or malignancy.

Differential Diagnosis

- Gastric metaplasia consists of foveolar epithelium lining the duodenal bulb in the setting of duodenitis. It lacks the ordered appearance of gastric heterotopias with oxyntic glands.
- Pyloric gland adenoma is formed of pyloric type rather than body type glands.
- Pyloric gland metaplasia is frequently noted in Crohn's disease. The background changes of mucosal disease, possibly granuloma, and the absence of body type glands allow distinction.

Treatment/Prognosis/Evolution

Gastric heterotopia typically causes no symptoms, thus treatment is not required. Biopsy should be performed to distinguish these from other neoplastic lesions.

Pancreatic Heterotopia (Synonyms Ectopic Pancreas, Pancreatic Rest)

Definition

This represents the localization of pancreatic parenchyma outside of the pancreas.

Clinical Features/Endoscopic Characteristics

Ectopic pancreas tissue is common but typically causes no symptoms. It usually presents as an incidental subepithelial nodule, which may have a small indentation at the site of pancreatic ductal tissue drainage. In rare cases, it can present as localized pancreatitis of the duodenal wall, which goes by the term "groove" pancreatitis as it occurs in the groove between the duodenum and pancreatic head or very rarely, pancreatic cancer.

Gastrointestinal Pathology: Correlative Endoscopic and Histologic Assessment, First Edition. Edited by Gregory Y. Lauwers and Michael B. Wallace.

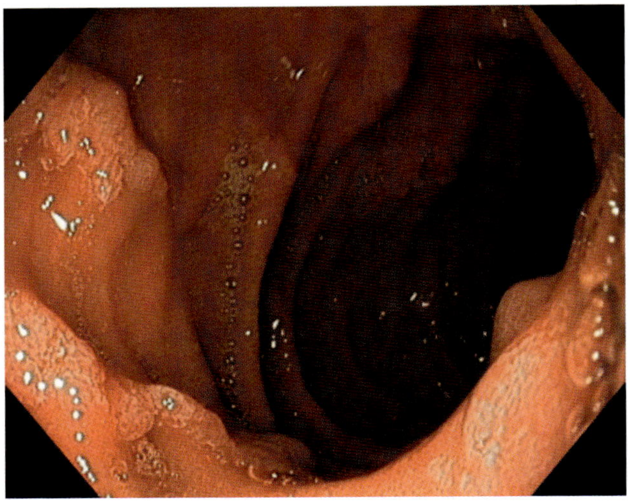

Figure 8.1 Gastric heterotopia of the proximal duodenal bulb. Note the surface pit pattern. *Source:* Image courtesy of Prof Miguel Munoz-Nava, Navarra Spain.

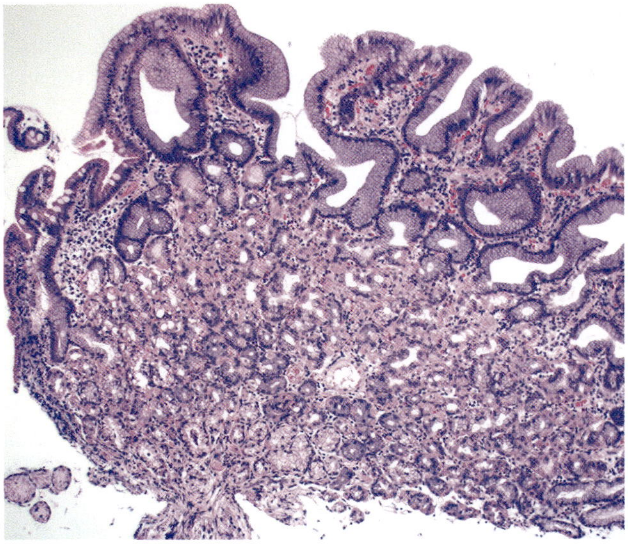

Figure 8.2 Gastric heterotopia. Note the surface foveolar epithelium and oxyntic glands.

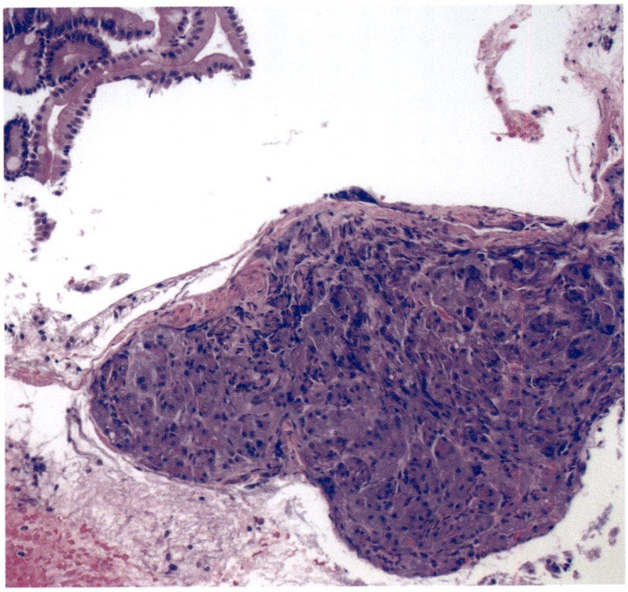

Figure 8.3 Pancreatic heterotopia. In this example, the heterotopia is uniquely composed of bland pancreatic acini.

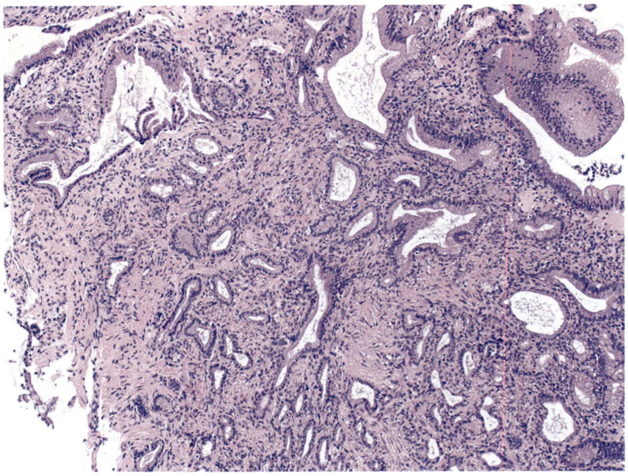

Figure 8.4 Ampullary adenomyoma. The lesion is composed of benign ductular elements entrapped within proliferating smooth muscle fascicle.

Microscopic Features

Pancreatic heterotopia can comprise various admixtures of non-neoplastic pancreatic ducts, pancreatic acini, and islets of Langerhans. It usually resides in the submucosa/base of mucosa, and endoscopic biopsies may not be diagnostic. A three-tier classification has been developed: Class I—all three elements present; Class II—acini and ducts but no islets (Figure 8.3); Class III—ducts with rare (or no) acini; and a fourth class, which is exceedingly rare, comprising endocrine elements only. The duct structures in Class III lesions may be associated with smooth muscle proliferation, and the term "adenomyoma" has been used.

Differential Diagnosis

- Ampullary adenomyoma has features similar to class III pancreatic heterotopias; so, knowledge of the site of biopsy is important for distinction. In general, ampullary adenomyoma is associated with more smooth muscle proliferation. Peribiliary glands indicate an ampullary location (Figure 8.4).
- Pancreatic metaplasia is very rare in the small intestine, and consists of a small lobulated collection of pancreatic acinar glands confined to the mucosa.
- Accessory pancreatic duct is found in the region of the ampulla.

Treatment/Prognosis/Evolution

Most lesions are benign. Cyst formation and development of PanIN in the ductal epithelium can occur. However, a few case reports of malignant transformation are known.

Hamartoma

Definition, General Features (Frequency), and Predisposing Factors

This benign tumor is composed of a disorganized collection of elements native to the site of occurrence. Several syndromes are associated with hamartomatous polyps throughout the gastrointestinal tract (discussed below). Solitary hamartomatous polyps of the small intestine are most frequently of Peutz–Jeghers, Brunner gland, or neuromuscular and vascular types.

Clinical Features/Endoscopic Characteristics

Hamartomas typically occur in patients with Peutz–Jeghers syndrome (PJS) and less commonly with Cowden syndrome, Bannayan–Riley–Ruvalcaba syndrome, and juvenile polyposis syndrome. Most experience is with PJS where half of patients are asymptomatic but they can present with small bowel obstruction, intussusception, or bleeding. The lifetime risk of symptomatic obstruction is nearly 70%. The polyps are typically large and pedunculated or semi-sessile and distributed throughout the small intestine. They may be diagnosed with cross sectional imaging (computed tomographic or magnetic resonance enterography) but management requires deep enteroscopy with balloon-assisted single or double balloon enteroscopes and polypectomy (Figure 8.5).

Microscopic Features

Peutz–Jeghers type polyps are discussed below and Brunner gland hamartomas are discussed in Chapter 9. Neuromuscular and vascular type hamartoma comprises an admixture of neural elements, both nerve bundles and ganglion cells, with smooth muscle proliferation. This is mostly within the submucosa and produces stricture formation rather than a discrete polyp. Ectatic vessels may be seen, particularly at the edge of areas of frequent mucosal ulceration. A clinical and histological overlap exists with NSAID-related diaphragm disease.

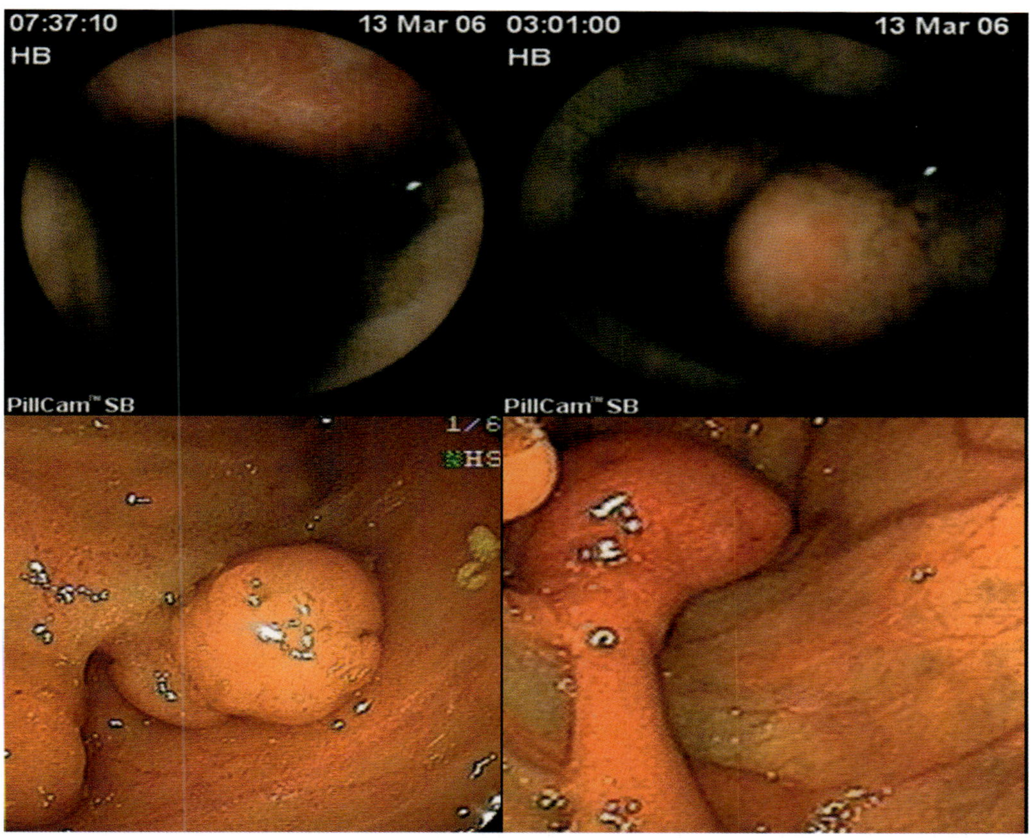

Figure 8.5 Hamartomatous polyps in a patient with Peutz–Jeghers syndrome. The upper panels are taken from a capsule endoscope (Pillcam) and the lower images from a double balloon enteroscope where the polyps were removed.

Differential Diagnosis

Neoplastic tumor is the major clinical differential diagnosis. In the case of neuromuscular and vascular type hamartoma, NSAID-related small bowel diaphragm disease and Crohn's disease need to be considered. A well-developed smooth muscle proliferation in the lamina propria and absence of granulomata are the most helpful features in excluding Crohn's disease.

Treatment/Prognosis/Evolution

Small bowel hamartomas should generally be removed due to the risk of obstruction. This is best accomplished by deep enteroscopy techniques and polypectomy using standard snare devices.

Endometriosis

Definition, General Features, and Frequency

Endometriosis refers to the presence of endometrial tissue (glands and stroma) outside of the endometrial cavity. Intestinal involvement is encountered in 4–37% of cases of pelvic endometriosis. The ileum is the most common site of small intestinal disease, but is less frequent than sigmoid or rectal involvement. It most often presents as a mural mass with stricture formation. The mucosa is involved in about 1/3 of cases with intestinal endometriosis. Mucosal polyps may occur with or without evident mural disease.

Clinical Features/Endoscopic Characteristics

Endometriosis of the small bowel presents with vague, nonspecific symptoms of abdominal pain, rarely with intestinal obstruction or bleeding.

Microscopic Features

The classic diagnostic triad is the presence of (i) endometrial glands and (ii) endometrial stroma, and (iii) evidence of hemorrhage. At least two of these elements are required for a confident diagnosis. Mucosal prolapse changes of lamina propria, fibrosis, smooth muscle proliferation, and crypt elongation may be associated. Acute and chronic inflammation and sometimes ulceration with mucosal distortion are possible, and can be a mimic for Crohn's disease. Finally, endometrial glands may be admixed with native intestinal glands and can be easily missed.

Immunochemical Features

A panel of estrogen receptor (ER; +), CK7(+), CK20(−), CDX-2(−), and PAX-8(+) immunohistochemical stains can distinguish endometriotic glands from native intestinal glands. Additionally stromal component of endometriosis can be highlighted by CD10 (+) immunohistochemistry.

Differential Diagnosis

The combination of chronic ulceroinflammatory changes and stricture can be mistaken for Crohn's disease.

Treatment/Prognosis/Evolution

The treatment is similar for endometriosis at other locations, hormonal therapy or laparoscopic ablation.

Pseudopolyp (Benign Mucosal Polyp, Inflammatory Pseudopolyp)

Definition, General Features, and Predisposing Factors

This term describes benign polypoid mucosal lesions characterized by stromal and epithelial expansion. Several processes fall under this generic designation. Local trauma or inflammation is a common predisposing factor. Inflammation may be related to Crohn's disease, or to medications, e.g. NSAIDs. Local mucosal ischemia is a rare cause.

Clinical Features/Endoscopic Characteristics

Pseudopolyps are most often found in inflammatory bowel disease and are a marker of chronic severe inflammation. They have a smooth surface and finger-like polypoid shape, which can usually distinguish them from adenomatous or hyperplastic polyps (Figure 8.6)

Microscopic Features

Expansion of the lamina propria by established fibrosis and/or a fibroblastic proliferation and inflammation is often present. Smooth muscle and neural hyperplasia and lymphangiectasia may occur, particularly in Crohn's disease. The crypt epithelium is frequently hyperplastic, and the glands may be dilated. Villi tend to be shortened. In some cases, there is ulceration and variable amounts of granulation tissue may comprise the polyp. Occasionally, only granulation tissue is noted: "granulation tissue polyp."

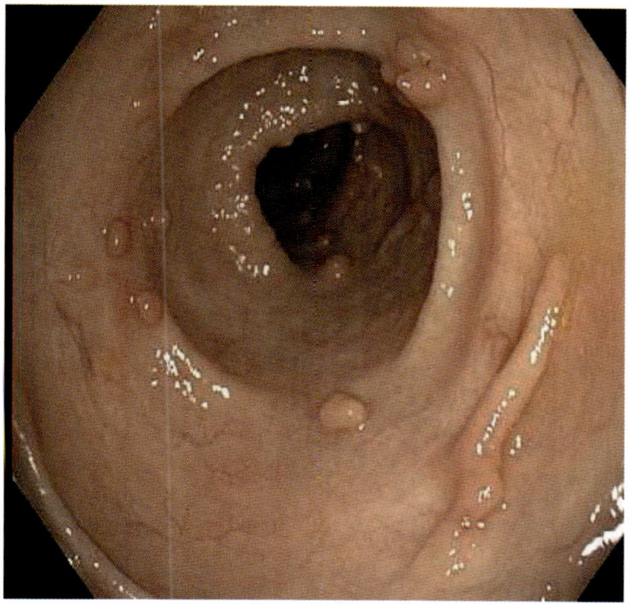

Figure 8.6 Intestinal pseudopolyps in a patient with inflammatory bowel disease. Note the bland pale color similar to background intestine.

Treatment/Prognosis/Evolution

No treatment is required of these benign polyps.

Mucosal Prolapse Type Polyps

Definition, General Features, and Predisposing Factors

These lesions are characterized by stromal and epithelial expansion induced by traction on the mucosa during peristalsis. Smooth muscle splaying is characteristic. Submucosal prolapse related to a submucosal lesion, anatomical abnormality (e.g. sharp angulation in the duodenum), or a mucosal tumor may predispose to that development. The mucosa may be normal and the polyps are due to expansion of the submucosa, a process akin to that described in the colon as colonic muco-submucosal elongated polyp.

Clinical Features/Endoscopic Characteristics

The clinical features are nonspecific with most lesions found incidentally. If these lesions become large, they may bleed or rarely cause obstruction.

Microscopic Features

The characteristic features are identical to those seen in the colon, with crypt elongation and stromal expansion by fibrosis and smooth muscle proliferation from the thickened muscularis mucosae. Inflammation and erosion can occur. These changes may be accompanied by a mucosal based neoplasm or overlie a submucosal lesion, so careful evaluation is necessary.

Treatment/Prognosis/Evolution

Therapy is indicated if these lesions cause bleeding or obstruction. In those cases, standard polypectomy can be performed. In some cases, polypectomy may be necessary to establish the diagnosis and distinguish from other small intestinal polyps.

Brunner's Gland Cyst

Definition

This represents the benign cystic dilatation of a main duct draining Brunner's glands.

Clinical Features/Endoscopic Characteristics

There are typically no clinical findings. They are found incidentally and confirmed by biopsy.

Microscopic Features

The cyst is present in the submucosa just beneath the muscularis mucosae. It is lined by a single layer of tall columnar mucinous epithelium with clear cytoplasm and basal nuclei. A micropapillary architecture is often present at least focally. There is no cytologic atypia or dysplasia, and the adjacent Brunner's glands appear normal (Figure 8.7)

Treatment/Prognosis/Evolution

No therapy is needed once a diagnosis is confirmed.

Polyposis Syndromes

Familial Adenomatous Polyposis

This is covered in more detail in the large intestine Chapter. Involvement of the small intestine is by way of multiple adenomatous polyps. As in the colon, there is an increased risk for malignant transformation.

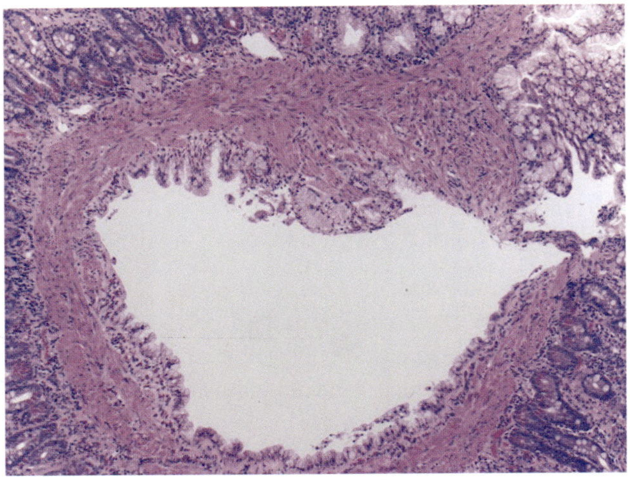

Figure 8.7 Brunner's gland cyst. The lesion is located underneath the mucosal surface. Notice the micropapillary architecture of the lining.

Peutz–Jeghers Syndrome (PJS)

Definition, General Features, and Predisposing Factors

This inherited syndrome is characterized by the development of mucocutaneous melanin pigmentation, hamartomatous gastrointestinal tract polyps, and neoplasia. Peutz–Jeghers Syndrome (PJS) is an autosomal dominant condition with high penetrance. Truncating germline mutations in the LKB1/STK11 gene on 19p13.3 are responsible for most cases. The LKB1 gene product appears to serve a variety of functions, one of which is involved in control of cellular growth and polarization. Disturbance of this function may be responsible for the disordered growth producing the polyps.

Clinical Features/Endoscopic Characteristics

Polyps may occur throughout the gastrointestinal tract, with the small intestine being the most common site. The jejunum predominates, followed by ileum and duodenum. The diagnostic criteria of PJS encompass multiple features:

1) Three or more histologically confirmed polyps.
2) Any number of polyps characteristic of PJS in patients with a family history.
3) Typical melanotic dermomucosal lesions in patients with a burdened family anamnesis.
4) Any number of typical PJS polyps and typical melanotic dermomucosal lesions.

Microscopic Features

PJS polyps are characterized by papillary architecture with an arborizing smooth muscle scaffold derived from the muscularis mucosa. The muscle core is covered by benign epithelial elements, including enterocytes, goblet cells, Paneth cells, and endocrine cells. Gastric metaplasia and/or gastric mucin expression often occurs. Lamina propria is not expanded. Inflammation is absent unless secondary ulceration occurs. This may be accompanied by reactive epithelial changes. Polyp torsion may cause epithelial misplacement into the submucosa ("pseudoinvasion"), which may mimic malignancy. True dysplasia and malignancy can develop.

Differential Diagnosis

Adenomatous polyp may enter the differential diagnosis when there are epithelial regenerative changes.

Treatment/Prognosis/Evolution

Treatment of PJS hamartomatous polyps is discussed under Section "Hamartoma."

Juvenile Polyposis Syndrome

Definition, General Features (Frequency), and Predisposing Factors

This autosomal dominant condition is characterized by the development of inflammatory hamartomatous polyps in the gut. The finding of a small intestinal juvenile type polyp is diagnostic of the syndrome. Juvenile polyposis syndrome occurs in 1 in 100 000 live births. Germline mutations in SMAD4 or BMPR1A are identified in approximately 60% of cases. Mutations in genes coding for proteins in the TGF-β/BMP signaling pathway may underlie the remaining cases.

Clinical Features/Endoscopic Characteristics

The diagnostic criteria are:

1) Either ≥3 juvenile polyps in the large bowel and the rectum; or
2) Any number of juvenile polyps in patients with a positive family history of the disease; or
3) Juvenile polyps outside the colon (stomach, small bowel).

Microscopic Features

The small intestinal lesions in JPS may vary from localized crypt elongation and/or reactive lymphoid hyperplasia to a fully developed pattern of cystic crypt dilation, edematous inflamed stroma, vascular congestion, and surface erosion. Inflammation is mixed with chronic inflammatory cells, eosinophils, and neutrophils typically present (Figure 8.8). SMAD4 mutation-related cases may be more cellular and show less stromal edema than BMPR1A mutation cases. Reactive epithelial changes are common, and need to be distinguished from dysplasia or invasive malignancy that may develop in the polyps.

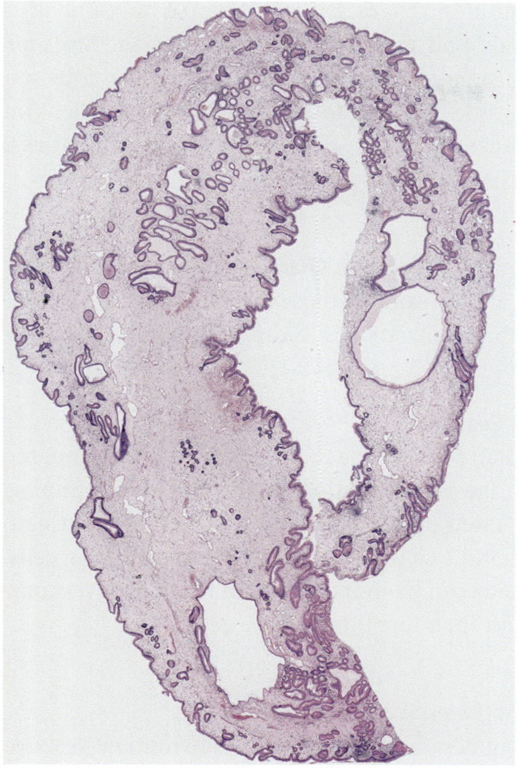

Figure 8.8 Juvenile polyp.

Treatment/Prognosis/Evolution

The most common indication for treatment is bleeding. Polyps can be removed with standard polypectomy techniques, although some may become very large and require endoscopic mucosal resection with injection of saline into the submucosal space below the lesion to safely remove them.

PTEN Hamartoma Tumor Syndrome (Syn. Cowden Syndrome)

Definition, General Features (Frequency), and Predisposing Factors

PTEN hamartoma tumor syndrome is a unifying name given to a heterogenous group of conditions that have in common germline mutations of the PTEN (phosphatase and tensin homolog) gene (10q22-q23). Cowden syndrome and Bannayan–Riley–Ruvalcaba syndrome are the most common forms. Cowden syndrome is inherited in autosomal dominant fashion and occurs in approximately 1 in 200 000 with the gastrointestinal tract being involved in up to 70% of cases. Cell cycle dysregulation, inhibition of apoptosis, and disordered cell migration and adhesion are most likely to underlie the development of hamartoma polyp.

Clinical Features/Endoscopic Characteristics

Clinical diagnostic criteria have been developed by an international consortium. Small intestinal hamartomas are a feature of Cowden syndrome. Clinical and endoscopic manifestations are similar to other hamartomas discussed.

Microscopic Features

The gastrointestinal manifestations are diverse. Hamartomatous polyps are the most characteristic lesion. They are typically <10–20 mm in diameter and found throughout the gut, with duodenal involvement reported in 37% of cases. They show lamina propria expansion that is more fibrous and less edematous or inflamed than in juvenile polyps. Crypts are expanded and dilated. Other manifestations include nodular lymphoid hyperplasia, adipose tissue in the lamina propria/true lipomas, ganglioneuromas (ganglioneuromatous hamartoma), and glycogenic acanthosis in the esophagus. A suggested increased risk for colorectal adenocarcinoma remains unproven.

Differential Diagnosis

Other hamartomatous lesions ought to be ruled out, in particular, juvenile polyps and the Cronkhite–Canada syndrome-related polyps. Ganglioneuromatosis may be considered if ganglioneuromatous hamartomas are evident. The spectrum of gastrointestinal lesions and the presence of extraintestinal lesions, particularly those affecting skin, help to make the diagnosis.

Treatment/Prognosis/Evolution

Treatment of small intestinal hamartoma is discussed in Section “Hamartoma.”

Cronkhite–Canada Syndrome

Definition and Predisposing Factors

This nonhereditary disorder, possibly the result of immune dysregulation, is characterized by gastrointestinal polyposis, protein losing enteropathy, and ectodermal changes.

Clinical Features/Endoscopic Characteristics

Cronkhite-Canada syndrome can present with confluent hamartomatous polyps throughout the stomach and small intestine; however, the primary symptoms are those of protein losing enteropathy with diarrhea and malnutrition.

Microscopic Features

Early features are total or subtotal villous atrophy accompanied by profound edema of the lamina propria along with a variable mixed inflammatory infiltrate. Active inflammation is common, and eosinophils are typically prominent, sometimes suggesting primary eosinophilic enteritis. Intraepithelial lymphocytes are not elevated. Later in the course of this disease, crypts become dilated, and together with the edema and inflammation produce the characteristic polyps (Figure 8.9).

Differential Diagnosis

The early inflammatory changes can be mistaken for eosinophilic enteritis, Crohn's disease, NSAID enteropathy, and celiac disease. The later polypoid phase may suggest a postinflammatory polyposis, juvenile polyposis, or PTEN hamartoma syndrome.

Treatment/Prognosis/Evolution

Treatment is typically with cromolyn sodium or prednisone. If hamartomatous polyps cause bleeding or are at risk of obstruction, they should be removed endoscopically.

Ganglioneuromatous Polyposis

Definition, General Features (Frequency), and Predisposing Factors

This condition is characterized by the presence, either in isolation or concurrently with other disease, of multiple intestinal tumors characterized by an admixture of a neuromatous and ganglion cell proliferation. Multiple ganglioneuromatous polyps are encountered in four settings: multiple endocrine neoplasia, type IIB, Von Recklinghausen disease, familial ganglioneuromatosis, and PTEN hamartoma syndrome.

Clinical Features/Endoscopic Characteristics

Symptoms are the same as those for other large polyp syndromes with obstruction or bleeding.

Microscopic Features

In a familial setting, the polyps may be encountered throughout the gastrointestinal tract. The polyps comprise a mucosal-based proliferation of cytologically bland neuromatous spindle cells and admixed mature ganglion cells. Ganglion cells can be infrequent, and multiple levels may be needed for their identification.

Immunohistochemical Features

Both neuromatous and ganglion cells are immunoreactive for S-100. Specific neuroendocrine stains such as chromogranin and synaptophysin will highlight the ganglion cell component, which may be sparse.

Differential Diagnosis

Several conditions ought to be excluded:

- Sporadic ganglioneuroma: This lesion is prevalent particularly in the colon. Extraintestinal syndromic

(a)

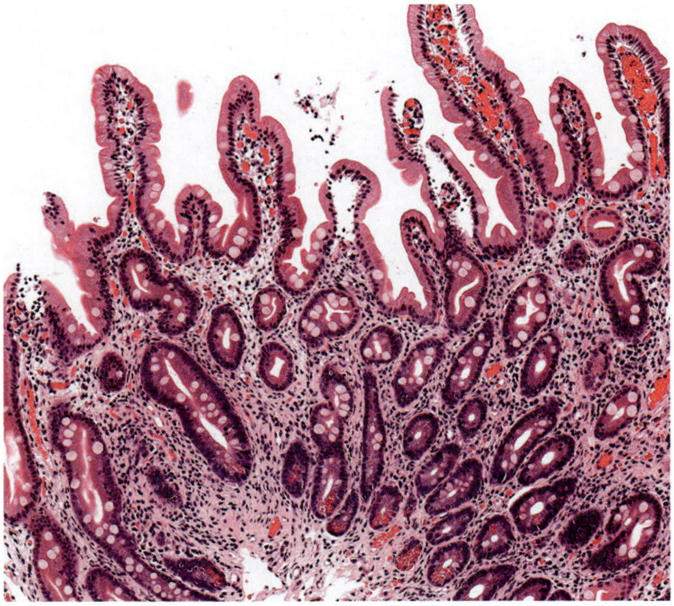

(b)

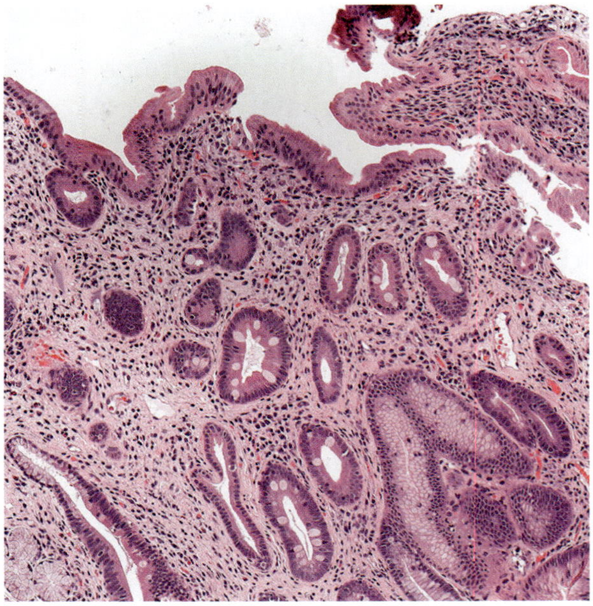

Figure 8.9 Examples of Cronkhite–Canada polyps showing a spectrum of changes with preserved mucosal architecture (a) and mucosal disarray (b).

manifestations and/or family history may help define an associated clinical syndrome.

- Benign nerve sheath neuroma: It presents as a cluster of uniform nerve bundles. The finding of ganglion cells is critical to the diagnosis of ganglioneuroma.
- Schwann cell hamartoma: The finding of ganglion cells is important to the diagnosis of ganglioneuroma.
- Schwannoma: The lesion is composed of short wavy cells. The finding of ganglion cells is critical to the diagnosis of ganglioneuroma.
- Perineurioma ("fibroblastic polyp"): Absence of staining for S-100 in perineurioma is the most helpful clue.
- Leiomyoma will express desmin and be nonreactive for S-100.
- Gangliocytic paraganglioma: The finding of a keratin-reactive neuroendocrine cell population is the most useful diagnostic feature.

Treatment/Prognosis/Evolution

Ganglioneuromas are typically benign and do not require resection unless causing symptoms or major deformity. Treatment is surgical resection when lesions become large and symptomatic.

Lymphoid Hyperplasia

Definition and Predisposing Factors

This represents the enlargement of preexisting lymphoid tissue in the Peyer's patches of the terminal ileum due to immune stimulation and reactive change. Small reactive lymphoid follicles also may be seen in the proximal small intestine, mainly as a response to food allergy in children or in primary immunodeficiency disorder (e.g. CVID). Viral infection, recent vaccination, and medication reaction are common predisposing factors.

Clinical Features/Endoscopic Characteristics

These are frequently encountered in the terminal ilium and present as nodular mucosa at endoscopy. They are confirmed by biopsy.

Microscopic Features

The normal ileal lymphoid tissue undergoes enlargement characterized by development of irregular reactive germinal centers and expansion of the mantle/marginal zone region. Follicle lysis may be seen when the process is marked. In pure form, there is no associated acute inflammation, ulceration, or granuloma formation.

Differential Diagnosis

- Lymphoma ought to be excluded. Features that raise concern include:
  - Lymphoepithelial lesions (lymphocytic destructive invasion of the epithelium with disappearance of glands).
  - Sheets of large lymphoid cells or any population of markedly atypical or enlarged lymphoid cells without germinal centers.
  - Atypical follicular architecture (i.e. no polarization, no tingible body macrophages, mantle/marginal zones absent or poorly seen, enlarged mantle/marginal zones, uniform cellular appearance).
- Crohn's disease may be another entity to exclude. The presence of active inflammation, granuloma formation, and architectural disturbance allows distinction.

Treatment/Prognosis/Evolution

No therapy is required.

Pneumatosis Intestinalis

Definition, General Features (Frequency), and Predisposing Factors

They include a condition characterized by the development of gas-filled cysts in the wall of the small intestine or colon. Occasionally, these may give a polypoid appearance to the mucosa. Two main theories of pathogenesis are debated: mechanical (mucosal disruption and increased intraluminal pressure) and microbiological (gas-forming bacteria).

Clinical Features/Endoscopic Characteristics

Most patients are asymptomatic. When symptomatic patients with small intestinal involvement do present to medical care, the most common manifestations are vomiting, distention, weight loss, diarrhea, and pain. Severe cases may present with abdominal catastrophe and infarction.

Microscopic Features

The gas cysts may be single or multiple, and vary from the size of adipocytes to several centimeters. Most cysts are located in the submucosa or subserosa. They often have no lining, appearing as a clear space surrounded by compressed or fibrotic tissue. Sometimes multinucleate giant cells surround the cysts, and, rarely, an apparent single cell lining is seen. Neutrophils, lymphocytes, plasma cells, and, predominantly, eosinophils may infiltrate the stroma around the cysts.

Differential Diagnosis

Lesions to rule out include

- Lymphangioma
- Fat necrosis
- Granulomatous inflammation, in cases with multinucleate giant cells
- Pseudolipomatosis

Treatment/Prognosis/Evolution

There are limited data on therapies. When patients present with intestinal infarction, laparotomy is required with resection of the affected small or large bowel. Other therapies that have been reported in small series include antibiotics, and hyperbaric oxygen.

Progressive fibrosis leads to involution of the cyst.

Nonneoplastic Vascular Lesions

Vascular abnormalities are discussed in this section, as they may occur as polypoid lesions. Vascular neoplasms are discussed in Chapter 9.

Pyogenic Granuloma

Definition, General Features, and Predisposing Factors

This represents a benign proliferation of capillary vessels originating from a feeding vessel. Pyogenic granuloma can cause significant blood loss. The etiology is often unknown. Trauma is responsible for at least some cases. Medications have been implicated, such as retinoids, the protease inhibitor indinavir, 5-fluorouracil, capecitabine, and some EGF receptor inhibitors.

Microscopic Features

Pyogenic granulomas are better termed lobulated capillary hemangioma, and are characterized by a raised, frequently ulcerated proliferation of capillary vessels in an edematous stroma. Variable numbers of acute and chronic inflammatory cells may be present. The vessels exhibit a characteristic branching pattern leading off a feeding vessel at the base.

Differential Diagnosis

The main differential diagnoses are exuberant granulation tissue and Kaposi's sarcoma. Inflammatory fibroid polyp and inflammatory myofibroblastic tumor may sometimes enter the differential diagnosis. Attention to the clinical setting will aid the differential diagnosis.

Vascular Abnormalities

Definition

Various non-neoplastic abnormalities in vascular architecture or vessel anatomy may give rise to gastrointestinal tract bleeding.

Clinical Features/Endoscopic Characteristics

These lesions present with both acute and more often, chronic bleeding (Figure 8.10).

Microscopic Features

The various conditions include

- ***Angiectasia***: This is characterized by dilated, thin-walled veins lacking an elastic lamina, which results from a regional or generalized increase in venous pressure.
- ***Hemodialysis associated telangiectasia***: Generalized angiectasia of the gastrointestinal tract can develop in patients on long-term hemodialysis. Changes in circulatory fluid volume may be a causative factor.
- ***Portal hypertensive enteropathy***: This form of generalized angiectasia results from portal hypertension. Thick-walled dilated vessels, along with edema of the lamina propria, fibromuscular proliferation, a decreased villous/crypt ratio, and thickened muscularis mucosae form a characteristic picture of portal hypertensive enteropathy. Occasionally, polyp formation or ulceration occurs.
- ***Dieulafoy's lesion***: This is defined by the presence of a "caliber persistent" submucosal vessel that projects into the overlying mucosa.
- ***Arteriovenous malformation***: This is characterized by an abnormal, frequently transmural collection of vessels displaying variable thickness of their vessel walls. An internal elastic lamina can be identified in some of the vessels.

Differential Diagnosis

Lymphangioma or lymphangiectasia also present as distended vessels. The presence of proteinaceous fluid rather than blood within the lumina is characteristic.

Treatment/Prognosis/Evolution

Treatment is typically endoscopic. Large vessel lesions such as varices or Dieulafoy's are treated with endoscopic band ligation or rarely injection of sclerosant or glue. Small vessel lesions such as arteriovenous malformation are treated with cautery such as argon plasma coagulation

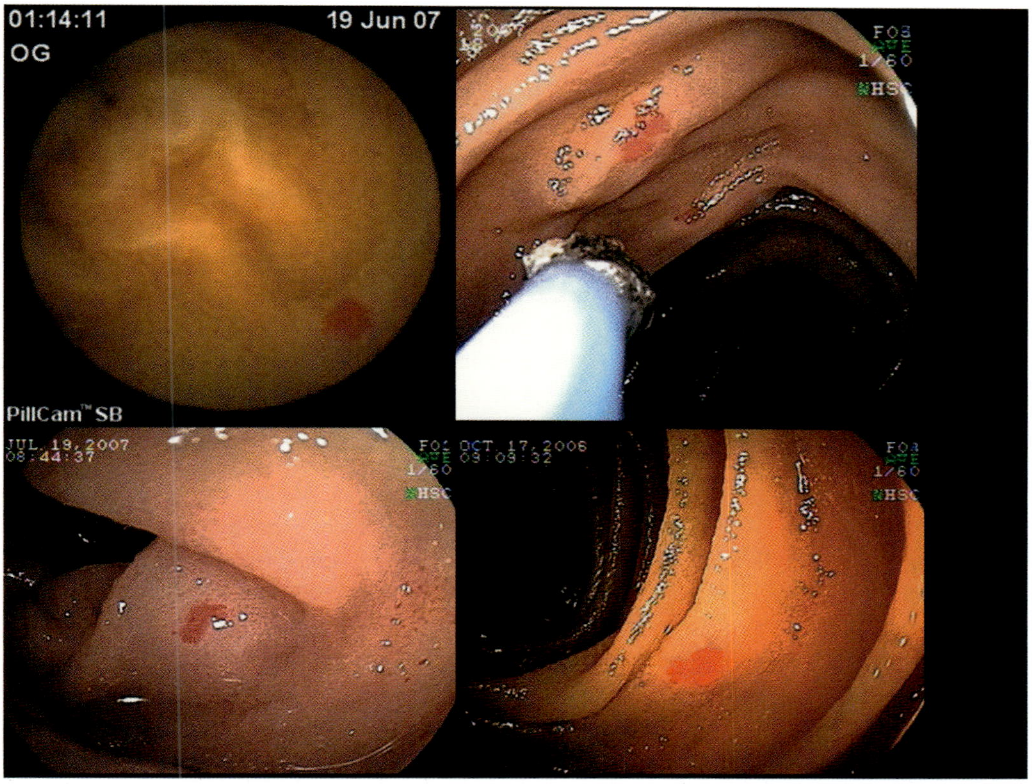

Figure 8.10 Arteriovenous malformations detected in small bowel on capsule endoscope (upper left panel) and double balloon enteroscopes (all other panels). The upper right panel shows an argon plasma coagulation catheter commonly used to ablate Arteriovenous malformations.

Primary Lymphangiectasia

Definition, General Features, and Predisposing Factors

This condition corresponds to the development of dilated intestinal lymphatics/lacteals with leakage of protein-rich material into the gut lumen, leading to protein losing enteropathy and malabsorption.

Clinical Features/Endoscopic Characteristics

These lesions present as white-colored villi in the small intestine and may be localized or diffuse depending on the underlying condition.

Microscopic Features

Dilated lymphatics appear through all layers of the intestine wall. They can appear empty or contain proteinaceous material with free-floating histiocytes. There is no associated inflammation (Figure 8.11).

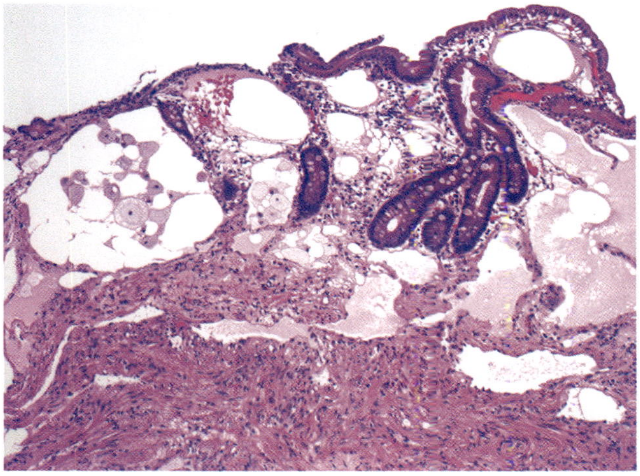

Figure 8.11 Lymphangiectasia. Note the dilated lymphatic channels containing proteinaceous material and floating histiocytes.

Differential Diagnosis

The main diagnostic considerations are lymphangioma, Whipple's disease, MAIC, and pneumatosis intestinalis.

Treatment/Prognosis/Evolution

No therapy is needed other than addressing any underlying causes.

Further Reading

Abramowsky, C., Hupertz, V., Kilbridge, P. et al. (1989). Intestinal lymphangiectasia in children: a study of upper gastrointestinal endoscopic biopsies. *Pediatr. Pathol.* 9: 289.

Aoyagi, K., Iida, M., Yao, T. et al. (1997). Characteristic endoscopic features of intestinal lymphangiectasia: correlation with histological findings. *Hepato-Gastroenterology* 44: 133.

Bettington, M., Brown, I., Kumarasinghe, M. et al. (2014). The challenging diagnosis of Cronkhite–Canada syndrome in the upper gastrointestinal tract: a series of 7 cases with clinical follow-up. *Am. J. Surg. Pathol.* 38 (2): 215–223.

Bromberg, S.H., Camilo Neto, C., Borges, A.F. et al. (2010). Pancreatic heterotopias: clinicopathological analysis of 18 patients. *Rev. Col. Bras. Cir.* 37 (6): 413–419.

Brosens, L.A.A., Jansen, M., Giardiello, F.M., and Offerhaus, G.J.A. (2010). Polyps of the small intestine. *Diagn. Histopathol.* 17 (2): 69–79.

Burke, A.P. and Sobin, L.H. (1989). The pathology of Cronkhite–Canada polyps. A comparison to juvenile polyposis. *Am. J. Surg. Pathol.* 13: 940–946.

Chen, H.M. and Fang, J.Y. (2009). Genetics of the hamartomatous polyposis syndromes: a molecular review. *Int. J. Color. Dis.* 24 (8): 865–874.

Cronkhite, L.W. Jr. and Canada, W.J. (1955). Generalized gastrointestinal polyposis; an unusual syndrome of polyposis, pigmentation, alopecia and onychotrophia. *N. Engl. J. Med.* 252: 1011–1015.

Di Giorgio, A., Sofo, L., Ridolfini, M.P. et al. (2007). Pneumatosis cystoides intestinalis. *Lancet* 369 (9563): 766.

Gammon, A., Jasperson, K., Kohlmann, W., and Burt, R.W. (2009). Hamartomatous polyposis syndromes. *Best Pract. Res. Clin. Gastroenterol.* 23 (2): 219–231.

Genta, R.M., Kinsey, S., Singhal, A., and Suterwala, S. (2010). Gastric foveolar metaplasia and gastric heterotopia in the duodenum: no evidence of an etiologic role for *Helicobacter pylori*. *Hum. Pathol.* 41: 1593–1600.

Hoedemaeker, P.J. (1970). Heterotopic gastric mucosa in the duodenum. *Digestion* 3: 165–173.

Jamart, J. (1979). Pneumatosis cystoides intestinalis. A statistical study of 919 cases. *Acta Hepatogastroenterol. (Stuttg)* 26 (5): 419.

Jiang, W., Roma, A.A., Lai, K. et al. (2013). Endometriosis involving the mucosa of the intestinal tract: a clinicopathologic study of 15 cases. *Mod. Pathol.* 26 (9): 1270–1278.

Kahn, E. and Daum, F. (1984). Pseudopolyps of the small intestine in Crohn's disease. *Hum. Pathol.* 15 (1): 84–86.

Kato, M., Mizuki, A., Hayashi, T. et al. (2000). Cowden's disease diagnosed through mucocutaneous lesions and gastrointestinal polyposis with recurrent hematochezia, unrevealed by initial diagnosis. *Intern. Med.* 39 (7): 559–563.

Koreishi, A., Lauwers, G.Y., and Misdraji, J. (2007). Pneumatosis intestinalis: a challenging biopsy diagnosis. *Am. J. Surg. Pathol.* 31 (10): 1469–1475.

Krauss, E., Konturek, P., Maiss, J. et al. (2010). Clinical significance of lymphoid hyperplasia of the lower gastrointestinal tract. *Endoscopy* 42 (4): 334–337.

Lessells, A.M. and Martin, D.F. (1982). Heterotopic gastric mucosa in the duodenum. *J. Clin. Pathol.* 35: 591–595.

Misra, V., Misra, S.P., Dwivedi, M., and Gupta, S.C. (1997). Histomorphometric study of portal hypertensive enteropathy. *Am. J. Clin. Pathol.* 108 (6): 652–657.

Mukhopadhyay, S., Harbol, T., Floyd, F.D., and Sidhu, J.S. (2004). Polypoid nodular lymphoid hyperplasia of the terminal ileum. *Arch. Pathol. Lab. Med.* 128 (10): 1186–1187.

Powers, M., Sayuk, G.S., and Wang, H.L. (2008). Brunner gland cyst: report of three cases. *Int. J. Clin. Exp. Pathol.* 1 (6): 536–538.

Riemann, J.F. and Schmidt, H. (1981). Synopsis of endoscopic and other morphological findings in intestinal lymphangiectasia. *Endoscopy* 13: 60.

Rondonotti, E., Villa, F., Signorelli, C., and de Franchis, R. (2006). Portal hypertensive enteropathy. *Gastrointest. Endosc. Clin. N. Am.* 16 (2): 277–286.

de Sanctis, S., Qureshi, T., and Stebbing, J.F. (2001). Clinical and pathological overlap in nonsteroidal anti-inflammatory drug-related small bowel diaphragm disease and the neuromuscular and vascular hamartoma of the small bowel. *Am. J. Surg. Pathol.* 25 (4): 539–541.

Shekitka, K.M. and Sobin, L.H. (1994). Ganglioneuromas of the gastrointestinal tract. Relation to Von Recklinghausen disease and other multiple tumor syndromes. *Am. J. Surg. Pathol.* 18 (3): 250–257.

Shepherd, N.A. and Jass, J.R. (1987). Neuromuscular and vascular hamartoma of the small intestine: is it Crohn's disease? *Gut* 28 (12): 1663–1668.

Shepherd, N.A., Bussey, H.J., and Jass, J.R. (1987). Epithelial misplacement in Peutz Jeghers polyps. A diagnostic pitfall. *Am. J. Surg. Pathol.* 11: 743–749.

Shirakawa, K., Nakamura, T., Endo, M. et al. (2007). Pyogenic granuloma of the small intestine. *Gastrointest. Endosc.* 66 (4): 827–828.

Stojcev, Z., Borun, P., Hermann, J. et al. (2013). Hamartomatous polyposis syndromes. *Hered Cancer Clin. Pract.* 11 (1) 4: 1–9.

Tan, C.L., Tan, S.H., So, J.B., and Petersson, F. (2013). Muco-submucosal elongated polyps of the gastrointestinal tract: a case series and a review of the literature. *World J. Gastroenterol.* 19 (11): 1845–1849.

Yano, T. and Yamamoto, H. (2009). Vascular, polypoid, and other lesions of the small bowel. *Best Pract. Res. Clin. Gastroenterol.* 23 (1): 61–74.

Yantiss, R.K., Clement, P.B., and Young, R.H. (2001). Endometriosis of the intestinal tract: a study of 44 cases of a disease that may cause diverse challenges in clinical and pathologic evaluation. *Am. J. Surg. Pathol.* 25 (4): 445–454.

Yuan, Z., Chen, J., Zheng, Q. et al. (2009). Heterotopic pancreas in the gastrointestinal tract. *World J. Gastroenterol.* 15 (29): 3701–3703.

Zbuk, K.M. and Eng, C. (2007). Hamartomatous polyposis syndromes. *Nat. Clin. Pract. Gastroenterol. Hepatol.* 4 (9): 492–502.

9

Epithelial and Nonepithelial Neoplasms of the Small Intestine

Ian Brown[1], *Michael B. Wallace*[2] *and Till S. Clauditz*[3]

[1] *Envoi Specialist Pathologists, Brisbane, Australia*
[2] *Mayo Clinic, Jacksonville, Florida, USA*
[3] *Department of Pathology, University-Medical-Center Hamburg-Eppendorf, Hamburg, Germany*

Adenoma

Brunner Gland Adenoma (Synonym: Brunner Gland Hamartoma)

Definition and Predisposing Factors (if Applicable)

This benign lesion is formed by proliferation of Brunner glands. It occurs in the proximal duodenum and, rarely, the proximal jejunum. The etiology is unknown, and the lesion may represent a hamartoma rather than a true neoplasm.

Clinical Features/Endoscopic Characteristics

Brunner gland adenomas are generally asymptomatic except in rare cases where bleeding can occur. The endoscopic appearance is usually a lobular sessile lesion similar to colorectal adenomas (Figure 9.1).

Microscopic Features

The lobulated proliferation of Brunner glands develops within the submucosa and basal mucosa. The lining cells, lacking atypia, are uniform and cuboidal and display pale cytoplasm containing neutral mucin. The gland architecture is regular, although cystic dilatation may occur. The overlying duodenal mucosa often displays reactive changes due to concomitant erosion. Brunner's glands may be admixed with a smooth muscle proliferation, adipose tissue, lymphoid tissue and/or heterotopic pancreatic acini and ducts (Figure 9.2).

Differential Diagnosis

- Brunner gland hyperplasia in peptic duodenitis: The distinguishing features are the finding of mucosal inflammation and less organized architecture.
- Pyloric gland adenoma: Cytoplasmic eosinophilia is usually appreciable. The lining cells typically exhibit some atypia with prominent nucleoli.

Treatment/Prognosis/Evolution

The lesion is benign and seldom causes clinical problems.

Pyloric Gland Adenoma

Definition and Predisposing Factors (If Applicable)

This neoplastic proliferation is composed of cells with differentiation toward gastric pyloric gland cells. Increases prevalence in both Lynch syndrome and Familial Adenomatous Polyposis has been suggested.

Clinical Features/Endoscopic Characteristics

Pyloric gland adenomas are commonly asymptomatic sessile similar to colorectal adenomas (Figure 9.3).

Microscopic Features

In the absence of dysplasia, pyloric gland adenoma is characterized by a proliferation of regular, tubular glands lined by cuboidal cells that have clear to eosinophilic cytoplasm and a round nucleus with generally small nucleolus. Dysplasia is characterized by architectural irregularity, increase in cell and nuclear size, and increased prominence of nucleoli. The progression to invasive carcinoma may be deceptive. A back-to-back gland pattern or infiltration by single tumor cells indicates malignancy (Figure 9.4).

Immunohistochemical and Molecular Features

As in normal pyloric gland epithelium, these lesions display cytoplasmic expression of MUC6. Expression of MUC5ac may be found in cells near the luminal aspect of the tumor.

Gastrointestinal Pathology: Correlative Endoscopic and Histologic Assessment, First Edition. Edited by Gregory Y. Lauwers and Michael B. Wallace.

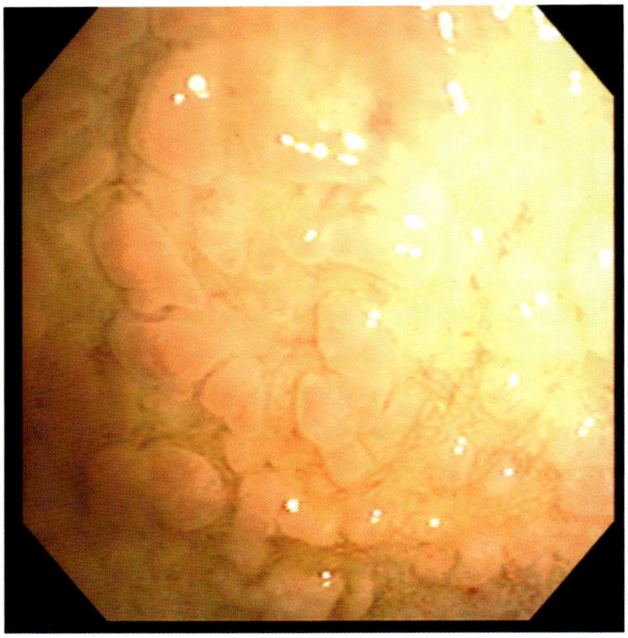

Figure 9.1 Endoscopic Brunner gland adenoma in the proximal duodenum.

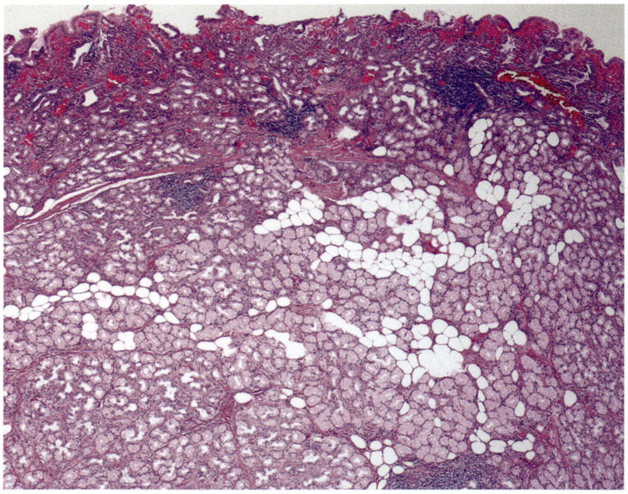

Figure 9.2 Brunner gland hamartoma.

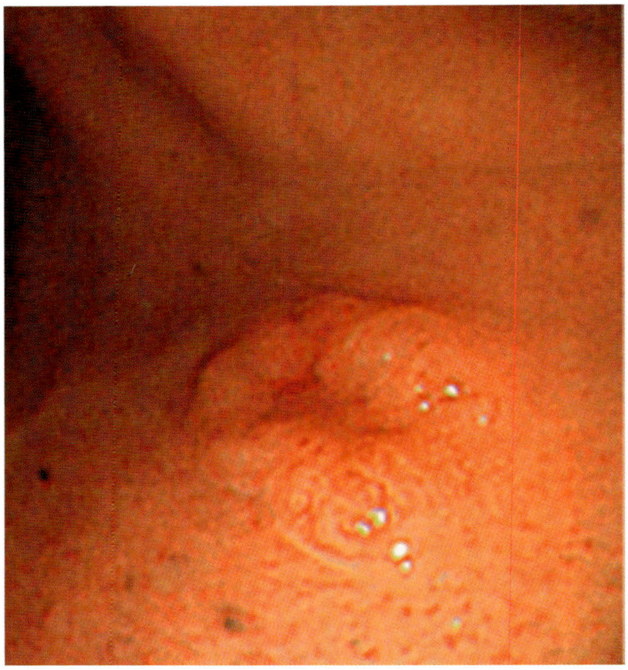

Figure 9.3 Endoscopic appearance of pyloric gland adenoma. *Source:* Reproduced with permission from Lee, S.E., Kang, S.Y., Cho, J. et al. (2014). Pyloric gland adenoma in Lynch syndrome. *Am. J. Surg. Pathol.* 38 (6): 784–792.

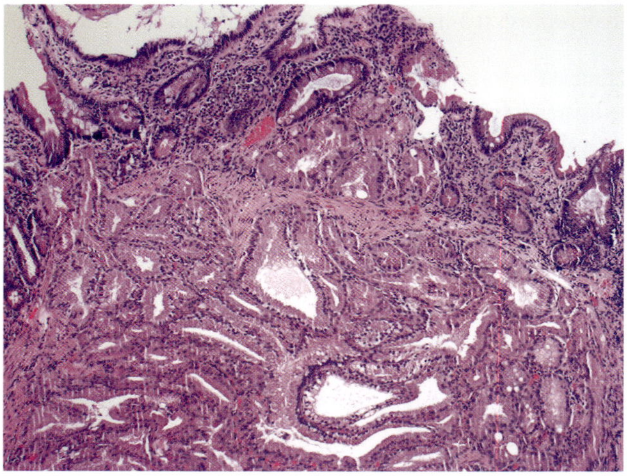

Figure 9.4 Pyloric gland adenoma of duodenum.

Differential Diagnosis

Gastric Heterotopias

This comprises specialized gastric mucosa, which is distinct from the neutral mucin-producing cells of pyloric gland adenoma.

Brunner Gland Hyperplasia/Adenoma

This distinction requires attention to the greater cytological and architectural atypia seen in pyloric gland adenoma. Brunner's gland adenoma will also express MUC6, so this stain is not helpful.

Well-Differentiated Adenocarcinoma

The possibility should be considered in all cases of pyloric gland adenoma. The distinction may require additional tissue to be examined. Persistent growth or large tumor size are concerning features.

Treatment/Prognosis/Evolution

These lesions are managed similar to other polypoid neoplasia, with endoscopic snare resection. Due to the rarity of these lesions, there is no consensus on prognosis and follow-up. In this authors' opinion, follow-up using colonic adenoma guidelines is likely appropriate.

Intestinal Type Adenoma

Definition

This represents a neoplastic, noninvasive proliferation of dysplastic intestinal lining cells.

Predisposing Factors

Familial adenomatous polyposis syndrome and Lynch syndrome are well-recognized predisposing conditions.

Clinical Features/Endoscopic Characteristics

Clinical and endoscopic features are similar to other adenomatous polyps of the small bowel. Most are asymptomatic. In FAP, specific guidelines suggest surveillance of the small bowel for adenomas based on the number, size, location, and histology. These have been codified into the Spigelman classification system.

Microscopic Features

These lesions are identical to their large intestinal counterparts. They may have tubular, tubulovillous or villous architecture, and accompanying dysplasia may be low grade or high grade. Serrated architecture, with a pattern resembling traditional serrated adenoma, may be observed (see below). Gastric surface metaplasia is present in 40% of cases and a distinctive clear cell change in the cytoplasm of the adenoma cells is present in some (Figure 9.5).

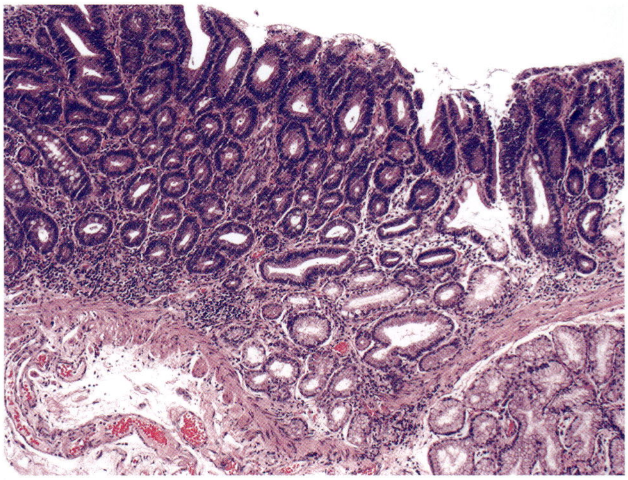

Figure 9.5 Tubular adenoma of duodenum.

Immunohistochemical and Molecular Features

Intestinal type adenomas arising in Lynch syndrome show a loss of nuclear immunohistochemical reaction for one or more of the mismatch repair proteins, MLH-1, MSH-2, MSH-6, and PMS-2, in approximately 70% of cases. Molecular studies demonstrate high levels of microsatellite instability in these cases.

Differential Diagnosis

Reactive Changes

These are seen commonly at the edge of an ulcer or secondary to acute inflammation. An abrupt change from normal to dysplastic epithelium of adenoma is a helpful distinguishing feature.

Adenocarcinoma

Intestinal type adenocarcinoma may arise from an adenoma, and the distinction on a biopsy rests on the finding of complex glandular architecture and stromal desmoplasia or infiltrating single cells. In the ampullary region, pancreatic or biliary tree neoplasia may mimic intestinal type adenoma, particularly on biopsy.

Treatment/Prognosis/Evolution

For non-ampullary adenomas, surgery is often the only definitive management but is reserved for patients with Spigelman class 4. Lower grade lesions can be removed endoscopically if feasible. Typically ampullary adenomas are removed endoscopically by ampullectomy, often in conjunction with temporary stenting of the pancreatic and bile ducts.

Serrated Polyps

Definition

It is defined as a polypoid glandular proliferation with serrated morphology of the gland architecture.

Clinical Features/Endoscopic Characteristics

The features are similar to other polyps. These lesions tend to be small, asymptomatic, and benign clinical behavior.

Microscopic Features

Small intestinal serrated lesions are poorly characterized compared to their colonic counterparts. A rare lesion resembling colonic hyperplastic polyp has been described. Lesions resembling traditional colonic serrated adenoma, either in pure form or as part of an otherwise conventional

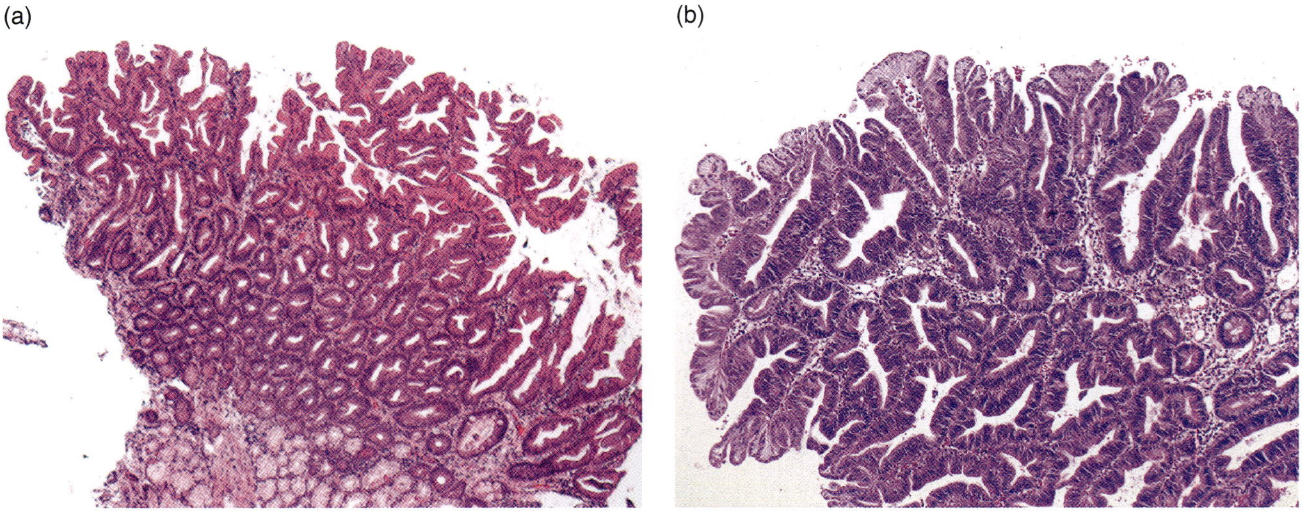

Figure 9.6 (a) Hyperplastic polyp of duodenum. (b) Serrated adenoma of duodenum.

intestinal type adenoma, are described but remain poorly characterized (Figure 9.6a, b).

Immunohistochemical and Molecular Features

BRAF mutation has been identified in hyperplastic polyp like lesions of the proximal small bowel.

Differential Diagnosis

Reactive Changes

In particular, mucosal regeneration after injury may acquire a serrated pattern. NSAID enteropathy is particularly likely to exhibit this pattern.

Treatment/Prognosis/Evolution

Lesions resembling colonic hyperplastic polyps are innocuous and do not require further treatments. Traditional serrated adenoma-like lesions most likely have a risk for development of malignancy similar to conventional adenomas. Hence, they should be treated and followed up accordingly.

Carcinoma

A broad spectrum of neoplasms is recognized. The WHO classification of small intestinal carcinoma is presented in Table 9.1. The most common subtypes will be discussed herein.

Table 9.1 WHO classification of small intestinal and ampullary tumors.

1) Adenocarcinoma NOS
2) Mucinous adenocarcinoma (greater than 50% mucinous)
3) Signet ring cell carcinoma (greater than 50% signet ring cells)
4) Medullary Carcinoma NOS
5) Adenocarcinoma, intestinal type
6) Pancreatobiliary-type carcinoma
7) Tubular adenocarcinoma
8) Neuroendocrine tumor (NET grade 1-3)
9) Neuroendocrine carcinoma (NEC; small and large cell)
10) Mixed neuroendocrine-non-neuroendocrine neoplasm (MiNEN)

Unusual subtypes include sarcomatoid, choriocarcinoma, and hepatoid variants.

Adenocarcinoma—Intestinal Type

Definition and Predisposing Factors (If Applicable)

This malignant neoplasm arises from the glandular epithelium of the small intestine. The major predisposing factors are inflammatory bowel disease (Crohn's) and hereditary syndromes (familial adenomatous polyposis and Lynch syndrome). Patients with non-syndromic colorectal cancer are also at slightly elevated risk.

General Features (Frequency)

Small bowel adenocarcinoma typically presents with occult bleeding (anemia) or obstruction.

An increased risk is noted in various conditions (Table 9.2).

Clinical Features/Endoscopic Characteristics

Clinical features of anemia are nonspecific but include fatigue and characteristic dietary cravings called pica (cravings for items such as ice chips or dirt). Obstruction may be subtle such as crampy abdominal pain or more obvious with distention and vomiting. Radiological features are classically a dilated small bowel, with air-fluid levels, and a focal transition point on enterography.

Table 9.2 Conditions associated with an increased risk of small intestinal carcinoma.

1) **Common:**
   - Polyposis syndromes
     - Familial adenomatous polyposis, Lynch syndrome (hereditary nonpolyposis colon cancer syndrome), juvenile polyposis syndrome, Peutz–Jeghers syndrome, and neurofibromatosis type 1
   - Crohn's disease
2) **Uncommon:**
   - Celiac disease
   - Congenital abnormalities: Meckel's diverticulum, heterotopic pancreas, duplication cysts
   - Chronic inflammation: ilecstomy, ileal pouch
   - Radiotherapy

Endoscopic features are similar to other malignant lesions with and ulcerated, sometimes bleeding mass.

Microscopic Features

These are identical to colorectal carcinoma with dysplastic cells in glandular or villoglandular arrangements invading the stroma of the mucosa or deeper layers of the small intestinal wall. Tumor cells are columnar with pencillate nuclei and eosinophilic cytoplasm. Desmoplasia is usually present, and is indicative of an invasive process. Necrotic debris ("dirty necrosis") is common within gland lumina. Rarely, tumors exhibit extensive extracellular mucin, are composed of signet ring tumor cells (more common in celiac disease), display cytoplasmic clear cell change, or exhibit deceptively well-differentiated cytoarchitectural features (well described in Crohn's disease-related carcinomas). A pre-existing adenoma may be evident (Figure 9.7).

Differential Diagnosis

- Adenocarcinoma of pancreaticobiliary type—see below.
- Adenocarcinoma of pyloric gland type—see below.
- Adenoma with high-grade dysplasia: The absence of definitive invasion of the lamina propria indicates the lesion is still an adenoma.
- Peutz–Jeghers polyp with pseudoinvasion: Distinction lies in the recognition of the underlying polyp and the absence of cytological dysplasia.
- Adenomyoma of ampulla and heterotopic pancreas devoid of acinar structures. No cytological atypia is seen in these.
- Endometriosis: The presence of endometrial stroma and the uniform benign cytology of the endometrial glands allow distinction. A panel of estrogen receptor (ER; +), CK7, CK20, CDX-2, and PAX-8 can be applied to difficult cases, with CK7 and PAX-8 positivity supporting a diagnosis of endometriosis. The stromal component of endometrioses can be confirmed by CD10 immunhistochemistry.

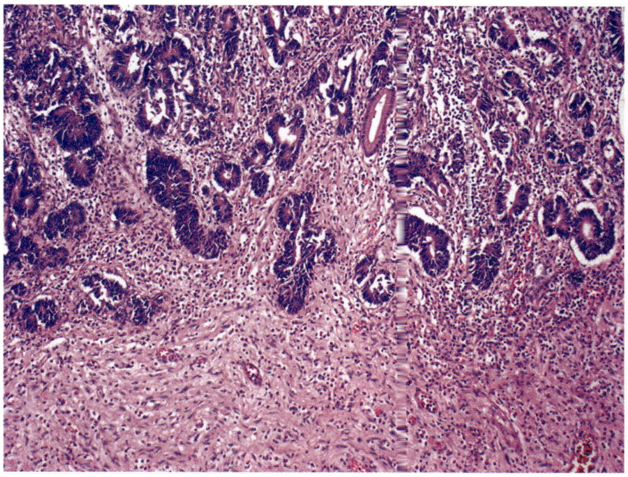

Figure 9.7 Adenocarcinoma of intestinal type arising in neurofibromatosis with background neurofibroma.

Spread

There may be direct invasion to involve the serosal surface, retroperitoneal structures (in the case of duodenal location) and into the pancreas. Most extraintestinal spread is via lymphatics to the regional lymph nodes. Extension via the portal venous system can lead to liver metastasis.

Treatment/Prognosis/Evolution

Treatment requires surgical resection to relieve symptoms, regardless of stage. In rare cases, palliation with enteral stenting may provide short-term relief.

Adenocarcinoma of Pancreaticobiliary Type

This neoplasm typically presents as a mass arising from the ampulla or in the periampullary region. In contrast to intestinal type adenocarcinoma, the neoplastic cells are more cuboidal and the glands tend to be smaller and lack "dirty necrosis." The prognosis of intestinal type adenocarcinoma is more favorable than pancreaticobiliary type adenocarcinoma, so it is important to make this distinction. A panel of immunohistochemical stains has been shown to be useful (Table 9.3; Figure 9.8).

Adenocarcinoma of Pyloric Gland Type

This usually arises from a pre-existing pyloric gland adenoma. Invasion can be difficult to establish on biopsy, with suspicion raised when complex cribriform or small gland patterns are present. The cuboidal tumor cells with clear or lightly eosinophilic cytoplasm are in contrast to the pencillate, brightly eosinophilic cells of intestinal type adenocarcinoma. Immunohistochemical stains aid differentiation

Table 9.3 Immunophenotypic classification of small intestinal adenocarcinoma.

Adenocarcinoma type	Immunohistochemical stain				
	MUC 1	MUC 2	CDX 2	CK7	CK20
Intestinal	−	+	+	±	+
Pancreaticobiliary	+	−	−	+	±
Pyloric[a]	−	−	−	Insufficient data	−

[a] Reactive for MUC 6.

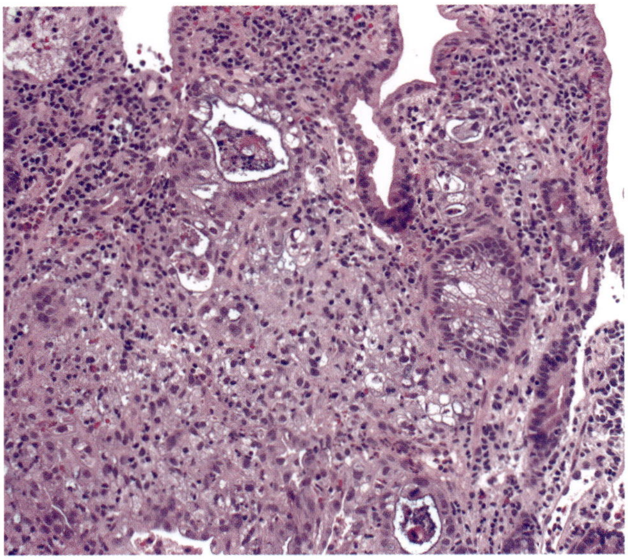

Figure 9.8 Pancreatic type adenocarcinoma in ampulla.

of Pyloric gland adenocarcinoma (MUC2−, MUC6+, CDX-2−, CK20−) from intestinal adenocarcinoma (MUC2+, MUC6−, CDX-2+, CK20+).

Neuroendocrine Neoplasms (Well-Differentiated Neuroendocrine Tumors (NET), Neuroendocrine Carcinoma (NEC), Mixed endocrine-non-endocrine neoplasms (MiNEN))

Definition, General Features, and Predisposing Factors

These tumors are derived from neuroendocrine cells native to the mucosa, and may be derived from the foregut (duodenum) or mid-gut (jejunum, ileum). They can either be of a specific type based on active hormone production and or particular morphology, or not exhibit a specific line of differentiation. This leads to a variety of terms. For instance in the duodenum/ampulla the following designations are applied to tumors with the similar morphology: gastrinoma, somatostatinoma, and nonfunctional neuroendocrine tumors (old "carcinoids"). Neuroendocrine tumors of the small intestine may arise in the setting of MEN1 and neurofibromatosis type 1 syndromes (see Table 9.4). Symptoms related to neuroendocrine tumors are usually related to metastases and associated hormonal effects but vary widely based on the hormone produces including carcinoid syndrome (5-HIAA), Zollinger Ellison syndrome (gastrin), or profound diarrhea from VIP secreting tumors.

Table 9.4 Features differentiating proximal and distal intestinal neuroendocrine tumors.

Proximal small intestine	Ileum
• 20% of all GIT NETs • 1–3% of duodenal neoplasms • Periampullary/ampullary in 20% • M : F = 2 : first, sixth decade • Syndromic MEN1 in 6%, NF1 rare • 90% nonfunctional • 10% functional (mostly gastrinoma of Zollinger Ellison sd. associated with MEN1 in 50%) • Multiple tumors in 10% • 75% are <2 cm (mucosa/submucosa) • Regional nodal metastases in 50% (early) • Liver metastases in 10% • Five-year survival Localized in 80–95% Regional LN in 65–75% Distant metastases in 5–10%	• 25% of all GIT NETs • 0.3–0.5% of all small intestinal neoplasms • M : F = 1.5 : 1, sixth/seventh decade • Non syndromic • 95% nonfunctional • 5% functional (carcinoid syndrome) • Multiple tumors in 20—50% • Nodal metastasis in 10–40% of tumors <10 mm diameter • Five-year survival If no metastasis ~100% If lymph node metastases ~75% If distant metastases ~50%

Clinical Features/Endoscopic Characteristics

Small low-grade neuroendocrine tumors are often found incidentally in the small bowel. They have "normal" overlying mucosal and thus the appearance of a submucosal tumor. Endoscopic biopsy may be falsely negative. Endoscopic ultrasound is the best modality to evaluate these and can be used to guide deep biopsy or fine-needle aspiration.

Microscopic Features

Features common to well-differentiated neuroendocrine tumor or carcinoma include architectural, cytomorphological, and stromal patterns.

1) **Architectural patterns**: Four characteristic patterns are recognized: (i) Type A—the *insular solid* pattern composed of small- to medium-sized tumor nests. Seemingly solid patterns may result from close packing of trabeculae and ribbons. (ii) Type B—the *trabecular* pattern typified by cell ribbons in single or, occasionally, double or multiple layers. (iii) Type C—the *glandular* pattern, comprising glandular patterns with either true glandular lumen or pseudoglands showing a cellular rim surrounding a central vessel. (iv) Type D—the *mixed* pattern, tumors with complex architecture resulting from combinations of two or more of the other patterns.
2) **Cellular morphology**: Well-differentiated neoplasms are characteristically composed of uniform round cells with variable amounts of eosinophilic cytoplasm and central nuclei with granular ("salt and pepper") chromatin pattern. Poorly differentiated neoplasms show more cytological variability, nuclear hyperchromasia, and may be of small cell or large cell type. Furthermore some cases show an additional adenocarcinoma component defined as MiNEN.
3) **Stroma**: Typically, a richly vascular fibrous stroma is present. Stromal elastosis may accompany ileal neuroendocrine tumors but is generally absent in biopsy specimens. Psammomatous dystrophic calcification may occur in somatostatinoma and amyloid deposition may be encountered in any functional neoplasm.

Well-differentiated lesions have a low mitotic activity, while poorly differentiated tumors have high mitotic rate, frequent apoptosis, and tumor necrosis.

The WHO classification of neuroendocrine tumors is based on tumor site, size, mitotic rate, and proliferation index, and the presence of angiolymphatic invasion (see Table 9.5; Figure 9.9a. b).

Immunohistochemical and Molecular Features

The neoplasms express cytokeratin and are reactive for at least two neuroendocrine markers. These include stains expressed in the following fashion: (i) cytoplasm or cell membrane (neuron-specific enolase [NSE], PGP9.5 and neural cell adhesion molecule [NCAM], CD56); (ii) synapse-like microvesicle reaction—synaptophysin and; (iii) large dense-core vesicle reaction—Chromogranin A, CD57.

Specific hormone production in tumor cells (which does not necessarily correlate with release into the bloodstream or with a specific clinical syndrome) can also be detected, e.g. insulin, gastrin, glucagon, and somatostatin. However, this is not necessary for histological classification. Furthermore, immunohistochemical evaluation of somatostatin receptor 2 (SSTR2) expression is useful for further therapy settings. Mutations for MEN1, DAXX and ATRX genes have been established in cases of NET. Alternatively, NECs show p53- and Rb1-mutations, which can be helpful in diagnostically challenging cases.

Differential Diagnosis

The main diagnostic considerations are as follows: (i) melanoma; (ii) gastrointestinal stromal tumor (GIST); (iii) neuroectodermal tumor; (iv) lymphoma; and (v) paraganglioma (and gangliocytic paraganglioma). A panel of

Table 9.5 Diagnostic criteria for NENs (including NET, NEC, MiNEN) adapted to the recent WHO Classification (5th Edition; 2019).

Terminology	Differentiation	Grade	Mitoses per $2mm^2$	Ki-67 proliferative index
NET				
G1		Low	<2	<3%
G2	Well	Intermediate	2–20	3–20%
G3		High	>20	>20%
NEC (small & large cell type)	Poor	High	>20	>20%
MiNEN	Variable	Variable	Variable	Variable

NEN (neuroendocrine neoplasm); NET (neuroendocrine tumor), NEC (neuroendocrine carcinoma), MiNEN (mixed neuroendocrine-non-neuroendocrine neoplasm).

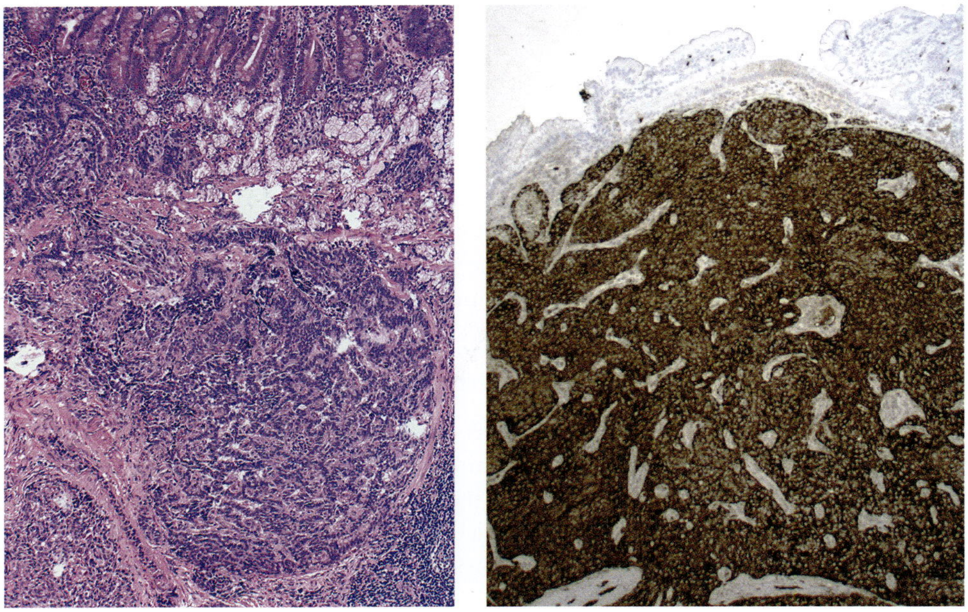

Figure 9.9 (a) NET of the duodenum. (b) Chromogranin IHC in duodenal NET.

immunohistochemical stains that includes neuroendocrine markers, keratin, CD117, S-100, and LCA usually allows distinction.

Treatment/Prognosis/Evolution

For lesions limited to the submucosal layer, endoscopic resection is feasible with the technique of submucosal injection and snare removal, or the more intensive endoscopic submucosal dissection although both carry significant risk of perforation or bleeding. Given these risks, consideration should be given to observation (for small low risk lesions) or surgical removal of larger high-risk lesions.

Gangliocytic Paraganglioma

Definition and General Features (Frequency)

This distinctive neuroendocrine neoplasm is characterized by divergent differentiation toward neuroendocrine cell, Schwann cell, and ganglion cell lineage. It is typically located at the ampulla, accounting for 20–25% of tumors with neuroendocrine differentiation at this site.

Clinical Features/Endoscopic Characteristics

These rare lesions present as asymptomatic small submucosal tumors in the second portion of the duodenum. Endoscopic ultrasound is helpful to identify the lesion and perform fine-needle aspiration or biopsy (Figure 9.10).

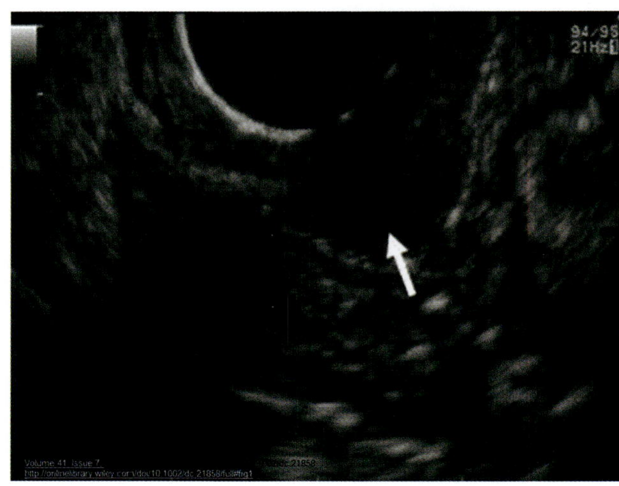

Figure 9.10 Endoscopic US image of GCPG. The lesion is hypoechoic (dark) arising in the submucosal layer of the duodenum.

Microscopic Features

Three cellular elements are required for the diagnosis:

1) Spindle-shaped Schwann cells, which form a background supporting stroma.
2) Ganglion cells, either clustered or dispersed in the Schwann cell stroma.
3) Well-differentiated neuroendocrine cells. These form nested or trabecular arrangements (Figure 9.11a).

Immunohistochemical and Molecular Features

The well-differentiated neuroendocrine component is immunoreactive for keratin and neuroendocrine stains (e.g. synaptophysin, chromogranin, CD56). The Schwann cells are decorated by S-100, and the ganglion cells are immunoreactive for S-100 and synaptophysin (Figure 9.11b, c).

Differential Diagnosis

In biopsies, one or sometimes two of the elements may be absent because of limited sampling, and deeper levels can be useful in identifying them. There may also be a predominance of spindle or epithelial elements in the tumor, directing the differential diagnosis, including:

- Nerve sheath tumor and GIST. The latter can be excluded on the basis of CD117 and/or DOG-1 reactivity.
- Neuroendocrine tumors are devoid of other elements. Paraganglioma does not contain ganglion cells and exhibits a sustentacular pattern of S-100 reactive cells around the tumor cell nests. Adenocarcinoma is typically nonreactive for S-100 and neuroendocrine markers.
- Ganglioneuroma: The presence of neuroendocrine elements is important to this distinction.

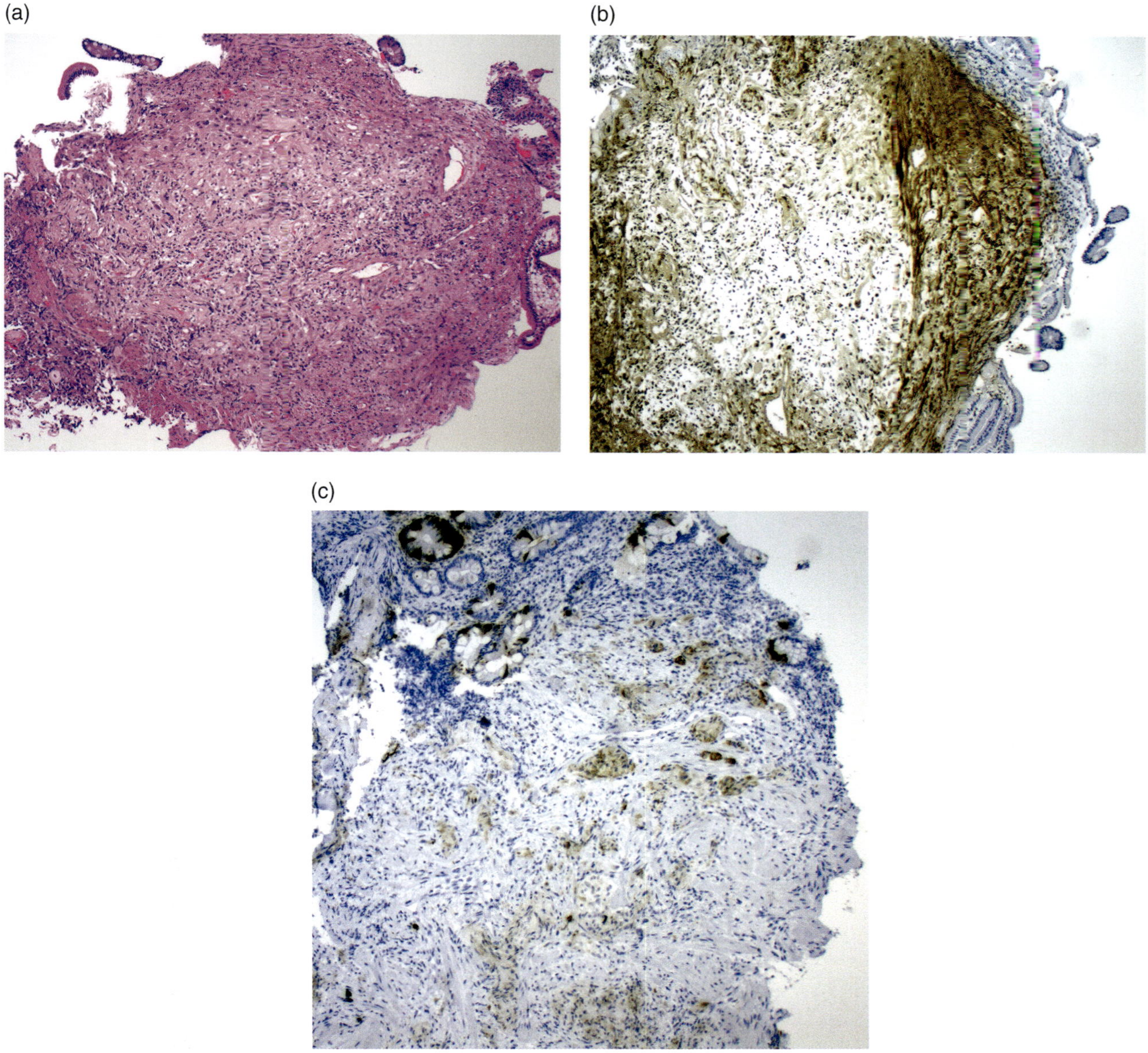

Figure 9.11 (a) Gangliocytic paraganglioma H&E MP. (b) Gangliocytic paraganglioma S-100 stain. (c) Gangliocytic paraganglioma Chromogranin stain.

Spread

Although rare reports of regional lymph node metastases exist, there have been no tumor-related deaths and the neoplasm is regarded as indolent.

Treatment/Prognosis/Evolution

Given the benign nature of these lesions, resection is typically not required.

Gastrointestinal Stromal Tumor (GIST)

A broad spectrum of mesenchymal neoplasms can affect the small bowel.

Definition, General Features (Frequency), and Predisposing Factors

GISTs are the mesenchymal neoplasms most commonly arising in the gastrointestinal tract. There is evidence of an origin from the interstitial cells of Cajal, a component of the gut autonomic nervous system, and most tumors harbor activating mutations of the tyrosine kinase receptors, e.g. c-KIT or platelet-derived growth factor receptor (PDGFR). In addition, mutation in exon 15 of BRAF and in genes encoding the enzyme complex of succinate dehydrogenase (SDH) have also been identified. Most GISTs develop as the result of sporadic mutations, but up to 5% have a hereditary basis, or occur in a multi-tumor syndrome (see Tables 9.6–9.9).

Clinical Features/Endoscopic Characteristics

Several settings are recognized: (i) in neurofibromatosis (NF-1), the tumors lack both c-KIT and PDGRA mutation; (ii) in Carney's triad (gastric GIST, pulmonary chondroma, and extra-adrenal paraganglioma), the neoplasms have dysfunction of SDH enzyme complex but do not have underlying gene mutation; (iii) in Carney–Stratakis syndrome (hereditary GIST and paraganglioma syndrome), they are caused by germline mutations in SDH and (iv) in familial GIST syndrome, the neoplasms have germline gain-of-function mutations in c-KIT (especially due to exon 11 mutation). PDGFRA mutation may also be found. At endoscopy, the lesions are rounded, submucosal, with overlying normal mucosa. Endoscopic ultrasound is the preferred method of evaluation. Lesions may arise from either the third echo layer (likely the muscularis mucosa) or fourth echo layer (muscularis propria). GIST lesions are hypoechoic, but more advanced lesions become large, with mixed areas of low and high density, and more irregular outer boarders (Figure 9.12).

It is uncommon in routine mucosal biopsy specimens to receive sufficient diagnostic tissue from a usually submucosa-based GIST. Direct sampling of the tumor via TUNNEL or SINK procedures yields more material.

Table 9.6 Gene mutational profile of c-KIT.

	Exon 9	Exon 11	Exon 13	Exon 17
Frequency (all GIST)	10–15%	65–70%	1%	1%
Histology	Usual pattern	Spindle > epithelioid		
Site predilection	Small intestine	Stomach	Insufficient data	Insufficient data
Imatinib response	++ (Often requires higher dose)	+++	Variable	Variable
Progressive disease	17%	3%	Insufficient data	Insufficient data

Table 9.7 Characteristics of PDGFA mutated GIST.

	Exon 12	Exon 14	Exon 18 (usually D842V)
Frequency (all GIST)	1.5%	0.5%	6%
Histopathology	• Epithelioid, multinucleate giant cells • Intermediate/high risk		
Site predilection	Stomach, omentum/peritoneal surface		
Imatinib response	Variable	Variable	Nil (D842V mutation is imatinib resistant)
Progressive disease	Overall less aggressive than c-kit mutant GIST		

Table 9.8 Characteristics of BRAF mutated GIST.

	Exon 15 (V600E)
Frequency	Rare (<1%), female > male
Histopathology	Spindle cell
Site	Small intestine > stomach
Imatinib response	Nil (BRAF inhibitors may be useful in advanced disease)
Progressive disease	Insufficient data

Microscopic Features

GISTs exhibit a variety of cellular and architectural patterns:

Cell type: This includes spindle (70%), epithelioid (20%), or mixed (10%) types. Spindle cells range from plump smooth muscle-like cells to thin wavy neural-like cells, sometimes with juxtanuclear vacuoles. Epithelioid cells are generally large and display cytoplasmic clearing (sometimes signet ring like). Nuclear variability and "floret"-like giant cells may be seen (Figure 9.13).

Architectural pattern: This includes short fascicles, palisading, nested (sometimes resembling neuroendocrine tumor), peritheliomatous, pseudovascular, pseudoglandular, hemangiopericytoma-like, linear streaming and sheeting/ frankly sarcomatous patterns.

Stroma: Variable patterns can be seen, including hyalinized collagen, myxoid areas, microcystic stromal degeneration, lymphocytic infiltration, and sometimes calcification and/or mature bone.

Immunohistochemical and Molecular Features

1) Immunohistochemistry:
   - CD117—positive in 95% of cases, decorating the cell membrane with a Golgi dot pattern of reaction in 45%. Negative staining is seen in between 35 and 80% of PDGFRA mutation GIST and is more common in epitheloid tumors. Positive reaction also is encountered in melanoma, seminoma, and occasionally desmoid tumor.
   - DOG-1—positive in >95%, it is as sensitive for c-KIT mutation spindle cell GISTs as CD117 and detects at least 1/3 of the CD117 nonreactive tumors. It also reacts with a higher proportion of epithelioid and/or PDGFRA mutation GISTs.
   - CD34—positive in 70%, and more likely in gastric sites than the small intestine.
   - SMA—positive in 30–40%.
   - S-100—positive in 5% of all GIST but up to 1/3 of NF1 associated GIST.
   - Desmin—positive in 1–2%.
   - Keratin—positive in 1–2%.

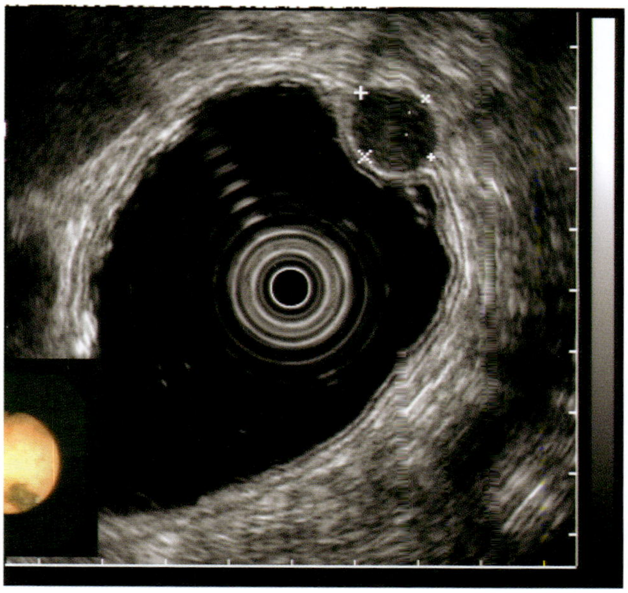

Figure 9.12 Small GIST (1–2 cm) at 1 o'clock. The lesion arises from the fourth echo layer corresponding to the muscularis propria. The size, regular shape, and smooth echo-texture suggest a low grade lesion.

Table 9.9 Characteristics of SDH deficient GIST.

	SDHB (also SDHA, SDHC, SDHD)
Frequency	Rare (<1%), often familial, young females
Histopathology	Multinodular/plexiform; epithelioid cells
Site	Stomach only
Imatinib response	Nil (inhibition of insulin-like growth factor 1 receptor shows promise)
Progressive disease	Traditional risk assessment is poorly predictive of progression risk 15% mortality (median 15 years follow-up) 20–25% develop liver metastases, however long-term survival is still possible

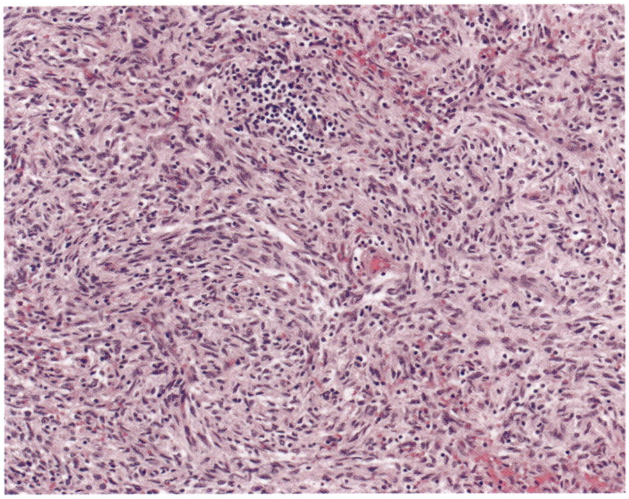

Figure 9.13 GIST composed of short fascicles.

- SDH subunits: SDHB is the commonly used stain, and may detect abnormalities in other subunits of the enzyme complex. There is loss of reaction in SDH mutation; hence, a good internal control (usually native gastric body mucosa) is required. SDH mutation is not expected in small intestinal GIST.

2) Gene mutation testing—testing for the common GIST-associated mutations of c-kit and PDGFR is widely available; this has potential diagnostic, prognostic, and therapeutic value (Table 9.6).

Differential Diagnosis

It primarily includes mesenchymal tumors (Table 9.6). Although broad, the differential diagnosis is usually easily established if the observers take fully into account the histologic characteristics of the neoplasms and apply various immunohistochemical stains wisely (Table 9.10).

Spread

GIST usually spreads to the peritoneal cavity in the first instance, with metastasis to the liver and extra-abdominal organs occurring later in many patients.

Treatment/Prognosis/Evolution

Treatment of localized GIST lesion can be surgical or more recently endoscopic removal. Treatment for progressive disease is with c-KIT targeted tyrosine kinase receptor inhibitors. Predictive factors for progressive disease after primary resection are based on tumor size, site, mitotic activity, and mutation background. These features are summarized in Tables 9.6–9.9 and 9.11.

Table 9.10 Mesenchymal neoplasms entering the differential diagnosis of GIST.

- Leiomyoma/leiomyosarcoma
- Schwannoma/neurofibroma/MPNST
- Solitary fibrous tumor
- Inflammatory myofibroblastic tumor
- Fibromatosis
- Synovial sarcoma
- Neuroendocrine tumor
- Glomus tumor
- Malignant mesothelioma
- Angiosarcoma
- Sarcomatoid carcinoma
- Follicular dendritic cell tumor
- Inflammatory fibroid polyp
- Dedifferentiated liposarcoma

In the stomach, glomus tumor and plexiform fibromyxoma enter the differential diagnosis.

Table 9.11 Risk of progressive disease in GISTs according to mitotic index, size, and site.

Mitotic index, HPF	Size, cm	Duodenum	Jejunum/ileum
≤5/50	≤2	None (0%)	None (0%)
≤5/50	2 to ≥5	Very low (3.8%)	Low (3.4%)
≤5/50	≥5 to >10	Insufficient data	Moderate (24%)
>5/50	>10	High (34%)	High (52%)
>5/50	≤2	Insufficient data	High (50%)
>5/50	2 to ≥5	High (50%)	High (73%)
>5/50	≥5 to >10	Insufficient data	High (85%)
>5/50	>10	High (86%)	High (90%)

Inflammatory Fibroid Polyp

Definition

This benign neoplasm limited to the luminal gastrointestinal tract is characterized by a spindle cell and small vessel proliferation typically accompanied by eosinophil rich inflammation.

Clinical Features/Endoscopic Characteristics

Like other small bowel polyps, these are typically asymptomatic until they become large enough to cause obstruction or rarely bleeding.

Microscopic Features

The lesion involves submucosa and mucosa and is characterized by a spindle tumor cell proliferation that may be paucicellular with fibromyxoid stroma or may be moderately cellular forming onion skin-like patterns around vessels and glands. The spindle cells may be thin and wavy, to plump and almost stellate. Sometimes a short fascicular pattern of growth is seen. Mitotic figures are rare. An inflammatory infiltrate rich in eosinophils and mast cells is common. Variable numbers of lymphocytes, plasma cells, and histiocytes are also present. Zones of stromal hyalinization can occur, but are infrequent in mucosal biopsy specimens (Figure 9.14).

Immunohistochemistry and Molecular Features

The cells are immunoreactive for CD34 and PDGFR, and occasionally for SMA, desmin, cyclin D1, CD68, and Factor XIIIa. They are not reactive to CD117, DOG-1, S-100, EMA, and keratin (e.g. AEI/AE3).

Mutations in the gene transcribing the α subunit of PDGFR (at exon 12 and 18 are most common) have been identified and confirm that the lesion is a true neoplasm and not a reactive inflammatory process. Exon 12 mutations are more commonly associated with small intestinal lesions while exon 18 mutation is most common in gastric lesions.

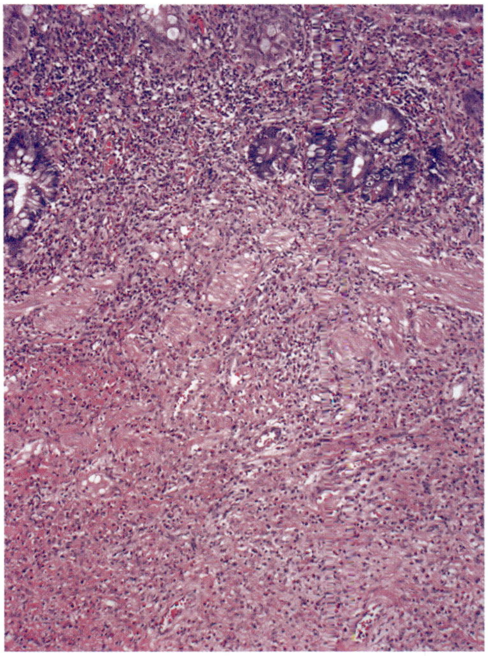

Figure 9.14 Inflammatory fibroid polyp of ileum LP.

Differential Diagnosis (See Table 9.12)

Treatment/Prognosis/Evolution

Treatment is required if symptomatic and includes endoscopic polypectomy or surgical resection.

Other Mesenchymal Tumors

Other mesenchymal tumors that may be encountered in mucosal biopsies of the small intestine may be seen in Table 9.13. A panel of immunohistochemical stains including smooth muscle actin, desmin, CD117, S-100, and EMA is beneficial in the initial workup of presumed mesenchymal lesions.

Lymphoma

The small intestine is a common site for gastrointestinal tract lymphoma. Follicular lymphoma and diffuse large B-cell lymphoma are most frequent. Other lymphomas encountered are listed in Table 9.14.

B-Cell Non-Hodgkin Lymphoma

Follicular B-Cell Lymphoma of the Gastrointestinal Tract

Definition and General Features (Frequency)

This distinctive subset of B-cell follicular lymphoma generally presents with an indolent behavior, developing particularly in the second part of duodenum.

Clinical Features/Endoscopic Characteristics

Abdominal pain is the most common presenting symptom, followed by bleeding, obstruction, and diarrhea.

Table 9.12 Histological differential diagnosis of inflammatory fibroid polyp.

- Differential diagnosis of inflammatory fibroid polyp
  1) GIST
  2) Inflammatory myofibroblastic tumor
  3) Exuberant healing ulcer site; granulation tissue
  4) Eosinophil-rich neoplastic process (e.g. Langerhans cell histiocytosis)
  5) Neoplasms with associated inflammation (e.g. Schwannoma)
  6) Myxoid tumors (e.g. liposarcoma, myxofibrosarcoma, myxoid solitary fibrous tumor, cellular myxoma)

Table 9.13 Other mesenchymal tumors entering the differential diagnosis of intestinal stromal neoplasms.

Mesenchymal cell of origin	Tumor type
Smooth muscle	Leiomyoma, leiomyosarcoma (rare)
Neural	Schwannoma, neurofibroma, MPNST[a], perineurioma
Fibroblastic/myofibroblastic	Solitary fibrous tumor, inflammatory myofibroblastic tumor, fibromatosis
Vascular	Glomus tumor, angiosarcoma
Adipose	Lipoma, liposarcoma
Unknown	Synovial sarcoma, clear cell sarcoma, PEComa

[a] MPNST, malignant peripheral nerve sheath tumor.

Table 9.14 Primary small intestinal non-Hodgkin lymphoma and frequency compared to all GIT lymphoma.

Tumor type	Frequency compared to all GIT lymphoma sites (%)
Diffuse large B-cell lymphoma	38
Follicular lymphoma	23
Enteropathy associated T-cell lymphoma	10
Post-transplant lymphoproliferative disorder	10
Burkitt lymphoma	8
MALT	5

Microscopic Features

The preservation of a follicular architecture is characteristic. The cells are small with irregular nuclear outline resembling centrocyte. Blastic cells resembling centroblasts are often seen as well. However, tingible body macrophages are conspicuously absent. Centrocyte like cells may extend in a diffuse fashion into the adjacent lamina propria appearing to fill the mucosa with a dense lymphoid infiltrate.

Immunohistochemical and Molecular Features

Duodenal follicular lymphoma exhibits the following:

Immunophenotype: CD10(+), B-cell lymphoma 2 (BCL-2)(+), BCL-6(+), and loose CD21(+) follicular dendritic cell network. CD10(+) cells extending in a sheet-like pattern into the lamina propria is particularly suggestive. The cell of origin may be a memory B cell, although previously, follicular lymphoma in the gut was likened to mucosa-associated lymphoid tissue (MALT) lymphoma. The combination of (i) expression of α-4-β-7 integrin (a mucosal homing receptor), (ii) VH gene deviation, and (iii) IgA production suggests that tumor cells are derived from mucosal B cells. Molecular analysis demonstrates a clonal restriction for Ig heavy- and light-chain genes, and Bcl-2 rearrangement (Figure 9.15a–c).

Differential Diagnosis

- Reactive lymphoid hyperplasia (discussed in Chapter 8).
- MALT lymphoma—the prominence of a follicular architecture and the finding of CD10-positive B cells, particularly when beyond the follicular structures, is in keeping with follicular lymphoma. (See Table 9.15 for immunohistochemical and molecular features of small bowel B-cell lymphoma.)

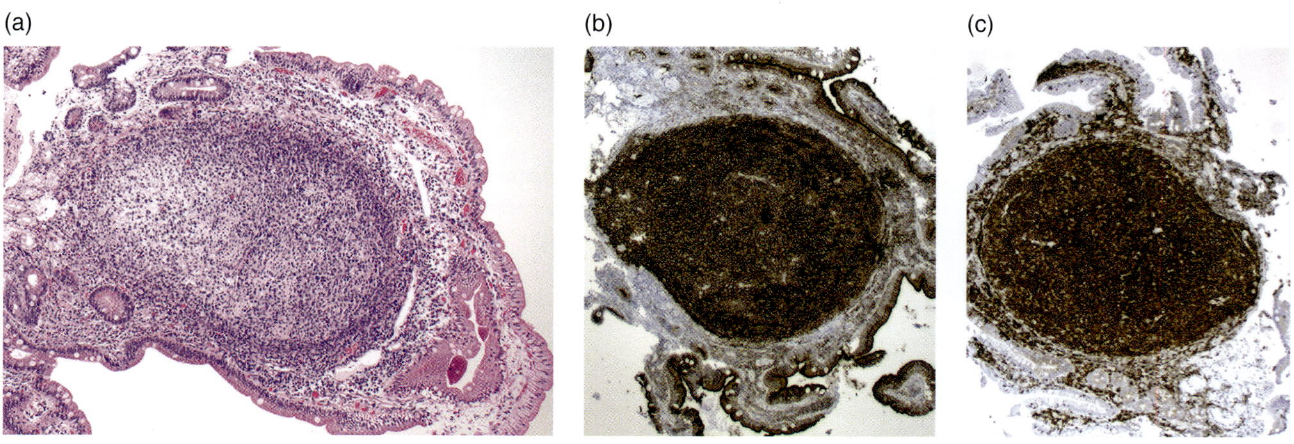

Figure 9.15 (a) Follicular lymphoma duodenum H&E. (b) Follicular lymphoma CD10. (c) Follicular lymphoma bcl2.

Table 9.15 B-cell lymphoma—immunohistochemical and molecular features.

	CD5	CD10	CD20	Other	Bcl-2	Bcl-6	Translocation
Follicular	−	+	+				Bcl-2t(14;18)(q34q21)
MALT	−	−	+	CD43−/+			MALT 1 t(11;18)(q21;q21) in1/3
IPSID	−	−	+	CD138 in plasmacytic cells; α-heavy chain			
Mantle cell	+	−	+	Cyclin D1, IgD(+)			Cyclin D1 (bcl-1) t(11;14)(q13;q32)
B-CLL/Small lymphocytic leukemia	+	−	+	CD23+	−		
Burkitt lymphoma	−	+	+	Ki-67 near 100%	−	+	Myc t(8;14)(q24;q32)
Diffuse large B-cell lymphoma	−	±	+		±	±	

Treatment/Prognosis/Evolution
FL is an indolent disease and is infrequently associated with spread beyond the intestinal wall.

Extranodal Marginal Zone Mucosa-Associated Lymphoid Tissue (MALT) Lymphoma

This subtype may present as a single mass or, rarely, as a lymphomatoid polyposis. The diagnostic features are discussed in the chapter on gastric tumor. A distinct subset presenting in the small intestine (IPSID) is discussed below.

Mantle Cell Lymphoma

Definition and General Features (Frequency)
This aggressive form of B-cell lymphoma has a predilection for the gut (facilitated by α-4-β-7 integrin expression), and frequently presents as multiple polyps.

Clinical Features/Endoscopic Characteristics
Clinical features are similar to other small bowel lymphomas discussed above.

Microscopic Features
Mantle cell lymphoma most commonly exhibits diffuse architecture with sheets of small to intermediate (and occasionally large "blastic") cells destroying native glands without lymphoepithelial lesion formation. Occasionally, a nodular pattern or a mantle zone pattern around reactive germinal centers may be seen. The presence of epithelioid histiocytes and perivascular sclerosis may be clues to the diagnosis (Figure 9.16).

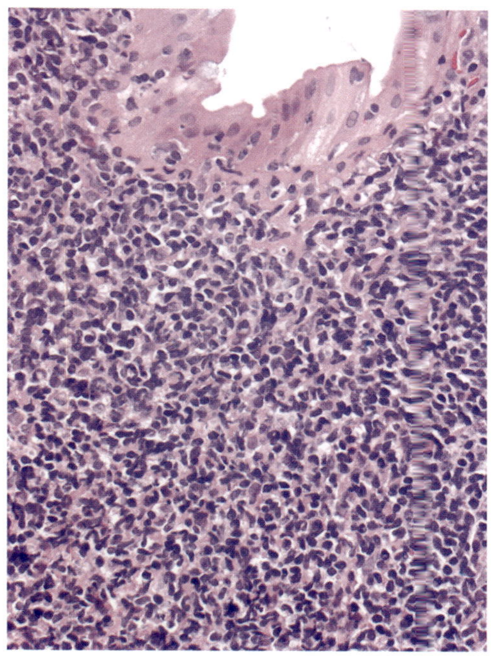

Figure 9.16 Mantle cell lymphoma ileum (HP 2).

Immunohistochemical and Molecular Features (See Table 9.15; Figure 9.17a–c)
Differential Diagnosis
1) Reactive lymphoid hyperplasia—particularly in the setting of lymphomatoid polyposis.
2) MALT lymphoma.
3) Follicular lymphoma.
4) B-CLL.

Treatment/Prognosis/Evolution
Mantle cell lymphoma is an aggressive tumor.

Diffuse Large B-Cell Lymphoma

As with other sites in the gastrointestinal tract diffuse large B-cell lymphoma may present as a solitary mass. It may arise de novo or as a result of transformation from another B-cell lymphoma (e.g. MALT). CD20 expression is typical unless the patient is undertaking treatment with anti-CD20 medication. CD10 expression is associated

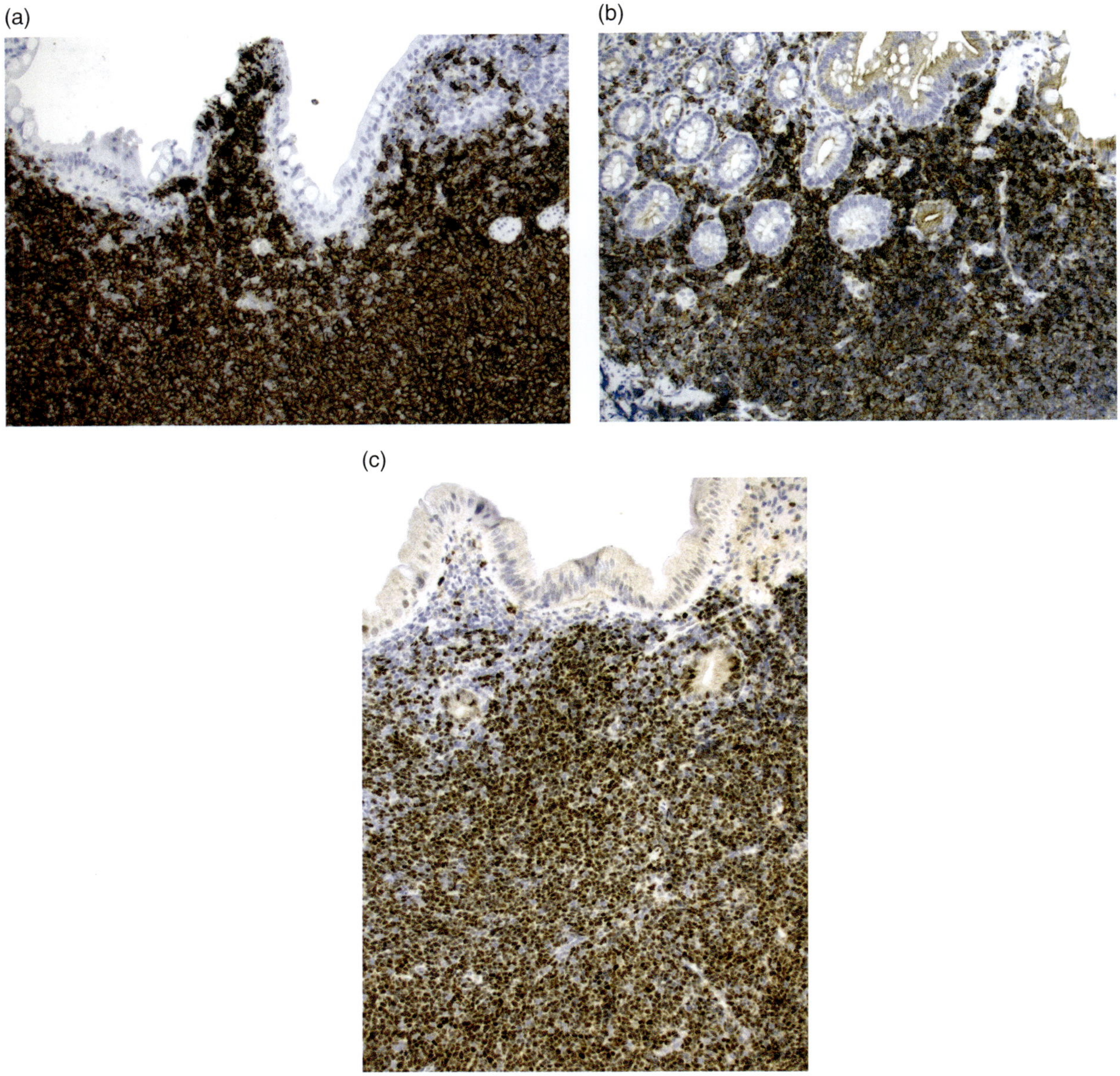

Figure 9.17 (a) Mantle cell lymphoma CD20. (b) Mantle cell lymphoma ileum CD5. (c) Mantle cell lymphoma ileum cyclin D1.

with a better prognosis than cases showing no expression. Mutations in Bcl-2 and Bcl-6 genes may be found. At least 10% of cases display a high proliferation index (>95%) by Ki67 stain. This is usually the result of additional mutations involving c-myc gene "double hit lymphoma." Rarely mutations of Bcl-2, Bcl-6 and c-myc occur, and these "triple hit" lymphomas are particularly aggressive.

Burkitt Lymphoma

Definition, General Features (Frequency), and Predisposing Factors

Burkitt lymphoma is an aggressive lymphoma occurring in both endemic (EBV infection associated) and sporadic forms. In both, gastrointestinal tract involvement has a predilection for the ileocecal region. Endemic areas are in Africa and the Middle East, with the latter region showing an increased predilection for intestinal disease. There is an increased risk for development in HIV-infected individuals.

Clinical Features/Endoscopic Characteristics

Clinical features are similar to other small bowel lymphomas discussed above.

Microscopic Features

Classical Burkitt lymphoma is characterized by a diffuse infiltrate of intermediate-sized cells with squared off cell borders, round nuclei, and 2–5 small- to medium-sized

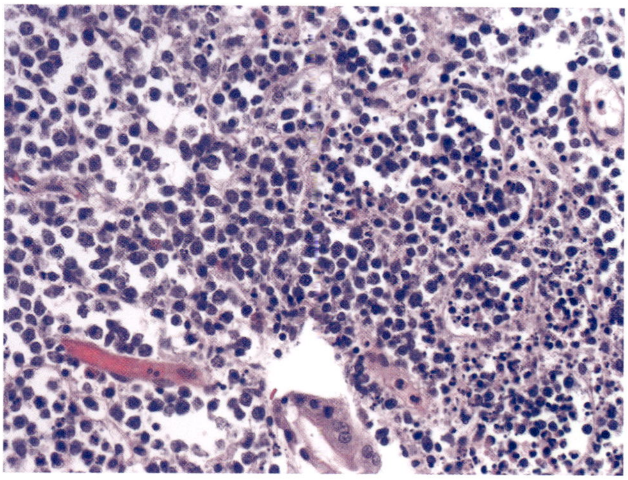

Figure 9.18 Burkitt lymphoma ileum.

paracentral nucleoli. Cytoplasmic vacuoles may be seen. Reflecting the high proliferation rate, numerous mitoses and apoptotic bodies are present, the latter being engulfed by histiocytes and imparting the characteristic "starry sky" appearance (Figure 9.18).

Immunohistochemical and Molecular Features (See Table 9.15; Figure 9.19a, b)

Differential Diagnosis

Other high-grade non-Hodgkins lymphomas of both B and T cell type. In practice, the most difficult separation is with diffuse, large B-cell lymphoma with c-myc-related double or triple hit mutation. Attention to the clinical setting, site of occurrence, and cell morphology are the most helpful features. Expression of EBV (EBVISH) is helpful in confirming endemic and immunodeficiency-related cases.

Treatment/Prognosis/Evolution

This is an aggressive tumor with rapid growth rate and high mortality if untreated. Perforation of the tumor site may occur after administration of chemotherapy.

Immunoproliferative Small Intestinal Disease (IPSID)/α-Heavy Chain Disease (Syn. Mediterranean Lymphoma)

Definition, Predisposing Factors (If Applicable)

This subtype of small intestinal MALT lymphoma predominantly occurs in young adults of Middle Eastern or Mediterranean origin. Infection with *Campylobacter jejuni* is associated with its development and early stage disease may respond to antibiotic therapy. Other risk factors include poor sanitation, concurrent parasitic infection, and low socioeconomic status.

Clinical Features/Endoscopic Characteristics

Clinical features are similar to other small bowel lymphomas discussed above.

Microscopic Features

Three stages of disease are recognized. In stage A, there is an infiltrate of essentially normal appearing lymphocytes and plasma cells in the mucosa without disturbance of villous architecture. In stage B, nodular collections of mildly

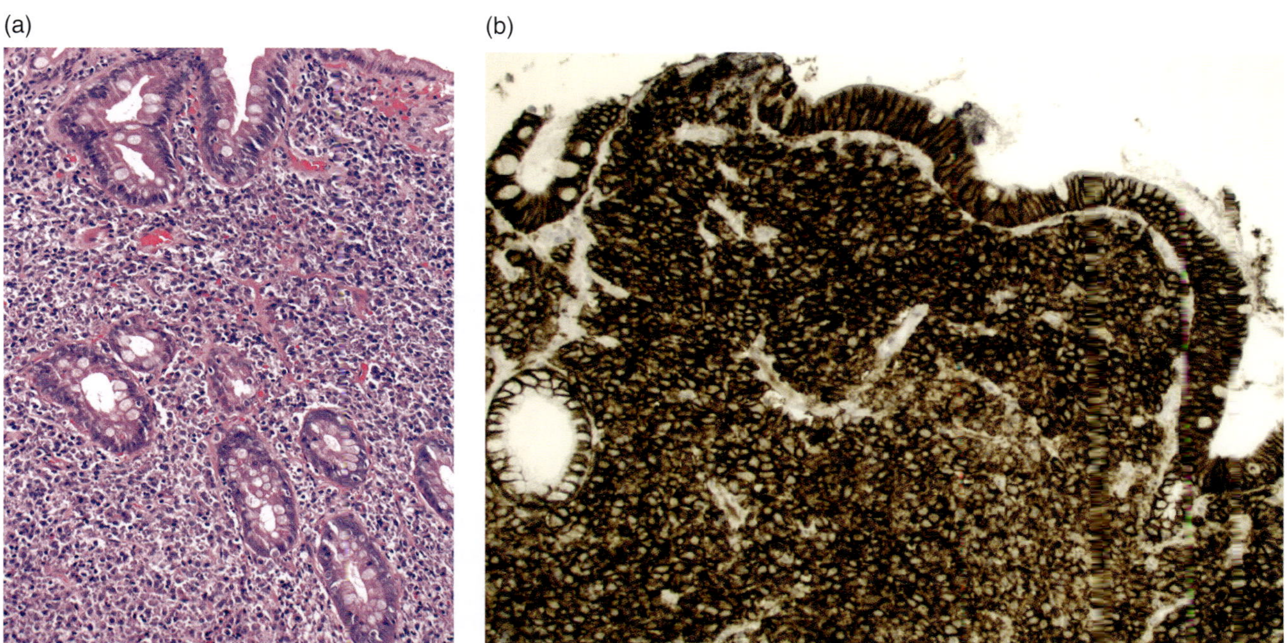

Figure 9.19 (a) IPSID. (b) IPSID CD138.

atypical lymphoid cells expand the lamina propria and cause villous blunting. Lymphoepithelial lesions and follicular colonization can be seen. Stage C disease is a fully developed malignancy with diffuse sheets of atypical, large cells, resembling immunoblasts or plasmablasts. Reed–Sternberg-like cells may be seen (Figure 9.19a).

Immunohistochemical and Molecular Features

The fully developed malignancy is characterized by positive staining for CD20, CD138 and α-heavy chain (but no light chain staining) (Figure 9.19b).

Differential Diagnosis

- Early in the disease, villous blunting and the plasma cell-rich infiltrate in the lamina propria can resemble celiac disease and other sprue conditions. The absence of intraepithelial lymphocytosis and the density of the infiltrate point to the diagnosis.
- Late, diffuse large B-cell lymphoma and plasmablastic lymphoma ought to be ruled out.

Spread

The disease commences in the proximal small intestine and spreads to involve the entire intestine, stomach, and colon.

Treatment/Prognosis/Evolution

Early stage disease often responds to antibiotic therapy (30–70% remission rate). Untreated IPSID progresses to lymphoplasmacytic and immunoblastic diffuse large cell lymphoma that invades the intestinal wall, involves mesenteric lymph nodes, and may metastasize to a distant organ. Later stage disease requires radiotherapy and chemotherapy.

B-Chronic Lymphocytic Leukemia/Small Lymphocytic Lymphoma

This lymphoma is uncommon in the small intestine and is generally only seen in advanced disease with poor prognosis. A diffuse small cell lymphoid infiltrate is seen. Sometimes there may be infiltration of the epithelium.

Post-transplant Lymphoproliferative Disorder

Definition, General Features, and Predisposing Factors

This lymphoproliferative disorder arises in immunosuppressed organ transplant recipients most often in association with EBV infection. Most cases are B-cell derived, although T-cell post-transplant lymphoproliferative disorder (PTLD) can be seen.

Immunosuppressive drugs required to prevent rejection are a predisposing factor. EBV infection is the main cofactor; however, it is not solely responsible for lymphomagenesis. Alterations in oncogenes and tumor suppressor genes and epigenetic changes, particularly hypermethylation, are important. Plasmacytoid dendritic cells that are activated by viral infections probably play a pathogenetic role, as do regulatory T cells, which modulate the immune reactions once incited by antigen.

Clinical Features/Endoscopic Characteristics

Clinical features are similar to other small bowel lymphomas discussed above.

Microscopic Features

There is a wide range of histopathologic findings from B-cell (plasma cell rich) hyperplasia to lymphoma. Table 9.16 provides a classification scheme. The lymphoma is most often polymorphic with an admixture of small lymphocytes, plasmacytoid cells, large immunoblastic cells, and occasional multilobated cells resembling Reed–Sternberg cells. Monomorphic lymphoma is usually a diffuse process with large immunoblastic or plasmoblastic cells. Geographic necrosis may be seen.

Immunohistochemical and Molecular Features

1) B-cell PTLD: The cells are immunoreactive with pan B-cell markers CD19, CD20, and CD79a. EBV in situ hybridization (EBV-ISH) is usually positive. Monoclonal expression of either kappa or lambda light

Table 9.16 Classification of post-transplant lymphoproliferative disorder (PTLD).

- **Early lesions**
  - Reactive plasmacytic hyperplasia
  - Infectious mononucleosis-like lesions
- **Polymorphic PTLD**
- **Monomorphic PTLD** (classified according to lymphoma they resemble)

B-cell neoplasms

- Diffuse large B-cell lymphoma (DLBCL)
- Burkitt's lymphoma
- Plasma cell myeloma
- Plasmacytoma-like lesions
- Others

T-cell neoplasms

- Peripheral T-cell lymphoma not otherwise specified
- Hepatosplenic T-cell lymphoma
- Others

- **Classical Hodgkin's lymphoma (HL)-type (HL-PTLD) and HL-like PTLD** chain is more common in monomorphic cases. PCR analysis of immunoglobulin gene rearrangement is often monoclonal.

2) T-cell PTLD: The tumor cells are immunoreactive with CD3 and CD5, and demonstrate clonal T-cell receptors $\alpha\beta$ or $\gamma\delta$ on PCR analysis.

Differential Diagnosis

In general the differential diagnosis may include a broad range of B- and T-cell NHL and also Hodgkin lymphoma, depending on the dominant morphologic pattern. The clinical setting should prompt consideration of the correct diagnosis.

Treatment/Prognosis/Evolution

Treatment of PTLD complex. Early polyclonal tumors and those associate with EBV may benefit from reduction in immunosuppression. Monoclonal tumors or tumors progressing after withdrawal of immunosuppression require additional treatment which may variously include chemotherapy, rituximab, radiotherapy, antiviral agents, and surgery.

T-Cell/NK-T Cell Non-Hodgkin Lymphoma

Ulcerative Jejunoileitis

Definition and Predisposing Factors (If Applicable)

This is a clinical syndrome of multiple intestinal ulcers, frequently complicated by hemorrhage, perforation, or obstruction, which is due to a celiac disease-related clonal T-cell proliferation.

Clinical Features/Endoscopic Characteristics

Clinical features are similar to other small bowel lymphomas discussed above.

Microscopic Features

There is a characteristic ulceration that extends into submucosa and occasionally deeper in the intestinal wall. Acute and chronic inflammation, fibrosis, and pseudopyloric gland metaplasia are present in preserved mucosa. Features of celiac disease are usually evident in the adjacent mucosa sometimes with superimposed changes of collagenous sprue.

Immunohistochemical and Molecular Features

The intraepithelial lymphocytes demonstrate an aberrant immunophenotype identical to RCD2 in the majority of cases. TCR monoclonality is present.

Differential Diagnosis

- This includes other causes of multifocal ulceration—drug injury (e.g. NSAIDs), vasculitis, and Crohn's disease. These lack a history or serological evidence of celiac disease and/or celiac disease enteropathy changes in the surrounding mucosa.
- Enteropathy-associated T-cell lymphoma—this forms a disease spectrum with ulcerative jejunitis and separation is based on the identification of a mass lesion.

Spread (Considered an In Situ Malignancy)

Ulcerative jejunitis may progress to enteropathy-associated T-cell lymphoma.

Treatment/Prognosis/Evolution

Surgical resection is often required to treat the complications of hemorrhage, perforation, or stricture formation.

Enteropathy-Associated T-Cell Lymphoma (Enteropathy-Type T-Cell Lymphoma, Intestinal T-Cell Lymphoma, ETTL)

Definition, General Features, and Predisposing Factors

This is a T-cell malignancy that usually, but not exclusively, arises in association with gluten-sensitive enteropathy.

The association of this lymphoma with celiac disease is based on the following evidence: (i) presence of celiac disease enteropathy in the adjacent mucosa; (ii) history of longstanding celiac disease in up to 10% of patients; (iii) enteropathy-associated T-cell lymphoma prevalence parallels celiac disease prevalence; and (iv) high prevalence of HLA DQ2 haplotype in both diseases.

Clinical Features/Endoscopic Characteristics

The clinical features are similar to other small bowel lymphomas discussed above.

Microscopic Features

Two morphological variants are recognized: (i) *monomorphic*—this variant is the more common, composed of intermediate to large cells with abundant pale eosinophilic cytoplasm and round or slightly irregular central nuclei with prominent nucleoli and (ii) *anaplastic*—this variant is composed of markedly pleomorphic multinucleated cells with abundant pale cytoplasm. There is an associated inflammatory infiltrate of histiocytes and eosinophils, the latter may be so marked as to obscure the tumor cells. Ulceration is frequent. The adjacent mucosa commonly shows features of celiac disease.

Immunohistochemical and Molecular Features

ETTL is a T-cell lymphoma. The typical immunophenotype is CD3+, CD5−, CD7+, CD4−, CD8− (occasional+),

CD103+, cytotoxic T-cell marker (TIA, granzyme, perforin) + and CD56− (rare +). In addition, the anaplastic variant is usually CD30+, but CD3− and CD8−.

PCR is clonal for TCRβ and TCRγ gene rearrangement.

HLA subtyping usually reveals HLA DQ2 and/or DQ8 haplotype. HLADQ2 homozygosity may occur and represents a genetic predisposition for ETTL

Chromosomal analysis displays gains at 1q32.2-q41, 5q34-q35.2, and 9q31.3-qter (most cases) and a loss at 16q12.1 (25%).

Differential Diagnosis

- Monomorphic CD56+ intestinal T-cell lymphoma—this neoplasm is also referred to as type II enteropathy-associated T-cell lymphoma because of its intestinal site of occurrence and the presence of villous blunting and conspicuous intraepithelial lymphocytosis in the adjacent mucosa. There is, however, no association with celiac disease either clinically or genetically. Tumor cells are characteristically CD8+ and CD56+. EBV is not detectable in this tumor excluding nasal type NK/T-cell lymphoma.
- Other T-cell lymphoma—in particular, anaplastic large cell lymphoma (CD30+ and ALK-1) and nasal type NK/T-cell lymphoma (CD56+, EBER+). No association with celiac disease is present with these lymphomas.
- B-cell lymphoma—diffuse large B-cell lymphoma is T-cell marker (CD3) negative and B-cell marker (CD20, CD79a) positive.
- Non-hematological malignancy—metastatic melanoma.

Spread

Systemic dissemination such as liver and spleen may be seen.

Treatment/Prognosis/Evolution

Prognosis is poor, resulting from severe malnutrition or complication of intestinal perforation.

Extranodal NK/T-Cell Lymphoma, Nasal Type (ENKTL)

Definition, General Features, and Predisposing Factors (If Applicable)

This mostly extranodal EBV infection-related lymphoma, known previously as polymorphic reticulosis or lethal midline granuloma, is usually of NK-cell origin but may be of T-cell origin. It is most commonly encountered in adult males of East Asian or South American origin. The gut is one of the more frequent sites of occurrence.

Clinical Features/Endoscopic Characteristics

Clinical features are similar to other small bowel lymphomas discussed above.

Microscopic Features

The lymphoma is pleomorphic with an admixture of small and large malignant cells together with a background of eosinophils, plasma cells, and histiocytes. Angioinvasive and angiodestructive growth is characteristic and is associated with zones of necrosis and prominent karyorrhectic debris. In some tumors there is predominance of small cells without necrosis.

Immunohistochemical and Molecular Features

Most cases have an NK-cell immunophenotype: CD2+, CD45RO+, CD43+, CD56+. Clonality for T-cell receptor is $\alpha\beta$− and $\gamma\delta$−. Surface CD3 is usually absent, but cytoplasmic CD3 may be detected on paraffin sections because of NK cells containing an epsilon (ε) chain of the CD3 molecular that is recognized by a CD3 immunohistochemical stain.

T-cell cases are characterized by surface CD3 expression and clonal T-cell receptor $\alpha\beta$+ or $\gamma\delta$+. EBV genome is demonstrable (EBV-ISH+).

Differential Diagnoses

- Reactive and infectious processes associated with extensive necrosis (e.g. *Mycobacterium tuberculosis* infection). Attention to atypia in the lymphoid cells allows distinction.
- Other large cell lymphomas, particularly those displaying angioinvasive growth. Immunophenotypic characterization separates most cases.
- Vasculitis—the finding of an extensive and atypical lymphoid infiltrate alerts to the possibility of lymphoma.
- NK-cell enteropathy—an expanding range of benign NK-cell proliferations is recognized. These may involve the gastrointestinal tract and be sufficiently dense as to cause concern for lymphoma. EBV infection is involved in the pathogenesis of some cases.

Treatment/Prognosis/Evolution

Aggressive with high mortality. Localized disease may respond to radiotherapy.

Hodgkin Lymphoma

Hodgkin lymphoma is overwhelmingly a nodal disease and is very unlikely to present in the small intestine in primary form. A primary enteric lymphoma with Reed–Sternberg-like cells is more likely to represent a form of T-cell lymphoma or PTLD.

Hematopoetic Disorders with Plasmacytic Differentiation

Primary enteric plasmacytoma is rare. Well-differentiated lesions may mimic a primary plasma cell-rich inflammatory process. The near absence of other inflammatory cells is a clue, and evaluation of Kappa and Lambda light chains is usually diagnostic, showing light chain restriction. Plasma cell-rich MALT lymphoma and IPSID are other diagnostic possibilities. Absence of reaction with the B-cell marker CD20 is a clue to excluding a form of B-cell lymphoma. The plasma cell nature of the tumor can be confirmed by CD38 and CD138 positivity. Poorly differentiated lesions ("anaplastic plasmacytoma") have a broad differential diagnosis including high-grade lymphoma, metastatic melanoma, and carcinoma. With respect to the latter, it should be remembered that some adenocarcinomas will express CD138 and plasmacytoma may express EMA.

Plasmablastic Lymphoma

Plasmablastic lymphoma is a rare aggressive B-cell lymphoproliferative disorder that is most commonly encountered in the oral cavity of HIV-positive patients. Small intestinal location is well described and non-immunosuppressed, but often elderly patients are being increasingly seen. Microscopically this is a large cell lymphoma with plasmacytic differentiation, and reactivity for CD79a, CD138, CD38, and CD10 is positive. EMA may also be expressed. The Ki67 proliferation index is typically high.

Lymphoplasmacytic Lymphoma

Lymphoplasmacytic lymphoma is a B-cell lymphoma with plasmacytic differentiation that underlies most cases of Waldenstrom's macroglobulinemia. The latter is characterized by deposition of IgM paraprotein producing eosinophilic, homogenous, and strongly PAS+, a process that begins within villous lymphatics and eventually fills the lamina propria.

Other

Extensive plasmacytic differentiation may be encountered in MALT lymphoma, IPSID and PTLD.

Other Hematopoetic Disorders

Mastocytosis

Definition/Clinical Features

Mastocytosis of the small intestine is part of a systemic process that seldom involves only the gastrointestinal tract; however, this may be the initial site of presentation of disease. The colon and terminal ileum are most commonly involved. Concurrent bone marrow involvement is typical and a leukemic form (mast cell leukemia) is sometimes encountered. In the intestine, lesions may be single and present as a polyp or multifocal and plaque like or indistinct.

Microscopic Features

The infiltrate is characterized by round to spindle-shaped cells expanding the lamina propria. The round cells frequently display cytoplasmic clearing leading to a "fried egg"-like appearance. The cells tend to collect around the glands and to form a dense superficial band. The process may be patchy. An associated eosinophil infiltrate is usual and can overwhelm the background mast cells, leading to an inaccurate diagnosis of eosinophilic enteritis. A rare pleomorphic tumor variant (mast cell sarcoma) has been described. Toluidine blue histochemical stain has been superseded by immunochemistry for c-kit and mast cell tryptase. CD25 reaction is highly specific for neoplastic Mast cells and confirms the diagnosis of systemic mastocytosis. Consensus criteria have been established and are presented in Table 9.17. Systemic mastocytosis is the result of a mutation of the gene encoding for the c-kit (tyrosine kinase) receptor (Figure 9.20a–c).

Table 9.17 Diagnostic criteria for systemic mastocytosis.

Major	
Multifocal dense aggregates of mast cells with more than 15 cells per aggregate in an extracutaneous tissue	
Minor	
1)	Greater than 25% of mast cells have morphologic abnormalities, e.g. spindle shape, irregular outline.
2)	Expression of CD25 with or without CD2 by mast cells.
3)	Detection of a codon 816 c-kit mutation by a sensitive technique in lesional tissue or peripheral blood.
4)	Serum baseline tryptase greater than 20 ng/ml.
Diagnosis = one major and one minor criterion or three minor criteria	

Source: Modified from Akin, C. and Valent, P. (2014). Diagnostic criteria and classification of mastocytosis in 2014. *Immunol. Allergy Clin. N. Am.* 34 (2): 207–218.

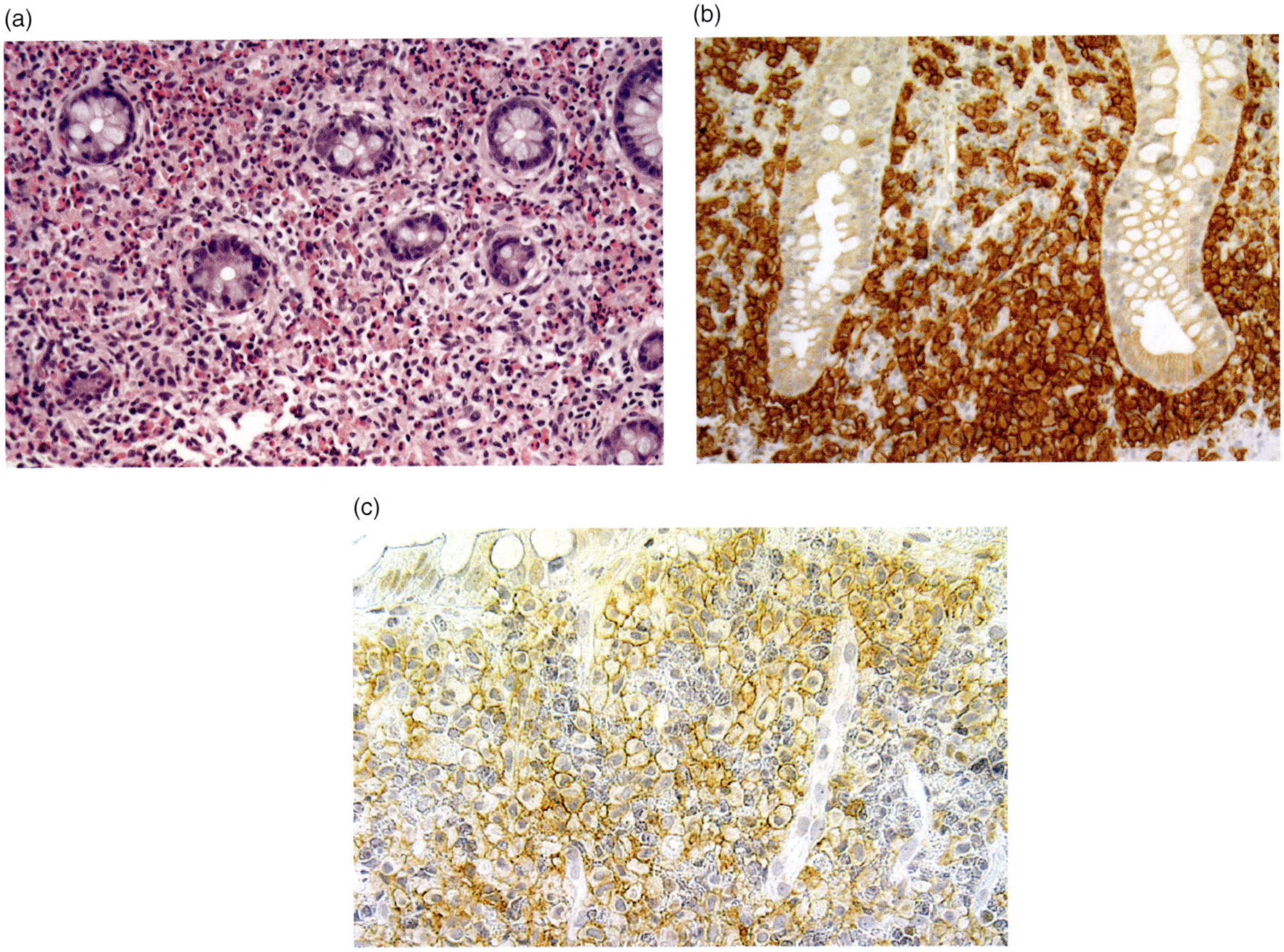

Figure 9.20 (a) Mastocytosis rich in eosinophils. (b) CD117 mastocytosis. (c) CD25 mastocytosis.

Treatment/Evolution/Prognosis

Mutation analysis of the c-kit gene may be beneficial as some mutations (except the common codon 816 mutation) are associated with a favorable response to tyrosine kinase receptor antagonists.

Leukemia

Leukemic infiltration of the small intestine is rare. When present there is generally evidence of systemic disease, although it may signal relapse following previous remission. Chronic lymphocytic leukemia, acute myeloid (myelogenous) leukemia, and acute lymphoblastic leukemia are most commonly encountered.

Granulocytic sarcoma refers to an extramedullary tumor of myeloblasts and/or immature myeloid cells. It is often a forerunner to the development of acute myelogenous leukemia, and may also signal impending blast crisis in the setting of a myeloproliferative disorder or leukemic transformation in myelodysplastic syndrome. It is sometimes a primary presentation of disease, and the small intestine is the most common site of occurrence in the gut. It tends to present as a polyp or larger sometime ulcerated mass. Microscopically, there is a diffuse infiltration of medium to large cells with occasional prominent nucleoli and minimal to moderate eosinophilic cytoplasm. A variable number of admixed maturing eosinophils and neutrophils are typically present in the more differentiated lesion. CD43 staining of tumor cells in the absence of CD3 staining lysozyme, CD34, CD117, and myeloperoxidase (MPO). Flow cytometry also is helpful. Characteristic cytogenetic abnormalities t(8; 21)(q22;q22) and inv(16)(p13q22) are often found. Treatment should consist of systemic chemotherapy tailored to the treatment of AML, possibly in conjunction with surgical resection or radiation.

Table 9.18 Histiocytic disorders of the small intestine.

Xanthogranulomatous inflammation
Infections rich in histiocytic cells (e.g. Whipple's disease, MAIC)
Neoplasms, e.g. Rosai–Dorfman disease, Langerhans cell histiocytosis, juvenile xanthogranuloma, Erdheim–Chester disease, crystal storing histiocytosis, histiocytic sarcoma
Malakoplakia

Histiocytic Disorders

Xanthoma

This collection of benign foamy histiocytes may form single or multiple tumors. These may involve the mucosa only or the full thickness of the intestinal wall. Xanthomas are asymptomatic unless large. Hyperlipidemia is an infrequent association in contradistinction to soft tissue xanthoma. A response to local mucosal injury is postulated as the etiology in most cases. The histiocytic nature of the cells is confirmed by immunoreactivity for histiocytic makers (e.g. CD68). The main diagnostic considerations are included Table 9.18.

Malakoplakia

This mass forming reactive process is caused by the accumulation of histiocytes unable to process bacterial products (usually derived from *Escherichia coli*). The mucosa of the terminal ileum is most commonly involved. Malakoplakia is characterized by sheets of histiocytes with abundant granular eosinophilic that contain basophilic, periodic acid—Schiff (PAS)-positive, diastase-resistant inclusions, and diagnostic targetoid Michaelis–Gutmann bodies. The latter are gray to blue with H&E and are positive for calcium von Kossa stain and iron Perls stain. The histiocytes are positive for CD68 antibody. Xanthogranulomatous inflammation is the main differential diagnosis but lacks the characteristic Michaelis–Gutmann bodies.

Langerhans Cell Histiocytosis

Small intestinal involvement is rare. It may affect adults as well as children and mostly presents as a polyp forming mucosal infiltrate measuring less than 10 mm diameter. The lesion is mostly well circumscribed and contains sheets of polygonal cells with moderate pink slightly granular cytoplasm. The nuclei are characteristically grooved and are occasionally folded. An infiltrate, sometimes prominent, of eosinophils and lymphocytes may accompany the tumor. Mucosal ulceration, reactive and/or entrapped epithelial elements, focal necrosis, and multinucleated giant cells can be seen. The lesions express S-100 protein and CD1a. Adult cases are typically solitary polyps that are cured by polypectomy. In contrast, pediatric cases are usually associated with systemic disease and a poor prognosis.

Metastases to the Small Intestine Mucosa

Definition

It is defined as tumor of the small intestinal wall that originated from a remote, typically extraintestinal site. Spread is via direct invasion, transcoelomic spread, or vascular/lymphatic permeation.

General Features (Frequency)

Intraluminal small intestinal metastases are very rare although extraluminal small bowel deposits are very common for many abdominal cavity tumors (colon, ovarian, appendiceal) as well as extra-abdominal (melanoma, lung, breast).

Clinical Features/Endoscopic Characteristics

The clinical and endoscopic features are nonspecific, typically bleeding and obstruction due to ulceration of the tumor.

Microscopic Features

Most small intestinal metastases are not diagnosed on endoscopic biopsies either because their complications such as obstruction, perforation, or hemorrhage require emergent surgical intervention or because they are located within the deep submucosa or muscularis propria and are therefore not accessible to biopsy forceps. Mostly, metastases are readily distinguished by distinctive morphology and lack of an in situ component. Immunohistochemistry may be required to determine the site of origin.

Differential Diagnosis

Melanoma is the most common metastatic tumor and causes the most diagnostic difficulty because of variable morphology. The major differential diagnostic considerations include:

- GIST
- Clear cell sarcoma
- Lymphoma
- Carcinoma

Treatment/Prognosis/Evolution

Metastatic disease in the small intestine is a marker of advanced disease.

Further Reading

Akin, C. and Valent, P. (2014). Diagnostic criteria and classification of mastocytosis in 2014. *Immunol. Allergy Clin. N. Am.* 34 (2): 207–218.

Al-Saleem, T. and Al-Mondhiry, H. (2005). Immunoproliferative small intestinal disease (IPSID): a model for mature B-cell neoplasms. *Blood* 105 (6): 2274–2280.

Arps, D.P. and Smith, L.B. (2013). Classic versus type II enteropathy-associated T-cell lymphoma: diagnostic considerations. *Arch. Pathol. Lab. Med.* 137 (9): 1227–1231.

Banks, P.M. (2007). Gastrointestinal lymphoproliferative disorders. *Histopathology* 50 (1): 42–54.

Chen, Z.M., Scudiere, J.R., Abraham, S.C., and Montgomery, E. (2009). Pyloric gland adenoma: an entity distinct from gastric foveolar type adenoma. *Am. J. Surg. Pathol.* 33 (2): 186–193.

Chu, P.G., Schwarz, R.E., Lau, S.K. et al. (2005). Immunohistochemical staining of pancreatobiliary and ampulla of Vater adenocarcinoma: application of CDX2, CK17, MUC1, and MUC2. *Am. J. Surg. Pathol.* 29 (3): 359–367.

Daum, O., Hatlova, J., Mandys, V. et al. (2010). Comparison of morphological, immunohistochemical, and molecular genetic features of inflammatory fibroid polyps (Vanek's tumors). *Virchows Arch.* 456: 491–497.

De Petris, G. and Leung, S.T. (2010). Pseudoneoplasms of the gastrointestinal tract. *Arch. Pathol. Lab. Med.* 134 (3): 378–392.

Detlefsen, S., Fagerberg, C.R., Ousager, L.B. et al. (2013). Histiocytic disorders of the gastrointestinal tract. *Hum. Pathol.* 44 (5): 683–696.

Doyle, L.A. and Hornick, J.L. (2014). Gastrointestinal stromal tumors: from KIT to succinate dehydrogenase. *Histopathology* 64 (1): 53–67.

Doyle, L.A. and Hornick, J.L. (2014). Pathology of extramedullary mastocytosis. *Immunol. Allergy Clin. N. Am.* 34 (2): 323–339.

Ferry, J.A. (2008). Extranodal lymphoma. *Arch. Pathol. Lab. Med.* 132: 565–578.

Gao, Y.P., Zhu, J.S., and Zheng, W.J. (2004). Brunner's gland adenoma of duodenum: a case report and literature review. *World J. Gastroenterol.* 10 (17): 2616–2617.

Ho-Yen, C., Chang, F., van der Walt, J. et al. (2009). Recent advances in refractory coeliac disease: a review. *Histopathology* 54 (7): 783–795.

Ibrahim, H.A. and Naresh, K.N. (2012). Posttransplant lymphoproliferative disorders. *Adv. Hematol.* 2012: 230173.

Khor, T.S., Brown, I., Kattampallil, J. et al. (2010). Duodenal adenocarcinoma arising from a pyloric gland adenoma with a brief review of the literature. *BMJ Case Rep.* https://doi.org/10.1136/bcr.10.2010.3385.

Klöppel, G., Rindi, G., Anlauf, M. et al. (2007). Site-specific biology and pathology of gastroenteropancreatic neuroendocrine tumors. *Virchows Arch.* 451 (Suppl 1): S9–S27.

Klöppel, G., Couvelard, A., Perren, A. et al. (2009). ENETS consensus guidelines for the standards of care in neuroendocrine tumors: towards a standardized approach to the diagnosis of gastroenteropancreatic neuroendocrine tumors and their prognostic stratification. *Neuroendocrinology* 90: 162–166.

Kohl, S.K. and Aoun, P. (2006). Granulocytic sarcoma of the small intestine. *Arch. Pathol. Lab. Med.* 130 (10): 1570–1574.

Lasota, J., Wang, Z.F., Sobin, L.H., and Miettinen, M. (2009). Gain of function PDGFRA mutations, earlier reported in gastrointestinal stromal tumors, are common in small intestinal inflammatory fibroid polyps. A study of 60 cases. *Mod. Pathol.* 22 (8): 1049–1056.

Lecuit, M., Abachin, E., Martin, A. et al. (2004). Immunoproliferative small intestinal disease associated with *Campylobacter jejuni*. *N. Engl. J. Med.* 350 (3): 239–248.

Levine, J.A., Burgart, L.J., Batts, K.P., and Wang, K.K. (1995). Brunner's gland hamartomas: clinical presentation and pathological features of 27 cases. *Am. J. Gastroenterol.* 90: 290–294.

Liu, T.C., Lin, M.T., Montgomery, E.A., and Singhi, A.D. (2013). Inflammatory fibroid polyps of the gastrointestinal tract: spectrum of clinical, morphologic, and immunohistochemistry features. *Am. J. Surg. Pathol.* 37 (4): 586–592.

Mansoor, A., Pittaluga, S., Beck, P.L. et al. (2011). NK-cell enteropathy: a benign NK-cell lymphoproliferative disease mimicking intestinal lymphoma: clinicopathologic features and follow-up in a unique case series. *Blood* 117 (5): 1447–1452.

Matysiak-Budnik, T., Jamet, P., Fabiani, B. et al. (2013). Primary intestinal B-cell lymphoma: a prospective multicentre clinical study of 91 cases. *Dig. Liver Dis.* 45 (11): 947–952.

Miettinen, M. and Lasota, J. (2013). Gastrointestinal stromal tumors. *Gastroenterol. Clin. N. Am.* 42 (2): 399–415.

Misdraji, J., Harris, N.L., Hasserjian, R.P. et al. (2011). Primary follicular lymphoma of the gastrointestinal tract. *Am. J. Surg. Pathol.* 35 (9): 1255–1263.

Neugut, A.I. and Santos, J. (1993). The association between cancers of the small and large bowel. *Cancer Epidemiol. Biomark. Prev.* 2 (6): 551–553.

Nielsen, S.L., Ingeholm, P., Holck, S., and Talbot, I. (2007). Xanthomatosis of the gastrointestinal tract with focus on small bowel involvement. *J. Clin. Pathol.* 60 (10): 1164–1166.

O'Malley, D.P., Goldstein, N.S., and Banks, P.M. (2014). The recognition and classification of lymphoproliferative disorders of the gut. *Hum. Pathol.* 45 (5): 899–916.

Rindi, G., Kloppel, G., Alhman, H. et al. (2006). TNM staging of foregut (neuro)endocrine tumors: a consensus proposal including a grading system. *Virchows Arch.* 449: 395–401.

Rosty, C., Buchanan, D.D., Walters, R.J. et al. (2011). Hyperplastic polyp of the duodenum: a report of 9 cases with immunohistochemical and molecular findings. *Hum. Pathol.* 42 (12): 1953–1959.

Rosty, C., Campbell, C., Clendenning, M. et al. (2014). Do serrated neoplasms of the small intestine represent a distinctive entity? Pathological findings and molecular alterations in a series of 13 cases. *Histopathology* 66 (3): 333–342.

Rubio, C.A. (2004). Serrated adenoma of the duodenum. *J. Clin. Pathol.* 57 (11): 1219–1221.

Said, J., Lones, M., and Yea, S. (2014). Burkitt lymphoma and MYC: what else is new? *Adv. Anat. Pathol.* 21 (3): 160–165.

Saurin, J., Gutknecht, C., Napoleon, B. et al. (2004). Surveillance of duodenal adenomas in familial adenomatous polyposis reveals high cumulative risk of advanced disease. *J. Clin. Oncol.* 22: 493.

Schildhaus, H.U., Caviar, T., Binot, E. et al. (2008) Inflammatory fibroid polyps harbour mutations in the platelet-derived growth factor receptor alpha (PDGFRA) gene. *J. Pathol.* 216 (2): 176–182.

Singhi, A.D. and Montgomery, E.A. (2011). Gastrointestinal tract langerhans cell histiocytosis: a clinicopathologic study of 12 patients. *Am. J. Surg. Pathol.* 35 (2): 305–310.

Soga, J. and Tazawa, K. (1971). Pathologic analysis of carcinoids; histologic re-evaluation of 62 cases. *Cancer* 28: 990–998.

Sundararajan, V., Robinson-Smith, T.M. and Lowy, A.M. (2003). Duodenal gangliocytic paraganglioma with lymph node metastasis: a case report and review of the literature. *Arch. Pathol. Lab. Med.* 127 (3): 139–141.

Takata, K., Sato, Y., Nakamura, N. et al. (2013). Duodenal follicular lymphoma lacks AID but expresses BACH2 and has memory B-cell characteristics. *Mod. Pathol.* 26 (1): 22–31.

Vieth, M., Kushima, R., Borchard, F., and Stolte, M. (2003). Pyloric gland adenoma: a clinico-pathological analysis of 90 cases. *Virchows Arch.* 442 (4): 317–321.

Wang, H.W., Yang, W., Sun, J.Z. et al. (2012). Plasmablastic lymphoma of the small intestine: case report and literature review. *World J. Gastroenterol.* 18 (45) 6677–6681.

WHO Classification of Tumors Editorial Board. Digestive System Tumors. Lyon (France): International Agency for Research on Cancer; 2019 (WHO classification of tumors series; 5th ed.; vol 1)

10

Inflammatory Conditions of the Colon

Tze Sheng Khor[1], Till S. Clauditz[2], Bence Kővári[3], Gregory Y. Lauwers[4], Michael B. Wallace[5] and Priyanthi Kumarasinghe[1]

[1] *Department of Anatomical Pathology, PathWest, QE II Medical Centre, Univ. of Western Australia, Perth, Australia*
[2] *Department of Pathology, University-Medical-Center Hamburg-Eppendorf, Hamburg, Germany*
[3] *Department of Pathology, University of Szeged, Szeged, Hungary*
[4] *Moffitt Cancer Center, Tampa, Florida, USA*
[5] *Mayo Clinic, Jacksonville, Florida, USA*

Non-Idiopathic Inflammatory Colitides

Infectious Colitis

Definition, General Features, and Predisposing Factors

Infectious colitis is commonly a self-limiting disease resolving within two to four weeks. The term "acute self-limiting colitis" is used to refer to a transient diarrheal illness and biopsy findings consistent with an infectious etiology but without microbiologic confirmation. Common risk factors include poor sanitation including poor food preparation standards, poor personal hygiene, and overcrowded conditions. Immunosuppressed individuals are also at increased risk.

Clinical Features and Endoscopic Features

Acute onset (sometimes bloody) diarrhea, abdominal cramps, and fever are common presentations. Colonoscopic findings include mucosal granularity and friability, erosions, and bleeding. Mass lesions and pseudomembranes may be seen occasionally. In most cases, the changes resolve rapidly and spontaneously.

Microscopic Features

A spectrum of histologic findings is suggestive of the diagnosis.

First, edema of the lamina propria, sometimes with focal hemorrhage, will develop. Synchronously, a mixed acute and chronic infiltrate can be noted in the superficial lamina propria, with neutrophils clustering adjacent to dilated capillaries. Scattered cryptitis and crypt abscesses can be noted. The mucosal architecture is generally preserved. Epithelial regenerative changes, including mucin depletion and increased mitoses, are usually detected. Flattening of the epithelium may be seen leading to dilatation of the luminal half of crypts, or may involve the crypt length with elliptical dilatation of the crypts ("withering" crypts), sometimes with epithelial bridging across the crypt lumen ("string of pearls").

In the second to third week of the disease, neutrophils disappear and the mononuclear cell population increases. If the infection persists, the mononuclear cells begin to expand in a pattern reminiscent of inflammatory bowel disease (IBD), with extension into the lower third. Lymphoid aggregates are occasionally observed. Finally, colonic lymphocytosis, i.e. patchy increased intraepithelial lymphocytes (IELs), may be seen during the resolution phase.

The etiologic diagnosis relies on laboratory tests as well as proper biopsy evaluation (Table 10.1). Ancillary studies that may aid in diagnosis include histochemical and immunoperoxidase stains, electron microscopy, in situ hybridization, and PCR-based molecular techniques. Fungi may be highlighted with either Gomori or PAS stains. Acid-fast bacillus (AFB) stains, including Ziehl–Neelsen and Wade–Fite, are useful in identifying tuberculosis or *Mycobacterium avium*. Microsporidia may be highlighted by Gram or Giemsa stains, while trichrome and PAS stains may help identify amebae. Ultrastructural examination aids in the identification of spirochetes, microsporidia, and some protozoans.

Differential Diagnosis

Infectious colitis needs to be distinguished from early IBD, acute self-limiting colitis (ASLC; Figure 10.1), ischemic colitis, and iatrogenic colitis. Excluding these conditions rests on good clinical judgment with thorough evaluation

Table 10.1 Selected antibodies and PCR assays useful in the diagnosis of infectious agents.

Organism	Antibody	PCR
Campylobacter	√	√
E. coli	√	
Shigella	√	
Salmonella	√	
Yersinia		√
Rotavirus	√	
Adenovirus	√	
Enterovirus		√

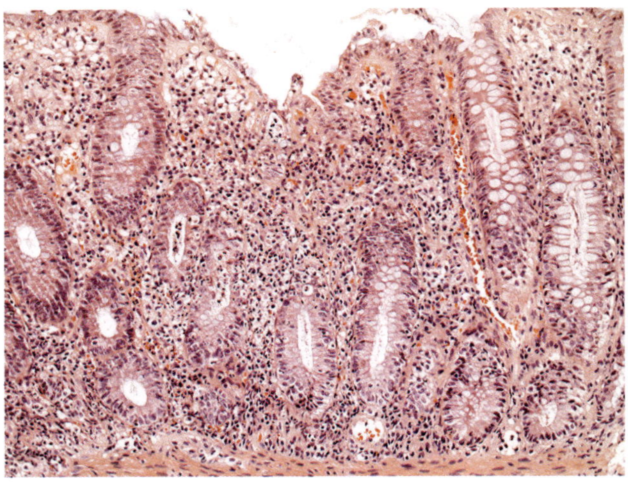

Figure 10.1 Biopsies of acute self-limiting colitis (ASLC) show a preserved mucosal architecture with a severe inflammation caused by neutrophils characterized by cryptitis and crypt abscesses.

of a combination of clinicopathologic features based on good communication between pathologists and clinicians. The key differential histologic features are summarized in Table 10.2.

Specific Etiologic Agents

A complete and exhaustive review of all pathologies and their characteristics goes beyond the scope of this work, and the reader is directed to specialized textbooks.

Bacterial

Common Enteric Bacterial Pathogens

Salmonella, Campylobacter, Enterohemorrhagic Escherichia coli O157:H7, Shigella and *Yersinia* are among the more common bacterial causes of infectious colitis. In general, mucosal invasive organisms produce more severe histological changes, while diseases caused by toxin production tend to produce less severe morphological changes. Common bacterial pathogens grouped according to their associated histologic patterns are summarized in Tables 10.2 and 10.3.

Mycobacterium tuberculosis

Most cases are due to *M. tuberculosis,* with *Mycobacterium bovis* being less common following pasteurization of milk (<1.5% of all cases). The latter, once rare in the West, has been associated with an increase in incidence because of the rush to non-pasteurized milk. The terminal ileum, cecum, and appendix are most frequently involved, whether primary or secondary. Three forms are reported: (i) ulcerative (~60% of cases); (ii) hypertrophic (10%), with fibrous scarring and mass-like lesions (mimicking Crohn's disease); and (iii) ulcerohypertrophic (30%), with thickening of the intestinal wall, ulceration, and formation of an inflammatory mass. It is noteworthy that pulmonary pathology and lymphadenopathy may not be detected. On colonoscopy, broad ulcers, strictures, and mucosal bridges, edematous or patulous ileocecal valve, and hypertrophic inflammatory masses can be seen.

The diagnosis can be easy when large caseating granulomas (aggregates of epithelioid cells and Langerhans giant cells with central caseation) and surrounding lymphoid cuff are detected (Figure 10.2). These can be found within the lamina propria or submucosa of intact mucosa or at the base of ulcers. The diagnostic yield is increased by having multiple biopsies and levels. The intact mucosa usually displays nonspecific chronic inflammation, and evidence of chronicity with architectural distortion and pyloric metaplasia. Aphthous ulcers over lymphoid follicles, cryptitis, and crypt abscess formation also are frequent.

Acid fast stains (AFB) may demonstrate typical organisms within granulomas. The highest positive yield for their detection is from an ulcer, especially if part of an ulcerated mass.

The differential diagnosis of granulomatous colitis is broad, but primarily includes Crohn's disease and Yersinia (see Table 10.4). Features that suggest TB include numerous or the presence of large (>400 µm) confluent granulomas with a lymphoid cuff, granulomas located in the submucosa or in granulation tissue often as palisaded epithelioid histiocytes, and disproportionate submucosal inflammation. Crohn's disease instead is characterized by infrequent (<5), discrete, and small (<200 µm in size) poorly organized mucosal granulomas. Aggregates of histiocytes, pericryptal granulomas, and focally active colitis are other features supporting a diagnosis of Crohn's disease.

Other Mycobacterial Infections

While *M. avium* complex (MAC) is usually restricted to the lung in immunocompetent individuals, disseminated infection is commonly observed in AIDS patients.

Table 10.2 Differential diagnosis of acute infectious-type (self-limiting) colitis (ASLC) from acute idiopathic inflammatory bowel disease (IIBD).

Feature	IIBD	ASLC	Ischemic colitis	Iatrogenic colitis
Architectural distortion	++	–	–/+	–/+[a]
"Withering crypts"	–	–/+[b]	++	–/+[c]
Lamina propria hyalinization	–	–/+[b]	++	–/+[c]
Fibrin platelet thrombi	–	–/+[b]	++	–/+[c]
Paneth cell metaplasia	+	–	–/+	–/+[c]
Villiform surface transformation	+	–	–	–
Basal plasmacytosis (in the lower fifth of mucosa)	++	–	–	–/+[a]
Basal lymphoid aggregates	++	–	–	–
Increased lamina propria lymphocytes and plasma cells	++	–/+	–	–/–[a]
Crypt abscesses	++	+/–	–/+	–/–
Giant cells	Basal	Superficial	–/+	–
Cryptitis	++	+	–/+	–/–
Edema	+/–	++	+	–/–
Pure neutrophil infiltrate/neutrophil predominance	–	+	–	–

[a] Histologic features of chronicity identical to that seen in IBD can sometimes be seen with certain medications, particularly NSAIDS.
[b] Withering crypts may sometimes be seen in ASLC but lacks other features of ischemia including focal crypt dropout, lamina propria hyalinosis, hemosiderin or fibrin platelet thrombi. In some forms of infectious colitis, however, such as EHEC colitis, there is a superimposed ischemic component and features of ischemia are mixed with an ASLC pattern.
[c] Certain medications, e.g. oral contraceptive, ergotamines, vasoconstrictors, cocaine, etc. may result in an ischemic pattern of injury.

Characteristically, a diffuse histiocytic infiltrate fills the lamina propria. Poorly circumscribed, noncaseating, epithelioid granulomas can be seen. The intracellular organisms are highlighted by using acid-fast stains (Ziehl–Neelsen) and sometimes arranged in distinctive stacks. The sheer number of organisms distinguishes *M. avium* from *M. tuberculosis*.

Other infections characterized by diffuse PAS-positive histiocytic infiltrates include Whipple's disease and histoplasmosis. In Whipple's disease, the causative actinobacterium *Tropheryma whipplei* is brightly stained, larger, and more coarsely granular than the weakly positive staining bacillary forms of MAC. MAC is acid-fast, whereas Whipple bacilli are not. *Histoplasma* are larger organisms and are highlighted by Grocott's methenamine silver stain.

Intestinal Spirochetosis

The clinical significance of intestinal spirochetosis, noted in 2–7% of colorectal biopsies in the general population and in up to 54% of biopsies in the homosexual population, is debated. Many individuals remain asymptomatic, but even in symptomatic patients, coinfection with other organisms should be excluded. *Brachyspira aalborgi* and *Brachyspira pilosicoli* are the two of the most common species causing intestinal disease. Of note, a mucosal invasive form with bacteremia has been recognized in immunocompromised hosts.

Microscopically, a thickened 2–3 μm basophilic fringe is present on the epithelial surface with sparing over goblet cells. PAS or Warthin–Starry stain highlights the colonization of the mucosal surface. The mucosa is usually normal, but focal increase in inflammation and cryptitis may be seen (Figure 10.3).

Viral

In most cases, diarrheal disease is self-limited. In practice, infection by *adenovirus, cytomegalovirus (CMV)*, and *herpes simplex virus (HSV)*, which is increased in immunosuppressed patients, are commonly investigated.

Cytomegalovirus (CMV)

CMV belongs to the herpes group of viruses. Three forms of infection can be observed: primary, reactivation, and superinfection. Primary infection is commonly subclinical and produces an infectious mononucleosis-like illness. CMV colitis commonly develop as part of disseminated disease, most likely due to reactivation of latent virus in the immunocompromised host (e.g. HIV/AIDS infection or post-transplantation). Finally, superinfection can occur, particularly in the setting of IBD. CMV colitis is associated with abdominal pain and diarrhea, which may be watery or bloody. On colonoscopy, ulcers (38%) or colitis (20%) or both (29%) may occur

Table 10.3 Range of histologic patterns on endoscopic biopsy of common bacterial pathogens causing infectious colitis.

Feature	Pathogens
Minimal or no inflammatory change	EPEC EAEC[a] ETEC *Staphylococcus aureus* Spirochates
Acute self-limited colitis pattern	Many viruses (often unidentified) *Shigella* sp. Campylobacter sp. Aeromonas Non-typhoid *Salmonella* sp. *Staphylococcus aureus*
Pseudomembranous colitis	EHEC[b] *Shigella* (occasionally)
Predominantly granulomatous	Yersinia sp.[c] Mycobacteria sp.
Predominantly lymphohistiocytic	*Salmonella* typhi[d]
Marked architectural distortion	*Salmonella* sp. *Shigella* sp. Aeromonas (occasionally) *Salmonella* typhi[d]
Ischemic pattern	EHEC[b] *Clostridium perfringens*
Prominent necrosis and ulceration	EHEC[b] *Clostridium perfringens*

EPEC, enteropathogenic *E. Coli*; EHEC, enterohemorrhagic *E. Coli*; EAEC, enteroadherent *E. Coli*; ETEC, enterotoxigenic *E. Coli*.
[a] EAEC: biopsy is typically relatively normal in appearance, may have mild edema and focal hemorrhage. Foci of epithelial denudation with adherent Gram-negative bacilli may be seen.
[b] EHEC: overlap features of ASLC and ischemic colitis. There are changes of ASLC but with fibrin thrombi, fibrin exudation, and disproportionate amount of lamina propria hemorrhage relative to the inflammation. Progression to more severe changes shows prominent submucosal edema, extensive hemorrhage, mucosal necrosis with ghost crypts filled with neutrophils with or without pseudomembranous.
[c] Yersinia: biopsy may show prominent lymphoid hyperplasia with aphthous ulceration over hyperplastic follicle, cryptitis, and epithelioid granulomas with central necrosis and prominent lymphoid cuffing.
[d] *Salmonella* typhi: biopsy findings vary depending on the stage of disease evolution (hyperplastic, necrotic, ulcerative, and healing): early in the hyperplastic phase, there is prominent lymphoid hyperplasia with progressive infiltration and obliteration by histiocytes with nuclear debris and erythrophagocytosis followed by edema, fibrinous exudate, and vascular thrombosis. Marked architectural changes may be seen. Continued histiocytic infiltration eventually obliterates lymphoid follicles with a diffuse infiltrate centrally and nodular infiltrate peripherally. Neutrophils are relatively sparse. Healing by granulation tissue and re-epithelialization occurs.

The diagnosis relies on detecting characteristic inclusions predominantly within stromal cells (Figure 10.4) (i.e. macrophages, endothelium, and fibroblasts). Typical infected cells show nuclear and cytoplasmic enlargement with a single dark amphophilic nuclear "owl's eye" inclusion that is pinkish-red on Giemsa stain. However, infected cells may have less distinctive smudged hematoxyphilic nuclei. The cytoplasm shows granular basophilic inclusions or may be foamy. CMV inclusions are often best detected in granulation tissue, and hence, it is important to obtain a biopsy directly from the ulcer base rather than the edges.

Background inflammation varies from mild to extensive acute and chronic inflammation with ulceration, often with ischemic features. The number of CMV inclusions generally parallels the severity of inflammation, but may be found in absence of significant inflammatory response.

The use of immunohistochemical stains is encouraged in any clinically suggestive case, even if the morphology is negative.

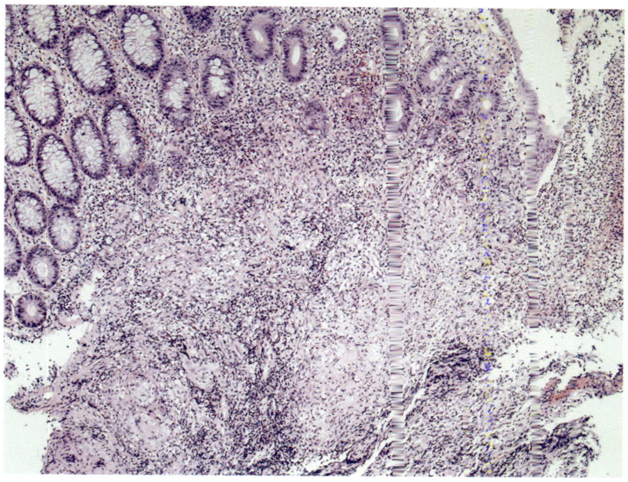

Figure 10.2 Colonic biopsy affected by *Mycobacterium tuberculosis* showing multiple epithelioid granulomas with central necrosis surrounded by a dense cuff of lymphocytes.

Table 10.4 Distinguishing features between TB, *Yersinia* and Crohn's disease.

Feature	Crohn's disease (CD)	*Yersinia*	Tuberculosis (TB)
Clinical/gross			
Ileal involvement	++	+	+
Ulcers	Linear (longitudinal) and aphthoid	Linear and aphthoid	Tend to be in transverse axis or circumferential
Edema	+	+	+
Pseudopolyps	+	+	+
Fistulae	+	+/−	+
Transverse fissures	+	−	+
Cobblestoning	+	−	−/+
Strictures	Generally long	+/−	Usually <3 cm
Anal lesions	Frequent	No	Rare
Serology for *Yersinia*	−	+	−
(PPD)	−	−	+
Stool culture	−	Often positive	30% positive
Microscopy			
Granulomas			
Number	Multiple	Few	Many and may be confluent
Size	Small (<200 μm)	Large	Large (50% over 200 μm)
Nature	Compact sarcoid-like; poorly organized, discrete, or isolated.	Epithelioid granulomas without foreign body giant cells with central necrosis and prominent lymphoid cuffing; stellate abscesses	Epithelioid granulomas with Langhans giant cells and central caseation
Location	Mucosal location more common than in other sites; granulomas may be associated with lymphatics	Mucosa; but also submucosa and deeper in bowel wall	Granulomas in submucosa (if present in biopsy) or in granulation tissue
Microgranulomas/histiocytic aggregates	+	−/+	−/+
Crypt centered inflammation/ pericryptal granuloma	+	−/+	−/+
Focally active colitis	+	−	−
Crypt architectural distortion	+; often unassociated with granulomatous inflammation	−/+	−/+

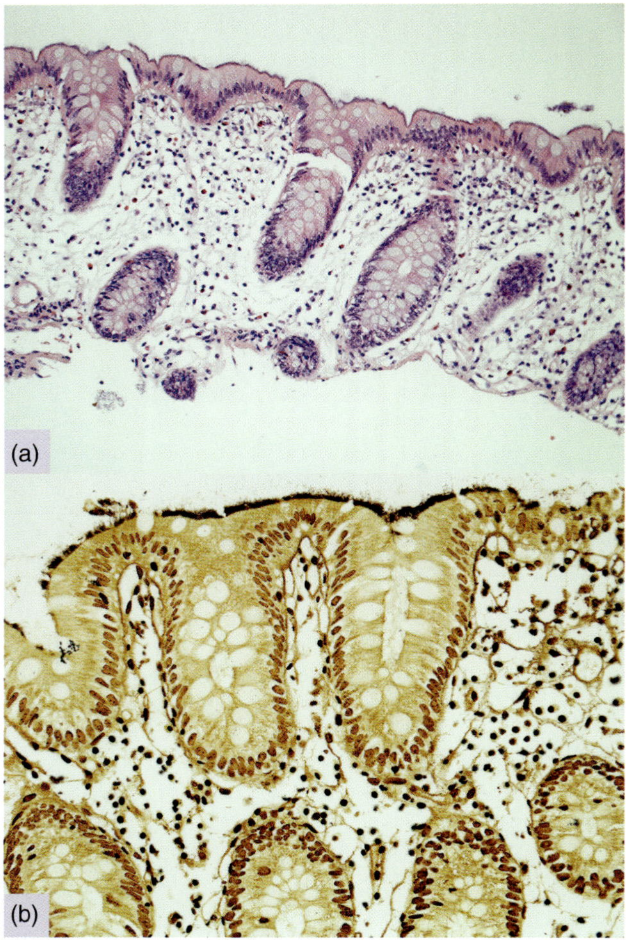

Figure 10.3 Typical appearance of a spirochetosis of the colon showing a purple fringe of the surface epithelium (a) typically sparing the deep crypts. The parasites can be highlighted with a silver stain, e.g. Warthin–Starry (b) and will appear black.

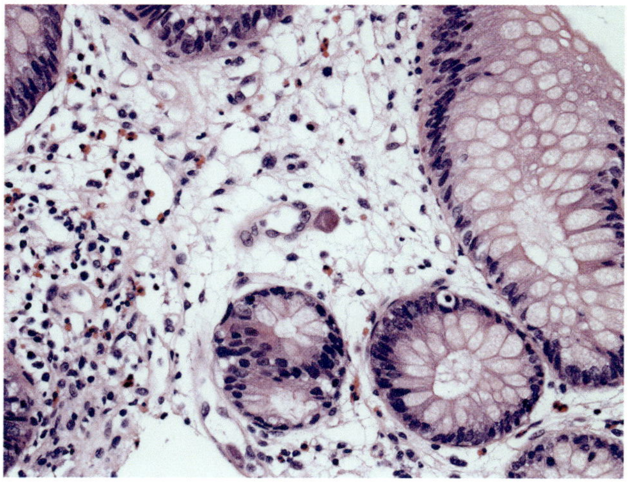

Figure 10.4 H.E. stain of the colon showing typical changes caused by CMV infection. In the center of the picture a infected fibroblast can be identified showing the typical pinkish nuclear inclusion also known as "owls eye."

Herpes Simplex

More common in immunosuppressed patients, primary herpetic colitis is rare, resulting from unprotected anal intercourse and oral-fecal contact.

The mucosa is commonly ulcerated with acute inflammation. Chronic inflammation with perivascular lymphocytic cuffing is sometimes observed. Viral cytopathic effect includes multinucleation, molding and margination of chromatin imparting a ground glass appearance. Typical Cowdry Type A inclusions may be seen. Immunohistochemistry is useful to confirm the diagnosis.

Adenovirus

This DNA virus infects goblet cells that display a crescentic to moderately enlarged irregular basal amphophilic smudgy nuclei associated with mucin containing vacuolated cytoplasm. The diagnosis can be confirmed by immunocytochemistry. Adenovirus is commonly responsible for diarrhea in children, but has also been recognized to produce colitis in immunocompromised patients, particularly with HIV/AIDS.

Pseudomembranous Colitis and Antibiotic-Associated Diarrhea and Colitis

Definition, General Features, and Predisposing Factors

Antibiotic-associated colitis (AAC) and antibiotic-associated diarrhea (AAD) occur during or following antibiotic therapy and are distinguished by biopsy findings. AAC demonstrates evidence of colitis without pseudomembranes, whereas AAD lacks evidence of colitis. Pseudomembranous colitis (PMC) is a severe complication of *Clostridium difficile* and its toxin, characterized by inflammatory pseudomembranes. It is frequently, but not invariably, associated with antibiotic therapy.

Diarrhea occurs in approximately 5–25% patients treated with antibiotics, and its occurrence varies influenced by several factors, including nosocomial outbreaks, patterns of antibiotic prescription, and individual susceptibility. All groups of antibiotics may result in AAD, the risk being greater with broad-spectrum antibiotics.

Most AAD are nonspecific. The mechanisms by which antibiotics cause diarrhea include alteration in composition of the intestinal flora resulting in altered metabolism of high-molecular weight carbohydrates and bile acids, leading to osmotic and secretory diarrhea. Direct allergic or toxic effects on the mucosa or pharmacologic effects on motility are alternative diarrheagenic mechanisms.

Disruption of the normal flora also promotes overgrowth of pathogenic bacteria, most commonly *C. difficile*, a Gram-positive anaerobic bacterium, accounting for 15–20% of all AAD cases. Other potential pathogens are less common (2–3%) and include enterotoxin-producing *Clostridium perfringens, Staphylococcus aureus, Klebsiella oxytoca,* and *Candida*. Although *C. difficile* and/or its toxin accounts for many cases of AAC and almost all instances of PMC, the latter is, however, a descriptive diagnosis, and not an etiologic one. Indeed, PMC may develop in association with other pathogens and/or toxins.

C. difficile exerts its pathogenic effects through the production of toxins, the most important being toxin A (an enterotoxin) and toxin B (a cytotoxin), which result in disruption of the cellular cytoskeleton, loosening of intercellular tight junctions, and profound secretory diarrhea. Most pathogenic strains produce both toxins, but 2–56% of *C. difficile* infection is attributable to strains producing toxin B alone. Between 2 and 5% of adults and up to 64% of healthy neonates are asymptomatically colonized with *C. difficile*. The prevalence of asymptomatic colonization rises to 20–30% in acute care hospitals, and may be as high as 50% in long-term care facilities. Notably, some patients after exposure to antibiotics and colonization by *C. difficile* develop PMC, while others will not. *C. difficile* is also a cause of exacerbation of IBD. It also has been noted as a causative agent of diarrhea in the community.

Clinical Features and Endoscopic Appearances

The clinical spectrum of *C. difficile* is wide, ranging from an asymptomatic carrier state to fulminant colitis. *C. difficile* infection usually causes mild to moderate diarrhea, with or without abdominal cramps. The average symptom duration is about a week, and the incubation period in early onset disease ranges from 1 to 10 days after the inciting antibiotic is started. Late onset disease with symptoms delayed for two to six weeks following antibiotic discontinuance is reported. Patients with severe colitis without pseudomembrane formation present with profuse debilitating diarrhea, abdominal pain and distension, and toxic megacolon. Common systemic manifestations include fever, nausea, anorexia, malaise, and dehydration. Peripheral leukocytosis and increased numbers of fecal leukocytes are common. Patients may experience occult colonic bleeding; rarely, frank hematochezia develops.

Other manifestations that can develop include protein-losing enteropathy and HUS. On colonoscopy, discrete raised indurated creamy yellow plaques are firmly attached to the underlying mucosa and separated from each other by congested mucosa. With more extensive involvement, the plaques may coalesce, and the necrotic membrane formed may then be indistinguishable from those seen in some cases of ischemic colitis. However, the disease can be patchy and the rectum and sigmoid colon can be spared, and thus, full colonoscopic examination is required. Occasionally, involvement of the terminal ileum is seen, and has been described.

Microscopic Features

In AAD, the biopsy may be normal or demonstrate minor changes only, whereas AAC resembles acute infectious colitis.

In PMC, the earliest changes consist of focal intercryptal surface erosion with a luminal spray of nuclear debris, neutrophils, and mucin. The surrounding lamina propria is edematous, with clusters of neutrophils and dilated capillaries. Focal cryptitis and a pink subepithelial exudate may be present. Intact surface epithelial cells may be tufted or appear crenated with infiltrating neutrophils.

The classical appearance of PMC corresponds to endoscopically identified discrete plaques. It is important the plaque be biopsied, as the intervening mucosa may be virtually normal. The epithelium of the affected crypts becomes flattened and progressively lost in a top to bottom pattern. The pseudomembrane corresponds to linear streaming of neutrophils and eosinophils within fibrin strands and mucus extending from distended crypts also known as volcano lesion. Fibrin thrombi may be identified in capillaries. Occasionally, signet ring cells corresponding to degenerate epithelial cells are confined to the basement membrane of the crypts. These cells are not infiltrative in any circumstances. The submucosa, if biopsied, is always edematous (Figure 10.5).

Differential Diagnosis

Pseudomembranes can be observed in ischemic colitis, which should be excluded on the basis of its characteristic features (see Table 10.5). When suspected, the diagnosis of PMC can be confirmed by toxin production (cytotoxic assay, sensitivity and specificity over 90%), or enzyme immunoassays, which can render diagnosis within four hours (sensitivity of 69–87%; specificity of 99–100%).

Treatment/Prognosis/Evolution

Treatment of *C. difficile* colitis has changed recently as evidence supporting fecal transplantation has emerged, although this is typically still reserved for recurrent cases. Some antibiotics are known to cause *C. difficile* colitis (clindamycin, amoxicillin) and should be discontinued when possible. Other antibiotics are used to treat *C. difficile*. First line antibiotics include oral vancomycin and fidaxomicin.

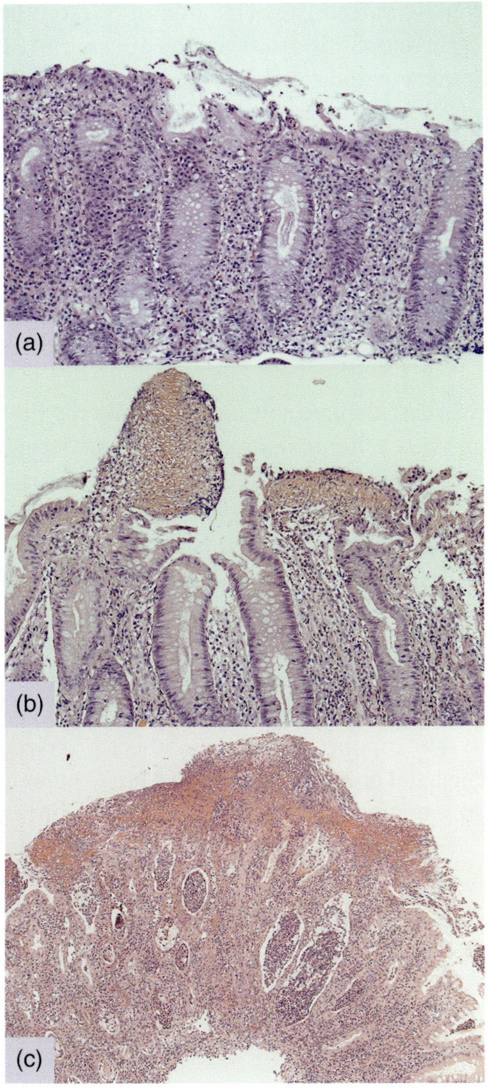

Figure 10.5 Biopsy specimens of pseudomembranous colitis showing the whole spectrum of the disease. The early stage (a) the colonic mucosa shows a severe active colitis with only sparse luminal debris. The intermediate (b) and late stage (c) of the disease show the typical debris, whereas the late stage additionally shows destruction or the mucosal architecture and volcano lesions.

Metronidazole remains effective and can be used orally, or intravenously (e.g. in a patient with fulminant colitis who cannot tolerate oral medication). Fecal microbial ("stool") transplantation (FMT) has emerged as the treatment of choice for recurrent disease. FMT can be delivered by colonoscopy infusion, small bowel (via upper endoscopy), and recently has been delivered in the form of frozen encapsulated tablets. The optimal methods are still not known. Surgery remains an option of last resort for patients with fulminant disease not responding to standard treatments.

Brainerd Diarrhea

Definition, General Features, and Predisposing Factors

This is an epidemic form of secretory diarrhea associated with patchy colonic lymphocytosis.

General Features

It is named after an outbreak of chronic diarrhea that occurred in Brainerd, Minnesota in 1983. The etiology remains elusive. Reported cases have been related to consumption of unpasteurized milk or contaminated water, and an infectious agent, possibly a virus or a chemical toxin, has been suggested.

Clinical and Endoscopic Features

Patients present with fecal urgency and incontinence, without systemic symptoms, after an incubation period of between 10 and 30 days.

The mucosa is either normal, or may show erythematous patches in the right colon, or scattered small whitish pustules.

Microscopic Features

Surface intraepithelial lymphocytosis is characteristic, mimicking lymphocytic colitis, although there is no surface epithelial injury, and the number of lymphocytes is usually more limited. Furthermore, there is no inflammatory expansion of the lamina propria.

Differential Diagnosis

The diagnosis is made from the presentation of an outbreak of diarrheal illness traceable to a point source but without an identifiable infectious cause, and with the appropriate histology. The histologic findings resemble colonic lymphocytosis and lymphocytic colitis (see Sections "Lymphocytic Colitis" and "Differential Diagnosis").

Prognosis, Evolution, and Clinical Management

Duration may be prolonged (median 15 months; range 1–19 months) and antibiotics are ineffective. Long-term prognosis is good with nearly 100% of cases resolving by three years. Preventative efforts include avoiding raw/unpasteurized milk and untreated drinking water.

Table 10.5 Differential diagnosis of acute ischemic colitis.

	Acute ischemia	Infectious colitis	Pseudomembranous colitis	Neutropenic colitis	Mucosal prolapse
Mucosal architecture	Preserved	Preserved	Preserved	Preserved	Preserved or mild distortion with "diamond" shaped crypts
Mucin depletion	+	+	+	+	+
Crypt withering	+	+/−	+	+	+/−
Surface/superficial crypt degeneration/sloughing	+	+/−	+	+	+/−
Pseudomembranes	+	−	+	+	−
LP inflammation	Minimal	Neutrophils, may have increased mononuclear cells at later stage	Neutrophils	None	Variable; generally mild
LP connective tissue alterations	Edema, hemorrhage, fibrin exudate/thrombi hyalinization and	Edema, focal hemorrhage	Edema, hemorrhage, fibrin exudate; fibrin thrombi	Edema, hemorrhage, fibrin exudate and hyalinization; fibrin thrombi	Fibromuscular obliteration
Cryptitis	−	+	+	−	+/−
Crypt abscesses	−	+/−	+	−	+/−
Comments	Distinction from PMC may be difficult. LP hemorrhage and hyalinization, atrophic microcrypts, full thickness mucosal necrosis, diffuse microscopic distribution of pseudomembranes, favor ischemia; endoscopic polypoid mucosa, favors ischemia; when complete mucosal necrosis with ulceration and granulation tissue occurs, unless intact mucosa is biopsied, the changes are indistinguishable from ulceration of any other cause	Some infections, e.g. EHEC, may result in ischemic pattern indistinguishable from ischemic colitis or mixed ischemic and acute infectious pattern; CMV may be associated with ischemia and identification of cytopathic effect is diagnostic	Endoscopic identification of diffuse pseudomembranes favors *C. difficile*; Stool toxin detection	Features are essentially of ischemia; however, the absence of neutrophils in the setting of significant cellular injury is the clue Knowledge of the clinical setting is important	Mucosal prolapse may have ischemic component; the lamina propria fibromuscular obliteration is important distinguishing feature

Parasites

Parasitic infections have the characteristic ability to elicit a brisk eosinophil infiltrate and sometimes granulomas.

Protozoan Infections

Amebiasis

Entameba histolytica infection is acquired through contaminated water and food but may also occur by direct fecal-oral contact or via anal intercourse.

The manifestations range through from asymptomatic infection to amebic dysentery. Some patients can present with extraintestinal disease including hepatic abscesses and, less commonly, systemic spread with abscesses in other organs. Current diagnostic tools include antigen detection in stool and PCR.

Several morphologic stages can be seen. Initially, a picture of typical infectious colitis can develop, with protozoa detected in the in the overlying exudate (Figure 10.6). Eventually, classic flask-shaped microulceration with tissue necrosis and ulceration extending to the submucosa develops, with a thick amorphous gray exudate separated from underlying viable tissue by a fibrinoid band. Chronic amebiasis demonstrates persisting ulceration and stricture, and mucosal architectural changes mimicking IBD. The trophozoites are usually found within the exudate, but may be seen invading mucosa. Erythrophagocytosis may be observed, and is highlighted by a Heidenhain's iron hematoxylin stain, while PAS reaction will highlight the cytoplasm of the organisms. Histiocytes tend to be smaller and are less intensely stained by PAS with a clearly identified nucleus.

Long-standing complications include transmural invasion with perforation and toxic megacolon. Mass-forming ameboma, invasion of perianal skin with granulomatous lesions, and amebic ulceration of the abdominal wall around colostomy openings can develop.

Differentiating amebiasis from IBD can be challenging; the focality of the inflammatory process together with positive identification is diagnostic. The absence of transmural lymphoid aggregates and granulomas helps distinguish it from Crohn's disease. However, amebiasis may coexist with and exacerbate pre-existing IBD.

Balantidium

Balantidium coli is a large and ciliated protozoan rarely causing dysentery in rural communities. This represents a zoonosis whose hosts are pigs, cows, and horses.

Cryptosporidia

Cryptosporidium is an intracellular protozoan acquired through drinking contaminated water and also may spread via contaminated food and person-to-person spread. In immunocompetent patients, mild self-limiting gastroenteritis or traveler's diarrhea is the typical presentation, while in immunocompromised individuals, a severe intractable diarrhea may develop and complicate with toxic megacolon. *Cryptosporidium parvum* is responsible for most human infections.

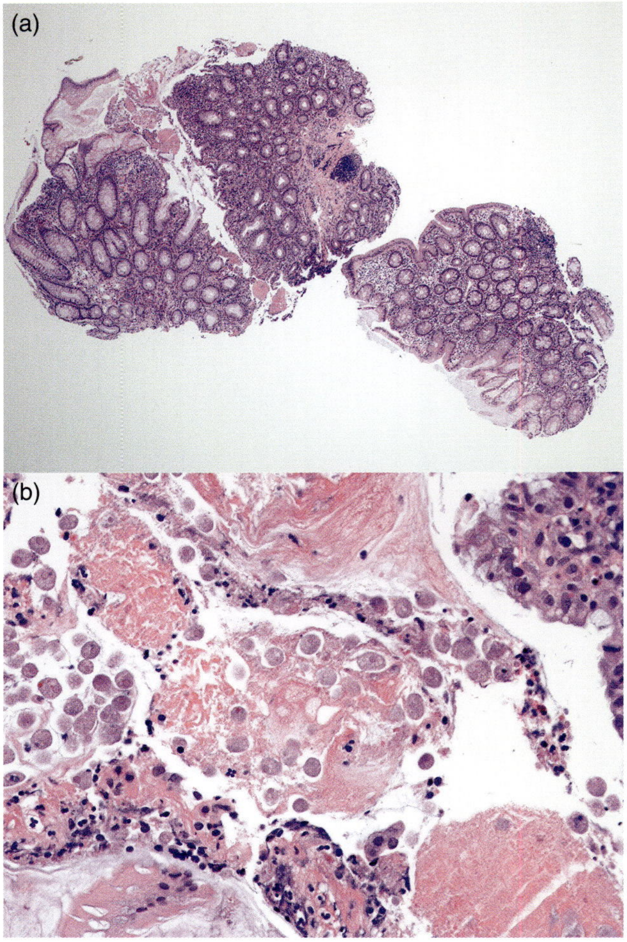

Figure 10.6 Example of a severe amebiasis showing a severe ulcerative colitis in the overview (a) and multiple trophozoites in the higher magnification (b). The trophozoites are round to oval in shape and measure up to 40 μm in size. They have a finely granular eosinophilic cytoplasm with a small pale nucleus with a central karyosome.

Cryptosporidia appear as uniform hematoxyphilic dots adherent to the apical membrane of epithelial cells within crypts (Figure 10.7). Special stains may aid in detecting the protozoa, which should not be mistaken for mucin droplets (positive for mucicarmine). Cryptosporidia are stained dark blue with Giemsa and are positive with PAS but negative with a Grocott's methenamine silver stain.

Visceral Leishmaniasis

This condition is related to the protozoan *Leishmania donovani*. Patients present with fever, loss of appetite, occasionally diarrhea, and eosinophilia. Splenomegaly,

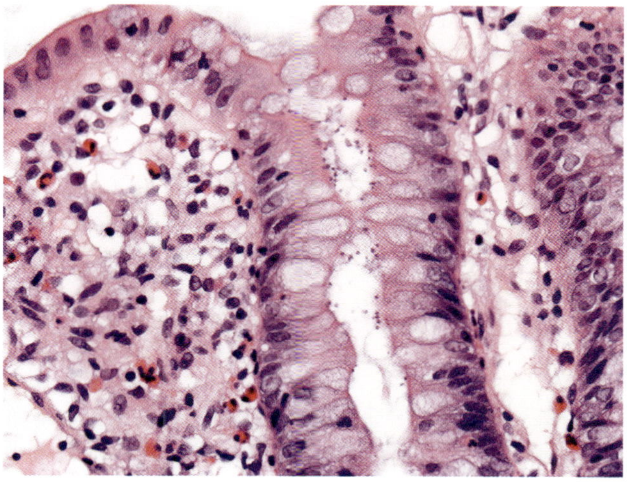

Figure 10.7 High magnification of a colon biopsy with a population of cryptosporidia characterized by uniform basophilic dots attached to the surface membrane.

hepatomegaly, anemia, and skin lesions (i.e. dermal leishmaniasis) may be detected. Kala azar is an important opportunistic infection in HIV/AIDS and may be associated with immune reconstitution disease. Diagnosis requires microscopic identification of characteristic *Leishmania* amastigotes, culture of the organism, or serologic positivity for the protozoan. However, chronic visceral leishmaniasis may first be diagnosed on a rectal biopsy. On biopsy, the lamina propria is obliterated by plasma cell, lymphocyte, and histiocyte infiltrate containing abundant amastigotes. Granulomas can be noted, but these granulomas are absent or poorly formed in immunocompromised patients.

Leishmaniasis must be differentiated from other infections resulting in dense histiocytic infiltrates of the mucosa (Table 10.6).

Helminthic Infections

Trematodes

Schistosomiasis

Intestinal infestation is commonly caused by *Schistosoma mansoni* (Africa and central South America) and *Schistosoma japonicum* (Asia) (Figure 10.8). Rectal and left-sided lesions are nearly always due to *S. mansoni,* whereas appendiceal and right-sided lesions are more commonly associated with *S. japonicum*.

An acute proctitis/colitis with edema and hemorrhage is noted in the acute stages of invasion. The biopsies show necrotic mucosa with oval ova, sometimes calcified, surrounded by a cellular infiltrate with eosinophilia. A surrounding granulomatous reaction can develop over time, with epithelioid histiocytes, giant cells, and eosinophils. At the chronic stage, a concentric fibrosis develops around the granuloma and the ova are commonly calcified. The species can be identified based on the terminal spine of the ova: *S. mansoni* possesses a subterminal lateral spine; *Schistosoma haematobium* a terminal spine; and *S. japonicum* an ill-defined subterminal knob with ova that are rounder.

Schistosomiasis is associated with an increased risk of colorectal carcinoma in chronic infection.

Table 10.6 Differential diagnosis of diffuse histiocytic infiltrates of the gastrointestinal tract.

Infections
Whipple's disease
MAC infection (immunocompromised host)
Leishmania
Histoplasma
Rhodococcus
Malakoplakia
Noninfectious
Xanthomatosis
Storage disorders
Neoplastic
Langerhans histiocytosis
"Histiocytic" lymphomas
Miscellaneous
Xanthogranulomatous colitis
Rosai–Dorfman disease
Erdheim–Chester disease

Nematode Infections

Usually affecting the small intestine, colonic involvement can be seen.

Strongyloidiasis

Strongyloidiasis stercoralis and *Strongyloidiasis fuelleborn* are the two species that cause strongyloidiasis in humans.

Microscopically, the rhabditiform larvae are identified in the crypts and the submucosa. The edematous mucosa usually contains numerous eosinophils and mononuclear cells. Necrotizing granulomas may develop. In severe cases, diffuse mucosal ulceration, edema, and hemorrhage can be observed. Strictures can develop in long-standing disease together with histological features of chronicity and granulomatous inflammation.

Trichuriasis

Humans acquire *Trichuris trichiura,* a whipworm that preferentially infects the cecum, by ingesting embryonated eggs from contaminated hands, soil, food, and water. In

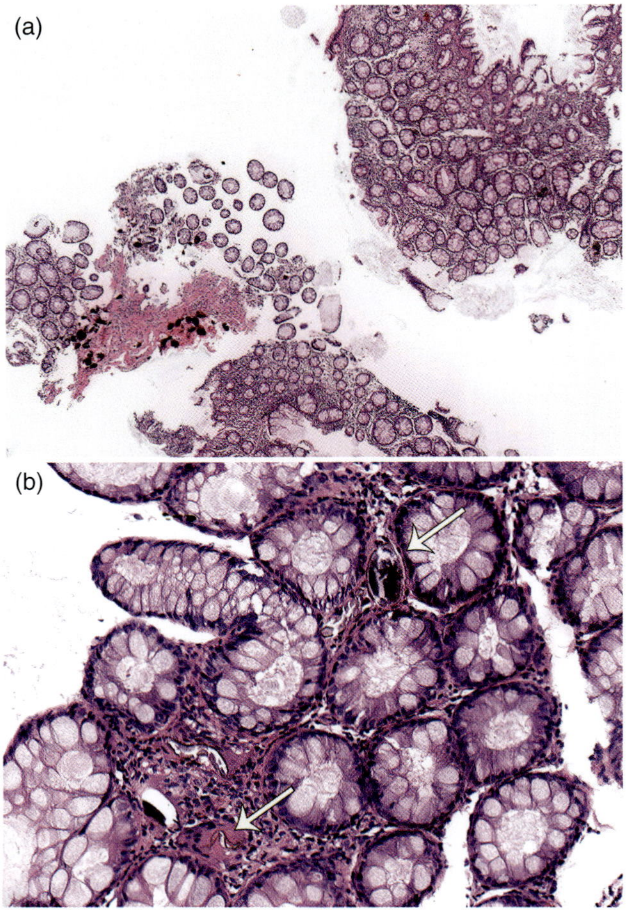

Figure 10.8 H.E. stain of a colonic biopsy with manifestation of *Schistosoma japonicum*. (a) Illustrates the mucosal changes in an overview perspective with several calcified eggs in the lower left and single eggs in the upper right biopsy fragments. Higher magnification (b) of the upper right biopsy fragment of (a) shows an additional giant giant cell around one egg (arrow bottom left).

severe cases, worms may be found in the appendix, terminal ileum, and rectum. *T. trichiura* worms are detected in the large intestine with their anterior ends deeply embedded in the mucosa, and can be removed endoscopically.

Adult worms embedded within mucosa may be associated with atrophy, necrosis, or focal crypt dilatation containing mucus, fibrin, and acute inflammatory cells. Subepithelial hemorrhage and increased lamina propria eosinophils, in addition to lymphocytes and plasma cells, may be observed.

Oxyuriasis

This infection is related to the pinworm *Enterobius vermicularis*. The infective ova, after ingestion, transforms to a larva that emerges in the small intestine and migrates to the cecum. The worms are commonly identified in appendectomy specimens, and rarely observed in colon biopsies. The secondary inflammatory infiltrate is nonspecific, but may be rich in eosinophils.

Fungi

Histoplasmosis, coccidioidomycosis, and paracoccidioidomycosis are endemic in regions of North and South America.

Candida

Candida glabrata is responsible for approximately 15% of mucosal and systemic candidiasis. In the immunocompromised host, there is a higher frequency of disseminated *Candida tropicalis* than *Candida albicans*.

Candida infection generally affects immunocompromised individuals or those with chronic debilitating disease (e.g. renal failure/hemodialysis, cancer), or receiving long-term antibiotherapy, or during severe postoperative complications, penetrating abdominal trauma, or indwelling vascular access devices. *Candida* organisms may also colonize blind loops and necrotic tissue.

Microscopically, the budding yeast-like forms (approximately 5 μm in size) are admixed with non-septate pseudohyphae that stain positively with PAS and Grocott's methenamine silver stains. In noninvasive disease, the fungi grow in devitalized tissues without invading underlying intact tissues. In the invasive form, the organism may invade the vessel walls, leading to ischemia, mucosal necrosis, and ulceration. The inflammatory reaction is primarily neutrophilic, and microabscesses can form. Histiocytes and giant cells may aggregate, and granulomas may form. The inflammatory response is usually limited in immunocompromised individuals.

Histoplasmosis

Histoplasmosis is the most common endemic systemic mycosis in several regions of the United States, ranging from the Gulf Coast to the Great Lakes, particularly along the Ohio and Mississippi River valleys. It is also endemic in the Caribbean and Central and South America. Even brief exposure through inhalation of spores may result in infection, and many inhabitants of these areas are infected. Infection can later be reactivated if the patient becomes immunosuppressed. The clinical syndromes include acute self-limited illness, disseminated histoplasmosis, and thoracic manifestations (chronic pulmonary histoplasmosis, mediastinal granulomata, and mediastinitis). Gastrointestinal histoplasmosis usually appears as part of disseminated disease by hematogenous spread, mostly in immunocompromised individuals, but rarely may occur in immunocompetent hosts or as isolated gastrointestinal histoplasmosis.

Microscopically, histoplasmosis is characterized by diffuse histiocytic collections expanding the lamina propria filled with small particulate organisms. The organisms may be highlighted with PAS and Grocott's methenamine silver (GMS) stains (Table 10.7). Occasionally, the organism lies within well-formed granulomas. Following therapy, degenerating and dead organisms are seen, and long after disease remission, there may be fungal cell wall remnants within macrophages.

Histoplasmosis should be distinguished from other diffuse histiocytic infiltrates and granulomatous reactions (Tables 10.6–10.8) including xanthomatosis, Whipple's disease, and atypical mycobacterial infections. Notably, Whipple's bacilli and *Mycobacteria* are negative for silver stain. Malakoplakia may also have abundant histiocytes admixed with lymphocytes and plasma cells but will show Michaelis–Gutmann bodies that may be highlighted by Perls Prussian Blue reaction, PAS, and Von Kossa stain. Other entities in the differential diagnosis include other fungi with yeast-like forms (Table 10.7). Histoplasmosis should also be distinguished from xanthoma/xanthomatosis, which is characterized by diffuse infiltrates of foamy lipid-laden histiocytes expanding the lamina propria.

Aspergillosis

Colonic involvement usually occurs with disseminated disease and secondary spread to gastrointestinal tract (GIT). Risk factors for aspergillosis include granulocytopenia, immunosuppression, broad-spectrum antibiotics, and steroids.

The diagnosis rests on the detection of typical dichotomously branched septate aspergillus hyphae in the tissues. Because the organism tends to invade vessels, causing vasculitis and thrombosis, the histologic picture is one of ischemia and infarction. The organisms may be detected on H&E slide, but methenamine silver and PAS stains highlight the organisms.

Blastomycosis

Blastomycosis occurs in the same areas as histoplasmosis. *B. dermatitidis* is a species of dimorphous, round, budding yeast, and begins with the inhalation of spores before it spreads, rarely, in the intestine by invading submucosal lymphoid tissue, in immunocompromised hosts. The infection is characterized by granulomatous inflammation with superimposed pyogenic inflammation.

Blastomyces are recognized as thick-walled, round, multinucleated celled structures measuring 8–15 µm in diameter that reproduce by broad-based budding. Multiple nuclei are seen in well-fixed sections. PAS and methenamine silver stains highlight the organisms.

Paracoccidioides

This infection, endemic in to South America, is usually seen in immigrants or travelers returning from endemic areas. Paracoccidioidomycosis is a systemic chronic granulomatous process that begins with an asymptomatic pulmonary infection following inhalation with subsequent dissemination to other organs. The disease has a long latency period of up to 30 years.

The fungi are easily seen in H&E-stained sections as large, round, oval cells measuring 5–15 µm in diameter that reproduce by single or multiple budding. The fungus can be highlighted by PAS and GMS. They are often surrounded by an ulcerative granulomatous reaction combined with pyogenic inflammation. Development of malakoplakia has been reported.

Clinically, it can mimic IBD; however, identification of the fungus will resolve the differential diagnosis. It should also be distinguished from other causes of granulomatous inflammation and distinguished from other spore-forming fungal organisms.

Mucormycosis

Mucormycosis is a ubiquitous and generally saprophytic fungus that may cause disease in diabetic patients and patients with acidosis secondary to uremia, diarrhea, or aspirin abuse. Gastrointestinal infection is usually rapidly fatal. Occasionally, the organisms colonize benign gastric ulcers without invading further.

The organisms have characteristic pleomorphic, broad, aseptate, irregularly right-angled, branched hyphae. Mucor is highlighted by PAS and methenamine silver stains. Hyphae also can be seen invading the surrounding tissues and blood vessels with local tissue destruction, vascular thrombosis, and ischemic necrosis.

Cryptococcus

Cryptococcus neoformans is diagnosed with increased frequency in immunocompromised patients, complicating AIDS and hematologic malignancies, or in patients on corticosteroids. The most important environmental source of infection is soil contaminated by bird droppings. Gastrointestinal cryptococcal infection is rare and usually a secondary involvement as part of disseminated disease initially arising within the lungs.

Microscopically, the yeast-like Gram-positive fungus are surrounded by an empty capsule appearing as a peripheral

Table 10.7 Fungal infections with spore formation in tissue sections.

	Predominantly spore forming					**Hyphae forming**	
	Histoplasma capsulatum* var. *capsulatum	***Blastomyces dermatitidis***	***Paracoccidioides brasiliensis***	***Candida* sp.**	***Cryptococcus neoformans***	**Aspergillosis**	**Mucormycosis**
Inflammatory reaction	Diffuse histiocytic infiltration ± granuloma, many intracellular organisms	Granulomatous ± suppuration	Granulomatous ± suppuration	Neutrophilic microabscesses ± histiocytic and granulomatous	Variable neutrophilic exudate ± granulomatous	Ischemic and infarcted with vasculitis and thrombosis, organism may invade vessels	Ischemic, and necrotic with thrombosis, may invade vessels
Size (μm)	2–4	7–15	5–60	3–6	2–20 μm	5–7	2–50
Shape	Spherical or oval	Spherical	Spherical	Spherical or oval	Spherical or oval	Hyphae	Hyphae
Number of buds	Single	Single	Multiple; "steering wheel" forms	Single; chains	Single, rarely multiple	–	–
Attachment of buds	Narrow	Very broad	Narrow	Narrow	Narrow	–	–
Thickness of cell wall	Thin	Thick	Variable	Thin	Thin	Mostly thin	Thick
Pseudohyphae and/or hyphae	Rare	Rare	Rare	Branched pseudohyphae	Rare	Septate, acute angle branching	Broad, ribbon like, pleomorphic, irregularly branching with rare cross walls
Spores	Yes	Yes	Yes	Yes	Yes	No	No
Number of nuclei	Single	Multiple	Multiple	Single	Single	–	–
PASD	−/+	−/+	+	+	+	+	+
Gomori's methanamine silver (GMS)	+	−/+		+	+	+	+
Mucicarmine reaction	–	−/+	–	–	+ (capsule)	–	–
Fontanna Masson stain	–	–	–	–	+ (cell wall)	–	–

Table 10.8 Causes of granulomatous inflammation in the colon and rectum.

Non infectious
Cell injury with mucin release
Crohn's disease
Feces due to perforation or fistulae
Foreign material (talc, sutures, barium)
Pneumatosis intestinalis
Pulse granulomas
Sarcoid
Medications
Infectious
Actinomyces
Brucella
Campylobacter
Histiocytosis
Histoplasmosis
Hyperinfective strongyloidiasis
Malakoplakia
Mycobacterium avium-intracellulare
Mycobacterium bovis
Salmonella
Schistosomiasis
Tuberculosis
Yersinia
Treponema pallidum, Chlamydia/Lymphogranuloma venereum (occasional, small ± mucin granulomas)

empty space. The polysaccharide capsule is a helpful diagnostic characteristic that can be highlighted by mucicarmine or Alcian blue. GMS fungal stain identifies the narrow-based budding yeast in tissue. A Fontana–Masson stain also may be helpful, as it stains the cell wall and will highlight capsule-deficient organisms.

Sexually Transmitted Infections

Diseases once seen predominantly in the homosexual population are increasingly prevalent in heterosexuals. Gonorrhea, chlamydia, herpes simplex, and syphilis are the most frequently recognized infections. However, *Salmonella*, *Campylobacter*, *Shigella*, and *Ameba* have also been reported to be sexually transmitted.

Gonorrhea

Rectal gonorrhea, related to the intracellular diplococcus *Neisseria gonorrhoeae*, is virtually always acquired by men having sex with men. Symptoms include anorectal discomfort, mucopurulent rectal discharge, or tenesmus, but a third of the infected individuals are asymptomatic, and many have a normal proctoscopic appearance and biopsy (84 and 68% respectively).

The biopsies show a mild to moderate increase in lymphoplasmacytic infiltrate of the lamina propria with preservation of the architecture. A minority of cases show acute inflammatory infiltrate with migration into surface epithelium and cryptitis reminiscent of an acute infectious colitis.

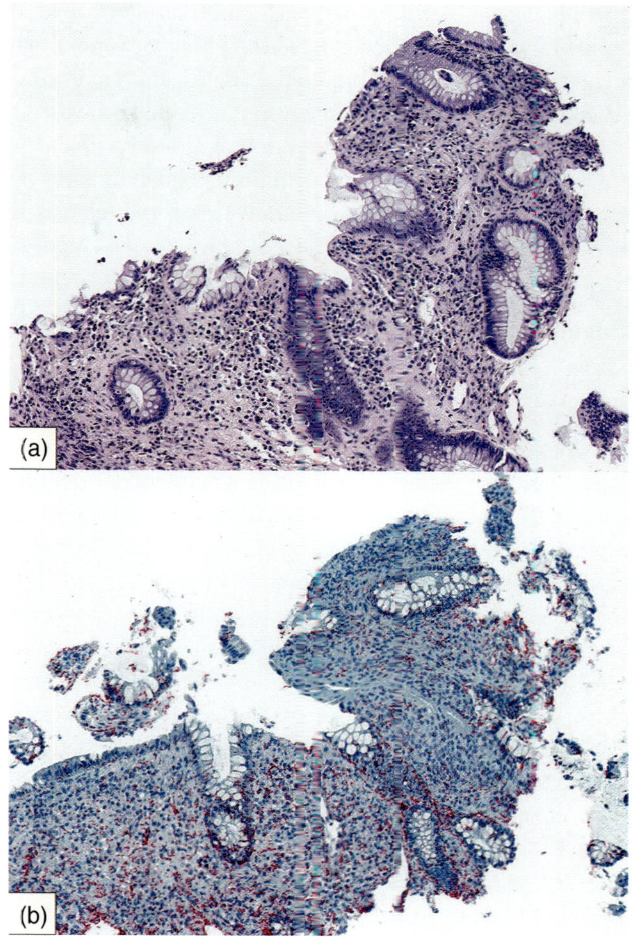

Figure 10.9 H.E. stain of Syphilitic colitis (a) with a predominant lymphoplasmacytic inflammatory infiltrate in the lamina propria and distorsion of the crypts. Immunhistochemically (b) Treponema pallidum appears red in epithelial and stromal portions of the biopsy.

Syphilis

Proctitis occurring during the secondary phase of syphilis is uncommon, and proctitis related to *Treponema pallidum* infection represents the primary lesion of syphilis (chancre).

The infection is characterized by a mixed dense inflammatory infiltrate variably rich in plasma cells (Figure 10.9) associated with proliferative vessels with plump endothelia, and possibly obliterative endarteritis. Cryptitis and ill-formed granulomas are also observed. In secondary syphilis, the proctitis resembles that of a typical bacterial infection, and small granulomas can be seen. Warthin–Starry, immunohistochemistry, or PCR are required to detect the organisms, although these may vary from few to many and be focal.

The lesion can mimic a carcinoma, solitary ulcer, or polyp. Warthin–Starry stain, immunohistochemistry, or PCR may detect the organisms; however, the diagnosis is often established by serologic tests.

Chlamydia/Lymphogranuloma Venereum

Chlamydia trachomatis, an obligate intracellular bacterium, causes this condition. Females are at risk of developing rectal and colonic lesions, presumably as the result of lymphatic spread from the vagina. When lymphogranuloma of the rectum occurs in males, it is invariably the result of anal sex, while heterosexual males usually develop buboes. Early in the course of the disease, it can be asymptomatic, or present as mild or chronic diarrhea due to distal proctocolitis. Biopsies show a mixed infiltrate with neutrophils, plasma cells, and lymphocytes infiltrating the mucosa. Crypt abscesses and occasional mucin granulomas may be present. The rectal mucosa is granular, nodular, and edematous with rigidity of the underlying tissues. Mild abnormality may extend up as far as the transverse colon. Although a pancolitis has been documented. There is a right to left gradient reverse to that of Crohn's disease, and severe macroscopic disease in the right colon is very unlikely to be due to lymphogranuloma venereum. Distally, there may be associated perianal abscesses and fistulae.

Strictures of the rectum, when they develop, present with an abrupt line of demarcation from the normal bowel. Microscopically, there is an inflammatory reaction with infiltration by lymphocytes and plasma cells together with transmural fibrosis. Neural hyperplasia is common. Epithelioid cell granulomas are rare in the chronic form, although it is well recognized in inguinal lymph nodes in the acute stage.

The diagnosis of lymphogranuloma venereum is confirmed by a direct demonstration on tissue sections using monoclonal antibodies or by serology showing seroconversion to particular immunotypes.

Both adenocarcinoma and squamous cell carcinoma have been reported as consequences of long-standing stricture of the rectum.

Chlamydia trachomatis Proctitis

The non-lymphogranuloma venereum immunotypes of *C. trachomatis* are mainly confined to infections of the genitourinary system, but can cause mild proctitis on occasion. Focal collections of neutrophils occur in the lamina propria. Occasionally, one may see granulomas with or without giant cells, or showing lymphoid follicular hyperplasia (follicular proctitis).

Etiology of Colitis with Pattern Recognition

Ischemic Colitis

Definition, General Features, and Predisposing Factors

Ischemic colitis results from hypoxia of the colonic tissue.

The incidence is reported as 4.5–44/100000 person-years. It is more common in the elderly and its frequency may be expected to increase with population aging. Ischemic colitis may be gangrenous or non-gangrenous, the latter either transient or chronic, with or without stricture formation, and rarely present as fulminant colitis.

The etiologies and risk factors are numerous (Table 10.9). "Watershed" areas are traditionally regarded as susceptible to ischemia, particularly with global hypoperfusion, and include the anastomosis between superior mesenteric and inferior mesenteric arteries (splenic flexure) and between inferior mesenteric and internal iliac arteries (rectosigmoid). The rectum is regarded as relatively resistant to ischemia given its dual splanchnic and systemic vascular supply. The right colon, with its less well-developed vasa recta, is also prone to ischemia. These areas, however, are not the only or most common sites involved (<14% involve the splenic flexure alone and <5% involve the rectosigmoid), and virtually any section of colon may be afflicted, with left colon most commonly involved, followed by transverse colon and splenic flexure, splenic flexure alone, right colon, and rectum.

Clinical and Endoscopic Features

Crampy abdominal pain and bright red or maroon-colored stool are the presenting symptoms. Nausea, vomiting, or abdominal distension can be reported. Transmural infarction is seen in 15% of cases. In 50% of cases, it is transient and reversible. Of those who initially recover, chronic non-reversible ischemic colitis may develop (20–25%) that may lead to stricturing disease (10–15%). Fulminant pancolitis is rare (1%). Isolated right-sided ischemic colitis has been reported as a distinctive entity, associated with chronic renal failure (hemodialysis), coronary artery disease, and atrial fibrillation, with a higher risk of mortality and need for surgery. The reason for this worse outcome has been explained by the common association of mesenteric ischemia.

In early ischemia, the mucosa appears pale and edematous with interspersed areas of hyperemia or petechial hemorrhage. Later, segmental erythema may be seen, with or without ulceration and bleeding. With more significant ischemia, submucosal edema and hemorrhage develop characterized as bluish-black blebs or nodules. In severe ischemia, the mucosa appears cyanotic, dusky, gray, or black. Pseudopolyps and pseudomembranes may be noted. In chronic ischemia, stricturing, decreased haustrations and mucosal granularity may be seen.

Table 10.9 Predisposing and etiologic factors for ischemic colitis.

Low flow states
Cardiac failure or dysrhythmias
Shock (sepsis, hemorrhagic, hypovolemic)
Ruptured ectopic pregnancy

Occlusive disease states
Arteriosclerosis
Arterial thrombus
Cholesterol emboli
Atrial myxoma
Inferior mesenteric artery thrombosis
Aortic dissection

Small vessel disease
Amyloidosis
Diabetes
Radiation injury

Mechanical colonic obstruction
Tumors
Adhesions
Volvulus
Strangulated hernia
Diverticulitis
Intestinal prolapse

Hypercoagulable states
Protein C and S deficiencies
Antithrombin III deficiency
Prothrombin 20210A mutation
Hyperhomocysteinemia
Anticardiolipin syndrome
Paroxysmal nocturnal hemoglobinuria

Hematologic disorders
Polycythemia vera
Sickle cell disease
Thrombotic thrombocytopenia purpura

Vasculitis and vasculopathy
Systemic lupus erythematosus
Polyarteritis nodosa
Wegner granulomatosis
Rheumatoid arthritis
Takayasu arteritis
Kawasaki's disease
Thromboangiitis obliterans
Fibromuscular dysplasia

Infection
Bacteria (*Escherichia coli* O157:H7)
Parasites (*Angiostrongylus costaricensis*, Schistosomiasis)
Viruses (hepatitis B virus, cytomegalovirus)
Intra-abdominal infections

Medications
Antihypertensive agents
Cocaine
Amphetamines
Diuretics
NSAIDs
Digoxin
Estrogens/oral contraceptives
Vasopressin
Pseudoephedrine
Alosetron
Danazol
Sumatriptans
Psychotropic drugs

Iatrogenic surgical/procedural causes
Aneurysmectomy
Aortic surgery
Coronary artery bypass surgery
Colonic surgery
Colonoscopy
Barium enema
Gynecologic surgery
Lumbar arteriography
Exchange transfusions
Hemodialysis

Airplane flights

Strenuous physical activity (long-distance runners)

Trauma

Microscopic Features

Early ischemia is characterized by mucin depletion and glandular withering with small glands lined by flattened epithelium with hyperchromatic nuclei. The surface epithelium may be sloughed off while the basal portions of crypts survive (Figure 10.10a). The lamina propria is edematous and hemorrhage may be seen, and classically has an eosinophilic hyalinized appearance. Fibrin thrombi may be detected within capillaries. Inflammation is generally minimal. The submucosa is edematous.

As lesions progress, complete epithelial loss with ghost-like crypt outlines and full thickness mucosal necrosis may ensue with ulceration (Figure 10.10b). Vascular anomalies (e.g. thrombi, muscular changes) can be noted and inflammation with neutrophils and mononuclear inflammatory cells. Vascular thrombi and an endophlebitis may be seen beneath these ulcers. Pseudomembranes may develop.

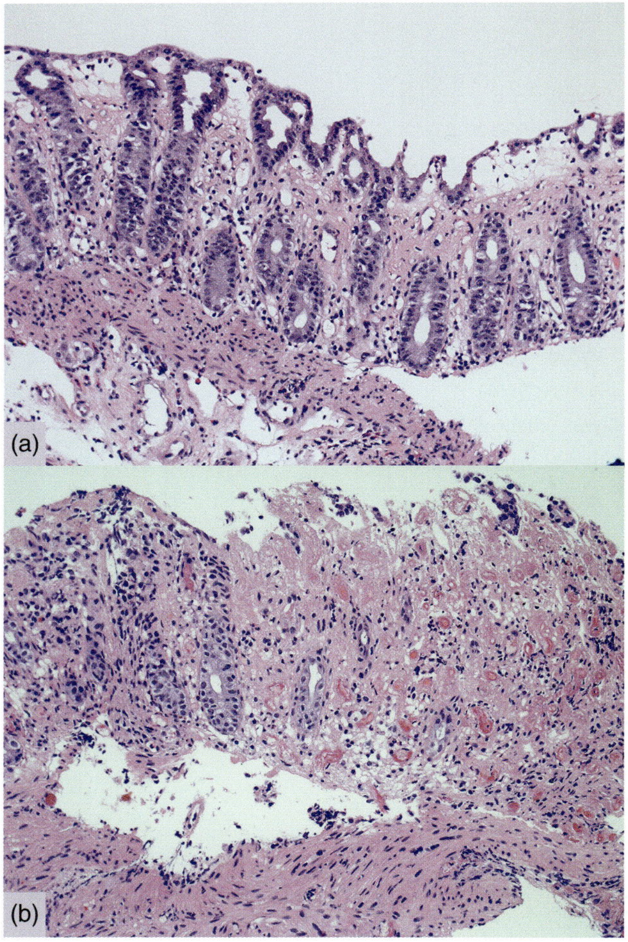

Figure 10.10 Typical histological appearance of an early (a) and a late (b) stage ischemic colitis. Picture (a) is a nice example of an early stage showing sloughing epithelium, hyalinization of the stroma and "preserved" architecture of the mucosa. Contrary the late stage (b) shows ulcerative changes with loss of crypts and fibrinoid thrombi in the small capillaries.

Mild ischemia may heal completely, but severe healed ischemia demonstrates marked, irregular atrophic glands set in a fibrous lamina propria containing siderophages. Pyloric gland and Paneth cell metaplasia may be seen. Rare exuberant reparative fibrosis processes that mimic carcinoma or strictures have been noted.

Differential Diagnosis

Distinguishing between acute ischemia and PMC may be challenging and requires synthesis of clinical and pathologic clues (Tables 10.10 and 10.11). Other potential considerations include infectious colitis, acute radiation injury, neutropenic colitis and mucosal prolapse. Chronic ischemia may need to be distinguished from chronic radiation proctitis and IBD (Table 10.10).

The necrotizing enterocolitic syndromes, such as necrotizing enterocolitis (pigbel) and neonatal necrotizing enterocolitis, are a heterogenous group of conditions that share common histologic features resembling ischemic colitis with extensive mucosal necrosis and hemorrhage. The small and large bowels are involved. The pathogenesis of these conditions is incompletely understood, although ischemia is thought to be an important component. Infection, particularly related clostridial species, is thought to play a role in some, although it may be difficult to separate primary infection from secondary infection subsequent to ischemia. These conditions, however, seldom impinge on biopsy practice as they are predominantly surgical emergencies and/or primarily involve small bowel.

Treatment/Prognosis/Evolution

Treatment of C. difficile colitis has changed recently as evidence supporting fecal transplantation has emerged, although this typically still reserved for recurrent cases. Some antibiotics are known to cause C. dif. colitis (clindamycin, amoxicillin) and should be discontinued when possible. Other antibiotics are used to treat C. dif. First line antibiotics include oral vancomycin and fidaxomicin. Metronidazole remains effective and can be used orally, or intravenously (e.g. in a patient with fulminant colitis who cannot tolerate oral medication). Fecal microbial ("stool") transplantation (FMT) has emerged as the treatment of choice for recurrent disease. FMT can be delivered by colonoscopy infusion, small bowel (via upper endoscopy) and recently has been delivered in the form of frozen encapsulated tablets. The optimal method is still not known. Surgery remains as an option of last resort for patients with fulminant disease not responding to standard treatments.

Table 10.10 Differential diagnosis of chronic ischemia.

Features	Chronic ischemia	IBD	Radiation
Mucosal architecture	Crypt distortion Atrophy	Crypt distortion Atrophy	Crypt distortion Atrophy
LP inflammation	Absent	"Empty" in quiescent disease or increased	Absent, empty appearance; eosinophils may be increased
Cryptitis	–	+/– (absent quiescent disease)	–
Crypt abscesses	–	+/– (absent quiescent disease)	–
LP connective tissue alterations	LP diffuse fibrosis ± submucosa fibrosis; may have thickening or splaying muscularis mucosa; hemosiderophages	LP fibrosis may occur, and may be deep band-like in mucosa; may have thickening or splaying muscularis mucosa	LP/submucosa fibrosis; may have thickening and splaying muscularis mucosa; Telangiectasia atypical fibroblasts; obliterative endarteritis and vascular hyalinization
Comments	Clinical history of prior episodes of ischemic colitis or risk factors for ischemia	Clinical history of IBD	Clinical history of prior radiation

Table 10.11 Risk factors for pseudomembranous colitis.

Host factors	Treatment factors	Environmental factors	*C. Difficile* factors
Older age (>65 years)	Recent antibiotic therapy	Recent hospitalization	Production of binary toxin in addition to toxins A and B
Prior antibiotic-associated diarrhea or *C. difficile* infection	Chemotherapy	Chronic care facilities	NAP1/BI/027 strain
Previous gastrointestinal surgery	Hematopoietic stem cell transplantation		Resistance to broad spectrum quinolones
Underlying gastrointestinal disease (e.g. inflammatory bowel disease, celiac disease)	Acid suppression		
Insufficient IgG antibody response to toxin A			
Severity of diarrhea			
Enteral feeding			

Focal Active Colitis (FAC)

Definition, General Features, and Predisposing Factors

Focal active colitis is characterized by focal cryptitis or crypt abscesses in the absence of any other significant abnormality.

This diagnosis refers to a microscopic pattern of inflammation, rather than a specific etiologic diagnosis. Its frequency is unknown, but estimates suggest up to 50 times per year in an average "general hospital" practice.

The diagnosis has been associated with multiple conditions (Table 10.12), with some differences between adult and pediatric populations. Broadly, focal active colitis may represent sporadic nonspecific changes, but may also be iatrogenic, or result from ischemic injury, or represent precursor lesions of IBD.

Clinical Features and Endoscopic Features

In some instances, a biopsy diagnosis of FAC may be an incidental biopsy finding in asymptomatic patients; however, most have diarrhea with or without abdominal pain. In others, the clinical presentation is consequent to the associated condition leading to endoscopy. The colonoscopic appearances include patchy erythema, or nonspecific findings including possible aphthous ulcers or vascular ectasia, or subepithelial hemorrhage, but may be essentially normal.

Microscopic Features

Isolated active neutrophilic crypt injury (cryptitis/crypt abscess) is characteristic (Figure 10.11). The number of crypts involved (from one to a few) is generally limited and

Table 10.12 Diseases associated with focal active colitis.

Diagnoses associated with FAC
Acute infectious/self-limiting colitis (adults 19–48%; pediatric 31%)
Ischemic colitis (adults 4–10%; pediatric 0%)
Crohn's disease (adults 0–13%; pediatric 27.6%)
Ulcerative colitis (adults 2%; pediatric ~7%)
Allergic (~6.5% pediatric)
Hirschsprung disease (~3% pediatric)
Irritable bowel syndrome (adults 14–33%; pediatric 0%)
Antibiotic associated diarrhea
Medications (adults 24–39%, esp. NSAIDS; pediatric 0%)
Bowel preparation (sodium phosphate)
Idiopathic/incidental finding (adults 29–40%; pediatric 27.6%)

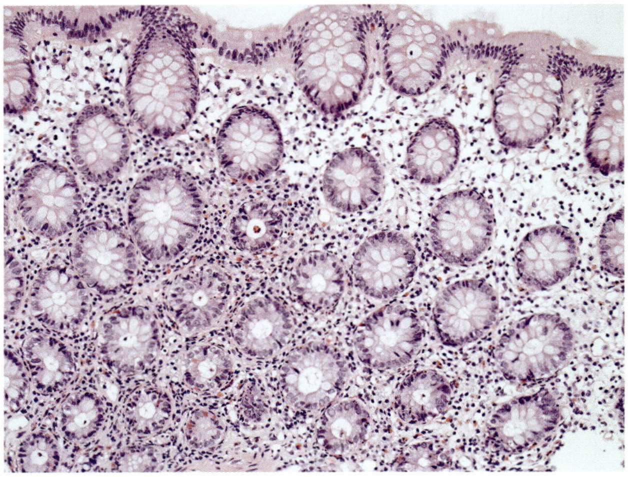

Figure 10.11 H.E. stain of FAC characterized by inflammation driven by neutrophils affecting only single crypts and showing crypt abscesses in some cases. The mucosal architecture is preserved.

should not exceed 50% of the biopsy specimen. Architectural changes and chronic inflammation are absent, and the remainder of the mucosa is essentially normal.

Differential Diagnosis

In practical terms, focal active colitis should be distinguished from *focal chronic active colitis*, in which architectural and other features of chronicity are observed. The pattern of "basal focal active colitis," especially if associated with apoptosis, may be predictive of an iatrogenic etiology.

Treatment/Prognosis/Evolution

In most instances, focal active colitis is an isolated incidental finding in asymptomatic patients or may be related to bowel preparation and have no significant clinical consequence. Knowledge of clinical setting, particularly medications, and associated findings is critical as these may point to a more specific diagnosis. In pediatric patients, FAC may herald the development of IBD, mostly Crohn's disease, and additional investigation or follow-up may be required.

Radiation Proctocolitis

Definition, General Features, and Predisposing Factors

This represents mucosal injury of the colorectum secondary to therapeutic ionizing radiation for malignancies. The regions most commonly affected are distal colon/rectum and ileum/cecum, following treatment of carcinomas of the rectum, anus, cervix, uterus, prostate, urinary bladder, and testes.

Acute radiation proctitis occurs during or within six weeks of irradiation. Chronic radiation proctitis is delayed; the symptoms commonly develop 9–14 months following irradiation, but can occur any time, sometimes up to 30 years later. The incidence of radiation proctitis is lower for brachytherapy (8–13%) than when irradiation is combined with other modalities (up to 21%). The incidence of chronic radiation proctitis is reported between 2 and 20%.

The predisposing features are shown in Table 10.13.

Clinical and Endoscopic Features

Early symptoms including diarrhea, mucoid discharge, bleeding, tenesmus, urgency, and incontinence are experienced by most patients by the middle of the second week of therapy.

Mucosal edema, friability, telangiectasia, duskiness, and loss of the normal vascular pattern are noted on colonoscopy. In some patients, the mucosa may appear granular and hemorrhagic, and multiple ulcers may be seen. In chronic radiation injury, pallor and telangiectasias are observed. Strictures, ulcerations, fistulas, and areas of mucosal hemorrhage may occur.

Between 1 and 12% of patients may develop complications, including strictures/stenosis, intestinal pseudo-obstruction, internal fistulae, perforation, hemorrhage, vascular obliteration, and mural fibrosis.

Microscopic Features

Acute Radiation Injury

Mucin depletion, regenerative nuclear atypia with loss of polarity, reduction in mitoses, and apoptosis are observed. Crypt withering and crypt loss or epithelial sloughing and mucosal ulceration may occur. The lamina propria is edematous, and eosinophilia is prominent, with cryptitis/abscesses. Vascular telangiectasia or fibrinoid necrosis may be present, and the submucosa may be edematous with a myxoid

Table 10.13 Risk factors for radiation colitis.

Therapy-related factors	Patient-related factors
Dose of radiation Dose <45 Gy are associated with few long-term effects; 45–70 Gy associated with increased complications; >70 Gy associated with significant and long-standing injury to surrounding tissues Multiple doses and accelerated fractionation increase incidence of toxicity	Comorbities Inflammatory bowel disease Immunosuppression, e.g. HIV/AIDS Diabetes Hypertension Atherosclerosis Prior surgery Empty intestinal lumen during therapy
Area of exposure	
Method of delivery Brachytherapy (radioactive implants) results in less exposure and injury to surrounding tissue compared to external beam radiation Newer modalities: Three-dimensional conformal radiation therapy (3D-CRT), intensity-modulated radiation therapy (IMRT), use of heavy particles (protons and neutrons) may have reduced risk of toxicity	
Combination therapy (chemoradiotherapy)	

quality. Sometimes inflammatory pseudopolyps develop. Usually, the damage resolves within one to three months.

Delayed Radiation Injury

This is characterized by crypt distortion and atrophy with variable loss of goblet cells and Paneth cell metaplasia. Epithelial atypia may be observed, with enlarged hyperchromatic nuclei with smudgy chromatin and maintained N : C ratio. Inflammation is usually absent. Mucosal erosion and ulceration can develop. Mucosal fibrosis or thickening of the collagen layer beneath the surface and crypt epithelium can develop, and vascular ectasia and lymphangiectasia are typical with perivascular hyalinization. Atypical "radiation" fibroblasts with enlarged hyperchromatic nuclei and basophilic cytoplasm are common. The muscularis mucosa is thickened and distorted, with focal discontinuity and glandular entrapment leading to colitis cystica profunda in some cases. Submucosa, if included, demonstrates arterial intimal proliferation, sometimes with foamy endothelial cells, mural hyalinization, and phlebosclerosis. Stromal fibrosis along with neuronal proliferation can be seen.

Differential Diagnosis

The differential diagnosis of acute and chronic radiation injury includes ischemic colitis. In addition, some features of acute radiation may overlap with eosinophilic colitis, whereas chronic radiation injury may mimic IBD. Collagenous colitis or amyloidosis also may be entertained, depending on the case (Table 10.14).

Treatment/Prognosis/Evolution

In mild cases, therapeutic measures are not absolutely necessary. However, if the symptoms are more pronounced, proctitis can be treated with drugs or interventional procedures. In the case of drug treatment anti inflammatory medication (e.g. sulfasalazine, sucralfate mesalamine, metronidazole etc.) is used. This treatment procedure may also help to stop possible bleeding. In addition, if there is an additional mechanical component (stenosis), stool softener can be given and possible dilatation can occur. In the case of severe mucosal damage with accompanying bleeding, removal of the damaged mucosa may be necessary, which can be performed by cryoablation, electrocoagulation or by using an argon laser (argon plasma coagulation; APC).

Diversion Proctocolitis

Definition, General Features, and Predisposing Factors

This mucosal inflammation results from diversion of the fecal stream, most commonly due to creation of an ileostomy or colostomy. The changes become apparent within 3–36 months of the diversion, and are related to alteration in the luminal flora with a loss of butyrate production, a short-chain fatty acid trophic to the epithelium. A theory of an underlying vascular or vasogenic abnormality has been proposed as well.

Table 10.14 Differential diagnosis of radiation.

	Differential diagnosis	Common features	Differentiating features
Acute radiation injury	Eosinophilic colitis	Tissue eosinophilia, eosinophilic cryptitis/crypt abscesses	Clinical history Epithelial atypia and lack of mitoses, vascular changes (telangiectasia and fibrinoid necrosis)
	Drug-induced colitis	Tissue eosinophilia, eosinophilic cryptitis/crypt abscesses, crypt apoptosis	
	Ischemic colitis	Withering crypts, surface necrosis and sloughing, ulceration	Clinical history Acute ischemic colitis often less inflammatory and prominent lamina propria hyalinization, with epithelial regenerative changes and mitosis, whereas radiation has prominent eosinophilia/eosinophilic cryptitis/abscess, epithelial atypia and reduced mitoses
Chronic radiation injury	Chronic ischemia	Crypt distortion and atrophy, Paneth cell metaplasia	Clinical history Identification of the vascular and connective tissue changes (telangiectasia, obliterative vascular changes and hyalinization, atypical fibroblasts)
	Inflammatory bowel disease		As above; IBD may show lamina propria chronic inflammation and active crypt inflammation
	Collagenous colitis	Subepithelial collagen band	Chronic radiation may occasionally demonstrate subepithelial collagen band; but lacks the inflammatory changes of CC and is associated with typical vascular and connective tissue alterations (see above)
	Mucosal prolapse	Crypt distortion, telangiectasia	Fibromuscular obliteration of lamina propria distinguishes mucosal prolapse; submucosal vascular changes and atypical fibroblasts characterize chronic radiation; clinical history
	Amyloidosis	Amyloid deposition may occasionally mimic lamina propria hyalinization or fibrosis in chronic radiation injury; amyloid in vascular walls may mimic vascular hyalinization	Clinical history; Congo red and trichrome stains will differentiate; typical vascular and connective tissue alterations of chronic radiation including telangiectasia and atypical fibroblasts

Clinical Features and Endoscopic Features

The patients with present with mucoid discharge or bloody discharge and crampy abdominal pain, but may be asymptomatic. Several mucosal patterns may be seen, including erythema, petechial hemorrhage, mucosal friability, mucosal nodularity sometimes surrounded by aphthous ulcers, nonspecific colitis, and inspissated mucus.

Microscopic Features

The pre-existing mucosal condition is important in determining the morphologic and clinical outcome. In pre-existing normal mucosa, development of marked lymphoid hyperplasia with or without focal overlying aphthous erosions/ulcers is characteristic. Crypt architecture is usually preserved, although the lymphoid hyperplasia may result in a degree of splaying or crypt distortion. There is expansion of the lamina propria by chronic inflammatory cells, mainly lymphocytes and plasma cells with some macrophages, and may be patchy or diffuse. Acute inflammation is minimal, but with time, focal neutrophilic infiltration, cryptitis, crypt abscesses, and ulceration may occur. Inflammatory pseudopolyps may develop.

The changes are somewhat different in previously diseased mucosa. Diversion exacerbates the inflammatory process in ulcerative colitis, and it may be difficult or impossible to determine how much is a result of diversion or exacerbation of the background IBD. Furthermore, fissuring ulceration and mucin crypt granuloma may obscure the picture. Transmural inflammation and lymphoid aggregates also may mimic Crohn's disease. In contrast, the histological appearances of diverted Crohn's disease typically show "burnt-out disease" with fibrosis and a lack of active inflammation. Granulomas become effete and hyalinized, and Schaumann bodies (unusual in Crohn's colitis) may be seen within these granulomas.

Differential Diagnosis

The changes may mimic follicular proctitis or ulcerative colitis, while the presence of aphthous lesions and focal active crypt inflammation may evoke Crohn's disease. Prominent follicular hyperplasia is a histologic clue and knowledge of the clinical setting is critical to the diagnosis. The presence of focal active colitis in a diverted segment in patients with CD should be regarded as diversion colitis as these resolve with restoration of the fecal stream. In a patient with UC and diversion, the presence of Crohn's disease-like features should not be taken to represent CD and the diagnosis should not be reversed without a thorough review of all histopathologic material (including index biopsies) in conjunction with clinical information.

Treatment and Prognosis

The changes of diversion colitis may resolve with butyrate enemas, although not invariably, but certainly with re-establishment of bowel continuity.

Neutropenic Enterocolitis (Typhlitis)

Definition, General Features, and Predisposing Factors

This is a segmental necrotizing and ulcerating inflammatory condition arising in neutropenic patients. It primarily affects the terminal ileum, cecum, and ascending colon, but can be more extensive. Patients usually have profound granulocytopenia (<500–1000/mm^3), for at least a week. Most cases have been associated with chemotherapy, predominantly for hematologic malignancies. Immunosuppression and other rare settings in which neutropenia arises also may predispose to neutropenic colitis.

The pathogenesis is thought to involve direct mucosal injury, secondary to chemotherapy (not a prerequisite), neoplastic infiltration, or neutropenia itself, resulting in loss of mucosal integrity. This allows pathogens such as *Pseudomonas* species or *E. coli* (in children), *C. septicum* (more common in adults), and *Candida* species (occasionally) to invade the wall with consequent sepsis. Bacterial invasion of vessels and toxin production results in disseminated intravascular coagulation with consequent ischemia. Sepsis, hypotension, and progressive bowel dilatation with increased mural pressure and further reduction in blood flow exacerbates the ischemia. The cecum is preferentially involved due to luminal stasis, higher mural pressure and relatively poor vascular supply, but may involve segments of small intestine. The predisposing factors are shown in Table 10.15.

Table 10.15 Risk factors for neutropenic colitis.

Chemotherapy
Paclitaxel
Docetaxel
Gemcitabine
Cytosine
Arabinoside
Vincristine
Doxorubicin
Cyclophosphamide
5-Fluorouracil
Leucovorin
Daunorubicin
Hematologic malignancies
Leukemia
Lymphoma
Non-hematologic malignancies
Breast
Lung
Colorectal
Ovarian cancer
Immune suppression
Transplantation
Stem cell or autologous bone marrow transplantation for hematologic and solid organ malignancies
Renal transplantation
AIDS
Miscellaneous causes of neutropenia
Aplastic anemia
Cyclic neutropenia
Idiosyncratic drug reactions

Clinical Features and Endoscopic Features

Patients present with dramatic onset with abdominal pain, fever, or watery or bloody diarrhea. Pain is often localized to right lower quadrant and may mimic appendicitis. Nausea and vomiting, progressive abdominal distension, rebound tenderness, right lower quadrant mass, and overt gastrointestinal bleeding may occur. The bowel appears thickened, edematous, congested, and hemorrhagic. Nodularity related to pneumatosis intestinalis may be seen.

Microscopic

The affected bowel shows hemorrhage and pronounced edema, ischemic changes with ulceration and necrosis, but with absence of neutrophils or inflammatory reaction. Pseudomembranes composed of fibrin and necrotic cells may coat luminal surface or ulcerated mucosa. In preserved areas of mucosa, crypt degeneration reminiscent of infection may be seen, but with no acute inflammatory reaction.

Gram stain may identify bacteria within the pseudomembranes, lamina propria, and submucosa, within and surrounding small vessels. PAS or silver stains may demonstrate *Candida* species organisms in some cases.

Differential Diagnosis

This includes ischemic colitis and PMC, but the absence of neutrophils and inflammation in conjunction with the clinical context points to the diagnosis (see Table 10.5, ischemic colitis).

Treatment /Prognosis / Evolution

Adjustment of dietary intake and parenteral nutrition are typically used in the presence of NE. Essential for the treatment of SD is the use of antibiotics, which is typically initiated with a monotherapy. If this is not effective, it is extended to a dual therapy. Antibiotics used in the treatment of NE are for example ß-lactamic antibiotics or cephalosporines. In case of perforation or ischemia of the intestine, surgical intervention would be necessary.

Microscopic Colitis (MC)

Two main forms of microscopic colitis are recognized, collagenous and lymphocytic colitis. They account for 10–20% of patients investigated for chronic watery diarrhea, with higher prevalence in those older than 70 years. Up to 25% of microscopic colitis cases occur under 45 years, but it is rarely reported in childhood. The incidence appears to be stabilizing following an initial rise, and presently approximates that of idiopathic IBD. Notably, microscopic colitis is less common, although increasingly reported, in Asia.

Several pathogenetic mechanisms have been suggested. Reports of familial clustering of microscopic colitis, associations with certain human leukocyte antigen (HLA) haplotypes (HLA-DQ2 or DQ1/3 and HLA-DR3DQ2 haplotype), polymorphisms in TNF-α gene and matrix metalloproteinase 9 gene, suggest an underlying genetic predisposition. Association with autoimmunity and response to steroids or immunosuppression supports an immune dysregulation basis. An abnormal response to a luminal or environmental agent has been suggested by the observation of improvement of collagenous colitis following institution of an elemental diet or diversion of the fecal stream. Finally, bacterial infection or toxin and bile salts also have been suggested. Subsequently, it is likely that the etiopathogenesis is multifactorial, with an abnormal immunological response to a luminal or environmental agent in a genetically susceptible host. A proportion of cases of collagenous and lymphocytic colitis appear to fulfill the criteria for drug-induced colitis.

Lymphocytic colitis and collagenous colitis share many clinicopathologic features, yet there are notable differences suggesting that they are likely two different, but perhaps related conditions. Furthermore, despite reports of cases transitioning from one form of MC to another, this is relatively rare, and patchiness of the subepithelial collagen in collagenous colitis potentially may account for variation in diagnoses within the same patient.

Table 10.16 Autoimmune disease associated with collagenous and lymphocytic colitis.

Autoimmune associations with lymphocytic and collagenous colitis
Common associations
Rheumatoid arthritis
Autoimmune thyroid disease
Diabetes
Less common reported associations
Psoriasis
Autoimmune gastritis
Sjogren syndrome
Raynaud disease
Polymyalgia rheumatica
Dermatomyositis
Mixed CTD
Systemic lupus erythematosus
Dermatitis herpetiformis
Sarcoidosis
CREST syndrome
Wegener granulomatosis
Behcet's syndrome

Collagenous Colitis

Definition, General Features, and Predisposing Factors

This is a clinicopathologic syndrome of chronic watery diarrhea associated with macroscopically near normal mucosa and characteristic histologic pattern of inflammation with thickened subepithelial collagen table.

The incidence of collagenous colitis ranges from 2.6–10.8/100 000, with the highest rates reported from United States, Canada, and Denmark. There is a suggestion of a north–south gradient, with lower incidence in more southern locations. The average age of diagnosis is 65 years, and there is a strong female predilection.

Increased risk is observed with smoking, history of polyarthritis or autoimmune disease (Table 10.16), celiac disease, and consumption of medications (Table 10.17). An increased risk has also been reported post solid-organ transplantation.

Clinical Features

The main symptom is chronic non-bloody diarrhea. Nocturnal diarrhea, fecal incontinence, and weight loss may occur. Serious dehydration and electrolyte disturbances

Table 10.17 Drugs that may be associated with microscopic colitis.

Analgesics
Nonsteroidal anti-inflammatory drugs (NSAIDs)[a]
Aspirin[a]
H_2-antagonist
Ranitidine[a]
Proton pump inhibitors
Lansoprazole[a]
Anti-androgen
Flutamide[a]
Selective serotonin reuptake inhibitor (SSRI)
Sertraline[a]
Paroxetine[b]
Anti-platelet (thienopyridine)
Ticlopidine[a]
Anti-diabetic (alpha-glucosidase inhibitor)
Acarbose[a]
HMG-CoA reductase inhibitor
Simvastatin[a]
Anti-epileptic
Carbamazepine[b]
Anti-parkinsonian
Madopar (levodopa and benserazide)[b]
Peripheral vasodilator
Vinburnine[b]
Anti-hypertensive
Lisinopril[b]
Migraine prophylaxis
Oxetorone[b]
Supplements
Tardyferon[b]

[a] Strong association.
[b] Possible association.

are rare. Abdominal pain is common and differentiation from irritable bowel syndrome (IBS) may be challenging. The onset is typically insidious, but may be sudden.

At colonoscopy, the mucosa is typically normal or shows minimal changes, including edema or an opalescent appearance, mild erythema, or diminished vascular pattern. Increasingly, colonoscopic abnormalities are being reported possibly related to improving colonoscopic technology, and may include pruning of mucosal vasculature, or crowded dilated tortuous capillaries; red spots, nodularity, or textural abnormalities (with or without chromoendoscopy); hemorrhagic lacerations or linear tears more commonly in ascending and transverse colon (either spontaneously or with insufflation) and fine linear cicatricial lines or thick scar-like ridges possibly due to healing of mucosal tears/defects. A mosaic or "honeycomb" pattern of the mucosa in the appropriate clinical context of chronic watery diarrhea has been reported by some as a distinguishing feature of collagenous colitis. Rarely, pseudomembranes may be seen in collagenous colitis.

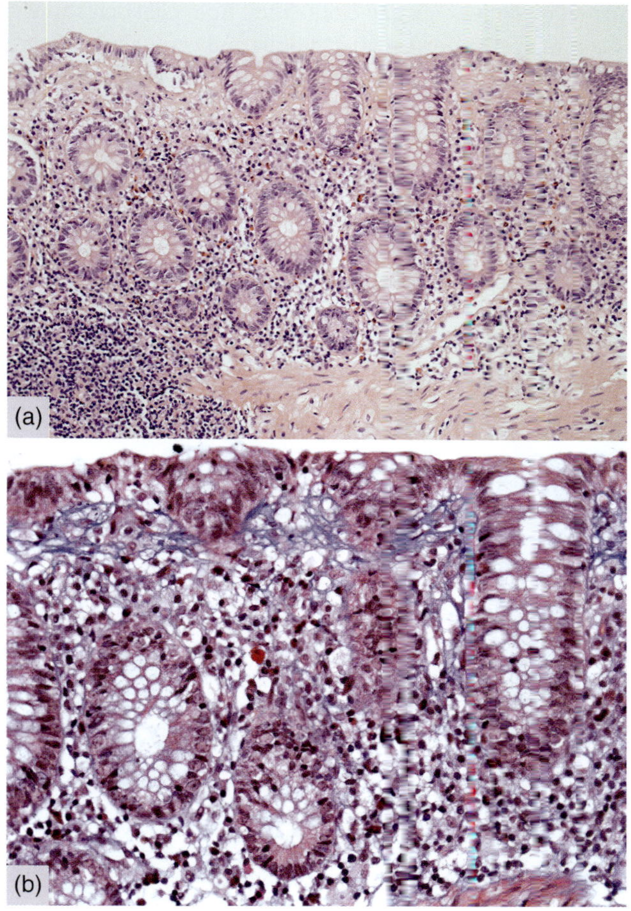

Figure 10.12 Typical finding in case of collagenous findings showing a thickened eosiniophilic collagen band (a) which can be highlighted with the trichorme stain (b). Furthermore this biopsy shows detached epithelium (a; upper left) as well as a prominent inflammatory background with a predominance of lymphoplasmocytic cells.

Multiple random colonic biopsies are recommended. Biopsies limited to the rectosigmoid alone may miss the diagnosis in up to 40% of cases. One study reported that the diagnostic yield was highest from biopsies of the transverse colon (83%) and right colon (70%) and lowest from the rectosigmoid (66%).

Microscopic Features

The mucosal architecture is normal, with hypercellular lamina propria secondary to lymphoplasmacytic infiltrate, and variable eosinophilia. There is also variable lymphocytic exocytosis with occasional intraepithelial eosinophils or neutrophils, and distinct epithelial damage with mucin depletion and regenerative cuboidal epithelium. Epithelial detachment is common (Figure 10.12a). Cryptitis and crypt abscesses are absent or rare. The characteristic thick collagen band is limited to the intercryptal zone, and does not extend alongside crypts (Figure 10.12b). The normal subepithelial collagen table is reported to be less than 7 μm, and a thickness of >10 μm is said to be diagnostic in the proper setting. However, more subtle features are diagnostic as well, such as presence of entrapped erythrocytes, inflammatory cells, and capillaries within the band, and an irregular jagged inferior margin. It should be noted that thickening of the subepithelial collagen band is nonuniform and may be more prominent proximally.

Variant Patterns of Collagenous Colitis have been Reported

- Pseudomembranes can rarely be seen superimposed on otherwise typical histology in cases with classic clinicopathologic and outcome characteristics. Some cases have been associated with CVID. However, coexistence of toxin-proven PMC with collagenous colitis has been reported, and therefore infectious, ischemic, and toxin/drug etiologies must be excluded.
- IBD-like features including crypt atrophy or irregularity (7.6%), Paneth cell metaplasia (44%), cryptitis/crypt abscesses (30%), and surface ulceration (2.5%) may be observed. However, these features are typically mild and focal (cryptitis/crypt abscesses in less than three crypts per biopsy specimen and architectural abnormalities limited to one portion of a single fragment), and lack other features of IBD. Importantly, clinical and endoscopic findings suggestive of IBD are lacking.
- Subepithelial macrophages or giant cells have been observed in otherwise typical collagenous colitis. These are of no significant clinical consequence.

Findings in Other Segments of the Gastrointestinal Tract

Associations with celiac disease, increased IEL in the ileal mucosa, collagenous ileitis, or collagenous gastroduodenitis have been reported.

Both Crohn's and ulcerative colitis also have been described in association with microscopic colitis (both LC and CC), either preceding it or developing after a diarrheal illness. It is not currently determined if these conditions are pathogenetically related or merely coincidental.

Ultrastructural examination has demonstrated that the subepithelial band is composed of collagen fibers with typical periodicity, closely grouped in a criss-cross manner beneath the basement membrane, which is not expanded, and may be focally deficient with epithelium resting directly on collagen.

Immunohistochemically, the collagen has been reported to stain for collagen types I, III, and VI, and tenascin. The latter can enhance appreciation of the abnormal jagged inferior margin and entrapped capillaries in the abnormally thickened subepithelial collagen plate.

Differential Diagnosis

See Table 10.18.

Treatment/Prognosis/Evolution

The clinical course is chronic with variable relapses, but overall, the long-term prognosis is good. Resolution of symptoms can occur spontaneously, with cessation of offending medication, or with treatment. Twenty percent of patients resolved spontaneously. Long-term cessation of diarrhea was observed in more than 70% of patients. Histologic features of inflammation may improve with treatment, as may the expanded subepithelial collagen; however, this is not invariable, and overall there is no correlation between treatment and change in symptoms or histological findings. Rarely, refractory disease may require diversion of fecal stream with ileostomy or colectomy. Collagenous colitis may rarely be associated with perforation. There is suggestion that Paneth cells and the degree of lamina propria inflammation may be associated with a more severe and prolonged course in collagenous colitis. However, overall, histologic features are not predictive of outcome. There is no increased risk of neoplasia.

Lymphocytic Colitis

Definition, General Features, and Predisposing Factors

Lymphocytic colitis encompasses a clinicopathologic syndrome of chronic watery diarrhea with macroscopically near normal colonic mucosa and a characteristic inflammatory pattern with increased IEL.

The reported incidence ranges from 2.2 to 14/100 000 persons per year. Female predominance is less consistently reported and less prominent compared to collagenous colitis, with equal incidence in males and females in some studies.

The predisposing factors are similar to collagenous colitis. The association of autoimmune disease and celiac disease is stronger.

Clinical Features

Chronic non-bloody diarrhea is the main symptom, with significant overlap with collagenous colitis, such that they are generally indistinguishable clinically (see Section

Table 10.18 Differential diagnosis of collagenous colitis (CC).

	Collagenous colitis	Ulcerative colitis	Amyloidosis	Radiation colitis	Mucosal prolapse	Chronic ischemia	Diverticulosis	Infectious colitis	Systemic sclerosis
Clinical	Chronic watery diarrhea	Chronic diarrhea ± blood ± mucus	Variable diarrhea or constipation (AL amyloidosis is more commonly associated with constipation, mechanical obstruction or chronic intestinal pseudoobstruction, while AA amyloidosis more is typically associated with diarrhea and malabsorption)	History of irradiation Diarrhea, mucus, urgency, tenesmus, bleeding	Constipation, rectal bleeding, mucus discharge, tenesmus, incontinence	May have history or previous episodes of ischemia	Diarrhea, constipation, PR bleeding, Pain	Diarrhea Pain History of travel or consumption of contaminated food/water	Involvement of the colon typically results in constipation, due to impaired motility, rather than diarrhea although this may occur as well
Endoscopy	Normal	Diffuse involvement beginning in rectum and extending for a variable distance proximally with loss of vascular markings, hyperemia, edema, granularity, friability, ulceration, pseudopolyps.	Normal; polypoid protrusions and thickening of the valvulae conniventes (AL amyloidosis); fine granular mucosa, mucosal friability and erosions (AA amyloidosis)	Pallor with friability, mucosal telangiectasia	Erythema, ulceration, polypoid masses	Scarring; may have other features of ischemia; involvement of "watershed" or ischemia-prone regions.	Diverticula	Variable, erythema, ulceration	Normal; telangiectasia; wide-mouthed diverticula, loss of haustration
Architectural distortion or chronicity and Paneth cell metaplasia	−/+[a]	++	−	+		−/+	+/−	−	−
Basal lymphoplasmacytosis	−[a]	++	−	−	−	−	−	−	−
Increased IEL	+	−/+	−	−	−	−	−	−/+ (resolving phase)	−

(Continued)

Table 10.18 (Continued)

	Collagenous colitis	Ulcerative colitis	Amyloidosis	Radiation colitis	Mucosal prolapse	Chronic ischemia	Diverticulosis	Infectious colitis	Systemic sclerosis
Surface epithelial damage and mucin depletion	++	++	– (lacks surface epithelial detachment seen in CC)	+	+	–/+	+/–	+	–
Expanded subepithelial collagen table	++	–/+	+[b]	+/–	+/–	–/+	+/–	–	–
Increased lamina propria chronic inflammatory cells	++	++	–	– (eosinophils) (Atypical fibroblasts, hyalinization of lamina propria)	– (muscle hyperplasia)	–/+	+	–/+ (late phase); Lamina propria neutrophils	–
Cryptitis/crypt abscesses	–/+[a]	++	–	+/– (eosinophilic cryptitis)	+/–	–	+/–	–/+	–
Vessels	No specific abnormality	No specific abnormality	Amyloid deposition in vessel walls. Deposits in lamina propria, muscualris mucosae or submucosa may be seen as well.	Telangiectasia, vascular hyalinization, fibrointimal expansion	Thickening, thrombosis	Arterio- and arteriolosclerosis; cholesterol emboli; organizing thrombus; (vasculitis)	–	–/+ (focal fibrin thrombi with certain infectious, e.g. *C. difficile*, EHEC)	Telangiectasia; mucoid intimal thickening of submucosal arteries ± vasculitis
Congo red	–	–	+	–	–	–	–	–	–
Trichrome	+ (highlights the subepithelial collagen thickening that is limited to the intercryptal zones)	–/+ (may highlight areas of subepithelial collagen thickening if present; lamina propria fibrosis may be seen particularly in areas of healed ulceration)	–	Lamina propria fibrosis; Radiation induced hyalinization less intense than collagenous colitis	Lamina propria fibrosis	May highlight more extensive lamina propria fibrosis than exclusively subepithelial	–/+	–	+ (subepithelial collagen thickening is not limited to the intercryptal zones but extends down crypts; there may be more diffuse lamina propria fibrosis)
Perl's	–	–	–	–	+/–	+	–	–	–

[a] Although IBD-like features have been reported in CC including chronic architectural changes, Paneth cell metaplasia, and cryptitis/crypt abscesses, these features are typically focal/limited.
[b] Amyloid involvement of the GI tract shows different patterns of deposition depending on the type of amyloid. AL (light chains) amyloid is more often associated with deposition in the muscularis mucosae, submucosa, muscularis propria and less likely to be detected on endoscopic biopsy. AA amyloid (serum amyloid A protein), on the other hand, is more common in the mucosa and submucosa. Amyloidosis related to hemodialysis (β_2-microglobulin) is similar to AL amyloid and mainly associated with deposition in the muscularis mucosae, submucosa, and muscularis propria. Senile amyloidosis tends to be found in the superficial vessels and submucosa. Familial amyloidotic polyneuropathy is typically associated with deposition in the nerves and seldom detected on mucosal biopsy. Amyloid deposition beneath the basement membrane may mimic collagenous colitis although this tends to involve both the surface epithelium and crypts.

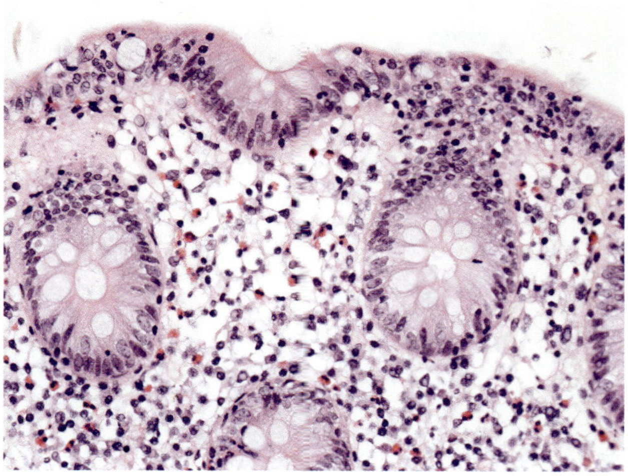

Figure 10.13 High magnification of lymphocytic colitis characterized by an increased amount of intraepithelial lymphocytes (IEL) and preserved mucosal architecture.

"Collagenous Colitis"). The symptoms of lymphocytic colitis may be milder. Typically, the mucosa appears near normal on colonoscopy, and mild nonspecific changes may be observed (see Section "Collagenous Colitis"). Recently, a furrowed or mosaic mucosal pattern has been reported.

Microscopic Features

This condition is characterized by increased IEL (Figure 10.13). The normal IEL count in the colon is less than 5 per 100 enterocytes. A threshold of >20/100 enterocytes has been used for the diagnosis, but in practice counting is generally unnecessary with obvious intraepithelial lymphocytosis. Epithelial injury with mucin depletion and attenuated surface epithelium is noted. Regenerative crypt changes may be seen with nuclear enlargement and increase in mitotic activity. The lamina propria is expanded by lymphocytes and plasma cells. The mucosal architecture usually is preserved.

Variant Patterns

1) *Lymphocytic Colitis with Giant Cells*
   Occasional cases may have subepithelial macrophages and giant cells, in otherwise typical background of lymphocytic colitis. These appear to behave like conventional lymphocytic colitis.
2) *Lymphocytic Colitis with IBD-Like Features*
   Some cases manifest IBD-like features including active crypt inflammation, architectural abnormalities, and Paneth cell metaplasia. Ulceration is generally absent.
3) *Paucicellular Lymphocytic Colitis*
   These are characterized by a lower density of surface intraepithelial lymphocytosis and patchiness, but the clinical profile is similar to classic cases. These cases lack CD25+FOXP3+ cells in the lamina propria compared to classic LC or CC, suggesting a different immunopathogenesis, and casting doubt on the validity of this pattern as a true variant.
4) *Cryptal Lymphocytic Colitis*
   The reason for the cryptal predominance of IELs is unknown, but may be related to antigens present within crypts rather than the lumen of the bowel. The clinicopathologic features and behavior are similar to classic cases.

Findings in Other Portions of Gastrointestinal Tract in Association with Lymphocytic Colitis

Lymphocytic colitis, like collagenous colitis, may be associated with celiac disease. A small subset of patients have been classified as "lymphocytic enterocolitis" and appear to be refractory to all therapy; however, it is not clear if a proportion of these may represent a lymphoproliferative disorder. Intraepithelial lymphocytosis involving the gut including gastric and small bowel (duodenum and ileal) mucosa can be associated with lymphocytic colitis. Enterocolic lymphocytic phlebitis, a rare process limited to the gut and characterized by lymphocytic infiltration of veins and venules, has been described in association and may be an iatrogenic manifestation.

A lymphocytic colitis-like pattern has been reported in association with Crohn's disease and may precede its onset. It is unclear if this represents coexistence of lymphocytic colitis and IBD, or whether this represents part of the histologic spectrum of a single disease process

The IELs are CD3+CD8+ T cells expressing TCR-$\alpha\beta$, in keeping with the phenotype of normal IEL. In contrast, the T cells in the lamina propria are CD4+.

Differential Diagnosis

See Tables 10.19 and 10.20 (Pitfalls and differential diagnosis).

In addition, LC and CC with giant cells should be distinguished from "granulomatous microscopic colitis." Although associated with watery diarrhea and normal colonoscopy, it does not share the typical histological features of either colitis, but displays increased chronic inflammation of the lamina propria with granulomas and crypt abscesses.

Treatment/Prognosis/Evolution

The prognosis and clinical course are similar to collagenous colitis, with minor variation. Lymphocytic colitis tends to have a shorter prediagnosis symptomatic period, milder symptomatology, and higher rates of remission.

Table 10.19 Differential diagnosis for lymphocytic colitis.

	Lymphocytic colitis	Non-specific colonic intraepithelial lymphocytosis	Brainerd diarrhea	Crohn's disease	Resolving colitis
Clinical	Chronic watery diarrhea	Nonspecific, may be asymptomatic or have symptoms related to associated conditions (e.g. celiac disease)	Acute onset, prolonged duration (~15 months) and features suggestive of point source of infection	Abdominal pain, weight loss, diarrhea	Diarrhea, abdominal pain
Intraepithelial lymphocytosis	++	+	+ (degree is less than lymphocytic colitis, similar to that in collagenous colitis)	−/+	+/−
Lamina propria chronic inflammation	+	−	−	+/− (patchy or discontinuous)	−/+ (mild increase lamina propria chronic inflammation, few neutrophils, may be patchy)
Epithelial damage and mucin depletion	++	−	−	−/+	+
Chronic architectural distortion/ Paneth cell metaplasia/Pyloric metaplasia	−/+ (focal)	−	−	+	−
Basal lymphoplasmacytosis/basal lymphoid aggregates	−	−	−	+	−
Cryptitis/crypt abscesses	−/+ (focal)	−	−	+	−/+
"Disproportionate" inflammation (submucosa)	−	−	−	+	−

Table 10.20 Pitfalls in the diagnosis of lymphocytic and collagenous colitis.

Lymphocytic colitis	Collagenous colitis
Normal variation *Epithelium overlying lymphoid follicles*: This normally has increased IELs. Step sections may help. *Right side of the colon:* This generally contains greater numbers of intraepithelial lymphocytes and lamina propria cells. Knowledge of the site is helpful.	*Artifactual thickening of "subepithelial collagen"*: Tangential sectioning may cause the basement membrane or subepithelial cytoplasmic zone to mimic a thickened subepithelial collagen table; fortuitous section of crypt sheath adjacent to surface epithelium. Assess only in well-orientated section (perpendicular section with ≥2–3 crypts full crypt lengths seen). In addition, consider associated features CC, i.e. epithelial damage, IELs, lamina propria inflammation and nature of subepithelial thickening, irregular inferior border with entrapped inflammatory cells and capillaries. Normal basement membrane has sharp inferior edge, even when artifactually "expanded" by tangential sectioning.
LC can be patchy: May be more severe in the right colon in 25% cases. Distal to the ascending colon but proximal to the rectosigmoid is the ideal location to maximize yield.	*Thickening of subepithelial collagen/basement membrane*: May be seen in many conditions, e.g. *C. difficile* infection, Crohn's, chronic ischemia, colon carcinoma, carcinoid, jejunoileal bypass, scleroderma, diabetes, hyperplastic polyps. These may be distinguished by the *context/associated features* and the nature of the subepithelial collagen expansion in CC, which is confined to the intercryptal epithelium and shows irregular inferior border with entrapped capillaries and inflammatory cells.
Colonic epithelial lymphocytosis: Increased IELs without epithelial injury and increased lamina propria inflammatory cells. This may be observed with gluten sensitivity or other allergic reaction to luminal antigens, medications (e.g. NSAID), in association with autoimmune or immunologic disease, or resolving colitis. The possibility that this may represent a mild or early form of lymphocytic colitis is not excluded, and some cases may overlap with "paucicellular" lymphocytic colitis.	*CC can be patchy*: Thickening of the subepithelial collagen may be more prominent proximally or rarely involve the right colon only and a proportion missed on left colon/rectal biopsies only. Emphasis should not be placed on absolute thickening of the subepithelial collagen but rather on the nature of the thickening, i.e. irregular inferior border with entrapped capillaries/inflammatory cells, as this feature is seen even in early thickening, which may be inconspicuous on HE, but may be highlighted with Trichrome stain.
Atypical presentation, e.g. colonoscopic abnormalities: Rare case of lymphocytic colitis associated with nodularity and loss of vascular markings. Experience is limited and caution is advised.	*Atypical presentation,* e.g. colonoscopic abnormalities: This may not necessarily exclude CC as it is becoming recognized that CC may have colonoscopic changes. However, careful clinicopathological correlation and exclusion of other conditions (e.g. IBD) are required and describing the changes as a "collagenous colitis pattern" with an explanatory note may be prudent.
Atypical features: e.g. IBD-like features. Careful clinicopathologic correlation and exclusion of other conditions required.	*Atypical features:* e.g. IBD-like features, pseudomembrane, ulcers (may be seen with NSAIDs). Careful clinicopathologic correlation and exclusion of other conditions required.

Colonic Diverticulosis and Diverticular Colitis

Definition, General Features, and Predisposing Factors

Diverticulosis is defined by the presence of diverticula, i.e. sac-like outpouchings of the colonic wall. Diverticular disease is defined as clinically significant and symptomatic uncomplicated or complicated diverticulosis. Diverticulitis is inflammation of a diverticulum, and segmental colitis associated with diverticula (SCAD, or diverticular colitis) is a complication characterized by inflammation in the interdiverticular mucosa without involvement of the diverticular orifices.

Diverticular disease is common in industrialized societies and is thought to be related to low-fiber diet. It affects half of the population over 60 years, and over 90% of cases involve the left colon, most commonly the sigmoid, but may extend proximally in severe disease and has several risk factors shown in Table 10.21. In contrast, diverticula in Asians, which tend to be right-sided and true diverticula composed of all layers of the bowel wall, occur at an earlier age and are thought to have a genetic basis.

Clinical Features

Most patients with uncomplicated diverticular disease remain asymptomatic. Between 10 and 25% may develop symptoms associated with diverticulitis or other

Table 10.21 Risk factors for diverticular disease.

Environmental and lifestyle	Associated or underlying conditions	Genetic predisposition
Low-fiber diet	Connective tissue disease (e.g. Ehlers–Danlos and Marfan syndrome)	Right-sided diverticula
Fat and red meat	Motility disorders and neuromuscular disease	
Low physical activity	Polycystic kidney disease	
Obesity (risk of diverticular bleeding and diverticulitis)	Inflammatory bowel disease (ulcerative colitis and Crohn's disease)	
Smoking (risk of perforated diverticulitis and diverticular abscess)		
NSAID, steroids, opiates (risk of diverticulitis and bleeding)		
Statin and vitamin D (may be protective for complicated diverticular disease)		

Table 10.22 Complications of diverticular disease.

Complications of diverticular disease
Inflammation
Diverticulitis
Peridiverticulitis
Diverticular disease-associated colitis
Bleeding
Mucosal
Erosion into penetrating vessels
Rupture
Perforation with peritonitis
Peridiverticular abscess
Inflammatory masses
Adhesions
Fistula
Strictures and obstruction
Giant diverticulum
Pylephlebitis and hepatic abscesses

complications (Table 10.22). Patients may present with left lower abdominal pain, fever, and leukocytosis. Constipation, nausea, vomiting, and diarrhea may also be reported.

Colonoscopic examination demonstrates diverticular openings and thickened haustral folds. Bleeding from diverticula may be observed. Purulent discharge or protruding granulation tissue may be seen with diverticulitis. Prolapsing folds, inflammatory polyps, and inverted diverticula may result in polypoid lesions. Diverticular colitis may demonstrate erythema, granularity, and friability similar in appearance to chronic IBD, confined to the segment affected by diverticula, and typically sparing the rectum. In severe cases, ulceration including linear ulceration and a cobblestone mucosal pattern resembling Crohn's disease (CD) may be seen.

Microscopic Features

Features pertinent to biopsy examination will reported here. Interested readers are referred to recent reviews for additional details. In uncomplicated disease, the biopsy is essentially normal. Redundant mucosal folds appear polypoid with increased mucosal height and crypt elongation or hyperplasia, edema, vascular congestion, and hemorrhage. Fibromuscular hyperplasia of the lamina propria resembling MP/SRUS is seen. Fibrin thrombi, hemosiderin, erosion, granulation tissue, and ischemic changes may occur. Variable lamina propria chronic inflammation, which may be associated with active inflammation, including cryptitis/crypt abscess, with or without mucosal prolapse changes, may be seen from biopsies around mouth of diverticula, particularly with associated diverticulitis.

SCAD demonstrates UC-like and CD-like variants. Architectural distortion, Paneth cell metaplasia, lamina propria mononuclear infiltration with basal lymphoid aggregates, and plasmacytosis can be noted, along with cryptitis, crypt abscesses, surface epithelial sloughing, and granulomatous cryptitis. Non-necrotizing granulomas can be seen as well.

Differential Diagnosis

Inflammation around diverticula may resemble infectious colitis and changes related to prolapse may mimic ischemic colitis (see Table 10.5). Thickening of the subepithelial collagen may be observed occasionally and mimic collagenous colitis (see Table 10.18 Differential diagnosis collagenous colitis).

SCAD may need to be differentiated from infectious colitis (*Shigella* and *Salmonella* may result in segmental colitis), although it tends to show features of chronicity. Knowledge of the clinical setting and stool cultures will be helpful. Differentiation of SCAD from IBD is difficult or impossible based on mucosal biopsies alone. Diagnostic clues include the restriction of inflammatory changes to the segment involved by diverticular disease with a normal rectum and colon proximal to the involved segment. However, ulcerative colitis with rectal sparing may still enter the differential diagnosis. The rectum is not involved in SCAD, whereas in ulcerative colitis, prior to medical treatment, it will show histologic changes despite a relatively normal macroscopic appearance (relative rectal sparing). In cases demonstrating Crohn's disease-like features, such a diagnosis should be avoided unless there is evidence of Crohn's disease elsewhere either concurrently or on follow-up. NSAID-associated colitis may show similar changes. Prominent crypt apoptosis is a histologic clue and knowledge of the clinical setting and anamnesis of the medication history will be helpful.

Treatment/Prognosis/Evolution

Compared with symptomatic diverticulosis without associated colitic changes, patients with SCAD are more likely to require surgical intervention. A small proportion of patients may progress to classic ulcerative colitis.

Mucosal Prolapse/Solitary Rectal Ulcer Syndrome (MPSRUS)

Definition, General Features, and Predisposing Factors

A chronic benign disorder of defecation characterized by histologic features of mucosal prolapse, it is an uncommon condition (incidence of 1/100 000) with a slight female predominance and a mean age of 49 years (range 14–76 years).

Typically associated with constipation, it is believed to be related to paradoxical contraction of the pelvic floor opposing the downward forces of defecation, resulting in prolapse of the colonic mucosa against the closed anal canal.

Clinical Features

The classic presentation includes rectal bleeding and passage of mucus, constipation, tenesmus, straining, or diarrhea. On sigmoidoscopy or colonoscopy, there may be typical solitary ulcer (35%) or multiple ulcers (22%), polypoid lesions (25%), or non-ulcerated lesions and erythema or hyperemic mucosa (18%). Evidence of rectal prolapse, either internal or external, with or without abnormal perineal descent may be detected on evacuation proctography. The lesions are most often found on the anterior or anterolateral wall of the rectum, typically 5–10 cm from the anal margin and centered on a rectal fold, but in some cases may be extensive and circumferential.

Microscopic Features

The histologic features include thickening of the mucosa with elongation, tortuosity, dilatation, and distortion of the crypts, particularly at the base. The crypt bases may become pointed and on cross-section "diamond-shaped." The epithelium may show hyperplastic changes, epithelial cells are commonly enlarged, and the goblet cells hypertrophied or elongated. Surface erosion is common, and degeneration of crypts reminiscent of ischemia may be seen (Figure 10.14). The lamina propria is edematous with congested superficial capillaries and a variable proliferation of fibroblasts can be seen. The muscularis propria is also hypertrophied with splaying of the fibers. A diagnostic feature is the presence of vertically oriented smooth muscle fibers extending upward between crypts. Epithelial misplacement with submucosal mucous cysts and localized colitis cystica profunda may occur. Finally, the inflammatory component is usually mild, but inflamed cases can be seen.

Differential Diagnosis

The differential diagnosis includes ischemia, early PMC (type I lesion), chronic radiation proctitis, and idiopathic IBD. Thickening of the subepithelial collagen may occur, raising the differential diagnosis of collagenous colitis. SRUS/MP may mimic carcinoma clinically, on endoscopy,

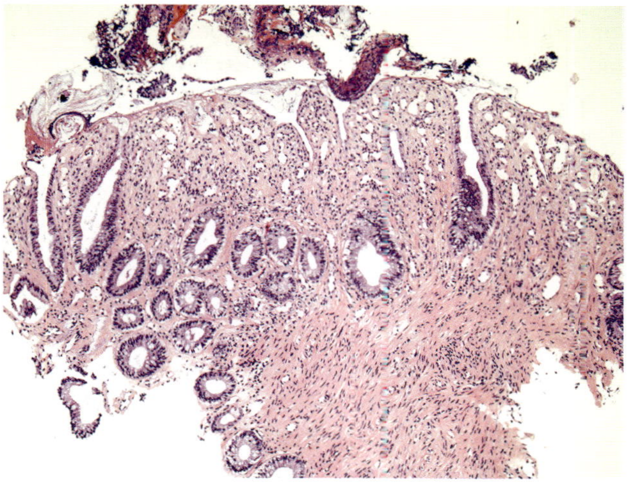

Figure 10.14 Characteristic changes in colonic biopsies caused by mucosal prolapse are distortion of the crypts, ulcerative changes, reactive changes of the epithelium and granulation tissue.

Table 10.23 Distinguishing misplaced glands from invasive adenocarcinoma.

	Misplaced glands	Invasive adenocarcinoma
Glandular profiles	Circumscribed	Irregular, infiltrative
Mucin pools (if present)	Circumscribed and rounded	Irregular, dissecting stroma
Relationship of epithelium to mucin pools (if present)	Around periphery of mucin pools, may be discontinuous	Floating within mucin pools
Epithelial architecture	Monolayer	Cellular crowding and piling up, complex glands, gland-in-gland configuration
Cytological features	Bland with basal nuclei, no dysplasia. May have regenerative/reactive features.	Atypia, may be marked.
Stromal reaction	No stromal desmoplasia. Granulation tissue, hemosiderin and hemorrhage.	True stromal desmoplasia
Presence of supporting lamina propria	Present (not invariably)	Absent

and histologically. The mimicry occurs particularly when there is gland displacement into submucosa, sometimes with mucin extravasation, mimicking mucinous adenocarcinoma (see Table 10.23).

Histologic changes of mucosal prolapse may arise in other clinical situations, such as internal intussusception, protruding lesions/masses including inflammatory cloacogenic polyp, inflammatory cap polyp, and inflammatory myoglandular polyp, redundant mucosal folds in the contracted colon of diverticular disease, and adjacent to stomal or diverticular openings.

Pneumatosis Coli

Definition, General Features, and Predisposing Factors

Pneumatosis coli represents the collection of gas in the colonic wall. It is not a single entity but rather represents a common end point of multiple conditions. It is uncommon and may be idiopathic (15%) or secondary to a range of predisposing processes. Three potential sources have been proposed for gas accumulation: (i) intraluminal, where increased intra-abdominal pressure may force intraluminal gas into the wall via minute mucosal defects; (ii) pulmonary, where air from ruptured bullae in obstructive pulmonary disease may track via tissue planes around great vessels and their abdominal branches; and (iii) bacterial translocation due to compromised mucosa, where intestinal necrosis allows gas-forming anaerobic bacteria to proliferate within intestinal wall. More than one contributing factor may be operating in an individual case. Depending on the associated condition, pneumatosis may be asymptomatic (often associated with obstructive pulmonary disease) or may have a fulminant presentation (often associated with ischemia and gas-forming bacteria).

Clinical and Endoscopic Features

The patients may be asymptomatic, or accompanied by constipation, diarrhea, abdominal pain, obstruction, intussusception, or even volvulus. Endoscopically, raised mucosal folds and soft rounded bluish cystic-nodular lesions mimicking polyps may be seen. In addition, features related to the underlying condition may be identified (Table 10.24).

Microscopic Features

The diagnosis can be challenging, since only the tops of the air cysts may be sampled, appearing as empty spaces with a few histiocytes or giant cells rimming the periphery and with an eosinophilic inflammatory infiltrate. The overlying mucosa may demonstrate architectural distortion and varying degree of active and chronic inflammation, as well as giant cells or granulomas. Pseudolipomatosis, i.e. collection of small air spaces in the lamina propria resembling fat, is a diagnostic clue. It is important to note that they are too large or confluent to be adipocytes, and occasionally may surround normal structures such as nerves.

Differential Diagnosis

The mucosal changes overlying pneumatosis coli may mimic IBD, but it also may complicate IBD. The knowledge of the clinical setting is therefore critical. Occasionally, the appearances may be mistaken for oleogranuloma or lymphangioma.

Treatment/Prognosis/Evolution

Pneumatosis coli can be treated with a diet plan, antibiotics and oxygen therapy. However, there is a risk of compromised bowel wall function with the development of an acute abdomen, massive dilatation of the bowel and

Table 10.24 Predisposing conditions for pneumatosis coli.

Intraluminal	Translocation of gas-forming bacteria through compromised mucosal barrier	Pulmonary
Trauma	Ischemic bowel disease	Chronic bronchitis
Endoscopy, endoscopic polypectomy	IBD	Emphysema
Blunt abdominal trauma	Neonatal necrotizing enterocolitis	Asthma
	Appendicitis	Bronchiectasis and cystic fibrosis
	AIDS	
	Drug-induced	
	Autoimmune and collagen vascular disease	
Mechanical		
Sigmoid volvulus		
Pyloric stenosis, bowel obstruction		

possible perforation requiring surgical exploration. In addition to an elevated lactate level, a leukocytosis or a lowered serum bicarbonate, a consultation with a question of a possible intervention should be performed.

Phlegmonous Colitis

Definition, General Features, and Predisposing Factors

This rare pathology is characterized by diffuse cellulitis of the submucosa. It can affect any portions of the gut, and most particularly the stomach. In the colon, variable lengths may be involved, and the entire small and large bowel may be affected.

Patients commonly have cirrhosis and portal hypertension. A variety of organisms have been implicated, including pneumococci, group B-hemolytic streptococci, and *E. coli*.

Clinical Features

The patients usually present with abdominal pain, diarrhea, and bleeding. Peritonitis and septic shock can complicate the clinical picture.

Microscopic Features

A marked acute inflammatory infiltrate is observed within an edematous submucosa, while the mucosa is intact. Focal mucosal ulceration or hemorrhage can develop. Thrombophlebitis and obliteration of vessels may be present. Gram stain may demonstrate organisms in the submucosa if included.

Differential Diagnosis

As the changes are centered in the submucosa, superficial biopsies may not be diagnostic or show only nonspecific changes including edema, hemorrhage, or focal ulceration.

Treatment/Prognosis/Evolution

The outcome is generally poor.

Obstructive Colitis

Definition, General Features, and Predisposing Factors

Obstructive colitis is consequent to the development of inflammation and ulceration proximal to an obstructed colonic segment. It occurs in 7% of patients with obstruction, from any cause, such as adenocarcinoma, volvulus, diverticular disease, or various motility disorders.

It develops more commonly in elderly patients and those with comorbidities including hypertension, diabetes, generalized atherosclerosis, and cardiac insufficiency.

Clinical Features and Endoscopic Features

Nausea, vomiting, abdominal pain, constipation, and, paradoxically, diarrhea may occur. The affected segment is usually separated from the site of obstruction by a segment of normal mucosa, often in excess of 10 cm. Endoscopically, there is dilatation with granular luminal surface and longitudinal or transverse ulcers, and closely mimic chronic IBD. The diffuse nature of the involvement and predominant mucosal pathology may suggest ulcerative colitis, while the focal nature of the disease, with a segment of normal mucosa beyond it, is reminiscent of Crohn's disease.

Microscopic Features

The mucosa may show a broad spectrum of changes from superficial foci of neutrophils with mucosal and submucosal edema, to a more diffuse acute inflammatory infiltrate to a broad ischemic type ulceration and may resemble necrotizing enterocolitis. In slowly developing obstruction, there is both acute and chronic injury, chronic superficial ulceration, and inflammatory pseudopolyps, mimicking IBD.

Differential Diagnosis

Since the histologic features are not specific, the key to the diagnosis is knowledge of the clinical setting.

Drug-Associated and Iatrogenic Colitis

Definition, General Features, and Predisposing Factors

This represents mucosal injury and inflammation caused by drugs or related to medical intervention or procedures.

Drug-induced injury of the GIT is common. The frequency of iatrogenic injury is reported at 3% of colonoscopic diagnoses of colitis.

Polypharmacy, particularly in elderly patients, predisposes to iatrogenic colonic injury, and a high index of suspicion should be maintained when evaluating biopsies for unexplained diarrhea or other gastrointestinal symptoms in this population.

The mechanism by which drugs cause injury to the colon is varied and may be multifactorial, including direct injury, apoptosis, ischemia, immunologic/hypersensitivity injury, and neuromuscular injury. Furthermore, exacerbation of an underlying condition or predisposition to infections has been reported.

The diagnosis is challenging, since to establish a causal relationship requires resolution of pathologic alterations and symptoms with withdrawal of the drug, followed by recrudescence of symptoms and pathologic alterations with reintroduction of the drug (criteria rarely fulfilled). An appropriate temporal sequence between the onset of symptomatology and administration of a drug is useful, although in some instances, a lag time of days up to weeks is present.

Furthermore, mucosal alterations and inflammation may also result from the bowel preparation or be secondary to the colonoscopic procedure proper and biopsy.

Clinical Features and Endoscopic Features

The clinical presentation may be varied with diarrhea, abdominal pain, rectal bleeding, nausea, vomiting, and constipation described. However, diarrhea is typically the leading presentation.

Colonoscopic findings are dependent on the particular drug and mechanism of injury. Appearances may be normal or show nonspecific features, including mucosal edema and erythema, these being the most common findings. Ulceration, strictures, multiple petechial hemorrhages, ischemic features, IBD-like features, or PMC may be seen in some patients. The finding of diaphragmatic disease, typically in the small intestine but well-recognized in the right side of the colon where it may be detected by colonoscopy, is considered pathognomonic of NSAIDs.

Microscopic Features

The histologic appearances of drug-induced injury is wide (Table 10.25, "Spectrum of reaction patterns in drug-associated colitis"). Various mucosal patterns are seen: (i) those that demonstrate relatively specific features that are suggestive of a particular offending drug or class of drugs; (ii) features that are suggestive of drug etiology but not a specific agent, particularly in combination (crypt apoptosis and eosinophilia); and (iii) those that result in reaction patterns that are not specific to drugs but instead mimic a wide range of colonic conditions (ischemic colitis, IBD).

(see Tables 10.25 and 10.26.).

Table 10.25 Spectrum of reaction patterns in drug-associated colitis.

Reaction patterns suggestive of a particular drug	Reaction patterns suggestive or a drug-induced pathology	Non-specific reaction patterns mimicking other inflammatory conditions of colon
Pseudomembranous colitis (antibiotics)	Apoptosis in deep crypts (apoptotic colopathy, GVHD-like)	Focal active colitis
Diaphragm disease (NSAIDs)	Eosinophilia (eosinophilic colitis), especially left-sided mucosal eosinophilia	Ischemic colitis
	Focal epithelial vacuolization (mainly a small intestinal feature)	Collagenous colitis
	Focal intraepithelial lymphocytosis	Lymphocytic colitis
	Melanosis coli	Idiopathic inflammatory bowel disease-like features
		Nonspecific ulceration

Table 10.26 Pattern of drug related injury and examples of associated drugs.

Pattern of injury	Drugs
Focal active colitis	NSAID, sodium phosphate, ipilimumab
Ischemic injury	Kayexalate, sevelamer, NSAID, estrogen, digitalis, diuretics, cocaine, oseltamivir, ergotamine, sumatriptan, methysergide, mycophenolate
Apoptosis (crypt base) ± dilated damaged crypts	NSAID, ipilimumab, mycophenolate, colchicine, taxol, 5-FU, sodium phosphate and other strong laxatives
Acute diffuse colitis	Fenemates, etodolac, diclofenac, naproxen, carbamazepine, rituximab
Chronic colitis	Mycophenolate, NSAIDS, ipilimumab, rituximab, anti-TNF
Pneumatosis coli	Glucosidase inhibitors, lactulose, sorbitol, bevacizumab
Pseudomembranous colitis	Antibiotics, chemical colitis secondary to hydrogen peroxide and glutaraldehyde
Eosinophilic colitis	NSAID, carbamazepine, clozapine, rifampicin, trimethoprim-sulfamethoxazole, tacrolimus, gold, cyclosporine, sulfasalazine, gemfibrozil, methylprednisolone, perazine, antiplatelet agents, estrogen/progestogen agents
Lymphocytic and microscopic colitis	(Refer to Table 10.17. Drugs associated with MC)

Differential Diagnosis

Iatrogenic colitis has the propensity to cause changes or reaction patterns mimicking other forms of inflammatory conditions, due to the limited repertoire of morphologic responses of the GIT to noxious stimuli. Certain features are useful in suggesting a drug-related etiology, including the presence of apoptosis in crypts, focal intraepithelial lymphocytosis, eosinophilia (particularly in the left colon), cytoplasmic vacuolation, and melanosis coli. An inflammatory pattern that does not fit a particular histologic pattern should also prompt the consideration of a drug-related injury. A high index of suspicion is required.

Table 10.27. lists common or important examples of drugs that may be associated with colonic injury. This is not meant to be an exhaustive or comprehensive list, and the number of drugs reported to cause gastrointestinal injury continues to grow.

Treatment/Prognosis/Evolution

Resolution is observed with the withdrawal of the offending drug.

Eosinophilic Conditions Affecting the Colon

Definition, General Features, and Predisposing Factors

These are a heterogenous group of conditions that share in common an eosinophil-rich infiltrate. They may be either primary or secondary (Table 10.28). Primary disorders affect the GIT in the absence of an identifiable cause for eosinophilia. These include eosinophilic gastroenteritis and eosinophilic colitis. In these conditions, the colon can be involved together with other parts of the gut or exclusively. A subset of patients (up to 75%) have associated allergic or atopic manifestations, such as eczema, allergic rhinitis, and asthma, and may exhibit increased total IgE and food-specific IgE levels.

Eosinophilic gastroenteritis is characterized by selective eosinophilic infiltration of the stomach, small bowel, or both, and variable involvement of the esophagus and large bowel. Eosinophilia may involve any layer(s) of the wall, and this forms the basis of subclassification into mucosal, muscularis, and serosal forms. Any age group may be affected, with most cases affecting adults in their thirties to fifties. The diagnosis is one of exclusion of other secondary causes of eosinophilia.

Eosinophilic colitis represents the eosinophilic infiltrates of the colon in the absence of known cause. It is more common in infants and adolescents than in any other age group. Most infantile cases are thought to be due to allergy to soy protein or cow's milk protein, but it also can occur in infants that are exclusively breast fed.

Clinical and Endoscopic Features

In eosinophilic gastroenteritis, mucosal and submucosal (57.5% of cases) infiltration represent the most common forms, and are characterized by diarrhea, vomiting, weight loss, abdominal pain, malabsorption, iron deficiency anemia, and protein losing enteropathy. Infiltration of the muscularis propria (30% cases) may lead to thickening of the bowel wall and obstruction. Serosal involvement (12.5%

Table 10.27 Important groups of drugs associated with colonic mucosal injury.

Agent	Sites of GIT affected	Usage/clinical setting	Clinical features/endoscopic	Histologic features	Differential diagnosis
Foreign material (crystalline) and nonabsorbable drugs in the gastrointestinal tract					
Sodium polystyrene sulfonate (kayexalate)	Upper GIT Lower GIT	Cation-exchange resin Treatment of hyperkalemia (renal failure, transplantation)	Ischemic necrotizing lesions in any segment of GIT, particularly SI and colon (within hours up to 11 days after intake)	Ulceration and mucosal ischemia Crystals are found in sloughed debris, on the surface or embedded in mucosa. These have angulated shape, basophilic (H&E) and nonpolarizable, and have a fish scale or mosaic texture	Cholestyramine Sevelamer Colesevelam
Cholestyramine	Generally not toxic	GI bile acid sequestrant Used to treat hyperlipidemia	—	Crystals are more opaque, deep red, more homogenous and lack fish-scale pattern	Kayexalate Sevelamer Colesevelam
Sevelamer	Colon Esophagus and small bowel	Anion-exchange resin Used to treat hyperphosphatemia	Ulceration	Ulceration, ischemia, and necrosis. Irregular shaped crystal with internal clefts resembling Kayexalate, two toned crystal with bright pink linear accentuations on a yellow background; may be deep eosinophilic to rusty brown at periphery when associated with ulcerated mucosa	Kayexalate Cholestyramine Colesevelam
Colesevelam	Generally thought to relatively non-toxic	Potent bile acid sequestrant, able to retain bound bile acids past ileum	May have associated mucosal abnormalities, but embedded resin or direct mucosal injury not observed	Angulated glassy crystal, rarely may have “washboard” cracking, red-drown shading from center to edge	Cholestyramine Kayexalate Sevelamer
Alpha-glucosidase inhibitor	Colon	Antidiabetic agent	Nodular/polypoid mucosa	Pneumatosis coli	
Drugs inducing mitotic arrest					
Colchicine	Most prominent in small bowel (duodenum) and antrum; any proliferative compartment of GIT	Inhibits tubulin polymerization and mitotic spindle formation Treatment of gout Effects on normal mucosa are only seen in toxicity, but effects may be seen in neoplastic mucosa at normal therapeutic levels	Symptoms of toxicity Vomiting, diarrhea, cholera-like syndrome	Increased mitosis in proliferative compartment of mucosa, with ring mitosis (mitotic arrest) Glandular apoptosis and pseudostratification	May mimic dysplasia Effects in hyperplastic polyp may mimic sessile serrated adenoma

Taxol	Favor esophagus, but any proliferative compartment of GIT (including colon)	Bind microtubules of mitotic spindle resulting in depolymerization Treatment of cancers (e.g. breast, esophagus, lung)	First 2–3 days of administration or in toxicity	Central nucleus of polymerized tubules with surrounding dispersed chromatin in metaphase Florid apoptosis Nuclear atypia	May result in changes mimicking dysplasia
Other chemotherapeutic agents: e.g. 5-FU Vinca alkaloids	Direct toxic effect on mitotically active cells	Inhibition of mitotically active cells	Nausea, vomiting, diarrhea Mucosal erythema, friability, ulceration	Random admixture of crypts in various stages of regeneration, some relatively normal although mucin depleted, some cuboidal to low columnar or lined by endothelial-thin epithelium. Marked apoptosis. Pyknotic and karyorrhectic nuclei Superficial necrosis and ulceration Restitution accompanied by cystic disorganized crypts with bizarre hypechromatic nuclei	May mimic dysplasia
Injury due to biologic agents					
Ipilimumab	Colon (stomach and duodenum)	Cytotoxic T lymphocyte antigen-4 (CTLA-4) monoclonal antibody. Blocking inhibitory signal of CTLA-4 augments T-cell response to tumor	Cramping, pain, and bloody diarrhea. Endoscopic findings vary from normal to segmental to diffuse erythema and ulceration of the mucosa (mimic inflammatory bowel disease).	Colon-mixed lamina propria infiltrate, intraepithelial lymphocytosis, apoptosis, cryptitis Lymphocytic colitis (rare) Stomach and duodenum show analogous features as colon	Associated villous blunting in duodenum may mimic celiac and autoimmune enteropathy Colonic changes may mimic IBD, but lacks basal lymphoplasmacytosis, architectural distortion and granulomas.
Adalimumab; Infliximab	Colon (esophagus)	Anti-TNF Treatment of inflammatory bowel disease, rheumatological disease	Colonic inflammation, mimicking IBD Esophageal inflammation	IBD Crohn-like (Etanercept, Infliximab, adalimumab) – results is so called "paradoxical" IBD (Lichenoid esophagitis with prominent dyskeratotic/apoptotic keratinocytes [Adalimumab])	Idiopathic inflammatory bowel disease (indistinguishable from conventional IBD) (Lichen planus and related dermatoses affecting esophagus)
Rituximab	Colon	CD20 monoclonal antibody Treatment of B cell lymphoma	New onset or exacerbation of IBD Crohn's-like (possibly related to Torovirus triggered)	UC-like Crohn's-like	Resembles conventional IBD

(*Continued*)

Table 10.27 (Continued)

Agent	Sites of GIT affected	Usage/clinical setting	Clinical features/endoscopic	Histologic features	Differential diagnosis
Mycophenolate	Upper and lower GIT	Inhibits de novo pathway of purine synthesis. B and T cells are selectively targeted as almost completely dependent on this, however, enterocytes, although less dependent, are still damaged.	Diarrhea, nausea, vomiting, ulcerations	GVHD-like: Apoptosis, dilated crypts lined by attenuated epithelial cells, crypt loss, and clusters of residual endocrine cells, empty lamina propria. IBD-like with lamina propria chronic inflammation, crypt abscess and crypt architectural distortion, Mixed pattern —GVHD and IBD-like Less commonly acute self-limiting colitis like or Ischemic-like pattern	GVHD – features favoring MPA include atrophic crypts with eosinophilic debris, greater number eosinophils, fewer apopototic microabscesses and endocrine ell aggregates. Involvement of squamous mucosae (skin and esophagus) favors GVHD. IBD Acute self-limiting colitis or ischemic colitis
Injury due to NSAIDS					
NSAIDS, aspirin	(Upper GIT) Lower GIT (colon, particularly right colon)	Cyclo-oxygenase inhibitor Widely used analgesic agent	Non-specific inflammatory changes Erosion/Ulcers Diaphragm disease	Focal Active colitis (basal type) Increased crypt apoptosis, focal mild non-specific lamina propria chronic inflammation, intraepithelial lymphocytosis Focal ulceration sharply demarcated with ischemic-like features (right colon) Diaphragm disease (right colon) IBD-like (UC or Crohn's) Eosinophilic colitis Microscopic colitis Ischemic colitis Granulomas (Sulindac)	May mimic IBD and other colitidies (e.g. ischemia)
Injury due to heavy metals					
Gold, mercury, silver	Colon	Direct toxic effect or hypersensitivity	Gold used to treat rheumatoid arthritis and is the most common. Multiple petechial hemorrhage, focal ulceration, pseudomembranes	Diffuse chronic mucosal inflammation rich in eosinophils Relative crypt preservation with occasional crypt dropout	May mimic eosinophilic colitis

Miscellaneous					
Potassium chloride	Colon	Direct toxic effect	Toxicity greater with slow release formulations Ulcers and strictures	Ulceration Fibrosis	Ulceration from any cause
Pancreatic enzyme replacement therapy	Colon; usually right side	High dose enteric coated pancreatic enzymes Historical interest; newer preparations do not cause these changes	Children or young adults with cystic fibrosis Watery diarrhea, abdominal distension, anorexia Strictures, mucosal ulceration and cobblestone appearance	Marked submucosal fibrosis with dense mature collage Mucosal may show non-specific acute or chronic inflammation or ulceration	May mimic inflammatory bowel disease (Crohn's) or ischemia
Artifacts/iatrogenic					
Sodium phosphate	Colon	Bowel preparation	Normal or mild erythema Aphthoid lesions	Focal active colitis Crypt apoptosis Aphthoid lesions	May be misinterpreted as Crohn's, infectious colitis, GVHD
Hypertonic enema	Colon	Bowel preparation	Normal or mild erythema	Flattened surface, focal surface etufting with PMN, edema, superficial hemorrhage, regenerating crypts	
Glutaraldehyde and hydrogen peroxide	Colon	Glutaraldehyde used as cleaning agent for colonoscopies Hydrogen peroxide used as a component of enemas, largely abandoned, although occasionally used as laxative	Symptoms usually 24–48 hours after exposure but can occur immediately after or during procedure	Resembles ischemic colitis May have pseudomembranes Nonspecific inflammatory patchy colitis	May mimic ischemic colitis and pseudomembranous colitis
Barium granuloma	Colon	Radiocontrast agent	Incidental finding Rarely form ulcerated mass	Grayish fine granular birefringent refractile material with giant cell reaction May have surrounding fibrosis	Other granulomastous conditions. Identifying particles is diagnostic
Oleogranuloma	Colon	Injected oil used as a vehice for sclerotherapy of hemorrhoids	Yellowish nodular mucosa	Large pale macropahges and multinucleate giant cells surrounding large lipid vacuoles. May have fibrosis. May involve mucosa and submucosa	Other granulomatous conditions.

Table 10.28 Classification of eosinophilic colitis.

Primary eosinophilic colitis
Atopic
Nonatopic
Secondary
Eosinophilic disorders
Eosinophilic gastroenteritis
Hypereosinophilic syndrome
Non-eosinophilic disorders
Inflammatory bowel disease
Celiac disease
Medication-induced
Infection/parasites
Vasculitis (Churg–Strauss syndrome) and connective tissue disease (scleroderma)
Radiation colitis
Systemic mastocytosis
Graft vs. host disease
Lymphoma/carcinoma

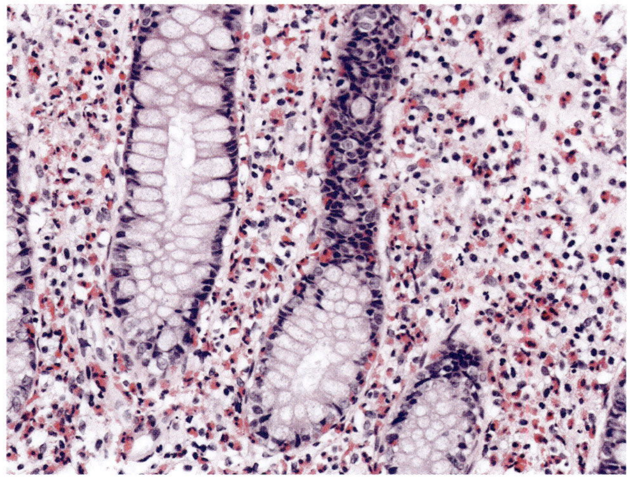

Figure 10.15 High magnification of a colonic biopsy with changes characteristically being found in the setting of eosinophilic colitis, preserved architecture and a dense infiltrate of eosinophils showing an epitheliotropism.

cases) leads to exudative ascites, and is often associated with higher peripheral eosinophilic counts. Peripheral eosinophilia is variable, and 25% of patients have normal eosinophil counts. Atopy and allergies are associated in 25–75% of cases. The evolution is variable, with permanent resolution in some patients; however, recurrent relapses are the norm. The endoscopic features are nonspecific, and include thickened folds, erythema, friability, nodularity, and abnormal peristalsis. Involvement may be patchy and segmental. Endoscopy may be normal in muscular or serosal disease, and imaging may be the only method to detect stenosis or thickening of the wall.

In eosinophilic colitis, diarrhea, which can be bloody, is the classic presentation. Other symptoms may include abdominal pain, anorexia, and weight loss. Most affected infants lack constitutional symptoms and are otherwise healthy. Peripheral blood eosinophilia and stool eosinophils may be present. The colonoscopic features are nonspecific, including erythema and loss of vascularity, friability, and nodularity.

Microscopic Features

In mucosal disease, a dense eosinophilic infiltrate or clustering with a preserved architecture is seen (Figure 10.15). Other suggestive features include eosinophilic degranulation, epithelial injury (e.g. mucin depletion), eosinophilic infiltration of epithelium, crypts or glands, and muscularis mucosa. In eosinophilic gastroenteritis with submucosal involvement, eosinophilic infiltration of submucosa may be seen if included in biopsies. Mast cells may be increased. As may be expected, mucosal biopsies may be normal in muscularis or serosal forms of eosinophilic gastroenteritis.

Knowledge of the biopsy site is important, as eosinophil numbers are greater in the proximal compared to distal colon, with the cecum having >30 eosinophils/HPF compared with the rectum <10 eosinophils/HPF. Although a threshold of >20 eosinophils per high-power field has been used by some in the diagnosis of eosinophilic colitis, it should be remembered that there is no established threshold above which a diagnosis of eosinophilic gastroenteritis or colitis should be rendered. Rather, a loss of the proximal–distal gradient of eosinophils, clustering or sheets of eosinophils to the exclusion of other inflammatory cells, eosinophil degranulation, epithelial infiltration accompanied by evidence of epithelial injury, and deep infiltration (muscularis mucosa, submucosa, muscularis propria or serosa) are more useful indicators of a pathologic increase.

Differential Diagnosis

The histologic features of eosinophilic gastroenteritis and colitis are not specific, and the diagnosis is one of exclusion (Table 10.29)

So-called *pericrypt eosinophilic enterocolitis* is an unusual condition in which many patients suffer from systemic connective tissue disease and chronic watery diarrhea. The colonoscopy is normal, and histologically, the eosinophils surround the deep crypts separating them from the muscularis mucosae and infiltrate muscularis mucosae.

Table 10.29 Differential diagnosis of eosinophilic colitis.

	Common feature(s) with eosinophilic colitis/gastroenteritis	Distinguishing feature(s)	Clinical
IBD	Increased mucosal eosinophils	Architectural distortion; LP CI, basal plasmacytosis and lymphoid aggregates; neutrophil cryptitis/abscesses; granulomas	Clinical features suggestive of inflammatory bowel disease
Parasites	Increased mucosal eosinophils; focal	May see parasite or ova	Clinical history and stool examination for ova/parasites; serology
Acute infectious (non-parasitic)	Increased mucosal eosinophils	Superficial LP neutrophils, neutrophil cryptitis/abscesses	Acute onset; stool microscopy and culture
Collagenous colitis	Increased mucosal eosinophils	Intraepithelial lymphocytosis, subepithelial collagen band, LP inflammation	Normal colonoscopy; chronic watery diarrhea
Vasculitis	Increased mucosal and tissue eosinophils	May have ischemia of the mucosa Inflammation in and around vessel walls (eosinophils, neutrophils, mononuclear cells), fibrinoid necrosis of vessel wall ± thrombi	Clinical features suggestive of vasculitic syndrome
Drug-induced colitis	Increased mucosal eosinophils	Apoptotis; melanosis; unusual mixed patterns	Medication history

Treatment/Prognosis/Evolution

In eosinophilic gastroenteritis, the mainstay of treatment of nonobstructive disease is corticosteroid therapy. Serosal disease appears to experience the greatest response to corticosteroids. The disease tends to relapse with cessation of therapy. Steroid-sparing treatments, such as dietary modification or montelukast, are preferred maintenance strategies. Immunosuppressive agents (e.g. azathioprine or mycophenolate mofetil) may be alternatives although clinical trials are lacking. Elimination or elemental diets may be helpful in patients with mucosal disease or identified allergic response to foods.

In eosinophilic colitis, most children with eosinophilic colitis will respond to withdrawal of the culprit antigen with resolution of the bloody diarrhea by one to three years of age and will be able to tolerate reintroduction of the culprit protein. Whether EC predisposes to subsequent development of IBD is debated. Adolescents and adults often require short course topical or systemic steroids (prednisolone and budesonide) or 5-ASA and in many, the disease runs a chronic waxing and waning course. Refractory cases may require immunomodulator therapy with azathioprine.

Mastocytic Enterocolitis

Definition, General Features, and Predisposing Factors

This condition is characterized by chronic diarrhea and increased benign mucosal mast cells (>20 / HPF) on mucosal biopsies (colonic or duodenal).

Whether this represents a true entity or a morphologic reaction pattern remains debated. Notably, systemic mastocytosis or cutaneous mastocytosis is absent, and serum tryptase is normal.

Clinical and Endoscopic Features

The patients, predominantly adult females, present with unexplained chronic diarrhea, defined as loose or liquid stools for up to several weeks. Others present with variable and intermittent abdominal pain resembling diarrhea-predominant IBS. Routine laboratory tests and stool analysis are unremarkable. Serum tryptase is normal. Colonoscopy and endoscopy are normal or show mild edema.

Microscopic Features

The mucosa may show a mild and focal increase in mixed inflammatory cells (Figure 10.16a). The diagnosis requires an immunohistochemical stain for mast cells, either mast cell tryptase, C-kit (Figure 10.16b) or CD25, as the mast cells are not easily detected on H&E slides. The normal number of mucosal mast cells is on average 13 per high-power field. The presence of greater than 20 mast cells per high-power field is diagnostic of mastocytic enterocolitis in this setting.

Differential Diagnosis

Increased mucosal mast cells may be seen in other conditions, including ulcerative colitis, collagenous colitis, gluten-sensitive enteropathy, radiation colitis, and all forms of

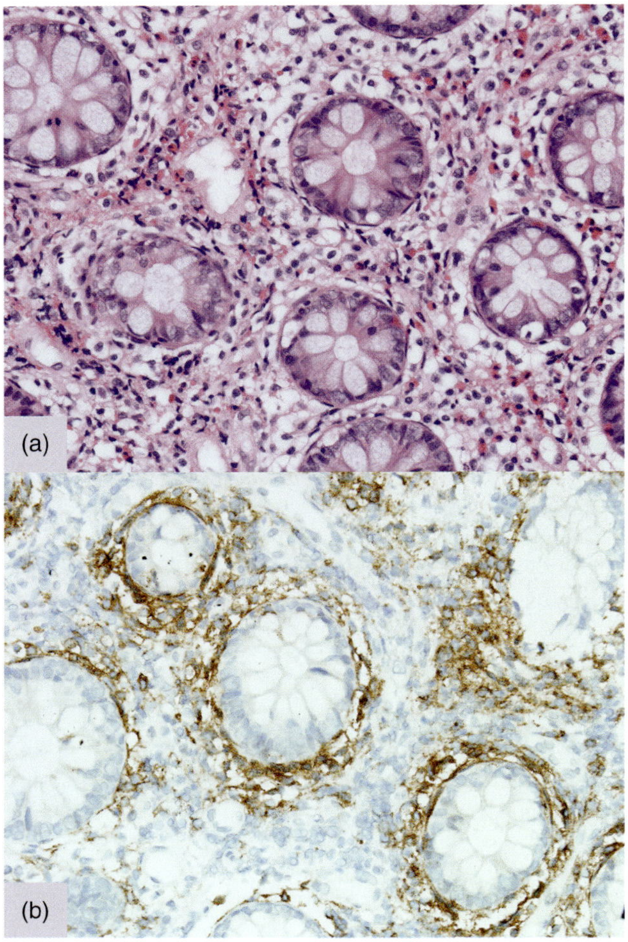

Figure 10.16 Example of mastocytic colitis showing a slightly increased mixed inflammation (a) and positivity of the mast cells for CD117 (b), surrounding the crypts.

IBS. But in these, the clinical history differs. Systemic mastocytosis and cutaneous mastocytosis with gastrointestinal symptoms may show marked mast cell infiltrate forming confluent sheets and aggregates, associated with increased eosinophils and mucosal distortion. The presence of mast cells greater than 15 per high-power field has been established as the diagnostic threshold of extracutaneous involvement. Furthermore, the immunophenotype is helpful, since neoplastic mast cells generally express CD25 and/or CD2. Importantly, we have observed few cases in which the gastrointestinal manifestation has represented the first clinical presentation of systemic or cutaneous mastocytosis.

Treatment and Prognosis

Up to 67% of patients may respond to antihistamines, mast cell stabilizers, or inhibitors of mediator release.

Graft Versus Host Disease (GVHD)

Definition, General Features, and Predisposing Factors

This immunologically mediated injury to the colonic mucosa is secondary to response of immunocompetent donor T cells to major and minor histocompatibility antigens of the host.

It commonly follows bone marrow transplantation, developing in approximately 30–50% of allogeneic bone marrow transplant recipients, while it rarely follows solid organ transplantation (small bowel approximately 5%; other solid organs <1%). Rare examples complicate maternal fetal cell transfer in immunodeficient children or transfusion of non-irradiated cells and blood products. Several other features affecting GVHD are summarized in Table 10.30.

Clinical and Endoscopic Features

A wide spectrum of symptoms is reported (see Table 10.31), including anorexia, nausea, vomiting, abdominal pain, and diarrhea. Endoscopically, the features may vary from subtle mucosal erythema and edema to diffuse ulceration and denudation.

Microscopic Features

The changes may be divided into acute and chronic GVHD. It should be noted that these so-called "chronic changes" may occur secondary to acute GVHD.

In early acute GVHD, there is edema of the lamina propria with increase in the number of lymphocytes and apop-

Table 10.30 Predictive factors for GVHD.

Donor characteristics
HLA mismatch
Females donors for male recipients
Unrelated donors
Multiparity in donors
Total body irradiation
Full donor chimerism vs. mixed chimerism
Intestinal flora (antibiotics can attenuate risk)
CMV status (if both donor and recipient are negative, risk is reduced; increased if one or both positive)
Older age (higher risk)
Poor performance status
Reduced intensity conditioning (results in less damage and less GVHD)
Umbilical cord blood (less likely to cause GVHD)

Table 10.31 Signs and symptoms of chronic GVHD.

Organ or site	Diagnostic[1]	Distinctive[2]	Other features[3]	Common[4]
Skin	Poikiloderma Lichen-planus like features Sclerotic features Morphea-like features Lichen sclerosus-like features	Depigmentation	Sweat impairment Ichthyosis Keratosis pilaris Hypo- or hyper-pigmentation	Erythema Maculopapular rash Pruritus
Nails		Dystrophy Longitudinal ridging, splitting or brittle features Onycholysis Pterygium unguis Nail loss (usually symmetrical; affects most nails)[a]		
Scalp and body hair		New onset scarring or nonscarring alopecia (following recovery from chemotherapy) Scaling, papulosquamous lesion	Thinning scalp hair, typically patchy, coarse, or dull (not explained by endocrine causes) Premature gray hair	
Mouth	Lichen type features Hypekeratotic plaques Restriction of mouth opening (secondary to sclerosis)	Xerostomia Mucocele Mucosal atrophy Pseudomembranes[a] Ulcers[a]		Gingivitis Mucositis Erythema Pain
Eyes		New onset dry, gritty, or painful eyes[b] Cicatricial conjunctivitis Keratoconjunctivitis sicca[b] Confluent areas of punctate keratopathy	Photophobia Periorbital hyperpigmentation Blepharitis	
Genitalia	Lichen planus-like features Vaginal scarring or stenosis	Erosion[a] Fissure[a] Ulcers[a]		
GIT	Esophageal web Strictures or stenosis in the upper to mid third of the esophagus		Exocrine pancreatic insufficiency	Anorexia Nausea Vomiting Diarrhea Weight loss Failure to thrive (infants and children)
Liver				Total bilirubin, alkaline Phosphatase >2 Upper limit of normal[a] ALT or AST >2 Upper limit of normal[a]
Lung	Bronchiolitis obliterans diagnosed with lung biopsy	Bronchiolitis obliterans diagnosed with PFTs and radiology[b]		BOOP

(Continued)

Table 10.31 (Continued)

Organ or site	Diagnostic[1]	Distinctive[2]	Other features[3]	Common[4]
Muscles, Fascia, Joints	Fasciitis Joint stiffness or contractures Secondary to sclerosis	Myositis or polymyositis[b]	Edema Muscle cramps Arthralgia or arthritis	
Hematopoietic and immune			Thrombocytopenia and eosinophilia Lymphopenia Hypo- or hypergammaglobulinemia Autoantibodies (AIHA and ITP)	
Other			Pericardial or pleural effusions Ascites Peripheral neuropathy Nephrotic syndrome Myasthenia gravis Cardiac conduction abnormality or cardiomyopathy	

GVHD, graft versus host disease; ALT, alanine aminotransferase; AST, aspartate aminotransferase; BOOP, bronchiolitis obliterans organizing pneumonia; PFTs, pulmonary function tests; AIHA, autoimmune hemolytic anemia; ITP, idiopathic thrombocytopenic purpura.
[a] In all cases, infection, drug effects, malignancy, or other causes must be excluded.
[b] Diagnosis of chronic GVHD requires biopsy or radiology confirmation (or Schirmer test for eyes).

Definitions
1) Diagnostic: Sufficient to establish diagnosis of chronic GVHD
2) Distinctive: Seen in chronic GVHD, but insufficient alone to establish a diagnosis of chronic GVHD
3) Other features: Can be acknowledged as part of the chronic GVHD symptomatology if the diagnosis is confirmed.
4) Common: Seen with both acute and chronic GVHD.

tosis within the crypts. The inflammatory infiltrate is generally scant, as many patients are leukopenic in the first few weeks following transplantation.

In established acute/active GVHD (Figure 10.17), numerous cryptic apoptotic bodies are noted, and cellular debris is observed in the dilated lumen. Increased IELs are also seen. As GVHD progresses, crypt abscesses, and numerous neutrophils develop, and crypt dropout, mucosal ulceration, and denudation may be seen. Endocrine cells may be more resistant and persist.

The severity of acute GVHD may be graded as Grade I (single cell apoptosis or crypt or gland epithelium), Grade II (destruction of single crypts or glands), Grade III (focal mucosal ulceration), and Grade IV (diffuse mucosal ulceration with denudation). However, this correlates poorly with clinical outcome. Current recommendations are the inclusion of a statement as to whether GVHD is absent or possibly, probably, or unequivocally present (Table 10.32).

There is presently no consensus on what constitutes chronic GVHD in the gut aside from finding of esophageal webs or strictures (upper to mid third). It is presently a clinicopathologic diagnosis, and requires at least one diagnostic clinical sign of chronic GVHD or presence of at least one distinctive manifestation (Table 10.31), with the diagnosis confirmed by pertinent biopsy or other relevant tests, as well as exclusion of other diagnoses. It encompasses classic chronic GVHD without features of acute GVHD, and an overlap syndrome in which diagnostic or distinctive features of chronic GVHD and acute GVHD appear together. Active and active and chronic GVHD may be better terms.

Chronic GVHD shows nonspecific findings. There is usually no ulceration, but structural distortion, Paneth cell metaplasia, and atrophy. Regenerative mucosal changes and apoptosis can be seen. Mild lymphoplasmacytic infiltration of the lamina propria may be found. There is fibrosis of the lamina propria and submucosa, and rarely, stricture and obstruction may result.

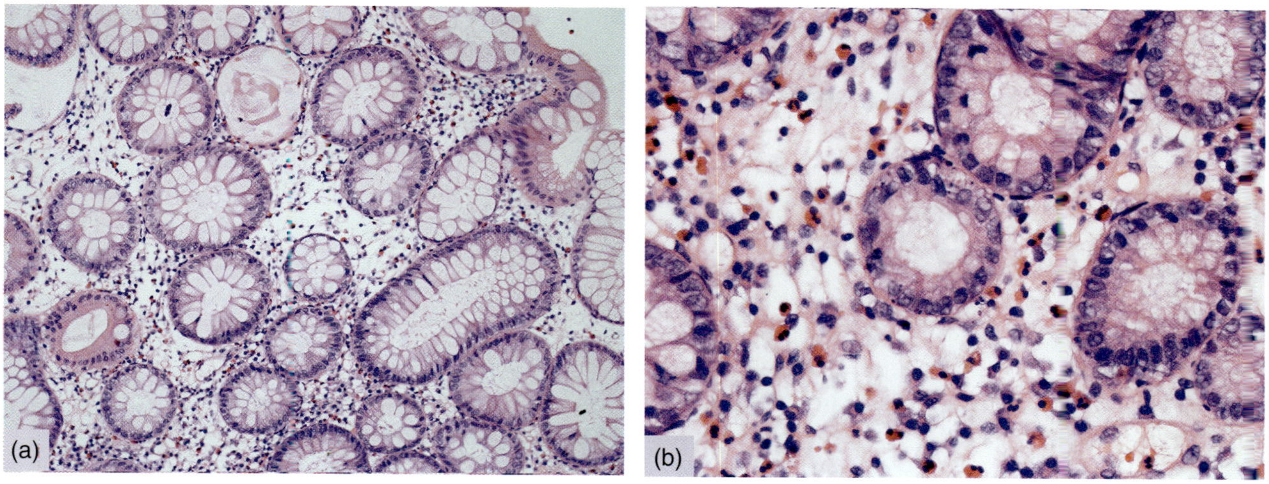

Figure 10.17 Mycrophenolate mofetil-related colitis is a pitfall mimicking changes of GvHD which are illustrated in this figure. In the H.E. overview (a) shows a sparse lymphoplasmacytic infiltrate a single crypt dorp out as well as single apoptosis in higher magnification (b).

Table 10.32 Recommendations for final diagnosis.

Category	Definition	Examples	Comments
Not GVHD	No evidence for GVHD	• Obvious CMV enteritis with inclusions near the apoptotic changes	Indicates possible alternate diagnoses and reasons for suspicion
Possible GVHD	Evidence for GVHD but other possible explanations	• Focal colonic ulcers with marked apoptotic cryptitis and destruction of crypts associated with use of MMF Coinfection with known active viral hepatitis • Clinical features suggest or favor drug reaction	
Consistent with GVHD	Clear evidence of GVHD but with mitigating factors	• Unequivocal evidence of CMV yet abundant apoptotic epithelial changes that are not associated with CMV infected cells by immunostaining • Single or rare apoptotic epithelial • Changes without other features of • Active GVHD and no alternative explanations • Limited sample or minimal or focal findings • Recent chemotherapy or radiotherapy	Equivalent to "probable," "favor," or "suggestive of" GVHD
GVHD	Unequivocal evidence of GVHD and no further comment necessary	• Inflammation may be minimal despite extensive destruction of the targeted epithelia	If extensive destruction of epithelium, ducts, or crypts or marked inflammation, may note "marked activity," but the features that define "marked" activity have not been prospectively defined and are highly dependent on the degree of secondary immunosuppressive treatment

GVHD, graft-vs-host disease; CMV, cytomegalovirus; MMF, mycophenolate mofetil.

Differential Diagnosis

In the first 20–30 days post transplantation, microscopic features associated with GVHD may be solely related to *chemoradiation* conditioning. GVHD usually manifests concurrently or shortly after skin involvement and rarely precedes it. Other conditions mimicking acute GVHD include infections, particularly CMV, adenovirus, and *Cryptosporidia* infection. Notably, CMV infection may coexist with and trigger GVHD. Apoptosis away from the vicinity of viral cytopathic changes may suggest coexisting GVHD. *Salmonella* infection with neutrophilic collections in crypt bases may also mimic GVHD. Many drugs, particularly mycophenolate mofetil, used to treat acute GVHD in solid organ transplant patients, may also mimic GVHD (Figure 10.17); thus, a detailed drug history is important. Anecdotally, the finding of cystic crypts lined by attenuated epithelium with luminal eosinophils is said to suggest mycophenolate. Other conditions associated with distinct apoptotic changes include autoimmune enteropathy, malignant thymomas, T-cell deficiencies, and common variable immunodeficiency.

Chronic GVHD

Injury secondary to chemoradiation may show overlap with chronic GVHD. However, other features will also be seen, including telangiectasia, atypical fibroblasts, and vascular hyalinization.

Treatment and Prognosis

Early diagnosis of acute GVHD and institution of appropriate treatment is important, since it has a high rate of mortality between 30 and 60%. Chronic GVHD may result in functional disturbances, stricturing, and bowel obstruction. GVHD prophylaxis or T-cell deletion of graft and genetic factors (e.g. homozygosity for common variant of promoter region of IL-10) are associated with a lower risk of GVHD.

Further Reading

Aggarwal, A. and Helper, D. (2014). Macroscopic findings in lymphocytic colitis. *Clin. Gastroenterol. Hepatol.* 12 (8): e65–e66.

Alt, B., Glass, N.R., and Sollinger, H. (1985). Neutropenic enterocolitis in adults. Review of the literature and assessment of surgical intervention. *Am. J. Surg.* 149: 405–408.

Alvares, J.F., Devarbhavi, H., Makhija, P. et al. (2005). Clinical, colonoscopic, and histological profile of colonic tuberculosis in a tertiary hospital. *Endoscopy* 37: 351–356.

Anagnostopoulos, I., Schuppan, D., Riecken, E.O. et al. (1999). Tenascin labelling in colorectal biopsies: a useful marker in the diagnosis of collagenous colitis. *Histopathology* 34: 425–431.

Andersen, T., Andersen, J.R., Tvede, M., and Franzmann, M.B. (1993). Collagenous colitis: are bacterial cytotoxins responsible? *Am. J. Gastroenterol.* 88: 375–377.

Anscombe, A.R., Keddie, N.C., and Schofield, P.F. (1967). Caecal tuberculosis. *Gut* 8: 337–343.

Arren BF, Dankwa EK, Davies JD. 'Diamond-shaped' crypts and mucosal elastin: helpful diagnostic features in biopsies of rectal prolapse. *Histopathology* 1990; 17: 129–34.

Ayata, G., Ithamukkala, S., Sapp, H. et al. (2002). Prevalence and significance of inflammatory bowel disease-like morphologic features in collagenous and lymphocytic colitis. *Am. J. Surg. Pathol.* 26: 1414–1423.

Baroco, A.L. and Oldfield, E.C. (2008). Gastrointestinal cytomegalovirus disease in the immunocompromised patient. *Curr. Gastroenterol. Rep.* 10: 409–416.

Bartlett, J.G. (2008). Historical perspectives on studies of *Clostridium difficile* and *C. difficile* infection. *Clin. Infect. Dis.* 46 (Suppl 1): S4–S11.

Beaugerie, L. and Pardi, D.S. (2005). Review article: drug-induced microscopic colitis – proposal for a scoring system and review of the literature. *Aliment. Pharmacol. Ther.* 22: 277–284.

Brandt, L.J., Feuerstadt, P., and Blaszka, M.C. (2010). Anatomic patterns, patient characteristics, and clinical outcomes in ischemic colitis: a study of 313 cases supported by histology. *Am. J. Gastroenterol.* 105: 2245–2252. quiz 53.

Bryant, D.A., Mintz, E.D., Puhr, N.D. et al. (1996). Colonic epithelial lymphocytosis associated with an epidemic of chronic diarrhea. *Am. J. Surg. Pathol.* 20: 1102–1109.

Buchman, A.L. and Rao, S. (2004). Pseudomembranous collagenous colitis. *Dig. Dis. Sci.* 49: 1763–1767.

Castellano, V.M., Munoz, M.T., Colina, F. et al. (1999). Collagenous gastrobulbitis and collagenous colitis. Case report and review of the literature. *Scand. J. Gastroenterol.* 34: 632–638.

Chadwick, V.S., Chen, W., Shu, D. et al. (2002). Activation of the mucosal immune system in irritable bowel syndrome. *Gastroenterology* 122: 1778–1783.

Chen, M.C., Chang, P.Y., Chuang, C.Y. et al. (1981). Colorectal cancer and schistosomiasis. *Lancet* 1: 971–973.

Chetty, R. and Govender, D. (2012). Lymphocytic and collagenous colitis: an overview of so-called microscopic colitis. *Nat. Rev. Gastroenterol. Hepatol.* 9: 209–218.

Chiang, J.M., Changchien, C.R., and Chen, J.R. (2006). Solitary rectal ulcer syndrome: an endoscopic and histological presentation and literature review. *Int. J. Color. Dis.* 21: 348–356.

Concha, R., Harrington, W. Jr., and Rogers, A.I. (2005). Intestinal strongyloidiasis: recognition, management, and determinants of outcome. *J. Clin. Gastroenterol.* 39: 203–211.

Cone, L.A., Woodard, D.R., Potts, B.E. et al. (1986). An update on the acquired immunodeficiency syndrome (AIDS). Associated disorders of the alimentary tract. *Dis. Colon Rectum* 29: 60–64.

Daley, A.J., Craven, P., Holland, A.J. et al. (2002). Herpes simplex virus colitis in a neonate. *Pediatr. Infect. Dis. J.* 21: 887–888.

Do, K.R., Cho, Y.S., Kim, H.K. et al. (2010). Intestinal helminthic infections diagnosed by colonoscopy in a regional hospital during 2001–2008. *Korean J Parasitol.* 48: 75–78.

Edwards, C.M., George, B., and Warren, B. (1999). Diversion colitis – new light through old windows. *Histopathology* 34: 1–5.

Edwards, C.M., George, B., and Warren, B.F. (1999). Diversion colitis: new light through old windows. *Histopathology* 35: 86–87.

Elder, K., Lashner, B.A., and Al Sclaiman, F. (2009). Clinical approach to colonic ischemia. *Cleve. Clin. J. Med.* 76: 401–409.

Erhan, Y., Zekioglu, O., Ozdemir, N., and Sen, S. (2000). Unilateral salpingitis due to enterobius vermicularis. *Int. J. Gynecol. Pathol.* 19: 188–189.

Fabio G Rodrigues, Giovanna Dasilva, and Steven D Wexner. Neutropenic enterocolitis. *World J Gastroenterol.* 2017 Jan 7; 23(1): 42–47. Published online 2017 Jan 7.

Fernandez-Banares, F., Salas, A., Esteve, M. et al. (2003). Collagenous and lymphocytic colitis. Evaluation of clinical and histological features, response to treatment, and long-term follow-up. *Am. J. Gastroenterol.* 98: 340–347.

Fernandez-Banares, F., Esteve, M., Espinos, J.C. et al. (2007). Drug consumption and the risk of microscopic colitis. *Am. J. Gastroenterol.* 102: 324–330.

Fernandez-Banares, F., Casalots, J., Salas, A. et al. (2009). Paucicellular lymphocytic colitis: is it a minor form of lymphocytic colitis? A clinical pathological and immunological study. *Am. J. Gastroenterol.* 104: 1189–1198.

Feuerstadt, P. and Brandt, L.J. (2010). Colon ischemia: recent insights and advances. *Curr. Gastroenterol. Rep.* 12: 383–390.

Filipovich, A.H., Weisdorf, D., Pavletic, S. et al. (2005). National Institutes of Health consensus development project on criteria for clinical trials in chronic graft-versus-host disease: I. Diagnosis and staging working group report. *Biol. Blood Marrow Transplant.* 11: 945–956.

Fine, K.D., Do, K., Schulte, K. et al. (2000). High prevalence of celiac sprue-like HLA-DQ genes and enteropathy in patients with the microscopic colitis syndrome. *Am. J. Gastroenterol.* 95: 1974–1982.

Fung, W.P., Monteiro, E.H., Ang, H.B. et al. (1972). Ulcerative postdysenteric colitis. *Am. J. Gastroenterol.* 57: 341–343.

Galiatsatos, P., Shrier, I., Lamoureux, E. and Szilagyi, A. (2005). Meta-analysis of outcome of cytomegalovirus colitis in immunocompetent hosts. *Dig. Dis. Sci.* 50: 609–616.

Gerding, D.N., Olson, M.M., Peterson, L.R. et al. (1986). *Clostridium difficile*-associated diarrhea and colitis in adults. A prospective case-controlled epidemiologic study. *Arch. Intern. Med.* 146: 95–100.

Goff, J.S., Barnett, J.L., Pelke, T., and Appelman, H.D. (1997). Collagenous colitis: histopathology and clinical course. *Am. J. Gastroenterol.* 92: 57–60.

Goldblum, J.R. and Wang, N. (2000). Lymphocytic and collagenous colitis as possible patterns of Crohn's colitis. *Am. J. Surg. Pathol.* 24: 755–756. author reply 56-7.

Goldstein, N.S. and Gyorfi, T. (1999). Focal lymphocytic colitis and collagenous colitis: patterns of Crohn's colitis? *Am. J. Surg. Pathol.* 23: 1075–1081.

Goodell, S.E., Quinn, T.C., Mkrtichian, E. et al. (1983). Herpes simplex virus proctitis in homosexual men. Clinical, sigmoidoscopic, and histopathological features. *N. Engl. J. Med.* 308: 868–871.

Gratama, S., Smedts, F., and Whitehead, R. (1995). Obstructive colitis: an analysis of 50 cases and a review of the literature. *Pathology* 27: 324–329.

Greenson, J.K., Stern, R.A., Carpenter, S.L., and Barnett, J.L. (1997). The clinical significance of focal active colitis. *Hum. Pathol.* 28: 729–733.

Guillemot, F., Colombel, J.F., Neut, C. et al. (1991). Treatment of diversion colitis by short-chain fatty acids. Prospective and double-blind study. *Dis. Colon Rectum* 34: 861–864.

Hahn, H.P. and Hornick, J.L. (2007). Immunoreactivity for CD25 in gastrointestinal mucosal mast cells is specific for systemic mastocytosis. *Am. J. Surg. Pathol.* 31: 1669–1676.

Hale, W.B. and NDSG (2008). Colonoscopy in the diagnosis and management of diverticular disease. *J. Clin. Gastroenterol.* 42: 1142–1144.

Haque, S., Eisen, R.N., and West, A.B. (1993). The morphologic features of diversion colitis: studies of a pediatric population with no other disease of the intestinal mucosa. *Hum. Pathol.* 24: 211–219.

Haque, R., Huston, C.D., Hughes, M. et al. (2003). Amebiasis. *N. Engl. J. Med.* 348: 1565–1573.

Harper, P.H., Lee, E.C., Kettlewell, M.G. et al. (1985). Role of the faecal stream in the maintenance of Crohn's colitis. *Gut* 26: 279–284.

Hasleton, P.S., Carr, N., and Schofield, P.F. (1985). Vascular changes in radiation bowel disease. *Histopathology* 9: 517–534.

Higgins, P.D., Davis, K.J., and review, L.L.S. (2004). The epidemiology of ischaemic colitis. *Aliment. Pharmacol. Ther.* 19: 729–738.

Hogenauer, C., Hammer, H.F., Krejs, G.J., and Reisinger, E.C. (1998). Mechanisms and management of antibiotic-associated diarrhea. *Clin. Infect. Dis.* 27: 702–710.

Holzer, T., Gervaz, P., Spahr, L. et al. (2009). Phlegmonous colitis: another source of sepsis in cirrhotic patients? *BMC Gastroenterol.* 9: 94.

Hulman, G. and Taylor, L.A. (1987). Entamoeba histolytica: demonstration by PAS/Martius yellow technique. *Med. Lab. Sci.* 44: 396–397.

Huppmann, A.R. and Orenstein, J.M. (2010). Opportunistic disorders of the gastrointestinal tract in the age of highly active antiretroviral therapy. *Hum. Pathol.* 41: 1777–1787.

Hurley, B.W. and Nguyen, C.C. (2002). The spectrum of pseudomembranous enterocolitis and antibiotic-associated diarrhea. *Arch. Intern. Med.* 162: 2177–2184.

Hussain, Z., Kelly, S., Clarke, A. et al. (2010). Colonic perforation in collagenous colitis: a systematic review of a rare complication and guidance on management. *Surg. Endosc.* 24: 2930–2934.

Idoate, M.A., Vazquez, J.J., and Civeira, P. (1993). Rectal biopsy as a diagnostic procedure of chronic visceral leishmaniasis. *Histopathology* 22: 589–590.

Jain, R. and Chetty, R. (2009). Enterocolic lymphocytic phlebitis and lymphocytic colitis: drug-related coexistent pathology. *Int. J. Color. Dis.* 24: 473–474.

Jakate, S., Demeo, M., John, R. et al. (2006). Mastocytic enterocolitis: increased mucosal mast cells in chronic intractable diarrhea. *Arch. Pathol. Lab. Med.* 130: 362–367.

Janoff, E.N., Orenstein, J.M., Manischewitz, J.F., and Smith, P.D. (1991). Adenovirus colitis in the acquired immunodeficiency syndrome. *Gastroenterology* 100: 976–979.

Jarnerot, G., Tysk, C., Bohr, J., and Eriksson, S. (1995). Collagenous colitis and fecal stream diversion. *Gastroenterology* 109: 449–455.

Jarnerot, G., Bohr, J., Tysk, C., and Eriksson, S. (1996). Faecal stream diversion in patients with collagenous colitis. *Gut* 38: 154–155.

Jarnerot, G., Hertervig, E., Granno, C. et al. (2001). Familial occurrence of microscopic colitis: a report on five families. *Scand. J. Gastroenterol.* 36: 959–962.

Jensen, L. and Munck, L.K. (2005). Elementary diet reduces diarrhoea associated with microscopic colitis. *Scand. J. Gastroenterol.* 40: 1495–1496.

Jokipii, L., Pohjola, S., and Jokipii, A.M. (1983). Cryptosporidium: a frequent finding in patients with gastrointestinal symptoms. *Lancet* 2: 358–361.

Joo, J.H., Ryu, K.H., Lee, Y.H. et al. (1998). Colonoscopic diagnosis of whipworm infection. *Hepato-Gastroenterology* 45: 2105–2109.

de Kantor, I.N., LoBue, P.A., and Thoen, C.O. Human tuberculosis caused by *Mycobacterium bovis* in the United States, Latin America and the Caribbean. *Int. J. Tuberc. Lung Dis.* 14: 1369–1373.

Kazal, H.L., Sohn, N., Carrasco, J.I. et al. (1976). The gay bowel syndrome: clinico-pathologic correlation in 260 cases. *Ann. Clin. Lab. Sci.* 6: 184–192.

Kazlow, P.G., Shah, K., Benkov, K.J. et al. (1986). Esophageal cryptosporidiosis in a child with acquired immune deficiency syndrome. *Gastroenterology* 91: 1301–1303.

Kennedy, G.D. and Heise, C.P. (2007). Radiation colitis and proctitis. *Clin. Colon. Rectal. Surg.* 20: 64–72.

Kimura, A.C., Mead, P., Walsh, B. et al. (2006). A large outbreak of Brainerd diarrhea associated with a restaurant in the Red River Valley, Texas. *Clin. Infect. Dis.* 43: 55–61.

Klotz, S.A., Drutz, D.J., Tam, M.R., and Reed, K.H. (1983). Hemorrhagic proctitis due to lymphogranuloma venereum serogroup L2. Diagnosis by fluorescent monoclonal antibody. *N. Engl. J. Med.* 308: 1563–1565.

Koreishi, A., Lauwers, G.Y., and Misdraji, J. (2007). *Pneumatosis intestinalis*: a challenging biopsy diagnosis. *Am. J. Surg. Pathol.* 31: 1469–1475.

Kotter, D.P., Gaetz, H.P., Lange, M. et al. (1984). Enteropathy associated with acquired immunodeficiency syndrome. *Ann. Intern. Med.* 101: 421.

Koulaouzidis, A. and Saeed, A.A. (2011). Distinct colonoscopy findings of microscopic colitis: not so microscopic after all? *World J Gastroenterol: WJG* 17: 4157–4165.

Kumar, N.B., Nostrant, T.T., and Appelman, H.D. (1982). The histopathologic spectrum of acute self-limited colitis (acute infectious-type colitis). *Am. J. Surg. Pathol.* 6: 523–529.

Lamps, L.W. (2007). Infective disorders of the gastrointestinal tract. *Histopathology* 50: 55–63.

Leupin, N., Curschmann, J., Kranzbuhler, H. et al. (2002). Acute radiation colitis in patients treated with short-term preoperative radiotherapy for rectal cancer. *Am. J. Surg. Pathol.* 26: 498–504.

Levine, T.S. and Price, A.B. (1994). Obstructive enterocolitis: a clinico-pathological discussion. *Histopathology* 25: 57–64.

Libbrecht, L., Croes, R., Ectors, N. et al. (2002). Microscopic colitis with giant cells. *Histopathology* 40: 335–338.

Lin, A.T., Lin, H.H., and Chen, C.L. (2005). Colonoscopic diagnosis of whipworm infection. *J. Gastroenterol. Hepatol.* 20: 965–967.

Liu, X., Xiao, S.Y., Plesec, T.P. et al. (2013). Collagenous colitis in children and adolescents: study of 7 cases and literature review. *Mod. Pathol.* 26: 881–887.

Lorenzetti, R., Campo, S.M., Stella, F. et al. (2003). An unusual endoscopic finding: *Trichuris trichiura*. Case report and review of the literature. *Dig. Liver Dis.* 35: 811–813.

Luvuno, F.M., Mtshali, Z., and Baker, L.W. (1982). Toxic dilatation complicating fulminant amoebic colitis. *Br. J. Surg.* 69: 56–57.

MacDonald, P.H. (2002). Ischaemic colitis. *Best Pract. Res. Clin. Gastroenterol.* 16: 51–61.

Maddox, A., Francis, N., Moss, J. et al. (1992). Adenovirus infection of the large bowel in HIV positive patients. *J. Clin. Pathol.* 45: 684–688.

Makapugay, L.M. and Dean, P.J. (1996). Diverticular disease-associated chronic colitis. *Am. J. Surg. Pathol.* 20: 94–102.

McMillan, A. and Lee, F.D. (1981). Sigmoidoscopic and microscopic appearance of the rectal mucosa in homosexual men. *Gut* 22: 1035–1041.

McMillan, A., Gilmour, H.M., Slatford, K., and McNeillage, G.J. (1983). Proctitis in homosexual men. A diagnostic problem. *Br. J. Vener. Dis.* 59: 260–264.

McMillan, A., Gilmour, H.M., McNeillage, G., and Scott, G.R. (1984). Amoebiasis in homosexual men. *Gut* 25: 356–360.

Meinhardt, P.L., Casemore, D.P., and Miller, K.B. (1996). Epidemiologic aspects of human cryptosporidiosis and the role of waterborne transmission. *Epidemiol. Rev.* 18: 118–136.

Melato, M. and Gorji, N. (1998). Primary intestinal cryptococcosis mimicking adenomatous polyp in an HIV-negative patient. *Am. J. Gastroenterol.* 93: 1592–1593.

Meyers, S., Mayer, L., Bottone, E. et al. (1981). Occurrence of *Clostridium difficile* toxin during the course of inflammatory bowel disease. *Gastroenterology* 80: 697–670.

Mintz, E. (2003). A riddle wrapped in a mystery inside an enigma: Brainerd diarrhoea turns 20. *Lancet* 362: 2037–2038.

Mintz, E.D., Weber, J.T., Guris, D. et al. (1998). An outbreak of Brainerd diarrhea among travelers to the Galapagos Islands. *J. Infect. Dis.* 177: 1041–1045.

de la Monte, S. and Hutchins, G.M. (1985). Follicular proctocolitis and neuromatous hyperplasia with lymphogranuloma venereum. *Hum. Pathol.* 16: 1025–1032.

Montoro, M.A., Brandt, L.J., Santolaria, S. et al. (2011). Clinical patterns and outcomes of ischaemic colitis: results of the Working Group for the Study of Ischaemic Colitis in Spain (CIE study). *Scand. J. Gastroenterol.* 46: 236–246.

van Mook, W.N., Koek, G.H., van der Ven, A.J. et al. (2004). Human intestinal spirochaetosis: any clinical significance? *Eur. J. Gastroenterol. Hepatol.* 16: 83–87.

Moriwaki, Y., Sugiyama, M., Toyoda, H. et al. (2009). Lethal obstructive colitis: how and when patients with colonic obstruction should be prevented from falling into a lethal condition. *Hepato-Gastroenterology* 56: 659–662.

Muller, S., Neureiter, D., Stolte, M. et al. (2001). Tenascin: a sensitive and specific diagnostic marker of minimal collagenous colitis. *Virchows Arch.* 438: 435–441.

Munch, A. and Langner, C. (2015). Microscopic colitis-clinical and pathologic perspectives. *Clin. Gastroenterol. Hepatol.* 13 (2): 228–236.

Munch, A., Aust, D., Bohr, J. et al. (2012). Microscopic colitis: current status, present and future challenges: statements of the European Microscopic Colitis Group. *J. Crohns. Colitis.* 6: 932–945.

Neut, C., Guillemot, F., and Colombel, J.F. (1997). Nitrate-reducing bacteria in diversion colitis: a clue to inflammation? *Dig. Dis. Sci.* 42: 2577–2580.

Nielsen, O.H., Vainer, B., and Rask-Madsen, J. (2008). Non-IBD and noninfectious colitis. *Nat. Clin. Pract. Gastroenterol. Hepatol.* 5: 28–39.

Nyhlin, N., Bohr, J., Eriksson, S., and Tysk, C. (2008). Microscopic colitis: a common and an easily overlooked cause of chronic diarrhoea. *Eur. J. Intern. Med.* 19: 181–186.

Odze, R.D., Wershil, B.K., Leichtner, A.M., and Antonioli, D.A. (1995). Allergic colitis in infants. *J. Pediatr.* 126: 163–170.

Offner, F.A., Jao, R.V., Lewin, K.J. et al. (1999). Collagenous colitis: a study of the distribution of morphological abnormalities and their histological detection. *Hum. Pathol.* 30: 451–457.

Ogilvie-McDaniel, C., Blaiss, M., Osborn, F.D., and Carpenter, J. (2008). Mastocytic enterocolitis: a newly described mast cell entity. *Ann. Allergy Asthma Immunol.* 101: 645–646.

Okpara, N., Aswad, B., and Baffy, G. (2009). Eosinophilic colitis. *World J. Gastroenterol.* 15: 2975–2979.

O'Sullivan, M., Clayton, N., Breslin, N.P. et al. (2000). Increased mast cells in the irritable bowel syndrome. *Neurogastroenterol. Motil.* 12: 449–457.

Padmanabhan, V., Callas, P.W., Li, S.C., and Trainer, T.D. (2003). Histopathological features of the terminal ileum in lymphocytic and collagenous colitis: a study of 32 cases and review of literature. *Mod. Pathol.* 16: 115–119.

Pampiglione, S., Rivasi, F., and Rubbiani, C. (1997). Cryptic infection by whipworm mimicking a sessile polyp of the colon. *Ital. J. Gastroenterol. Hepatol.* 29: 365–366.

Pardi, D.S. and Kelly, C.P. (2011). Microscopic colitis. *Gastroenterology* 140: 1155–1165.

Patel, N., Amarapurkar, D., Agal, S. et al. (2004). Gastrointestinal luminal tuberculosis: establishing the diagnosis. *J. Gastroenterol. Hepatol.* 19: 1240–1246.

Patterson, M. and Schoppe, L.E. (1982). The presentation of amoebiasis. *Med. Clin. N. Am.* 66: 689–705.

Pittman, F.E. and Hennigar, G.R. (1974). Sigmoidoscopic and colonic mucosal biopsy findings in amebic colitis. *Arch. Pathol.* 97: 155–158.

Prata, A. (1978). Schistosomiasis mansoni. *Clin. Gastroenterol.* 7: 49–75.

Price, A.B. (2003). Pathology of drug-associated gastrointestinal disease. *Br. J. Clin. Pharmacol.* 56: 477–482.

Price, A.B. and Day, D.W. (1981). Pseudomembraneous and infective colitis. In: *Recent Advances in Histopathology* (eds. P.P. Anthony and R.N.M. MacSween), 99. Edinburgh: Churchill Livingstone.

Pulimood, A.B., Amarapurkar, D.N., Ghoshal, U. et al. (2011). Differentiation of Crohn's disease from intestinal tuberculosis in India in 2010. *World J. Gastroenterol.* 17: 433–443.

Quinn, T.C., Lukehart, S.A., Goodell, S. et al. (1982). Rectal mass caused by Treponema pallidum: confirmation by immunofluorescent staining. *Gastroenterology* 82: 135–139.

Rabinowitz, M., Bassan, I., and Robinson, M.J. (1988). Sexually transmitted cytomegalovirus proctitis in a woman. *Am. J. Gastroenterol.* 83: 885–887.

Rasmussen, M.A. and Munck, L.K. (2012). Systematic review: are lymphocytic colitis and collagenous colitis two subtypes of the same disease – microscopic colitis? *Aliment. Pharmacol. Ther.* 36: 79–90.

Riddell, R.H., Tanaka, M., and Mazzoleni, G. (1992). Non-steroidal anti-inflammatory drugs as a possible cause of collagenous colitis: a case-control study. *Gut* 33: 683–686.

Riggs, M.M., Sethi, A.K., Zabarsky, T.F. et al. (2007). Asymptomatic carriers are a potential source for transmission of epidemic and nonepidemic *Clostridium difficile* strains among long-term care facility residents. *Clin. Infect. Dis.* 45: 992–998.

Robert, M.E., Skacel, M., Ullman, T. et al. (2004). Patterns of colonic involvement at initial presentation in ulcerative colitis: a retrospective study of 46 newly diagnosed cases. *Am. J. Clin. Pathol.* 122: 94–99.

Roe, A.M., Warren, B.F., Brodribb, A.J., and Brown, C. (1993). Diversion colitis and involution of the defunctioned anorectum. *Gut* 34: 382–385.

Rompalo, A.M. (1999). Diagnosis and treatment of sexually acquired proctitis and proctocolitis: an update. *Clin. Infect. Dis.* 28 (Suppl 1): S84–S90.

Rosen, Y. and Won, O.K. (1978). Phlegmonous enterocolitis. *Am J Dig Dis* 23: 248–256.

Rubio, C.A. and Lindholm, J. (2002). Cryptal lymphocytic coloproctitis: a new phenotype of lymphocytic colitis? *J. Clin. Pathol.* 55: 138–140.

Salas, A., Fernandez-Banares, F., Casalots, J. et al. (2003). Subepithelial myofibroblasts and tenascin expression in microscopic colitis. *Histopathology* 43: 48–54.

Satoh, T., Sasatomi, E., Wu, L., and Tokunaga, O. (2000). Phlegmonous colitis: a specific and severe complication of chronic hepatic disease. *Virchows Arch.* 437: 656–661.

Saurine, T.J., Brewer, J.M., and Eckstein, R.P. (2004). Microscopic colitis with granulomatous inflammation. *Histopathology* 45: 82–86.

Seppala, K., Hjelt, L., and Sipponen, P. (1981). Colonoscopy in the diagnosis of antibiotic-associated colitis. A prospective study. *Scand. J. Gastroenterol.* 16: 465–468.

Shaikh, Z.H., Ueno, N.T., and Kontoyiannis, D.P. (2001). Fatal Salmonella group G enteritis mimicking intestinal graft-versus-host disease in a bone marrow transplant recipient. *Transpl. Infect. Dis.* 3: 29–33.

Shaz, B.H., Reddy, S.I., Ayata, G. et al. (2004). Sequential clinical and histopathological changes in collagenous and lymphocytic colitis over time. *Mod. Pathol.* 17: 395–401.

Shetty, S., Anjarwalla, S.M., Gupta, J. et al. (2011). Focal active colitis: a prospective study of clinicopathological correlations in 90 patients. *Histopathology* 59: 850–856.

Shulman, H.M., Kleiner, D., Lee, S.J. et al. (2006). Histopathologic diagnosis of chronic graft-versus-host disease: National Institutes of Health Consensus Development Project on Criteria for Clinical Trials in Chronic Graft-versus-Host Disease: II. Pathology Working Group Report. *Biol. Blood Marrow Transplant.* 12: 31–47.

Singh, B., Mortensen, N.J., and Warren, B.F. (2007). Histopathological mimicry in mucosal prolapse. *Histopathology* 50: 97–102.

Smith, D. (1965). Infectious syphilis of the rectum. Report of a case. *Dis. Colon Rectum* 8.

Sung, A.D. and Chao, N.J. (2013). Concise review: acute graft-versus-host disease: immunobiology, prevention, and treatment. *Stem Cells Transl. Med.* 2: 25–32.

Surawicz, C.M. and Belic, L. (1984). Rectal biopsy helps to distinguish acute self-limited colitis from idiopathic inflammatory bowel disease. *Gastroenterology* 86: 104–113.

Surawicz, C.M. and Myerson, D. (1988). Self-limited cytomegalovirus colitis in immunocompetent individuals. *Gastroenterology* 94: 194–199.

Talley, N.J., Shorter, R.G., Phillips, S.F., and Zinsmeister, A.R. (1990). Eosinophilic gastroenteritis: a clinicopathological study of patients with disease of the mucosa, muscle layer, and subserosal tissues. *Gut* 31: 54–58.

Taylor, N.S., Thorne, G.M., and Bartlett, J.G. (1981). Comparison of two toxins produced by *Clostridium difficile*. *Infect. Immun.* 34: 1036–1043.

Theodoropoulou, A. and Koutroubakis, I.E. (2008). Ischemic colitis: clinical practice in diagnosis and treatment. *World J. Gastroenterol.* 14: 7302–7308.

Toner, M., Condell, D., and O'Briain, D.S. (1990). Obstructive colitis. Ulceroinflammatory lesions occurring proximal to colonic obstruction. *Am. J. Surg. Pathol.* 14: 719–728.

Tursi, A., Elisei, W., Giorgetti, G.M. et al. (2011). Inflammatory manifestations at colonoscopy in patients with colonic diverticular disease. *Aliment. Pharmacol. Ther.* 33: 358–365.

Ullery, B.W., Pieracci, F.M., Rodney, J.R., and Barie, P.S. (2009). Neutropenic enterocolitis. *Surg. Infect.* 10: 307–314.

Unal, A., Guven, K., Yurci, A. et al. (2008). Is increased colon subepithelial collagen layer thickness in diabetic patients related to collagenous colitis? An immunohistochemical study. *Pathol. Res. Pract.* 204: 537–544.

Ung, K.A., Kilander, A., Willen, R., and Abrahamsson, H. (2002). Role of bile acids in lymphocytic colitis. *Hepato-Gastroenterology* 49: 432–437.

Vaizey, C.J., van den Bogaerde, J.B., Emmanuel, A.V. et al. (1998). Solitary rectal ulcer syndrome. *Br. J. Surg.* 85: 1617–1623.

Vesoulis, Z., Lozanski, G., and Loiudice, T. (2000). Synchronous occurrence of collagenous colitis and pseudomembranous colitis. *Can. J. Gastroenterol.* 14: 353–358.

Vigren, L., Olesen, M., Benoni, C., and Sjoberg, K. (2012). Are collagenous and lymphocytic colitis different aspects of the same disease? *Scand. J. Gastroenterol.* 47: 1448–1453.

Villanacci, V., Casella, G., and Bassotti, G. (2011). The spectrum of drug-related colitides: important entities, though frequently overlooked. *Dig. Liver Dis.* 43: 523–528.

Volk, E.E., Shapiro, B.D., Easley, K.A., and Goldblum, J.R. (1998). The clinical significance of a biopsy-based diagnosis of focal active colitis: a clinicopathologic study of 31 cases. *Mod. Pathol.* 11: 789–794.

Warren, K.S. (1978). Schistosomiasis japonica. *Clin. Gastroenterol.* 7: 77–85.

Warren, B.F., Shepherd, N.A., Bartolo, D.C., and Bradfield, J.W. (1993). Pathology of the defunctioned rectum in ulcerative colitis. *Gut* 34: 514–516.

Washington, K., Gottfried, M.R., and Wilson, M.L. (1991). Gastrointestinal cryptococcosis. *Mod. Pathol.* 4: 707–711.

Weller, I.V. (1985). The gay bowel. *Gut* 26: 869–875.

Williams, J.J., Kaplan, G.G., Makhija, S. et al. (2008). Microscopic colitis-defining incidence rates and risk factors: a population-based study. *Clin. Gastroenterol. Hepatol.* 6: 35–40.

Williams, J.J., Beck, P.L., Andrews, C.N. et al. (2010). Microscopic colitis – a common cause of diarrhoea in older adults. *Age Ageing* 39: 162–168.

Wren, B., Heard, S.R., and Tabaqchali, S. (1987). Association between production of toxins A and B and types of *Clostridium difficile*. *J. Clin. Pathol.* 40: 1397–1401.

Wu, T.T. and Hamilton, S.R. (1999). Lymphocytic gastritis: association with etiology and topology. *Am. J. Surg. Pathol.* 23: 153–158.

Xin, W., Brown, P.I., and Greenson, J.K. (2003). The clinical significance of focal active colitis in pediatric patients. *Am. J. Surg. Pathol.* 27: 1134–1138.

Yamamoto-Furusho, J.K. and Torijano-Carrera, E. (2010). Intestinal protozoa infections among patients with ulcerative colitis: prevalence and impact on clinical disease course. *Digestion* 82: 18–23.

Yan, B.M. and Shaffer, E.A. (2009). Primary eosinophilic disorders of the gastrointestinal tract. *Gut* 58: 721–732.

Ye, H., Losada, M., and West, A.B. (2005). Diverticulosis coli: update on a "Western" disease. *Adv. Anat. Pathol.* 12: 74–80.

Yoshida, M., Kutsumi, H., Ogawa, M. et al. (1996). A case of *Trichuris trichiura* infection diagnosed by colonoscopy. *Am. J. Gastroenterol.* 91: 161–162.

Yuan, S., Reyes, V., and Bronner, M.P. (2003). Pseudomembranous collagenous colitis. *Am. J. Surg. Pathol.* 27: 1375–1379.

Inflammatory Bowel Disease

Definition, General Features, Predisposing Factors

Inflammatory bowel diseases (IBD), i.e. Crohn's disease (CD) and ulcerative colitis (UC) are idiopathic chronic inflammatory conditions. The term "unclassified" (Inflammatory Bowel Disease Unclassified, IBDU) can be used when a distinction between CD and UC is not possible on biopsy specimens, while the terminology "Indeterminate colitis" is reserved for when a definitive diagnosis of CD or UC cannot be made following colectomy with full pathological examination.

IBD can first develop in childhood or adolescence. In adults, UC is slightly more common in males, while CD occurs more frequently in females. This gender distribution is reversed in children. Over the last 50 years, the incidence and prevalence of both UC (peak age 30–40 years) and CD (peak age 20–30 years) has been increasing.

Geographic and ethnic differences exist with a north–south gradient observed in Europe and North America. Higher incidences are observed in Ashkenazi Jews and Caucasians. Lower incidences are reported in Hispanics and Asians.

Smoking is associated with reduction in symptoms and risk of developing UC, whereas in CD, it increases the risk or exacerbates the disease. Appendectomy, particularly before age 20, may reduce the risk of UC, or delay disease onset and produce a milder phenotype, although disease extent may be greater. Food antigens, infection, or dysbiosis are also potential contributing factors.

Genetic factors predispose to the development of IBD as well. Twin studies show concordance rates of 36% for CD and 16% for UC. A family history of IBD increases the risk for UC and CD, and is the strongest risk factor for IBD, the influence being greater for CD. The risk is greatest for first degree relatives (1 in 10–20 lifetime risk), The risk is increased for either type of IBD, but is greater for the same phenotype of IBD as the affected proband.

IBD-susceptibility genes have been identified, with a third associated with both UC and CD, and the remainder specific to either UC or CD. Mutations in the *NOD2* (Chromosome 16), which encodes an intracytoplasmic bacterial sensor protein involved in innate immunity via NF-κB activation, was the first described susceptibility gene for CD and predisposes to ileal CD. The HLA regions contain several disease-susceptibility loci, including HLA DRBI*0103 and HLA DRB*07, associated with UC and ileal CD, respectively. Other candidate genes predominately involve immune-related molecules, for example TLR4, MDR1, NOD1/CARD4, IL-10 signaling and TNF-α. Epigenetic influences likely modulate associated gene expression with important implications for IBD development.

Current evidence suggests a complex interplay of environmental factors with various contributions of genetic susceptibility, mucosal barrier defects, dysregulated innate, and adaptive immune responses, infections, dysbiosis, and other environmental agents. However, no single pathogen has been consistently associated with IBD. The favored hypothesis is that IBD results from an aberrant immune response and loss of tolerance to the normal intestinal flora, leading to chronic inflammation of the gut, in a genetically susceptible individual.

Clinical and Endoscopical Features

Clinical Presentation

Most patients with UC complain of bloody diarrhea; colicky abdominal pain, urgency, or tenesmus. It is often characterized by episodic exacerbations and remissions. Less commonly, patients present with low grade disease or a severe form with toxic megacolon.

The presentation in Crohn's disease is more heterogenous and symptoms vary, largely according to location of disease such as small bowel obstruction in ileal disease, or colitic symptoms similar to UC in Crohn's colitis. Malaise, anorexia, and fever are more common than in UC. Crohn's colitis usually presents with diarrhea, rectal bleeding, or perianal disease; recurrent abdominal pain Anal and perianal disease, including edematous skin tags, ulcers, fissures, fistulae, abscesses are observed in up to 75% of patients with colonic CD at some point during the course of their illness (Figure 10.18).

Extraintestinal Manifestations

Between 20 and 40% of IBD patients present with extraintestinal manifestations particularly affecting the skin, eyes, hepatobiliary, and musculoskeletal systems.

Primary sclerosing cholangitis (PSC), i.e. a fibrosing and structuring inflammation of intra- and extrahepatic bile ducts is a particularly debilitating complication since some may develop cirrhosis. PSC also increases the risk of cholangiocarcinoma, with 10–15% lifetime risk and is associated with cumulative risk of colorectal cancer estimated at 9% after 10 years, 30% after 20 years, and 50% after 25 years of colitis.

PSC has an established strong association with IBD, particularly UC. At least 85–90% of PSC patients have coexisting UC and 10–15% CD. On the other hand, 5% of UC patients and 3% of CD patients develop PSC. Patients with

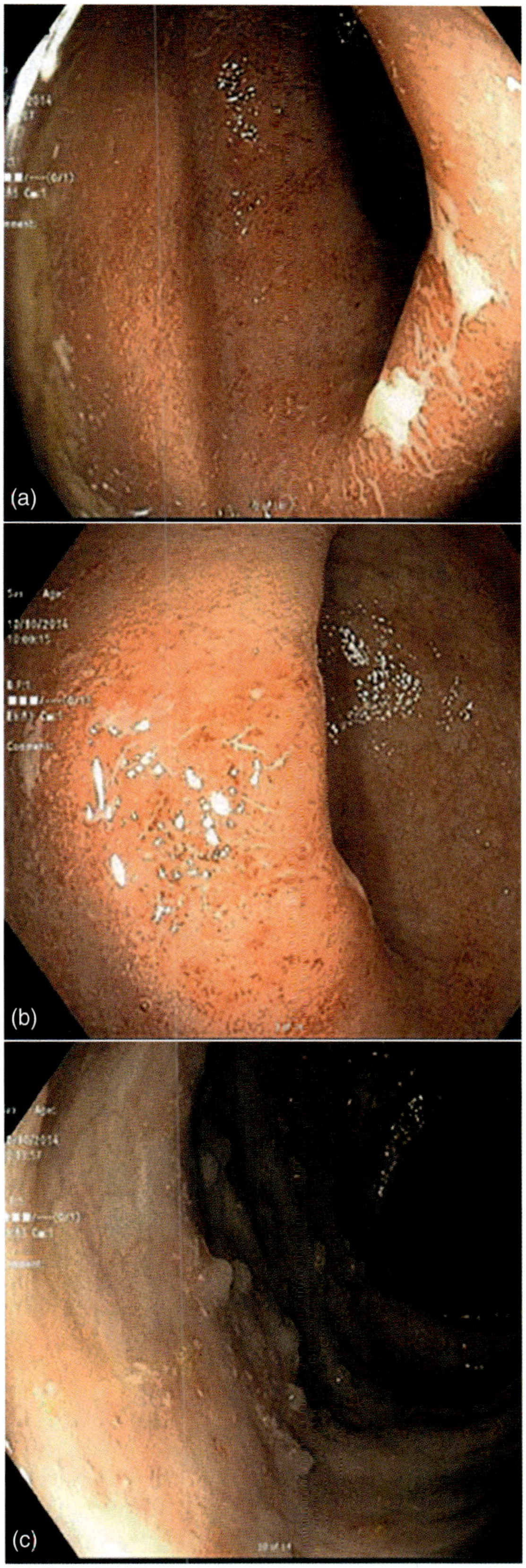

Figure 10.18 Endoscopic appearance of severe Crohn's disease. (a) Deep ulceration. (b) Multifocal superficial and deep ulceration. (c) Nearly confluent deep ulceration with pseudopolyps and near complete loss of mucosa.

UC and extensive colonic involvement with or without backwash ileitis are more likely to develop PSC than patients with only left colon involvement. PSC is most common in patients 30–40 years of age, and there is a male predominance (M : F = 2 : 1). The clinical course of PSC bears no relationship to underlying bowel disease, and PSC can develop either years before or after the development of bowel symptoms.

Endoscopy

Although some features are highly suggestive of IBD, there are no specific lesions pathognomonic of this diagnosis. The endoscopic impression may underestimate the extent and severity of IBD. Initial endoscopy with biopsy is the standard of care for diagnosis of IBD. It is especially critical to exclude other causes of diarrhea such as IBS, microscopic colitis, and infections such as *C. difficile*. There is increasing evidence that endoscopic activity (even in the absence of clinical symptoms) is predictive of relapse and is increasingly used to guide therapy ("treat to target")

As such, endoscopic evaluation combined with biopsy and histology has become increasing important to assessment of treatment outcomes, typically at the time of suspected clinical remission, or at times of symptom flares. In the immunosuppressed patient who flares, exclusion of non-IBD causes, especially CMV colitis, is important.

Ulcerative Colitis

UC typically begins in the rectum and progresses proximally in a contiguous fashion without obvious skip lesions. The earliest recognizable form of mucosal damage is redness with a prominent vascular pattern and erosion with purulent foci. The proximal limit of the disease most frequently shows an abrupt transition from disease to normal mucosa. In the untreated patient, the disease is typically worse distally. The mucosa has a granular or velvety surface appearance and is extremely friable, and when ulcers are present, the deep (circular) muscle coats may be visible. Full-thickness ulceration of the mucosa is usually patchy but any intact intervening mucosa is always diseased. Severe disease may become transmural and toxic dilatation or perforation may occur. Involvement of the terminal ileum in ulcerative colitis, so-called backwash ileitis, with patchy inflammation without ulceration extending few centimeters into the ileum may be seen. Severe involvement is rare but can be associated with a tendency to dilatation, rigidity, and muscular thickening of the bowel wall, which when present raises the possibility of CD, which should always be considered. Intubation and biopsy of the terminal ileum should be attempted in all patients with suspected IBD as significant ileal involvement with ulceration, stenosis, or distortion of the ileocecal valve favors CD.

Inflammatory polyps or pseudopolyps are noted in 12–20% of cases resulting from previous severe mucosal damage. Inflammatory polyps are both mucosal excrescences and sometimes re-epithelialized granulation tissue. These may be present in large numbers and fuse to one another to form mucosal bridges across the lumen. Pseudopolyps are raised mucosal islands resulting from surrounding ulceration of the mucosa and usually submucosa. Typical images from the colon in UC are shown in Figure 10.19.

Crohn's Disease

Colonic CD may occur with terminal ileal involvement together with right-sided disease, or it may be limited to the colon (in 14–32% of patients).

Colonic Crohn's disease can present in three patterns:

(i) Discontinuous, patchy, or focal disease, the hallmark of colonic Crohn's disease. Ulceration may vary from early aphthoid ulcers surrounded by normal or mildly edematous mucosa to deep serpiginous fissuring ulcers. Cobblestoning is due to areas of marked edema of the mucosa and submucosa separated by narrow fissuring ulcers. However, it is observed less commonly than in the small bowel disease. Fistulae, perforations, and abscesses may develop at base of ulcers. (ii) Diffuse colitis that may be difficult to distinguish from ulcerative colitis and in which rectal sparing and the presence of anal or perianal inflammation are useful distinguishing features. (iii) Stricturing disease resulting from transmural inflammation, fibrosis, and fibromuscular proliferation, and Crohn's proctitis. These patterns may coexist or evolve from one to another during the course of the disease. The rectum is macroscopically normal in about 50% of cases of Crohn's colitis. Typical endoscopic images are shown in Figure 10.19.

Microscopic Findings

Ulcerative Colitis

In untreated patients, a key feature is the diffuse mucosal inflammation, only sometimes extending to involve superficial submucosa. However, the features depend on whether the biopsies are taken during an active, resolving, or remission phase.

A hallmark of UC is the architectural distortion, i.e. evidence of chronicity. The crypts may initially appear elongated but as the disease progresses, crypt irregularity with

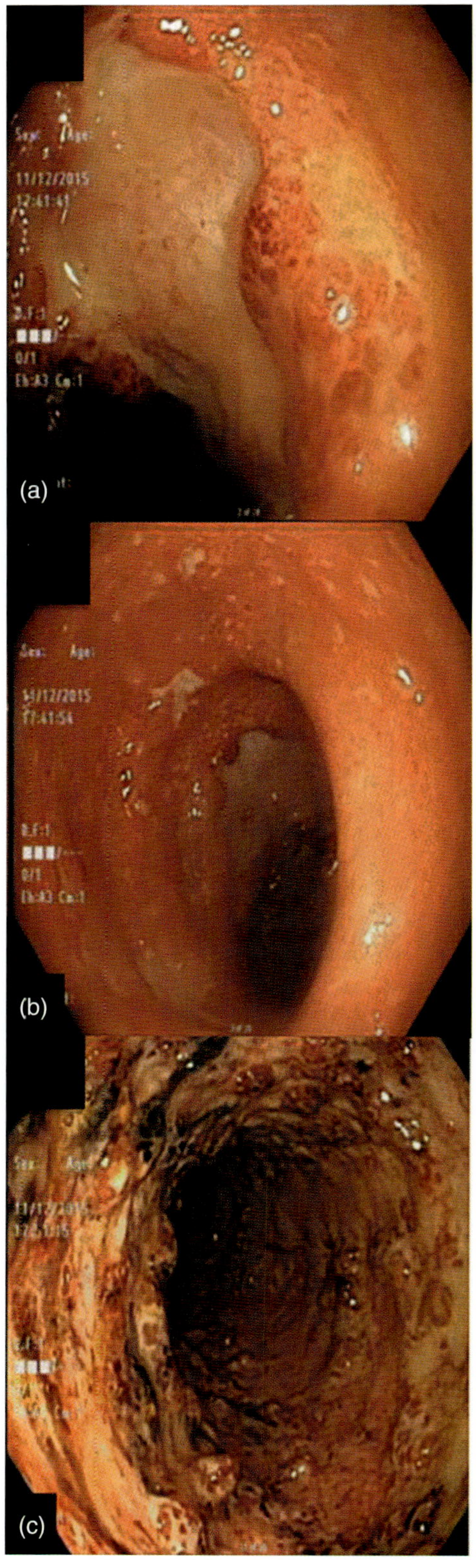

Figure 10.19 Endoscopic appearances of ulcerative colitis: (a) severe ulceration on the right side of image; (b) moderate inflammation with granular, friable mucosa, and mucous exudate; (c) pseudopolyps in otherwise quiescent disease. All three images are from patients with ulcerative colitis.

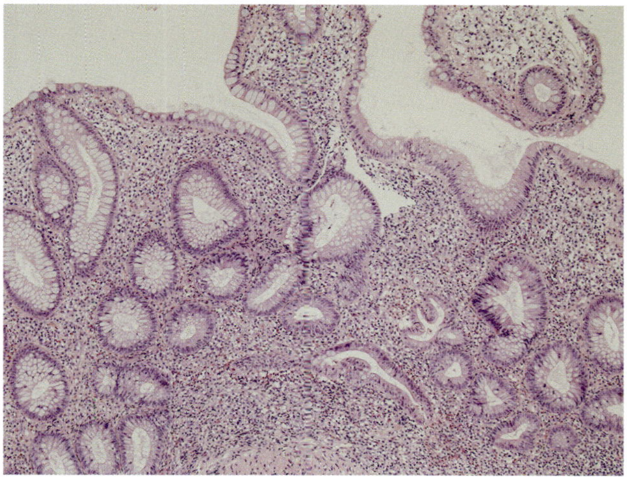

Figure 10.20 Colonic mucosa with typical architectural disarray caused by UC showing branching irregularity of the crypts, branching, and loss of parallelism.

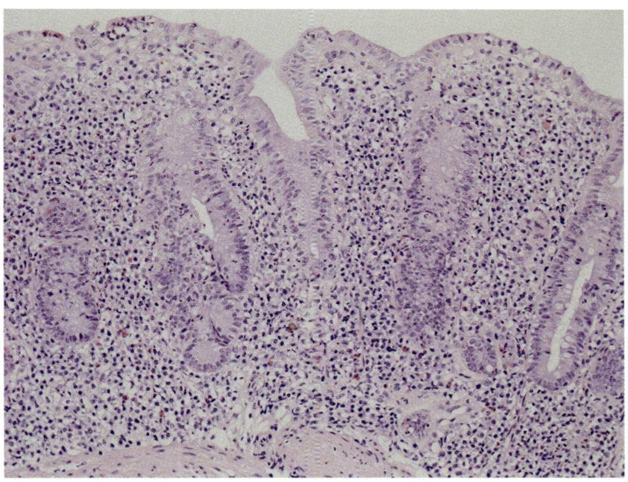

Figure 10.21 Colonic mucosa of UC showing a dense lymphoplasmacytic infiltrate and loss of crypts.

branching, loss of parallel arrangement, and shortening develop (Figure 10.20). Over time, atrophy and loss of crypts may be seen. Paneth cell metaplasia in the left colon is another feature of chronicity (Figure 10.21). Pyloric metaplasia can be detected as well. Increased numbers of endocrine cells may also be noted at the base of the crypts. The lamina propria is expanded by a mixed inflammatory infiltrate throughout, extending into the lower third. Basal plasmacytosis separating the base of crypts from the muscularis mucosa (MM) is detected. One should be watchful of mucin granulomas related to crypt rupture and reaction to extravasated mucin. These are located adjacent to acutely inflamed destroyed crypts and step levels may be necessary to exclude Crohn's granulomas. Mucin depletion of goblet cells and varying degrees of epithelial regeneration are present.

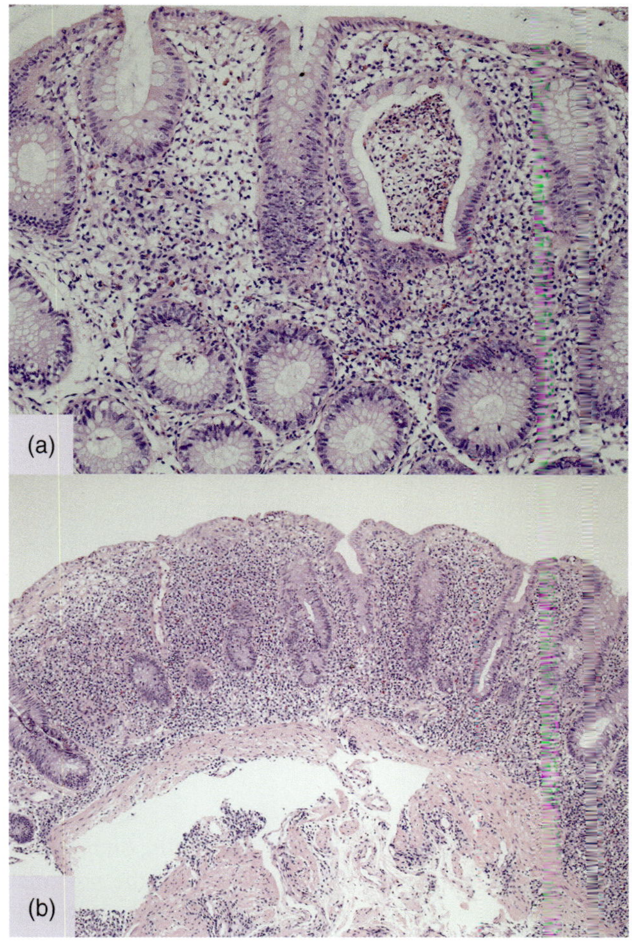

Figure 10.22 Typical inflammatory changes of an active UC showing crypt abscesses (a) as well as loss of crypts and erosive changes (b).

The degree of activity relies on identifying active inflammation, i.e. cryptitis and crypt abscess (Figure 10.22a), surface epithelial neutrophils, erosion, or ulceration (Figure 10.22b). Lamina propria neutrophils may be seen, however, their presence is not usually included in assessing activity (Figure 10.23). Activity may be graded into mild (cryptitis in ≤25% of crypts and/or crypt abscesses in ≤10% of crypts), moderate (cryptitis in >25% of crypts and/or crypt abscesses in >10% of crypts, and/or sparse small foci of erosions), and severe (ulceration or multiple foci of erosions).

In the resolving phase, cellular and architectural restitution can be noted and in some cases, an apparently normal colonic mucosa will be noted in endoscopic biopsies. However, most often some degree of architectural distortion and atrophy with flattened mucosal surface will be detected with various degrees of residual chronic inflammation and even in some cases hypocellularity of the lamina propria as evidence of medical therapy (Figure 10.23).

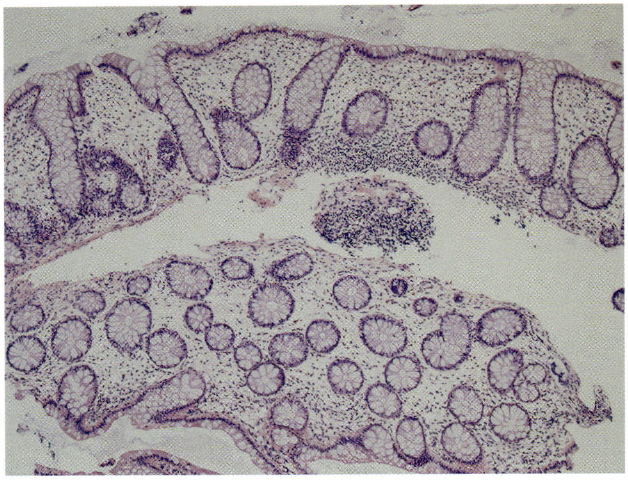

Figure 10.23 Specimen of a long-standing UC under therapy showing scattered lymphoplasmacytic infiltrate embedded in a hypocellular lamina propria and only discrete architectural changes.

Endocrine cell hyperplasia and hypertrophy or duplication of the muscularis mucosae may be detected.

Crohn's Disease

The diagnosis of CD colitis can be challenging on biopsies. The patchy distribution of the alterations in the proximal colon and ileocecal region with rectal sparing is diagnostically useful. The mucosal inflammation consists of focal aggregate of lymphocytes, plasma cells, and macrophages that varies from place to place, even within a small biopsy, both vertically and longitudinally in the affected mucosa. Mucin depletion is also focal and less marked than in UC. Similarly, architectural changes are not as marked, sometimes subtle, and may be focal or discontinuous (Figure 10.24a). Focal cryptitis or crypt abscesses (less common than in UC) are evidence of active disease (Figure 10.24b). This characteristic pattern of "focally enhanced" colitis must be distinguished from "isolated" focal active colitis, which is not associated with background chronic inflammation. Basal lymphoid aggregates found alongside the bases of crypts may be seen.

Granulomas comprised of collections of epithelioid histiocytes and a cuff of lymphocytes with or without Langerhans cells are detected in 15–30% of the biopsies. They may be seen in inflamed mucosa and in endoscopically normal mucosa. Compared to tuberculosis, Crohn's granulomas are small (<200 μm) and usually few or single (<5) and rarely cluster or become confluent (Figure 10.25). They should be searched for particularly in the submucosa, if included in the biopsy, as these are easily distinguishable from mucin crypt granulomas. In addition,

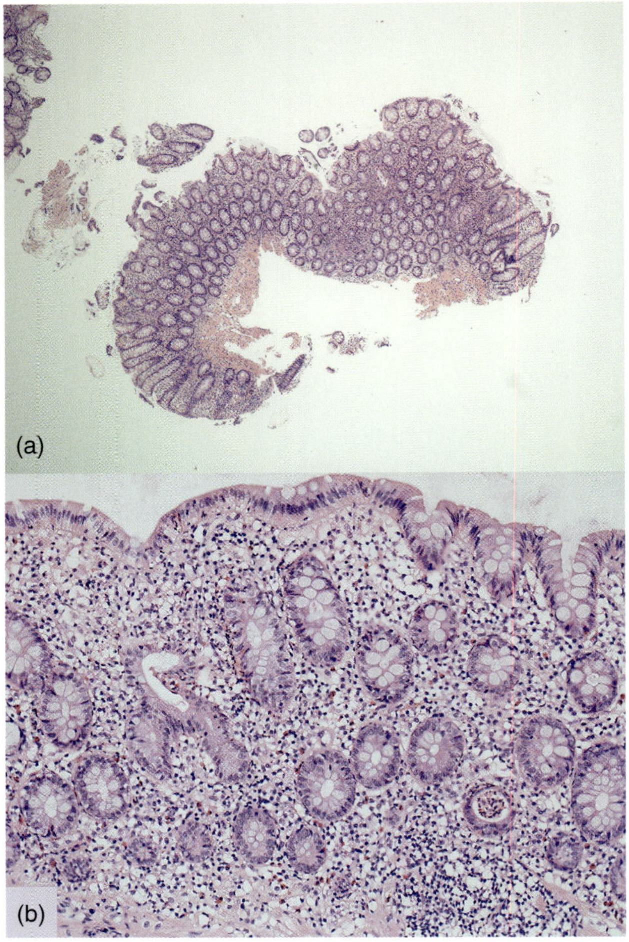

Figure 10.24 Hisological appearance of a Crohn's patient showing a dense inflammatory infiltrate in the overview with preserved architecture of the colonic mucosa (a). Furthermore, focal cryptitis and small abscesses may be a sign of active inflammation (b).

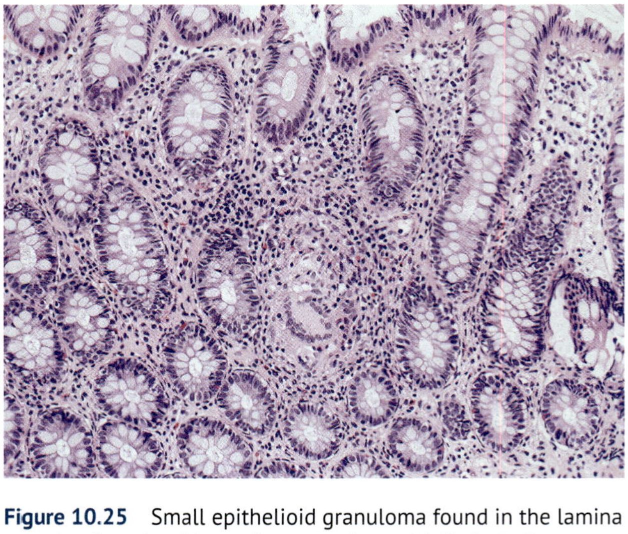

Figure 10.25 Small epithelioid granuloma found in the lamina propria of a colon biopsy from a patient with Crohn's disease.

Table 10.33 Features of Ulcerative colitis (UC) vs. Crohn's disease (CD).

	Classic	Less common but compatible	Incompatible
UC	• Chronic active colitis with architectural dissarray, basal lymphoplasmacytosis, distal Paneth cell metaplasia • Inflammation limited to mucosa • Continuous involvement, including rectum • No extracolonic involvement	• Deeper or transmural inflammation in fulminant colitis • Cecal/appendiceal and right-sided discontinuous inflammation • Backwash ileitis • Duodenitis or gastritis	• True non-pericryptic granulomas (stand-alone) • Small bowel involvement (excluding backwash ileitis) • Transmural lymphoid aggregates/disproportionate inflammation on biopsy • Perianal granulomatous inflammation.
CD	• Patchy/discontinuous chronic active ileitis or colitis with intervening zones of normal bowel • Chronic active ileitis, villous blunting and crypt distortion, pyloric metaplasia • Granulomas • Fissuring ulceration, stricture, and fistula formation	• Continuous mucosal inflammation and limited submucosal inflammation in older patients with isolated Crohn's colitis	

ill-defined histiocytes aggregates and few inflammatory cells or giant cells can be observed.

Aphthous ulcers characterized by superficial erosions overlying lymphoid follicles are characteristic of Crohn's disease, but may also be seen in infectious colitides (*Campylobacter*, *Shigella*, *Salmonella*, Yersinia), Behcet's disease, drugs, diverticular disease, diversion colitis, bowel preparation, or even ulcerative colitis.

When submucosa is present, the presence of "disproportionate inflammation" is a useful diagnostic feature in CD particularly when the overlying mucosa is intact.

In addition, Paneth cells or pseudopyloric metaplasia (ulcer-associated cell lineage) can be detected although the latter is less common in colonic CD than in the small bowel.

The main histomorphologic differences of UC and CD are summarized in Table 10.33.

Morphologic Variants of UC and CD

Over time, morphologic variants of both UC and CD have been recognized making the distinction of both diseases at times particularly challenging.

Ulcerative Colitis

Skip Lesions and Rectal Sparing

Once believed to be characteristic of Crohn's disease, mucosal skip lesions and rectal sparing (either relative or definite) can be noted in UC during successful therapy or spontaneously during *resolving phase*. Thus, it is crucial to review the entire set of biopsies, including those obtained before any treatment was instituted.

Patchiness of disease and relative (normal endoscopy with microscopic inflammation) or absolute (normal endoscopy and microscopy) rectal sparing commonly occur in the pediatric patients particularly under 10 years of age and possibly in children with associated PSC. Early pediatric UC has also less severe inflammatory and architectural changes. Furthermore, relative rectal sparing may occur in up to about 30% of patients.

Discontinuous Disease in the Setting of Fulminant UC

Fulminant colitis is observed in 5–13% of UC patients, either as a first presentation or an acute relapse. Although the mucosal alterations may be diffuse, the mucosa may also show CD-like histologic features, including relative, or complete rectal sparing and patchy, fissuring, or linear ulceration.

Cecal (or Ascending Colon) Patch in the Setting of Ulcerative Colitis

UC patients with either rectal or left-sided colitis frequently show patchy right sided (involving cecum and/or appendix) chronic-active inflammation, which may be falsely interpreted as CD.

Table 10.34 Differential diagnosis of inflammatory bowel disease.

	UC	CD	Infectious colitis (ASLC)	Diversion colitis	SCAD[a]	Microscopic colitis	Ischemia	Radiation	MP/SRUS
Architecture	**Villiform surface** **Diffuse/severe crypt distortion**	**Patchy/mild/ discontinuous crypt distortion**	**Preserved**	Generally preserved	Variable architectural distortion	**Preserved**[b]	May be abnormal if chronic/previous episodes of ischemia	**Variable crypt distortion**	May be preserved or mildly distorted, may observe pointed or "diamond" shaped crypts
Epithelial alterations	**Diffuse goblet cell depletion**	Relative preservation of goblet cell population	Goblet cell depletion	Variable mucin depletion	Variable mucin depletion	**Mucin depletion; epithelial injury**; **increased IEL**	Goblet cell depletion, **withering crypts**, degeneration/ necrosis of surface and superficial crypts	May have mild epithelial nuclear atypia	Variable mucin depletion, epithelial serrations
Metaplasia	Paneth cell metaplasia; pseudopyloric metaplasia rare	Pseudopyloric or Paneth metaplasia (rarely squamous)	—	—	May have Paneth cell metaplasia	Absent[b]	Paneth cell metaplasia may be seen in chronic ischemia	Paneth cell metaplasia may occur	—
LP inflammation	**Diffuse heavy mixed LP inflammation**, with **basal plasmacytosis**	**Patchy/ discontinuous LP inflammation**, basal lymphoid aggregates, basal plasmacytosis	**Neutrophils** **Edema** (increased chronic inflammatory cells may be seen late stage)	**Diffuse LP inflammation with prominent follicular hyperplasia**	LP mixed inflammation	**LP inflammation** (lymphoplasmacytic, variable eosinophils – may be prominent in CC)	Typically **pauci-inflammatory**; may have increase inflammation with reperfusion injury or superimposed infection	Typically not increased	Significant inflammation not typical; inflammation associated with surface erosions may be observed
Cryptitis/crypt abscesses	**Prominent**, "generalized active crypt inflammation"	**Focal/patchy**	Cryptitis, often superficial; crypt abscesses may be seen	May be seen	Variable	Absent[b]	Absent	Typically absent	Absent; may be seen in association with erosions/ ulceration
Granulomas	**Absent** (except cryptolytic granulomas)	**Present**; non-caseating granulomas, microgranulomas	Typically absent. Granulomas may occur (*Yersinia*, TB, *Campylobacter*, fungal, parasitic)	Absent/Rare	Absent/rare	Absent	Absent	Absent	Absent

Connective tissue alterations	May have thickening of MM LP fibrosis, occasionally band-like in deep mucosa	**Thickening and reduplication MM**, lymphangiectasia, **submucosal fibrosis, neural hypertrophy** (occasionally vasculitis)	Absent	—	Prolapse changes Focal thickening of subepithelial collagen, Thickening muscularis mucosa	**Thickened subepithelial collagen in CC**	**Hyalinization of LP** Fibrin thrombi	**Telangiectasia, atypical fibroblasts, LP fibrosis or focal thickening subepithelial collagen**	**Fibromuscular obliteration of the lamina propria**
Other	Knowledge of distribution ie rectal with variable proximal continuous extension	**Disproportionate (submucosal) inflammation** Knowledge of clinical/endoscopic (e.g. skip lesion and distribution, fissuring ulcers, involvement of other portions of GIT)	**Acute onset/ short history**	**Occurs in diverted colon**	**Limited to segment involved by diverticula (sigmoid)**	**Normal colonoscopy** **History of chronic non-bloody diarrhea**	Cholesterol emboli or vasculitis in submucosal vessels Pseudomembranes LP fibrosis and hemosiderin (chronic)	**Thickened/ hyalinized vessels**	–

Important differentiating features are highlighted in **Bold.**

CC, collagenous colitis; MM, muscularis mucosa; MP/SRUS, mucosal prolapse/solitary rectal ulcer syndrome; UC, ulcerative colitis; CD, Crohn's disease; SCAD, segmental colitis associated with diverticular disease; ASLC, acute self-limiting colitis.

[a] The histologic appearance on biopsy may mimic UC or CD closely.

[b] Rarely, microscopic colitis may be associated with IBD-like changes. These include crypt distortion, although typically limited and focal (one portion of a single fragment of tissue). Paneth cell metaplasia may occur (often limited; and more common in CC). Cryptitis/crypt abscesses can be seen but are always focal (less than three crypts per biopsy specimen in all affected cases).

Ulcerative Proctitis

This term refers to a chronic idiopathic localized inflammation of the rectal mucosa. The changes are those seen in classic UC but less commonly a pattern of follicular proctitis can be observed, although some investigators believe that follicular proctitis may represent an entity distinct from the spectrum of UC.

Crohn's Disease

Crohn's Colitis

Patients with colonic CD tend to be older compared with patients with ileocolonic disease. In about 15% of patients, continuous mucosal inflammation and limited submucosal inflammation makes the distinction from UC difficult. In such cases, granulomas and more subtle changes such as limited mucin depletion and architectural damage are helpful.

Differential Diagnosis

One of the most important differential diagnosis when considering the possibility of IBD is acute self-limiting colitis (ASLC). The other possibilities to consider would be sexually transmitted disease-related proctitis, especially in the setting of ulcerative proctitis. Table 10.34 provides the features that would distinguish UC and CD from other mimics.

Treatment/Prognosis/Evolution

Clinical management of IBD is complex and beyond the scope of this review, however general principles are discussed. The goal of all IBD therapies is to achieve sustained clinical and histological remission and to prevent complications of disease and therapy. Corticosteroids have been the mainstay of inducing remission for many decades but are increasingly replaced by targeted biological therapies. This includes suppression of pro-inflammatory cytokines such as TNF and IL-6, as well as activation of anti-inflammatory cytokines such as IL-10 and IL-11. Biological therapies are now used for both UC and CD. Other agents typically used for mild to moderate disease include mesalamine, which comes in a wide variety for form, and immune modulators such as Imuran and azathioprine. The latter two are especially effects for steroid sparing and to maintain remission. For fistulizing CD, antibiotics, and enteral diversion (with total parenteral nutrition) may be necessary adjuncts to biological therapy. With modern medical therapy, surgery is less and less needed, typically reserved for fulminant colitis and dysplastic lesions that cannot be removed endoscopically.

Further Reading

Agrawal, D., Rukkannagari, S., and Kethu, S. (2007). Pathogenesis and clinical approach to extraintestinal manifestations of inflammatory bowel disease. *Minerva Gastroenterol. Dietol.* 53: 233–248.

Ahuja, V. and Tandon, R.K. (2010). Inflammatory bowel disease in the Asia-Pacific area: a comparison with developed countries and regional differences. *J. Dig. Dis.* 11: 134–147.

Auvin, S., Molinie, F., Gower-Rousseau, C. et al. (2005). Incidence, clinical presentation and location at diagnosis of pediatric inflammatory bowel disease: a prospective population-based study in northern France (1988–1999). *J. Pediatr. Gastroenterol. Nutr.* 41: 49–55.

Bernstein, C.N., Shanahan, F., Anton, P.A., and Weinstein, W.M. (1995). Patchiness of mucosal inflammation in treated ulcerative colitis: a prospective study. *Gastrointest. Endosc.* 42: 232–237.

Bouguen, G. et al. (2015). Treat to target: a proposed new paradigm for the management of Crohn's disease. *Clin. Gastroenterol. Hepatol.* 13 (6): 1042–1050. e2.

Braegger, C.P., Ballabeni, P., Rogler, D. et al. (2011). Epidemiology of inflammatory bowel disease: is there a shift towards onset at a younger age? *J. Pediatr. Gastroenterol. Nutr.* 53: 141–144.

Broome, U., Lofberg, R., Veress, B., and Eriksson, L.S. (1995). Primary sclerosing cholangitis and ulcerative colitis: evidence for increased neoplastic potential. *Hepatology* 22: 1404–1408.

Carbonnel, F., Jantchou, P., Monnet, E., and Cosnes, J. (2009). Environmental risk factors in Crohn's disease and ulcerative colitis: an update. *Gastroenterol. Clin. Biol.* 33 (Suppl 3): S145–S157.

Cosnes, J., Gower-Rousseau, C., Seksik, P., and Cortot, A. (2011). Epidemiology and natural history of inflammatory bowel diseases. *Gastroenterology* 140: 1785–1794. e4.

D'Haens, G., Geboes, K., Peeters, M. et al. (1997). Patchy cecal inflammation associated with distal ulcerative colitis: a prospective endoscopic study. *Am. J. Gastroenterol.* 92: 1275–1279.

Farmer, R.G. (1987). Nonspecific ulcerative proctitis. *Gastroenterol. Clin. N. Am.* 16: 157–174.

Faubion, W.A. Jr., Loftus, E.V., Sandborn, W.J. et al. (2001). Pediatric “PSC-IBD”: a descriptive report of associated inflammatory bowel disease among pediatric patients with PSC. *J. Pediatr. Gastroenterol. Nutr.* 33: 296–300.

Fazio, V.W. (1980). Toxic megacolon in ulcerative colitis and Crohn’s colitis. *Clin. Gastroenterol.* 9: 389–407.

Feakins, R.M. and British Society of Gastroenterology (2013). Inflammatory bowel disease biopsies: updated British Society of Gastroenterology reporting guidelines. *J. Clin. Pathol.* 66: 1005–1026.

Fefferman, D.S. and Farrell, R.J. (2005). Endoscopy in inflammatory bowel disease: indications, surveillance, and use in clinical practice. *Clin. Gastroenterol. Hepatol.* 3: 11–24.

Flejou, J.F., Potet, F., Bogomoletz, W.V. et al. (1988). Lymphoid follicular proctitis. A condition different from ulcerative proctitis? *Dig. Dis. Sci.* 33: 314–320.

Frisch, M., Pedersen, B.V., and Andersson, R.E. (2009). Appendicitis, mesenteric lymphadenitis, and subsequent risk of ulcerative colitis: cohort studies in Sweden and Denmark. *BMJ* 338: b716.

Gledhill, A., Hall, P.A., Cruse, J.P., and Pollock, D.J. (1986). Enteroendocrine cell hyperplasia, carcinoid tumours and adenocarcinoma in long-standing ulcerative colitis. *Histopathology* 10: 501–508.

Glickman, J.N., Bousvaros, A., Farraye, F.A. et al. (2004). Pediatric patients with untreated ulcerative colitis may present initially with unusual morphologic findings. *Am. J. Surg. Pathol.* 28: 190–197.

Hanby, A.M. and Wright, N.A. (1993). The ulcer-associated cell lineage: the gastrointestinal repair kit? *J. Pathol.* 171: 3–4.

Hirschfield, G.M., Karlsen, T.H., Lindor, K.D., and Adams, D.H. (2013). Primary sclerosing cholangitis. *Lancet* 382: 1587–1599.

Jalan, K.N., Walker, R.J., Sircus, W. et al. (1969). Pseudopolyposis in ulcerative colitis. *Lancet* 2: 555–559.

Kaser, A., Zeissig, S., and Blumberg, R.S. (2010). Genes and environment: how will our concepts on the pathophysiology of IBD develop in the future? *Dig. Dis.* 28: 395–405.

Kelly, J.K. and Gabos, S. (1987). The pathogenesis of inflammatory polyps. *Dis. Colon Rectum* 30: 251–254.

Khor, B., Gardet, A., and Xavier, R.J. (2011). Genetics and pathogenesis of inflammatory bowel disease. *Nature* 474: 307–317.

Kim, B., Barnett, J.L., Kleer, C.G., and Appelman, H.D. (1999). Endoscopic and histological patchiness in treated ulcerative colitis. *Am. J. Gastroenterol.* 94: 3258–3262.

Kleer, C.G. and Appelman, H.D. (1998). Ulcerative colitis: patterns of involvement in colorectal biopsies and changes with time. *Am. J. Surg. Pathol.* 22: 983–989.

Kuchazik, T., Maaser, C., Lugering, A. et al. (2006). Recent understanding of IBD pathogenesis: implications for future therapies. *Inflamm. Bowel Dis.* 12: 1068–1083.

Larsen, S., Bendtzen, K., and Nielsen, O.H. (2010). Extraintestinal manifestations of inflammatory bowel disease: epidemiology, diagnosis, and management. *Ann. Med.* 42: 97–114.

Lee, Y.M. and Kaplan, M.M. (1995). Primary sclerosing cholangitis. *N. Engl. J. Med.* 332: 924–933.

Longman, R.J. and Warren, B.F. (2000). Is the colonic reparative cell lineage yet to be discovered? *Gut* 47: 307–308.

Lumb, G., Protheroe, R.H., and Ramsay, G.S. (1955). Ulcerative colitis with dilatation of the colon. *Br. J. Surg.* 43: 182–188.

Magro, F., Langner, C., Driessen, A. et al. (2013). European consensus on the histopathology of inflammatory bowel disease. *J. Crohns Colitis* 7: 827–851.

Markowitz, J., Kahn, E., Grancher, K. et al. (1993). Atypical rectosigmoid histology in children with newly diagnosed ulcerative colitis. *Am. J. Gastroenterol.* 88: 2034–2037.

Meuwissen, S.G., Feltkamp-Vroom, T.M., De La Riviere, A.B. et al. (1976). Analysis of the lympho-plasmacytic infiltrate in Crohn’s disease with special reference to identification of lymphocyte-subpopulations. *Gut* 17: 770–780.

Mowat, C., Cole, A., Windsor, A. et al. (2011). Guidelines for the management of inflammatory bowel disease in adults. *Gut* 60: 571–607.

Mutinga, M.L., Odze, R.D., Wang, H.H. et al. (2004). The clinical significance of right-sided colonic inflammation in patients with left-sided chronic ulcerative colitis. *Inflamm. Bowel Dis.* 10: 215–219.

Navaneethan, U. (2014). Hepatobiliary manifestations of ulcerative colitis: an example of gut-liver crosstalk. *Gastroenterol. Rep.* 2 (3): 193–200.

Odze, R. (2003). Diagnostic problems and advances in inflammatory bowel disease. *Mod. Pathol.* 16: 347–358.

Odze, R., Antonioli, D., Peppercorn, M., and Goldman, H. (1993). Effect of topical 5-aminosalicylic acid (5-ASA) therapy on rectal mucosal biopsy morphology in chronic ulcerative colitis. *Am. J. Surg. Pathol.* 17: 869–875.

Okawa, K., Aoki, T., Sano, K. et al. (1998). Ulcerative colitis with skip lesions at the mouth of the appendix: a clinical study. *Am. J. Gastroenterol.* 93: 2405–2410.

Pulimood, A.B., Ramakrishna, B.S., Kurian, G. et al. (1999). Endoscopic mucosal biopsies are useful in distinguishing granulomatous colitis due to Crohn’s disease from tuberculosis. *Gut* 45: 537–541.

Radford-Smith, G.L. (2008). What is the importance of appendectomy in the natural history of IBD? *Inflamm. Bowel Dis.* 14 (Suppl 2): S72–S74.

Radford-Smith, G.L., Edwards, J.E., Purdie, D.M. et al. (2002). Protective role of appendicectomy on onset and severity of ulcerative colitis and Crohn's disease. *Gut* 51: 808–813.

Robert, M.E., Skacel, M., Ullman, T. et al. (2004). Patterns of colonic involvement at initial presentation in ulcerative colitis: a retrospective study of 46 newly diagnosed cases. *Am. J. Clin. Pathol.* 122: 94–99.

Russell, R.K. and Satsangi, J. (2004). IBD: a family affair. *Best Pract. Res. Clin. Gastroenterol.* 18: 525–539.

Satsangi, J., Silverberg, M.S., Vermeire, S., and Colombel, J.F. (2006). The Montreal classification of inflammatory bowel disease: controversies, consensus, and implications. *Gut* 55: 749–753.

Schmidt, C. and Stallmach, A. (2005). Etiology and pathogenesis of inflammatory bowel disease. *Minerva Gastroenterol. Dietol.* 51: 127–145.

Scoville, E.A. and Schwartz, D.A. (2017). Endoscopy in inflammatory bowel disease: advances in disease management. *Gastrointest Endosc.* 86 (6): 952–961.

Soucy, G., Wang, H.H., Farraye, F.A. et al. (2012). Clinical and pathological analysis of colonic Crohn's disease, including a subgroup with ulcerative colitis-like features. *Mod. Pathol.* 25: 295–307.

Thompson, A.I. and Lees, C.W. (2011). Genetics of ulcerative colitis. *Inflamm. Bowel Dis.* 17: 831–848.

Tsaitas, C., Semertzidou, A., and Sinakos, E. (2014). Update on inflammatory bowel disease in patients with primary sclerosing cholangitis. *World J. Hepatol.* 6: 178–187.

Warren, B.F. (2004). Classic pathology of ulcerative and Crohn's colitis. *J. Clin. Gastroenterol.* 38: S33–S35.

Washington, K., Greenson, J.K., Montgomery, E. et al. (2002). Histopathology of ulcerative colitis in initial rectal biopsy in children. *Am. J. Surg. Pathol.* 26: 1441–1449.

Weersma, R.K., van Dullemen, H.M., van der Steege, G. et al. (2007). Review article: inflammatory bowel disease and genetics. *Aliment. Pharmacol. Ther.* 26 (Suppl 2): 57–65.

Xavier, R.J. and Podolsky, D.K. (2007). Unravelling the pathogenesis of inflammatory bowel disease. *Nature* 448: 427–434.

Yang, S.K., Jung, H.Y., Kang, G.H. et al. (1999). Appendiceal orifice inflammation as a skip lesion in ulcerative colitis: an analysis in relation to medical therapy and disease extent. *Gastrointest. Endosc.* 49: 743–747.

Yantiss, R.K., Farraye, F.A., O'Brien, M.J. et al. (2006). Prognostic significance of superficial fissuring ulceration in patients with severe "indeterminate" colitis. *Am. J. Surg. Pathol.* 30: 165–170.

Dysplasia in Inflammatory Bowel Disease

Definition, General Features, Predisposing Factors

Patients with inflammatory bowel disease are at high risk for developing colorectal carcinoma (CRC), which represent the cause of death in 15–20% of these patients. Dysplasia, which is defined as unequivocal neoplastic epithelial change confined by the basement membrane, is both a precursor and a marker of risk for CRC. A meta-analysis reported a 3.7% prevalence of CRC in UC with cumulative probability of 2, 8, and 18% after 10, 20, and 30 years, respectively. However, recent data suggest this risk may have been overestimated or is declining, possibly related to colonoscopic surveillance, anti-inflammatory chemoprophylaxis, early surgical intervention, or diet/environmental factors. The risk of CRC in CD relates to the presence and extent of colitis, and this risk approaches the risk in UC of similar duration and severity.

The strongest association of risk for CRC includes duration (greater than eight years) and extent of colitis (highest risk with pancolitis, intermediate with left-sided colitis, and minimal to none with proctitis/proctosigmoiditis). Other factors include primary sclerosing cholangitis, a family history of CRC, severity of histologic inflammation, and young age at onset (less than 15 years). Backwash ileitis has been inconsistently reported as a risk factor. The finding of a stricture during colonoscopy is associated with heightened risk.

Clinical Features/Endoscopic Characteristics

The spectrum of gross/endoscopic changes includes polypoid lesions, resembling adenomas and slightly raised and plaque-like lesions resembling flat adenomas. They can be villous, or have a velvety/chamois leather-like mucosal appearance. Dysplasia occasionally occurs in flat and otherwise unremarkable mucosa. Even in flat dysplastic mucosa, the pit pattern may be abnormal. These changes are better detected by using chromoendoscopy with magnification. It has been shown that surveillance using this technique has doubled the number of dysplastic lesions identified, so it has a much higher yield of dysplasia than random biopsies, which it could replace. It can be estimated that 320 regularly spaced biopsies are required to ensure to detect a 2 cm patch of flat dysplasia in a large bowel of 100 cm in length and 10 cm in diameter. Chromoendoscopy, narrow-band imaging, or confocal endomicroscopy, which allows visualization of nuclei in crypts, all may have roles to play.

Microscopic Features

The diagnosis of IBD-associated dysplasia is frequently hindered by superimposed inflammatory and regenerative processes and may cause significant diagnostic difficulties considering differentiation from reactive atypia. The dysplastic epithelium most commonly resembles typical "sporadic" adenomatous epithelium and is recognized by both cytological and architectural criteria (Figure 10.26).

Architectural Features

Dysplastic epithelium colonizes the pre-existing crypt architecture, often with features of crypt architectural distortion, but with closely packed crypts rather than the sparse crypt pattern observed in atrophic non-dysplastic IBD mucosa (Figure 10.26). Like in adenomas, various degree of crypt budding may be observed. When extreme, the distinction from early lamina propria invasion is subjective and poorly reproducible. Fortunately, for management purposes, this distinction is of little importance. In some instances, a villous or serrated architecture may be observed. Of note, serration may occur in both non-dysplastic regenerative and dysplastic mucosa, however, and attention to cytologic features is important.

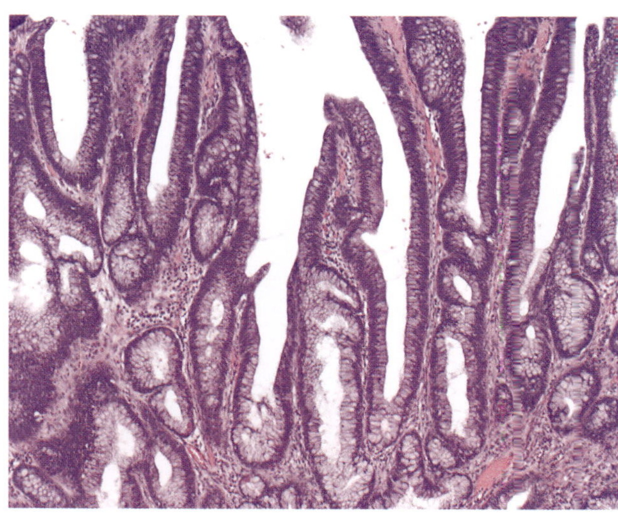

Figure 10.26 Low-grade IBD-associated dysplasia. This lesion shows a conventional intestinal (adenomatous) morphology with tubulovillous architecture, nuclear stratification with maintained cell polarity and mild cytologic atypia.

Cytological Features

Most cases show increased severity of cytological atypia as the lumen is approached. This *loss of basal-luminal maturation* is a criterion for establishing a diagnosis of dysplasia.

The spectrum includes nuclear stratification, abnormal nuclear chromatin from dense and hyperchromatic to open with variably prominent nucleoli, irregular nuclear contours, pleomorphism, increased nuclear: cytoplasmic ratio, and loss of polarity. The severity increases with the grade of dysplasia (Figures 10.26 and 10.27). Mitoses are variably increased, including atypical forms, and mitoses in the upper third of crypts suggest possibility of dysplasia. A sharp transition with adjacent non-neoplastic epithelium usually denotes the presence of dysplasia.

Variant Patterns

Several rare and incompletely characterized variants of IBD-associated dysplasia have been recently reported. These infrequent variants should not be neglected, as they have comparable tendency to be associated with underlying carcinoma. The non-conventional subtypes are possibly underdiagnosed, and, owing to the lack of established diagnostic criteria, interobserver agreement is poor. No specific surveillance guidelines are currently available for these lesions, as their natural history and clinical significance are largely unclear at this time.

The most commonly diagnosed non-conventional subtype is the endoscopically frequently polypoid *villous hypermucinous dysplasia* with tall mucin-rich cells lining rigid villous structures and low-grade atypia progressively increasing towards the crypt base (Figure 10.28).

IBD-associated *serrated dysplasia* is also usually polypoid and histologically shows a saw-toothed or stellate architecture. This category comprises further subtypes, analogous to the sporadic serrated dysplasia variants, including *traditional serrated adenoma (TSA)-like* (Figure 10.29) and *sessile serrated lesion (SSL)-like* dysplasias, as well as *serrated dysplasia not otherwise specified*. In a recent study,

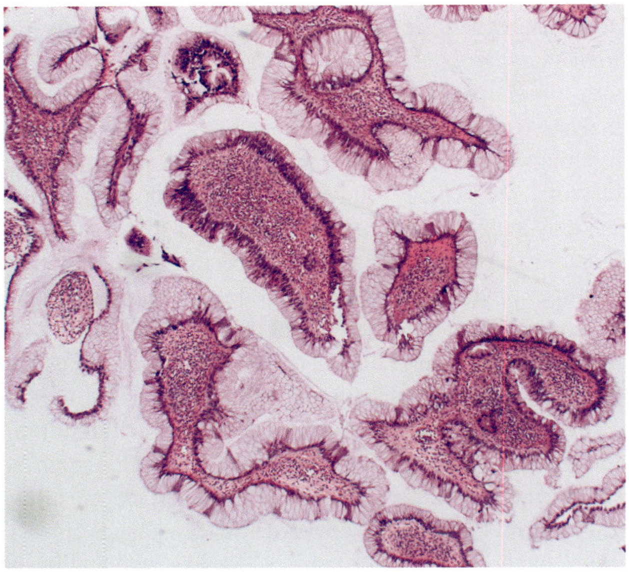

Figure 10.28 Hypermucinous dysplasia typically shows a villous/tubulovillous pattern. The cells are reminiscent of gastric foveolar cells with prominent mucinous cytoplasm with mild nuclear enlargement, and hyperchromasia at the tip of the villi and progressively increasing nuclear atypia at the base of the crypts.

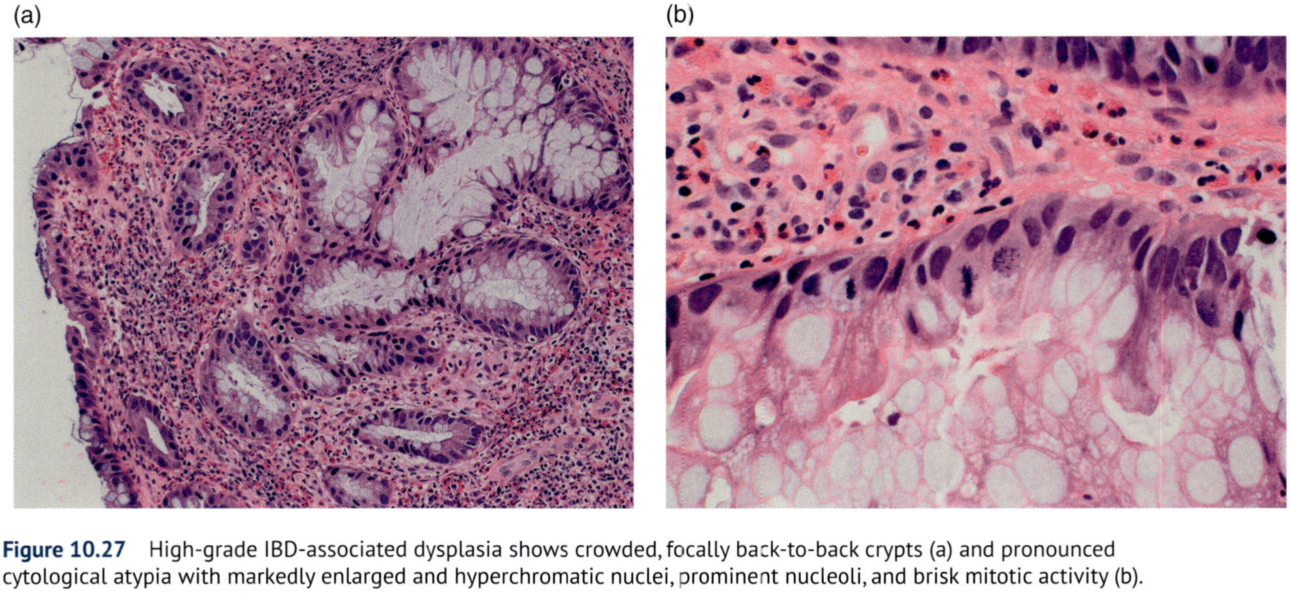

Figure 10.27 High-grade IBD-associated dysplasia shows crowded, focally back-to-back crypts (a) and pronounced cytological atypia with markedly enlarged and hyperchromatic nuclei, prominent nucleoli, and brisk mitotic activity (b).

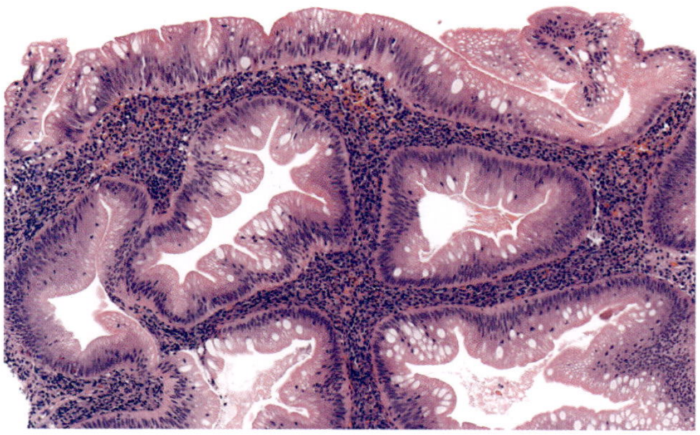

Figure 10.29 IBD-associated TSA-like dysplasia presents with narrow, slit-like serrations, tall columnar cells, eosinophilic cytoplasm, and penicillate nuclei. A few abortive ectopic crypts may also be noticed.

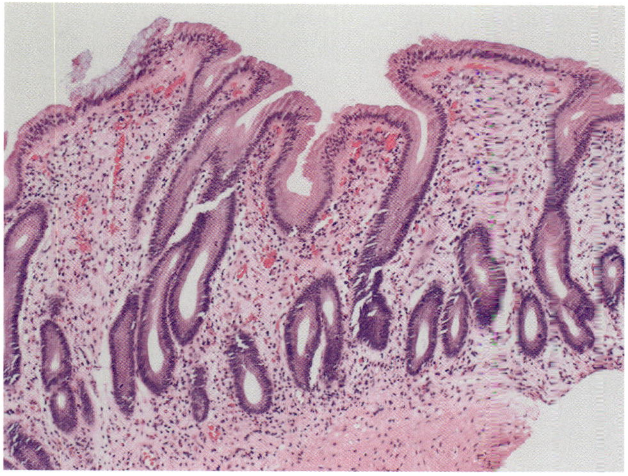

Figure 10.30 Example of goblet cell-deficient dysplasia (GCD) with tubular crypts lined by enlarged, hyperchromatic, and penicillate nuclei. This lesion is characterized by the complete or near complete absence of goblet cells.

the incidence of high-grade dysplasia and carcinoma for low-grade serrated dysplasia was similar to that for conventional low-grade dysplasia.

Crypt cell dysplasia is typically endoscopically flat, often invisible. Microscopically it is characterized by a non-crowded crypt pattern with mildly enlarged, hyperchromatic, slightly irregular, mostly non-stratified nuclei limited to the crypt base, showing maturation towards the surface. High-grade dysplasia or colorectal cancer have been reported to develop in 86% of patients within a mean follow-up time of 27 months.

Goblet cell deficient dysplasia (GCD) and *dysplasia with Paneth cell differentiation* (DPD) typically show tubular growth pattern. The crypts are lined by enlarged, hyperchromatic, and penicillate nuclei. DPD is defined by increased Paneth cell differentiation, that exceeds what is present in surrounding mucosa, involving at least two adjacent crypts in two foci. GCD is characterized by the absence of goblet cells (Figure 10.30). Although the number of goblet cells may be reduced in other dysplasia subtypes, they are not absent or nearly absent.

The Classification and Grading of Dysplasia

This is based on the notion that increasing grade of dysplasia is associated with heightened malignant potential.

The classification is subjective, with the two grades, low and high, and the term "indefinite" used to qualify equivocal cases, in which regenerative atypia and dysplasia cannot be definitely differentiated (Table 10.1). The two-tier classification system of high- or low-grade dysplasia yields higher reproducibility compared to a three-tier categorization and forms the basis of patient surveillance (Figures 10.26 and 10.27). For lesions classified as "indefinite," repeat colonoscopy with generous biopsy sampling of any challenging area is advised to ensure that unequivocal dysplasia or worse is excluded.

High-grade dysplasia is characterized by severe architectural and/or cytological changes. There are no established criteria related to the extent of the changes before the lesion is deemed high or low grade. However, in practice, the most severely dysplastic area, even if it is small, determines the final grade.

Differential Diagnosis

None of the cytological or architectural features are unique to dysplasia, and each can be seen in isolation in inflamed or regenerating colonic mucosa.

Distinction from Reactive Changes

The presence of an acute inflammatory infiltrate, whether in the lamina propria or, especially, within the epithelium, calls for prudence. The presence of either cuboidal (regenerative) epithelium, or surface maturation with hyperchromatic nuclei at the base suggests that the changes are reactive, and under these circumstances, a diagnosis of dysplasia should be made only when other features make it absolutely certain. Importantly, in the setting of reactive changes, the nuclei are enlarged, often vesicular with prominent nucleoli, with little or no overlap of nuclei, especially toward the surface. In addition, some degree of pseudostratification can be seen, especially at crypt bases.

In some situations, the distinction between reactive and dysplasia may be extremely difficult, necessitating a diagnosis of "indefinite for dysplasia." This diagnosis may be applied when any one or a small number of features of genuine dysplasia are seen but insufficient to warrant a confident opinion. Other situations in which such a diagnosis is rendered include limited sampling, damaged tissue, suboptimal orientation with limited or no surface epithelium, cytological changes in the presence of severe active inflammation (e.g. ulcerated mucosa), and, finally, low-grade "bottom up" atypia limited to the crypt bases with maturation as the surface is approached.

Drug-Induced Changes

Immunosuppressive drugs such as cyclosporin may cause cellular atypia mimicking dysplasia. The induced changes include villiform mucosal transformation and epithelial regenerative changes, which are severe with marked nuclear enlargement, sometimes extending to the mucosal surface, but usually with plentiful eosinophilic cytoplasm. Perhaps, the most distinctive feature is that the "pseudodysplasia" induced by cyclosporin is strikingly diffuse, with many and sometimes all crypts showing similar changes, a pattern not usually associated with dysplasia.

Distinction of Regenerative Changes from Dysplasia Originating in Inflammatory Polyps

Fortunately, dysplasia in inflammatory polyps is distinctly uncommon. An important concept for the colonoscopist is that no polypoid lesion in IBD patients should be biopsied or removed in isolation and must always be accompanied by generous sampling of adjacent flat mucosa. This is cardinal, since it can assist the pathologist in making the distinction between regenerative atypia and dysplasia.

Role of Immunohistochemistry

Several adjunctive markers have been sought to help improve the diagnosis of dysplasia. Importantly, the result of these ancillary reactions should never be interpreted as the sole argument in favor or against dysplasia, thus should only be used to confirm the morphological interpretation. Of these, p53 and Ki-67 have been studied most extensively. Although p53 expression increases progressively from low- to high-grade dysplasia, some lesions considered indefinite for dysplasia or negative may occasionally be positive, limiting its utility. Ki-67, which ordinarily stains replicative basal colonocytes, exhibits abnormal surface staining pattern in most dysplastic lesions; however, much overlap between reactive epithelium and dysplasia is observed, therefore evaluation of cell proliferation is not useful in individual cases to distinguish these lesions. Recently, AMACR has been suggested as a potentially useful marker, particularly in combination with p53. AMACR was not expressed in any mucosal biopsy in UC that was considered negative for dysplasia, but was increased significantly in foci of low-grade dysplasia (96%), high-grade dysplasia (80%), and adenocarcinoma (71%) in one study. In the authors' experience, however, routine use of ancillary markers has not been useful, as the results are inconsistent.

Treatment and Prognosis

The proper use of terminology for dysplastic lesions must be underscored when considering treatment. Dysplasia in IBD may be endoscopically visible or invisible (Table 10.2), with different management implications. The term DALM dysplasia-associated lesion or mass should be abandoned.

Elevated/polypoid dysplastic lesions, that are amenable to endoscopic removal, including those regarded as sporadic adenomas within non-diseased colorectum, or lesions within colitic areas that are pedunculated with histologically confirmed non-dysplastic pedicles, and a lack of dysplasia in adjacent flat mucosa and elsewhere in the colorectum, may be managed conservatively with polypectomy and continued surveillance. This is maintained even when resected polyps contain HGD. The endoscopic, histologic, and prognostic similarities between polypoid dysplasia in IBD and sporadic adenoma suggest that some, if not all, may represent fortuitous adenomas, a hypothesis that is supported by limited molecular-based evidence. Both "flat" HGD and elevated/polypoid dysplastic lesions (low or high grade) not amenable to endoscopic resection carry a high risk of carcinoma, and colectomy is recommended. In contrast, the management of "flat" LGD is more controversial. Some recommend colectomy, even for unifocal "flat" LGD, but particularly if multifocal or persistent on follow-up. Alternatively, especially in cases with endoscopically invisible dysplasia, intensified surveillance involving an IBD expert endoscopist using high-definition chromoendoscopy is suggested. Table 10.35 summarizes the recommendations of the recent SCENIC guidelines for surveillance and management of IBD-associated dysplasia.

Table 10.35 Summary of recommendations for management of IBD-associated dysplasia discovered on surveillance colonoscopy according to the SCENIC guidelines.

Following complete removal of endoscopically resectable polypoid dysplastic lesions, endoscopic surveillance is recommended rather than colectomy
Following complete removal of endoscopically resectable nonpolypoid dysplastic lesions, endoscopic surveillance is recommended rather than colectomy
For patients with endoscopically invisible dysplasia (confirmed by a GI pathologist), referral is suggested to an endoscopist expert in IBD surveillance using high-definition chromoendoscopy

Further Reading

Aust, D.E., Willenbucher, R.F., Terdiman, J.P. et al. (2000). Chromosomal alterations in ulcerative colitis-related and sporadic colorectal cancers by comparative genomic hybridization. *Hum. Pathol.* 31: 109–114.

Averboukh, F., Ziv, Y., Kariv, Y. et al. (2011). Colorectal carcinoma in inflammatory bowel disease: a comparison between Crohn's and ulcerative colitis. *Colorectal Dis.* 13: 1230–1235.

Bernstein, C.N., Blanchard, J.F., Kliewer, E., and Wajda, A. (2001). Cancer risk in patients with inflammatory bowel disease: a population-based study. *Cancer* 91: 854–862.

Blackstone, M.O., Riddell, R.H., Rogers, B.H., and Levin, B. (1981). Dysplasia-associated lesion or mass (DALM) detected by colonoscopy in long-standing ulcerative colitis: an indication for colectomy. *Gastroenterology* 80: 366–374.

Choi, P.M. and Zelig, M.P. (1994). Similarity of colorectal cancer in Crohn's disease and ulcerative colitis: implications for carcinogenesis and prevention. *Gut* 35: 950–954.

Choi, W.T., Yozu, M., Miller, G.C. et al. (2020). Nonconventional dysplasia in patients with inflammatory bowel disease and colorectal carcinoma: a multicenter clinicopathologic study. *Mod. Pathol.* 33: 933–943.

Dawson, I.M. and Pryse-Davies, J. (1959). The development of carcinoma of the large intestine in ulcerative colitis. *Br. J. Surg.* 47: 113–128.

van Dekken, H., Wink, J.C., Vissers, K.J. et al. (2007). Wnt pathway-related gene expression during malignant progression in ulcerative colitis. *Acta Histochem.* 109: 266–272.

Dorer, R. and Odze, R.D. (2006). AMACR immunostaining is useful in detecting dysplastic epithelium in Barrett's esophagus, ulcerative colitis, and Crohn's disease. *Am. J. Surg. Pathol.* 30: 871–877.

Downs-Kelly, E., Mendelin, J.E., Bennett, A.E. et al. (2008). Poor interobserver agreement in the distinction of high-grade dysplasia and adenocarcinoma in pretreatment Barrett's esophagus biopsies. *Am. J. Gastroenterol.* 103: 2333–2340. quiz 41.

Eaden, J.A., Abrams, K.R., and Mayberry, J.F. (2001). The risk of colorectal cancer in ulcerative colitis: a meta-analysis. *Gut* 48: 526–535.

Ekbom, A., Helmick, C., Zack, M., and Adami, H.O. (1990). Ulcerative colitis and colorectal cancer. A population-based study. *N. Engl. J. Med.* 323: 1228–1233.

Granqvist, S., Gabrielsson, N., Sundelin, P., and Thorgeirsson, T. (1980). Precancerous lesions in the mucosa in ulcerative colitis. A radiographic, endoscopic, and histopathologic study. *Scand. J. Gastroenterol.* 15: 289–296.

Gupta, R.B., Harpaz, N., Itzkowitz, S. et al. (2007). Histologic inflammation is a risk factor for progression to colorectal neoplasia in ulcerative colitis: a cohort study. *Gastroenterology* 133: 1099–1105. quiz 340-1.

Gyde, S.N., Prior, P., Allan, R.N. et al. (1988). Colorectal cancer in ulcerative colitis: a cohort study of primary referrals from three centres. *Gut* 29: 206–217.

Harpaz, N. and Polydorides, A.D. (2010). Colorectal dysplasia in chronic inflammatory bowel disease: pathology, clinical implications, and pathogenesis. *Arch. Pathol. Lab. Med.* 134: 876–895.

Haskell, H., Andrews, C.W. Jr., Reddy, S.I. et al. (2005). Pathologic features and clinical significance of "backwash" ileitis in ulcerative colitis. *Am. J. Surg. Pathol.* 29: 1472–1481.

Heuschen, U.A., Hinz, U., Allemeyer, E.H. et al. (2001). Backwash ileitis is strongly associated with colorectal carcinoma in ulcerative colitis. *Gastroenterology* 120: 841–847.

Huang, Q., Fukami, N., Kashida, H. et al. (2004). Interobserver and intra-observer consistency in the endoscopic assessment of colonic pit patterns. *Gastrointest. Endosc.* 60: 520–526.

Hyde, G.M., Thillainayagam, A.V., and Jewell, D.P. (1998). Intravenous cyclosporin as rescue therapy in severe ulcerative colitis: time for a reappraisal? *Eur. J. Gastroenterol. Hepatol.* 10: 411–413.

Hyde, G.M., Jewell, D.P., and Warren, B.F. (2002). Histological changes associated with the use of intravenous cyclosporin in the treatment of severe ulcerative colitis may mimic dysplasia. *Colorectal Dis.* 4: 455–458.

Issa, J.P., Ahuja, N., Toyota, M. et al. (2001). Accelerated age-related CpG island methylation in ulcerative colitis. *Cancer Res.* 61: 3573–3577.

Itzkowitz, S.H. and Present, D.H. (2005). Consensus conference: colorectal cancer screening and surveillance in inflammatory bowel disease. *Inflamm. Bowel. Dis.* 11: 314–321.

Jess, T., Loftus, E.V. Jr., Velayos, F.S. et al. (2006). Risk of intestinal cancer in inflammatory bowel disease: a population-based study from olmsted county, Minnesota. *Gastroenterology.* 130: 1039–1046.

Karlen, P., Lofberg, R., Brostrom, O. et al. (1999). Increased risk of cancer in ulcerative colitis: a population-based cohort study. *Am. J. Gastroenterol.* 94: 1047–1052.

Kelly, J.K., Langevin, J.M., Price, L.M. et al. (1986). Giant and symptomatic inflammatory polyps of the colon in idiopathic inflammatory bowel disease. *Am. J. Surg. Pathol.* 10: 420–428.

Kiesslich, R., Fritsch, J., Holtmann, M. et al. (2003). Methylene blue-aided chromoendoscopy for the detection of intraepithelial neoplasia and colon cancer in ulcerative colitis. *Gastroenterology* 124: 880–888.

Kornfeld, D., Ekbom, A., and Ihre, T. (1997). Is there an excess risk for colorectal cancer in patients with ulcerative colitis and concomitant primary sclerosing cholangitis? A population based study. *Gut* 41: 522–525.

Laine, L., Kaltenbach, T., Barkun, A. et al. (2015). SCENIC international consensus statement on surveillance and management of dysplasia in inflammatory bowel disease. *Gastrointest Endosc.* 81: 489–501. e26.

Lakatos, L., Mester, G., Erdelyi, Z. et al. (2006). Risk factors for ulcerative colitis-associated colorectal cancer in a Hungarian cohort of patients with ulcerative colitis: results of a population-based study. *Inflamm. Bowel Dis.* 12: 205–211.

Lennard-Jones, J.E., Morson, B.C., Ritchie, J.K. et al. (1977). Cancer in colitis: assessment of the individual risk by clinical and histological criteria. *Gastroenterology* 73: 1280–1289.

Lichtiger, S., Present, D.H., Kornbluth, A. et al. (1994). Cyclosporine in severe ulcerative colitis refractory to steroid therapy. *N. Engl. J. Med.* 330: 1841–1845.

Loftus, E.V. Jr. (2006). Epidemiology and risk factors for colorectal dysplasia and cancer in ulcerative colitis. *Gastroenterol. Clin. North Am.* 35: 517–531.

Lundqvist, K. and Broome, U. (1997). Differences in colonic disease activity in patients with ulcerative colitis with and without primary sclerosing cholangitis: a case control study. *Dis. Colon. Rectum.* 40: 451–456.

Lyda, M.H., Noffsinger, A., Belli, J., and Fenoglio-Preiser, C.M. (2000). Microsatellite instability and K-ras mutations in patients with ulcerative colitis. *Hum. Pathol.* 31: 665–671.

Maia, L., Dinis, J., Cravo, M. et al. (2005). Who takes the lead in the development of ulcerative colitis-associated colorectal cancers: mutator, suppressor, or methylator pathway? *Cancer Genet. Cytogenet.* 162: 68–73.

Manning, A.P., Bulgim, O.R., Dixon, M.F., and Axon, A.T. (1987). Screening by colonoscopy for colonic epithelial dysplasia in inflammatory bowel disease. *Gut* 28: 1489–1494.

Marx, A., Wandrey, T., Simon, P. et al. (2009). Combined alpha-methylacyl coenzyme A racemase/p53 analysis to identify dysplasia in inflammatory bowel disease. *Hum. Pathol.* 40: 166–173.

Mathy, C., Schneider, K., Chen, Y.Y. et al. (2003). Gross versus microscopic pancolitis and the occurrence of neoplasia in ulcerative colitis. *Inflamm. Bowel. Dis.* 9: 351–355.

Moriyama, T., Matsumoto, T., Nakamura, S. et al. (2007). Hypermethylation of p14 (ARF) may be predictive of colitic cancer in patients with ulcerative colitis. *Dis. Colon. Rectum.* 50: 1384–1392.

Morson, B.C. and Pang, L.S. (1967). Rectal biopsy as an aid to cancer control in ulcerative colitis. *Gut* 8: 423–434.

Odze, R. (2006). Pathology of dysplasia and cancer in inflammatory bowel disease. *Gastroenterol. Clin. N. Am.* 35: 533–552.

Odze, R.D., Brown, C.A., Hartmann, C.J. et al. (2000). Genetic alterations in chronic ulcerative colitis-associated adenoma-like DALMs are similar to non-colitic sporadic adenomas. *Am. J. Surg. Pathol.* 24: 1209–1216.

Pereira, D., Kővári, B., Brown, I. et al. (2020). Non-conventional dysplasia of the tubular gut: a review and illustration of their histomorphologic spectrum. *Histopathology.*

Potack, J. and Itzkowitz, S.H. (2008). Colorectal cancer in inflammatory bowel disease. *Gut Liver.* 2: 61–73.

Riddell, R.H. and Morson, B.C. (1979). Value of sigmoidoscopy and biopsy in detection of carcinoma and premalignant change in ulcerative colitis. *Gut* 20: 575–580.

Riddell, R.H., Goldman, H., Ransohoff, D.F. et al. (1983). Dysplasia in inflammatory bowel disease: standardized classification with provisional clinical applications. *Hum. Pathol.* 14: 931–968.

Rubio, C.A. (2007). Serrated neoplasias and de novo carcinomas in ulcerative colitis: a histological study in colectomy specimens. *J. Gastroenterol. Hepatol.* 22: 1024–1031.

Rutter, M., Saunders, B., Wilkinson, K. et al. (2004). Severity of inflammation is a risk factor for colorectal neoplasia in ulcerative colitis. *Gastroenterology* 126: 451–459.

Shetty, K., Rybicki, L., Brzezinski, A. et al. (1999). The risk for cancer or dysplasia in ulcerative colitis patients with primary sclerosing cholangitis. *Am. J. Gastroenterol.* 94: 1643–1649.

Srivastava, A., Redston, M., Farraye, F.A. et al. (2008). Hyperplastic/serrated polyposis in inflammatory bowel disease: a case series of a previously undescribed entity. *Am. J. Surg. Pathol.* 32: 296–303.

Velayos, F.S., Terdiman, J.P., and Walsh, J.M. (2005). Effect of 5-aminosalicylate use on colorectal cancer and dysplasia risk: a systematic review and metaanalysis of observational studies. *Am. J. Gastroenterol.* 100: 1345–1353.

Vucelic, B. (2009). Inflammatory bowel diseases: controversies in the use of diagnostic procedures. *Dig. Dis.* 27: 269–277.

Walsh, S., Murphy, M., Silverman, M. et al. (1999). p27 expression in inflammatory bowel disease-associated neoplasia. Further evidence of a unique molecular pathogenesis. *Am. J. Pathol.* 155: 1511–1518.

Warren, S. and Sommers, S.C. (1949). Pathogenesis of ulcerative colitis. *Am. J. Pathol.* 25: 657–679.

Winther, K.V., Jess, T., Langholz, E. et al. (2004). Long-term risk of cancer in ulcerative colitis: a population-based cohort study from Copenhagen County. *Clin. Gastroenterol. Hepatol.* 2: 1088–1095.

Wong, N.A., Mayer, N.J., MacKell, S. et al. (2000). Immunohistochemical assessment of Ki67 and p53 expression assists the diagnosis and grading of ulcerative colitis-related dysplasia. *Histopathology* 37: 108–114.

11

Polyps of the Large Intestine

Christophe Rosty[1], Michael B. Wallace[2] and Till S. Clauditz[3]

[1]*Envoi Specialist Pathologists, Brisbane, Australia*
[2]*Mayo Clinic, Jacksonville, Florida, USA*
[3]*Department of Pathology, University-Medical-Center Hamburg-Eppendorf, Hamburg, Germany*

Polyps of the large intestine are broadly defined as any projections of the mucosa into the lumen of the bowel. A wide range of mucosal and submucosal lesions can result in polyp formation. The vast majority originate from the epithelial component of the mucosa, and are divided into conventional adenomas and serrated polyps. Non-neoplastic polyps of the large bowel comprise inflammatory polyps and hamartomatous polyps. Other, less common colorectal polyps include mesenchymal polyps and lymphoid polyps.

Epithelial Polyps

Conventional Adenoma

Definitions and General Features

Conventional adenomas, also called adenomatous polyps, are primarily defined by the presence of adenomatous dysplasia in the colonic epithelium and are further subclassified according to their histologic architecture (tubular, tubulovillous, villous) and the degree of dysplasia (low grade, high grade). Advanced adenomas are defined as conventional adenomas with one or more of the following features: >10 mm in size, presence of high-grade dysplasia, or presence of a villous component (tubulovillous or villous adenoma) (Figure 11.1).

Conventional adenoma is one of the lesions of the large bowel most frequently encountered in practice. The prevalence of adenomas detected during screening colonoscopy ranges from 11.9 to 22.8%, of which 25% are advanced lesions.

Predisposing factors for individuals to develop conventional adenomas are similar to those of colorectal cancer, comprising genetic predisposition and environmental risk factors. Familial adenomatous polyposis (FAPs) and *MUTYH*-associated polyposis are two well-defined genetic syndromes characterized by the occurrence of multiple conventional adenomas at a young age (discussed in detail in Chapter 13). Advancing age is strongly associated with adenoma formation, with a sharp increase in prevalence observed after 50 years, which is taken into account by most colorectal cancer screening programs worldwide. Other strong risk factors include male gender, family history of colorectal neoplasia, and geographic location, with the highest prevalence of adenomas in western countries such as the United States and Australia. Lifestyle risk factors include abdominal obesity; cigarette smoking; alcohol consumption; type 2 diabetes; low physical activity; and dietary habits such as consumption of processed or grilled red meat, high fat, and low fibers. Prolonged use of non-steroidal anti-inflammatory drugs, estrogen replacement therapy in women, and high calcium and folate intake have been reported to have a protective effect on adenoma formation.

Clinical Features and Endoscopic Characteristics

Most adenomatous polyps are asymptomatic unless they become very large and cause bleeding or anemia. Most are found on screening or surveillance colonoscopy. Endoscopic features that help detect and characterize adenomatous lesion are now highly advanced. With the advent of advanced endoscopic resection methods such as endoscopic mucosal resection (EMR) and endoscopic submucosal dissection (ESD), which can provide curative resection of even T1 invasive cancer, it has become increasingly important to classify these lesions by optical inspection in vivo ("optical biopsy") followed by appropriate therapy (simple snare polypectomy vs. EMR vs. ESD). This differentiation is made based on the shape (which is codified by the Paris classification system) and surface pattern (which is codified by either

Gastrointestinal Pathology: Correlative Endoscopic and Histologic Assessment, First Edition. Edited by Gregory Y. Lauwers and Michael B. Wallace.

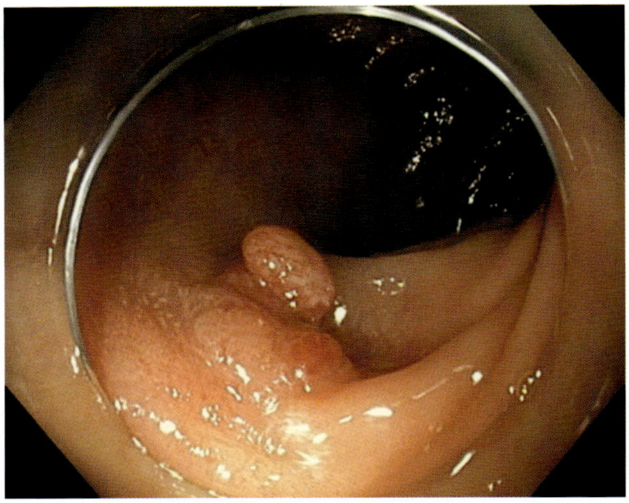

Figure 11.1 Tubulovillous adenoma with high-grade dysplasia. Features suggestive of villous and high-grade histology include the highly irregular and dilated surface vessels.

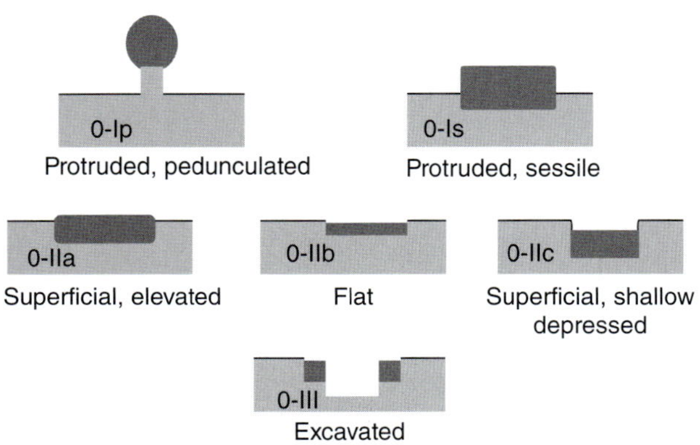

Figure 11.2 Paris Classification of polyp shape. 0–1p refers to pedunculated polyps, 0–1s to sessile. Flat polyps, defined as having <2.5 mm vertical elevation are subclassified as 0-IIa slightly elevated, 0-IIb flat, and 0-IIc depressed and 0-III as ulcerated. Invasive cancer is seen primarily in 0-IIc and deeply (beyond the superficial submucosa) in 0-III. *Source:* From Larghi, A. and Waxman, I. (2005). Endoscopic mucosal resection: treatment of neoplasia. *Gastrointestinal Endoscopy Clinics of North America* 15 (3): 431–454. © 2005 Elsevier.

the Kudo (for use with topical dye spray) or Sano/Narrow Band Imaging International Classification for Endoscopy (NICE) classifications (Figure 11.2).

The surface pattern is also valuable for endoscopic classification of polyps. The most widely accepted system is the NICE classification, which is based on viewing the polyp with optical enhancement such as narrow-band imaging (Figure 11.3).

Microscopic Features

By definition, conventional adenomas show a dysplastic epithelium characterized by enlarged hyperchromatic nuclei with a pencillate shape, crowding, and variable degrees of nuclear pleomorphism. The dysplastic changes are present throughout the crypts with loss of maturation at the surface epithelium, referred to as top-down dysplasia. Conventional adenomas are categorized into low-grade or high-grade dysplasia, depending on the degree of architectural complexity and of cytologic atypia. In adenoma with low-grade dysplasia, crypts are arranged in a parallel fashion with no complex architecture such as back-to-back glands or cribriform configuration. The cytologic atypia are mild, with uniform nuclei mostly confined to the basal half of the cells, preservation of nuclear polarity, and minimal pleomorphism. Adenomas with high-grade dysplasia (Figure 11.4) typically display a cribriform configuration, more pseudostratification, loss of nuclear polarity, and more prominent nuclear pleomorphism, identical to what is found in invasive colorectal adenocarcinoma. However, the degree of dysplasia in an adenoma is not always uniform but, rather, represents a spectrum of cytologic and architectural changes ranging from very mild to "adenocarcinoma in situ." The latter term should not be used and should be replaced by "adenoma with high-grade dysplasia" due to the lack of metastatic potential of adenocarcinoma confined to the large bowel mucosa (i.e. which does not invade beyond the muscularis mucosae into the submucosa). The use of "adenocarcinoma" for these lesions may be confusing and lead to unnecessary overtreatment by surgical resection. A malignant polyp refers to the presence of an invasive adenocarcinoma in, usually, a pedunculated adenoma, or to a polypoid adenocarcinoma (see Chapter 13).

Two main architectural patterns are seen in conventional adenomas: tubular and villous architecture. Tubular adenomas are defined by the presence of more than 75% of tubular structures in the polyp. The villous component of a conventional adenoma is significant if comprising at least 25% of the polyp: If between 25 and 75% of the polyp, this is diagnostic of a tubulovillous adenoma, and if >75% of the polyp, this is a villous adenoma. These cutoff values for villosity are arbitrary and not always straightforward to apply. Moreover, no solid diagnostic criteria have been defined for what represents a villous component in an adenoma. This likely explains why some studies have emphasized the poor interobserver agreement in the histologic evaluation of the villous component by pathologists. The same issue of poor reproducibility has been reported for the histologic diagnosis of high-grade dysplasia. This may not necessarily affect patient management for colonoscopy interval in the case of polyps >10 mm in size. However, a recent study showed poor interobserver agreement among five gastrointestinal pathologists reporting the degree of villosity and of dysplasia in conventional adenomas

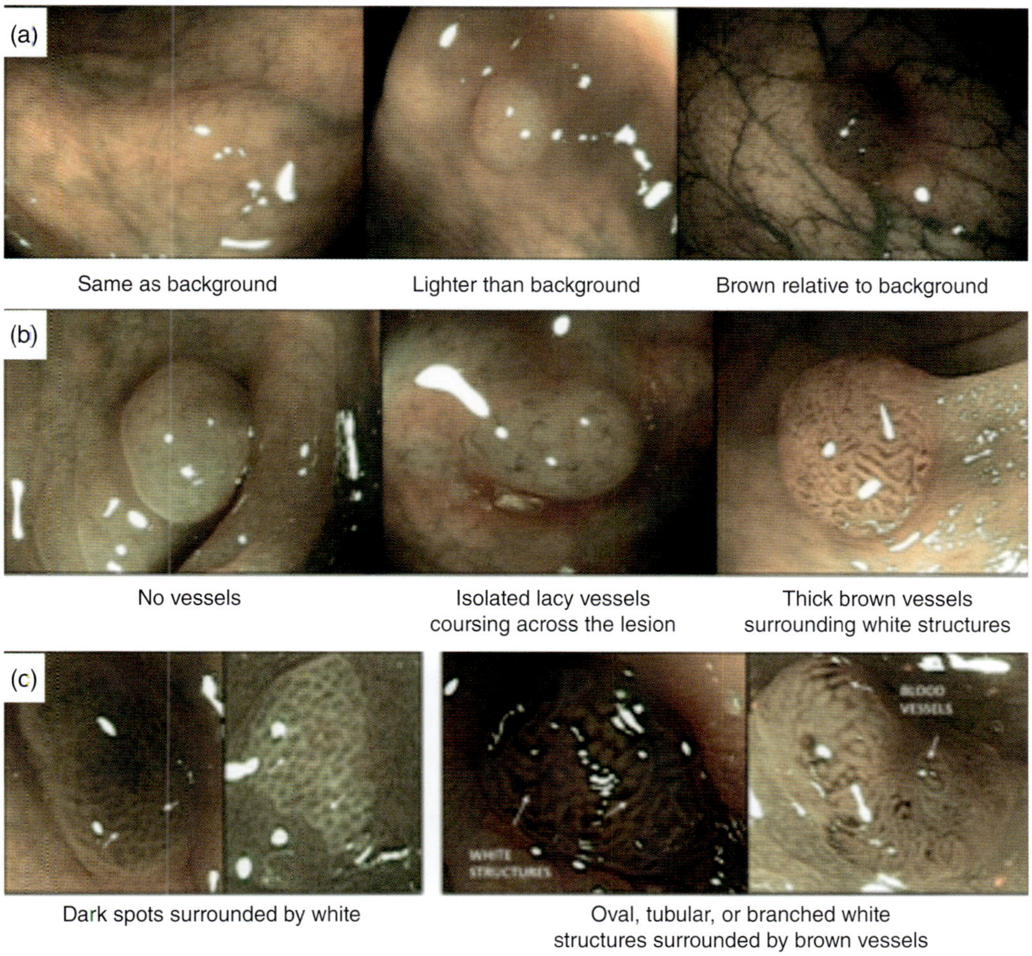

Figure 11.3 Narrow-band imaging International Classification for Endoscopy (NICE). Hyperplastic polyps have a color similar to or lighter than background mucosa, no vessels, and dark spots surrounded by white. Adenoma features are shown.

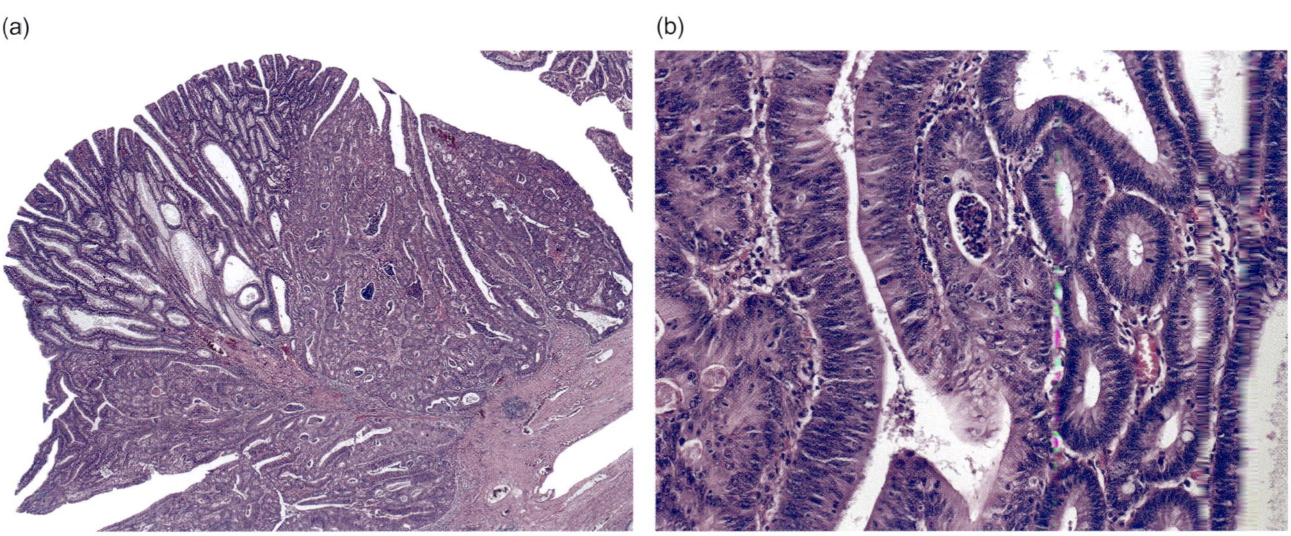

Figure 11.4 Hematoxylin–Eosin stain of a tubulovillous adenoma with high-grade dysplasia. Note the architectural complexity in panel 4A (left); panel 4B (right) shows low and high-grade cytologic atypia.

<10 mm, calling into question the validity of determining interval surveillance guidelines based on these subjective histologic features.

Immunohistochemical Studies and Molecular Features

No ancillary test is necessary to establish a diagnosis of conventional adenoma. In the context of patients fulfilling the clinical Amsterdam criteria for hereditary nonpolyposis colorectal cancer (HNPCC) syndrome, immunohistochemistry for mismatch repair (MMR) proteins could be performed to identify Lynch syndrome patients. However, a normal expression of MMR proteins in adenomas does not exclude Lynch syndrome. Adenomas with a villous component and/or high-grade dysplasia are more likely to demonstrate loss of MMR proteins in Lynch syndrome patients compared to adenomas showing no advanced features.

Differential Diagnosis

The diagnosis of conventional adenoma is straightforward in the vast majority of cases. It may be difficult to separate conventional adenoma from the dysplastic component of a sessile serrated adenoma. If there are fragments of sessile serrated adenoma admixed with fragments showing conventional dysplasia from a single large polyp resected piecemeal, the correct diagnosis should be sessile serrated adenoma with cytological dysplasia. Good communication between gastroenterologists and pathologists is paramount to establish the diagnosis. Pathologists should be aware that the correct diagnosis of a polyp may require analysis of deeper sections when no obvious histologic changes are identified in the first analyzed sections.

Prognosis, Evolution, and Clinical Management

Adenomatous polyps are considered premalignant with a genomic pathway well described as the adenoma-carcinoma sequence. Colonoscopy with removal of adenomas has been shown to reduce the risk of colorectal cancer death by approximately 50%. The current standard of care is to screen for adenomas beginning at age 50 in average-risk individuals, and to remove all detected polyps with histological confirmation. Various methods of removal have been reported including cold forceps polypectomy, snare polypectomy with or without electrocautery, and EMR or ESD. For small polyps, the risk of invasive malignancy is extremely low. Removal with snare is preferred of cold forceps, which has been shown to be incomplete. For small polyps (<1 cm), cold snare is preferred due to lower risk of thermal injury and better histological sample without cautery artifact. For larger polyps, snare with cautery is typically needed to cut through tissue and cauterize blood vessels. For very large (>2 cm) lateral spreading polyps, and any polyp with features of invasive cancer, EMR, or ESD is preferred. ESD is a very advanced and time-consuming procedure, which is limited to those polyps that are predicted to be superficially invasive (Paris II-c) and cannot be removed en bloc with EMR.

Serrated Polyps

Definitions and General Features

Serrated polyps are a group of epithelial polyps that share a common architectural pattern of "sawtooth" or serrated crypts. Up to 47% of colonic polyps resected during colonoscopy are serrated polyps. In a prospective study, 21% of asymptomatic individuals had at least one hyperplastic polyp (HP) identified by colonoscopy. The World Health Organization (WHO) 2019 classification recognizes five subgroups of serrated polyps: HP, sessile serrated lesion (SSL; former SSA/P), sessile serrated lesion with dysplasia (SSLD), traditional serrated adenoma (TSA) and Unclassified serrated adenoma. Individuals who develop serrated polyps often have conventional adenoma, and there is an overlap between the risk factors for serrated polyps and conventional adenoma. There is evidence of a strong role for cigarette smoking in association with SSL and a subtype of colorectal carcinoma arising from SSL.

Clinical Features and Endoscopic Characteristics

Like adenomas, serrated polyps are typically asymptomatic. SSL has a predilection for the proximal colon whereas TSAs have a predilection for the distal colon. TSAs appear similar to adenoma with a reddish, often semi-pedunculated shape. SSLs are typically sessile, with a pale surface color, adherent mucous cap, small "lacy" vessels on the surface, and indistinct borders (Figure 11.5).

Recognition of these lesions is challenging and only recently has there been a concerted effort to detect and completely remove these. Studies suggest that standard snare polypectomy may be insufficient to completely remove SSLs with at least 1/3 being incompletely removed. While still being studied, methods such as EMR with submucosal injection of blue dye may facilitate complete resection (Figures 11.5a–d).

Microscopic Features

The histologic diagnosis of serrated polyps is based on the growth pattern of the lesion (sessile in HP and SSL exophytic in TSA); the architecture of the crypts, which differs from HP to SSL; and the cytologic features in TSA.

Typical HPs are small flat polyps in the distal colon that represent 70–80% of all serrated polyps. HPs have virtually no risk of progression to more advanced neoplasm. The crypts of HP are elongated and retain their normal

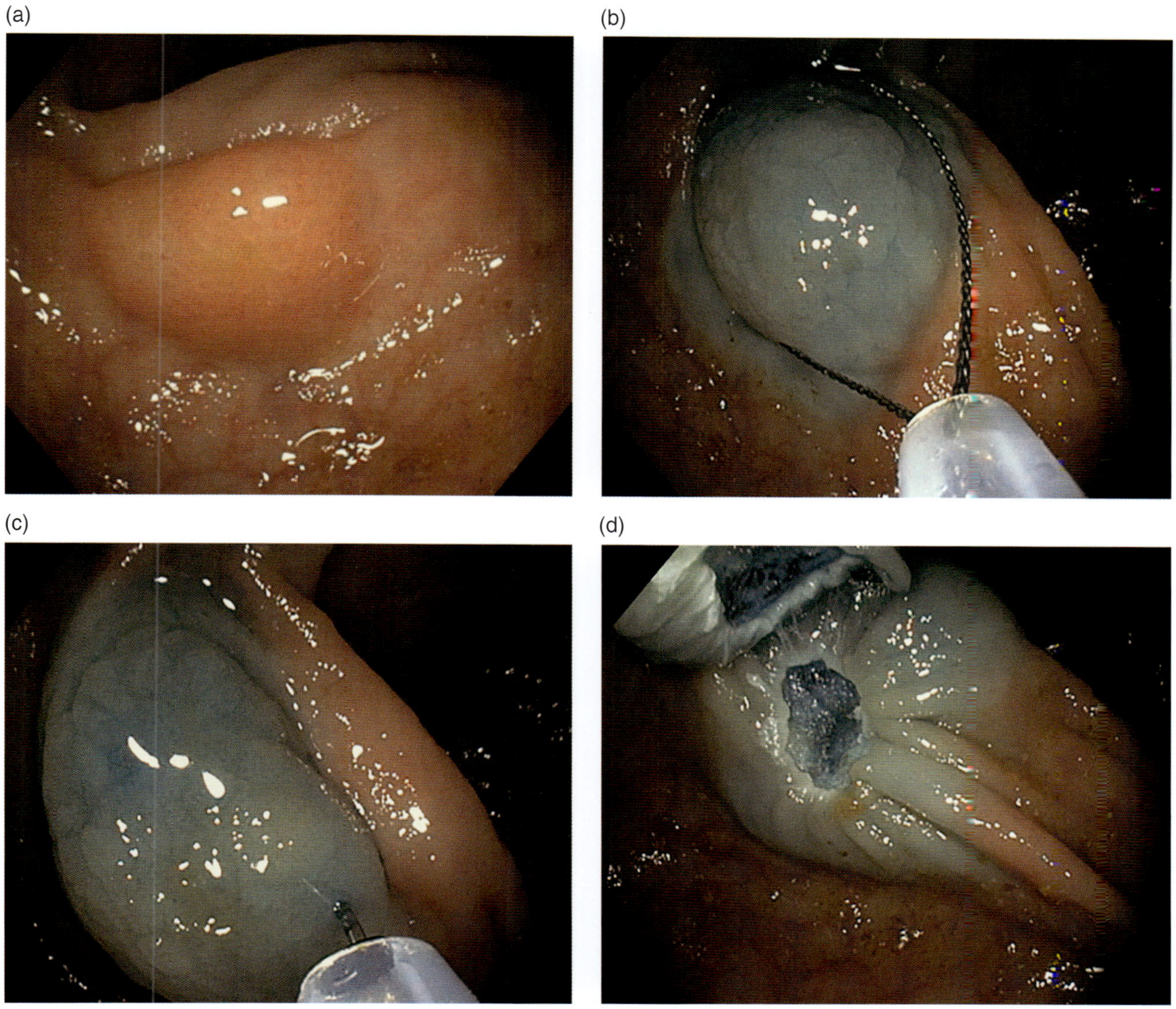

Figure 11.5 Endoscopic resection of sessile serrated polyp (a) with standard view, (b) after injection of submucosal saline-methylene blue, (c) large snare placed around the polyp, and (d) after snare resection.

architecture, with a narrow base where the proliferative cells lie (Figures 11.6 and 11.7).

The serration is more evident in the upper half of the crypts. Cytologic dysplasia is absent. Microvesicular HPs demonstrate more obvious serration, and are composed predominantly of epithelial cells with microvesicular mucin. On the other hand, goblet cell HPs may display very subtle serration limited to the surface epithelium, and are composed predominantly of goblet cell mucin, contrasting with the adjacent normal mucosa. In pathology reports, subdivision of HP between the microvesicular and the goblet cell subtypes is not necessary.

SSLs are increasingly recognized lesions representing up to 25% of serrated polyps and 15% of all colonic polyps. SSLs are well-documented precursor lesions of colorectal carcinoma with *BRAF* mutation and CpG island methylator phenotype (CIMP). More common in the proximal colon and usually >10 mm in size, SSLs are characterized by abnormal crypts showing a dilated base resulting in an L-shaped or inverted T-shaped pattern (Figure 11.8). It is now widely accepted that in a flat serrated polyp, the presence of at least one unequivocal architecturally distorted, dilated, and horizontally branched crypt is sufficient for a diagnosis of SSL. Cytologic dysplasia can develop in SSL, which is now diagnosed as SSLD and may portend a rapid step toward malignant transformation (Figures 11.9 and 11.10).

The dysplastic component is sharply demarcated from the adjacent SSL, which previously led these lesions to be called "mixed polyps," a terminology that should no longer be used.

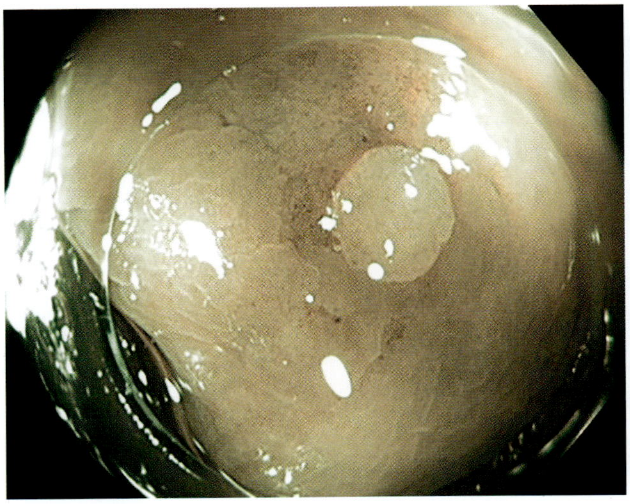

Figure 11.6 Hyperplastic polyp as seen in narrow-band imaging model. Note the pale color, small stellate surface pattern, and small size typical of this lesion.

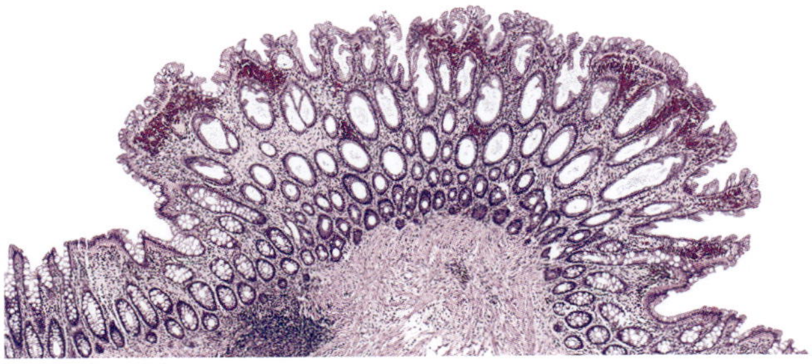

Figure 11.7 Hyperplastic polyp presenting as a localized projection of the colonic mucosa with preserved basal crypt architecture and serration (jig saw pattern) in the upper part of the crypts.

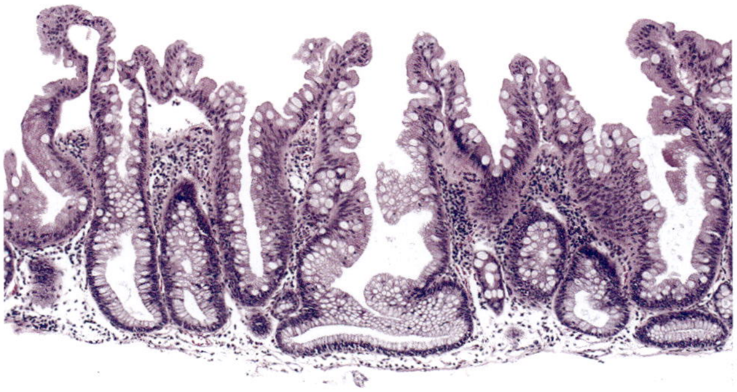

Figure 11.8 Sessile serrated lesion displaying horizontally shaped crypt bases, prominent serration throughout the crypts, and goblet cells in the bases of the crypts.

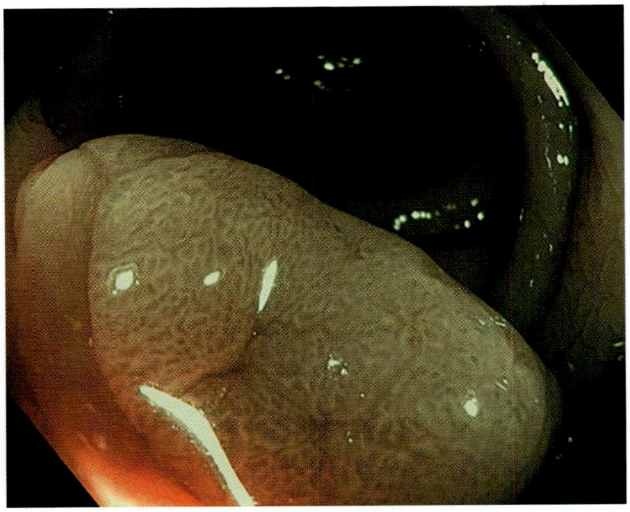

Figure 11.9 Sessile serrated lesion with dysplasia. This lesion was atypically located in the sigmoid with more dilated irregular surface pattern.

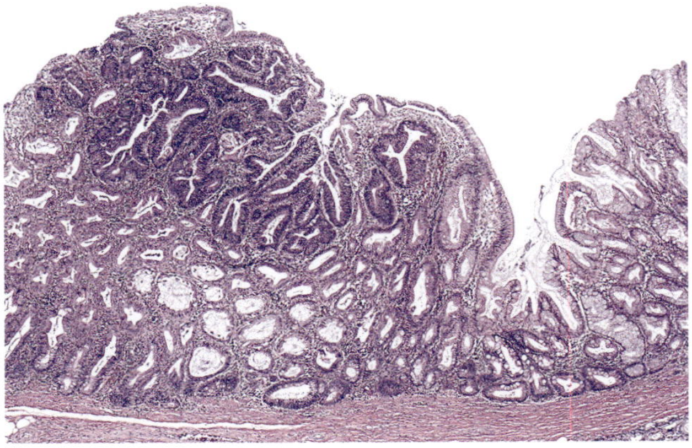

Figure 11.10 Sessile serrated lesion with dysplasia. There is a clear demarcated area showing complex architecture and hyperchromasia resembling conventional adenomatous dysplasia.

The least common subtype of serrated polyp is the TSA, an exophytic polyp frequently seen in the distal colon, with a villiform growth pattern, ectopic crypt formations, and characteristic eosinophilic cells with regular pencillate nuclei (Figures 11.11 and 11.12). An adjacent flat component of SSL sometimes can be found. TSA is a heterogeneous polyp subtype that can progress to advanced lesions with serrated or adenomatous dysplasia and to colorectal carcinoma with aggressive histologic features and a microsatellite stable phenotype.

Immunohistochemical Studies and Molecular Features

The histological diagnosis of each subtype of serrated polyps is established on the morphologic characteristics of the polyp. The majority of serrated polyps (except goblet cell HP and a subset of TSA) harbor the $BRAF^{V600E}$ mutation, for which a specific antibody is now commercially available to detect cells with this mutation using immunohistochemistry.

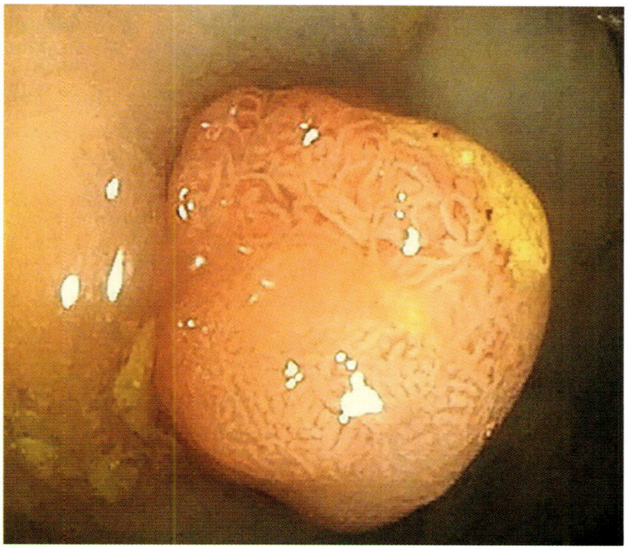

Figure 11.11 Endoscopic appearance of a rectal polyp being diagnosed as a traditional serrated adenoma (TSA), showing morphologic overlap of the mucosal surface with tubular adenoma, being described in the literature.

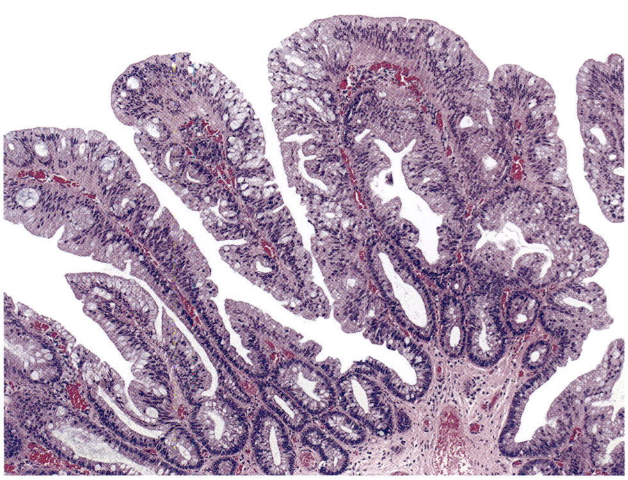

Figure 11.12 Traditional serrated adenoma with villous projections, ectopic crypt formations, and eosinophilic cells.

However, there is no need in diagnostic practice to use the $BRAF^{V600E}$ mutation-specific antibody. It may be helpful to document the loss of MLH1 expression in the dysplastic component of SSL, but this abnormality is not present in all SSLs with cytological dysplasia, and a normal retained expression of MLH1 in overtly dysplastic cells does not exclude the diagnosis. On the other hand, advanced TSAs only rarely demonstrate loss of MLH1 expression.

Differential Diagnosis

The WHO histologic criteria for the diagnosis of serrated polyp subtypes were first published in 2010. Before this time, most published studies reported poor interobserver agreement in the diagnosis of SSA/P. While there are still issues in the pathology community on differentiating SSL from HP, some recent studies demonstrated a significant increase in SSL diagnosis due to better awareness by pathologists.

Treatment/Prognosis/Evolution

Sessile serrated and traditional serrated polyps are thought to have a more aggressive natural history compared with adenomas. On the other hand, small, distal HPs are thought to have little, if any, malignant potential. This view continues to evolve, particularly with regard to proximal HP. Current recommendations are to remove all polyps with the exception of diminutive (<5 mm) rectosigmoid polyps with obvious hyperplastic features. Evolving issues include the optimal method for removal of SSA, and optical diagnosis with non-removal of small distal HP, and optical diagnosis with removal but not histological confirmation of small low-grade adenomas; a so-called "resect and discard" strategy.

Inflammatory Polyps

Inflammatory polyps are non-neoplastic lesions, which develop secondary to local injury to the colonic mucosa. The majority of cases are associated with mucosal prolapse and inflammatory bowel disease.

Mucosal Prolapse Polyps

Prolapse of the mucosa can occur anywhere in the large bowel, with a predilection for the distal colon and the rectum. Diverticular disease and constipation are often associated with mucosal prolapse. Reactive changes in the mucosa may lead to polyp formations that can mimic endoscopically neoplastic polyps. The salient microscopic features of mucosal prolapse polyps are:

- Expanded lamina propria with solidification by fibromuscular proliferation and various degrees of inflammation and hemorrhage
- Distortion of colonic crypts with branching, elongation, and serration
- Superficial erosion with reactive cytologic changes

Depending on the predominance of one of these microscopic features, mucosal prolapse polyps have been given a variety of names: Inflammatory cap polyp when ulceration is prominent with a cap of granulation tissue; inflammatory cloacogenic polyp when located in the anorectal junction; inflammatory myoglandular polyp when the stromal proliferation is dominant with cystically dilated crypts; and prominent mucosal fold or polypoid prolapsing fold for small lesions with subtle regenerative changes and fibrosis in the lamina propria.

Possibly related to mucosal prolapse polyp is the colonic muco-submucosal elongated polyp, which can measure up to 150 mm and is characterized by the presence of submucosa in the stalk and the absence of architectural changes and inflammation in the mucosa.

Difficulties in the Diagnosis of Mucosal Prolapse Polyps May Occur in the Following Settings

- Prominent regenerative changes secondary to ulceration mimicking dysplasia and conventional adenoma.
- Serration in mucosal prolapse polyps may mimic serrated polyps; careful examination of changes in lamina propria should be sought to distinguish these entities.
- Difficulty in distinguishing some forms of prolapse polyps from hamartomatous polyps, as both lesions may have a similar histologic appearance; clinical context may help.
- Superimposed prolapse changes on polyps of a different nature: Prolapse changes in HPs may look like a SSA/P.

Inflammatory Bowel Disease-Associated Polyps

Non-neoplastic polyps arising in the context of ulcerative colitis and Crohn's disease are commonly named inflammatory pseudopolyps. Compared with mucosal prolapse polyps, these polyps frequently display an increased number of inflammatory cells in the lamina propria, granulation tissue, and crypt architectural changes similar to what is seen in inflammatory bowel disease (Figure 11.13). Filiform polyposis refers to a condition in which multiple long inflammatory pseudopolyps are present. A common difficulty in inflammatory pseudopolyps is the distinction between reactive cytologic atypia and dysplasia. The use of ancillary studies such as p53 immunohistochemistry may help in the diagnosis.

Hamartomatous Polyps

Hamartomas of the large bowel are defined by overgrowths of the stromal and epithelial components of the mucosa, which often arise in the setting of hamartomatous polyposis syndromes: juvenile polyposis, Peutz–Jeghers polyposis, and *PTEN* hamartomatous tumor syndrome (see Chapter 13 for detailed description of polyposis syndromes). There is significant overlap in the histologic appearance of these different subtypes of hamartomatous polyps with mucosal prolapse polyps.

Juvenile Polyps

Most juvenile polyps are diagnosed in children between 2 and 10 years of age with a slight male predominance, and are solitary lesions, not part of juvenile polyposis syndrome. The majority of juvenile polyps (80–90%) are located in the distal colon and the rectum, but a proximal location is not uncommon. Typically, juvenile polyps are pedunculated lesions with surface ulceration, marked expansion of the lamina propria showing edematous and inflamed stroma, and cystically dilated crypts filled with mucin and inflammatory cells (Figure 11.14). Dysplasia and carcinoma do not develop in solitary juvenile polyps. Reactive changes adjacent to ulceration are frequently encountered and should not be interpreted as dysplasia.

Peutz–Jeghers Polyps

Peutz–Jeghers polyps are usually part of Peutz–Jeghers polyposis syndrome, although rare cases of sporadic Peutz–Jeghers polyps have been reported. Macroscopically, Peutz–Jeghers polyps are sessile when small, or pedunculated when large, with risk of intussusception. Their classical appearance is that of arborizing bundles of smooth muscle separating lobules of epithelial component (Figure 11.15). Dysplasia and carcinoma can occur. The lobular configuration and the lesser degree of edema and inflammatory infiltrate in the stroma are helpful in differentiating Peutz–Jeghers polyps from juvenile polyps.

PTEN Hamartomatous Tumor Syndrome Polyps

PTEN hamartoma tumor syndrome includes Cowden syndrome and Bannayan–Riley–Ruvalcaba (also called Bannayan–Zonana) syndrome. Colonic polyps of patients with this syndrome include hamartoma with a prominent stroma and cystically dilated crypts resembling juvenile polyps. Outside the known context suggestive of *PTEN* hamartoma tumor syndrome, a diagnosis is difficult to make from the histology of hamartomatous polyps. Potential clues may come from other associated lesions in the gastrointestinal tract: glycogenic acanthosis in the esophagus, hyperplastic-like polyps in the stomach, ganglioneuromas, lipomas, and benign lymphoid polyps in the large bowel.

Mesenchymal Polyps

Mesenchymal polyps comprise cell proliferations from the stromal component of the large bowel wall, including smooth muscle, neural component, adipose tissue, blood vessels, and

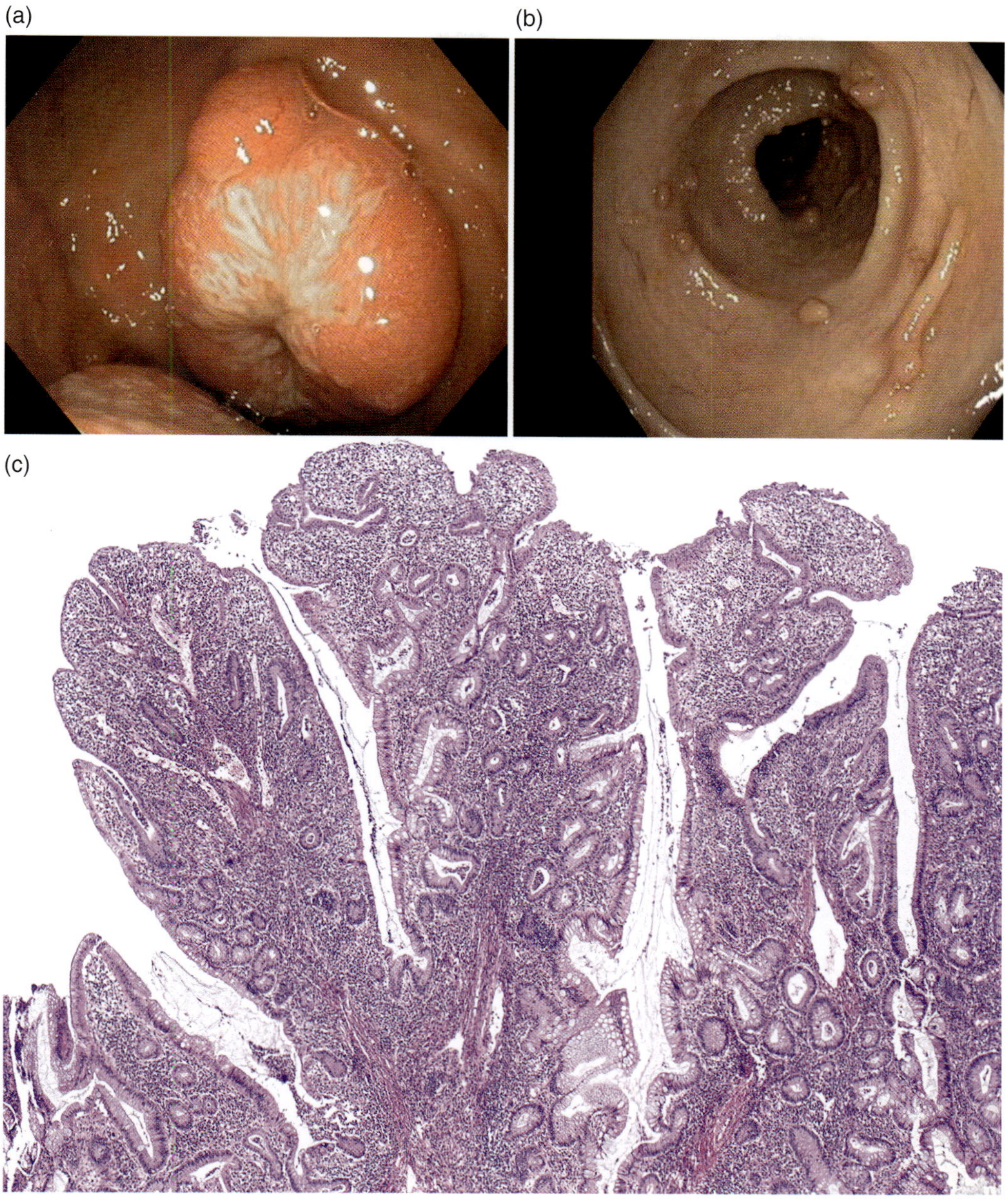

Figure 11.13 Endoscopic examples of (a) inflammatory and (b) filiform pseudopolyp. Note the fibrin exudate with linear ulceration topping the inflammatory pseudopolyp in (a). Typical histological appearance of an inflammatory pseudopolyp is shown in (c).

other stromal lesions of unclear origin. Immunohistochemistry can be helpful in the diagnosis, including S100, desmin, CD34, CD117, and GLUT-1 markers. The most common types of mesenchymal polyps are discussed here.

Leiomyoma of the Muscularis Mucosae

This is the most common mesenchymal tumor of the large bowel, and is usually found incidentally in patients undergoing screening colonoscopy. Leiomyomas are small lesions (median 4 mm) arising from the muscularis mucosae and predominantly located in the rectosigmoid region. The overlying mucosa is sometimes attenuated. The smooth muscle differentiation with proliferation of eosinophilic spindle is usually evident (Figure 11.16); positivity for desmin and negativity of other markers can be used to confirm the diagnosis.

Lipoma

Lipomas are the most common submucosal mesenchymal tumor in the large bowel, and are usually incidental findings

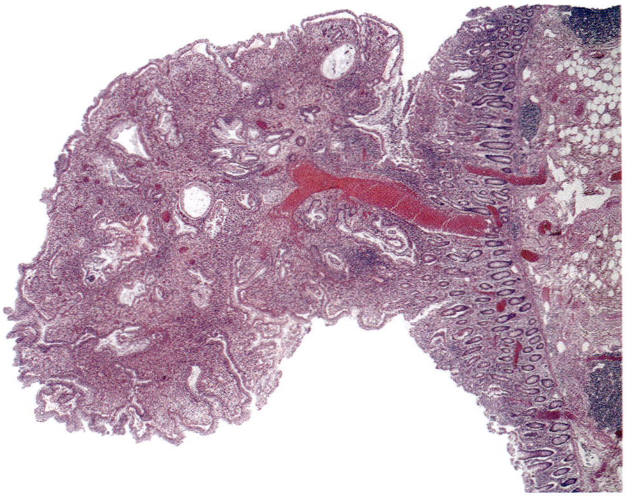

Figure 11.14 Typical histomorphology of a juvenile polyp with haphazardly cystically distended crypts embedded in inflamed lamina propria.

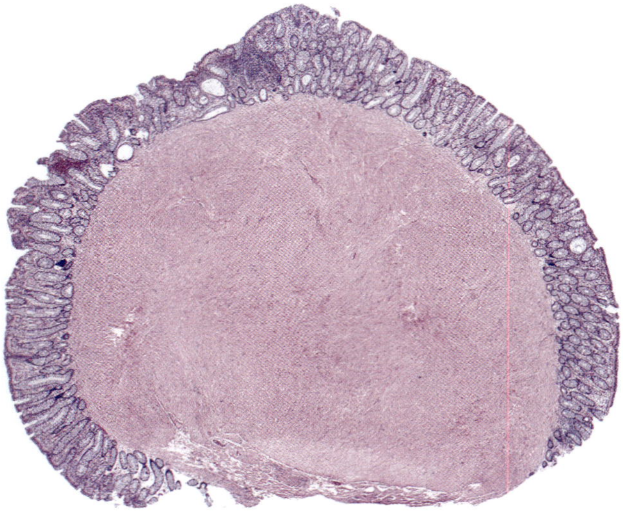

Figure 11.16 Microscopic appearance of a colonic mucosal leiomyoma with its typical red fibrillar cytoplasm and fascicular arrangement.

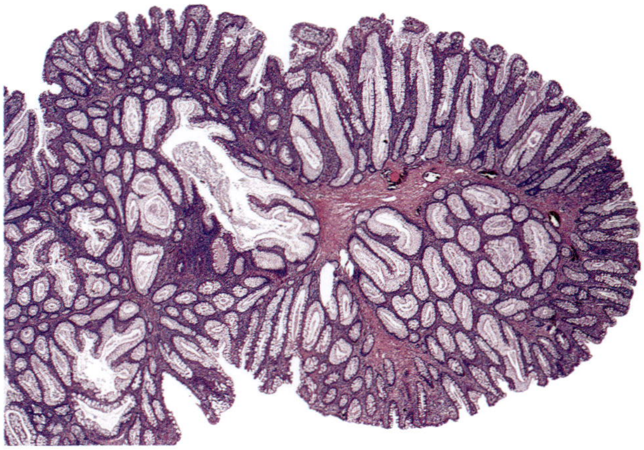

Figure 11.15 Hamartomatous polyp in a patient with Peutz–Jeghers syndrome characterized by its broad dissected bands of muscularis mucosa smooth muscle with a "tree like" appearance.

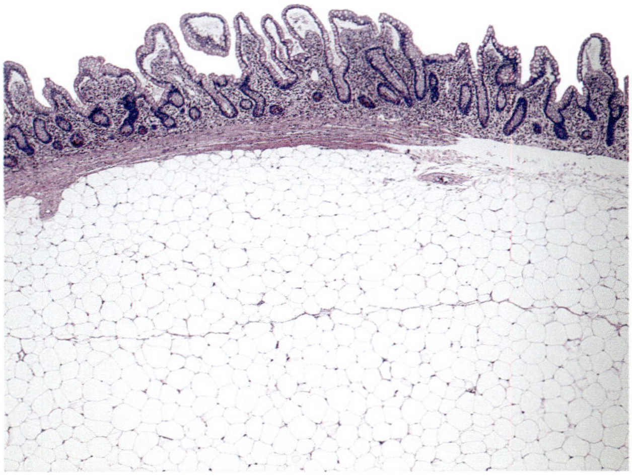

Figure 11.17 Histology of a submucosal lipoma with benign well-circumscribed adipose tissue.

in adults (Figures 11.17 and 11.18). Large lipomas can present with bowel obstruction or intussusception. Their yellow appearance and submucosal location make the diagnosis straightforward. When multiple lipomas are diagnosed, the possibility of *PTEN* hamartomatous tumor syndrome should be raised. Lipomatous changes/hypertrophy frequently occur at the ileocecal valve and are sometimes biopsied; it most likely represents prolapsed submucosa and should not be called lipoma.

Fibroblastic Polyp

Also called perineuriomas, fibroblastic polyps are benign, small, solitary, and incidental lesions frequently located in the distal colon and the rectum. When associated with serrated polyps (HP or SSA/P), they are reported as combined fibroblastic/serrated polyps (Figure 11.19). Fibroblastic polyps are composed of bland spindle cells in the lamina propria that express perineurial markers (GLUT-1 or EMA).

Neural Tumors

Neural tumors are small, benign, and usually solitary lesions with a predilection for the distal colon and the rectum. Ganglioneuromas are composed of spindled S-100-positive Schwann cells and ganglion cells. Multiple ganglioneuromas can be seen in the setting of ganglioneuromatosis polyposis associated with FAP, or in the setting of diffuse ganglioneuromatosis associated with

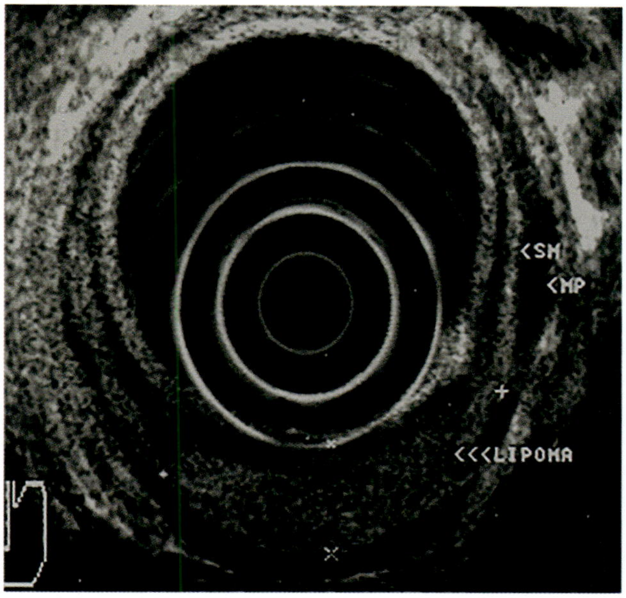

Figure 11.18 Endoscopic ultrasound (EUS) image of a lipoma arising in the submucosa. Note that it is bright on EUS due to the echogenicity of fatty tissue.

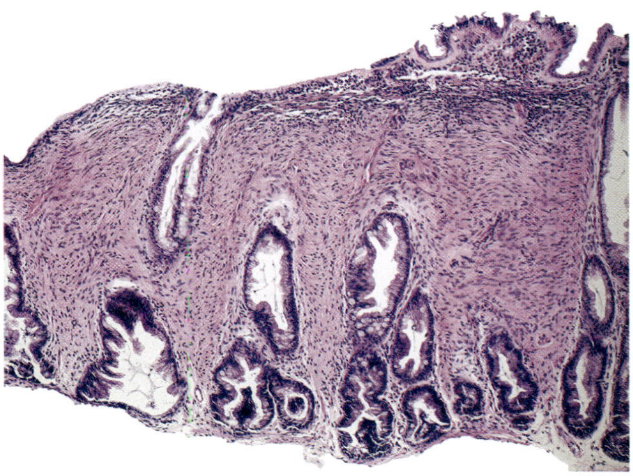

Figure 11.19 Combined fibroblastic polyp and SSL with fibrotic changes of the lamina propria and serrated appearance and distention of the crypts.

neurofibromatosis type 1 (NF1) and multiple endocrine neoplasia (MEN) type IIB.

Schwann cell hamartoma is an ill-defined proliferation of S-100-positive spindle cells in the lamina propria entrapping colonic crypts. Ganglion cells are absent. They should be distinguished from neurofibroma, as Schwann cell hamartomas are not associated with NF1.

Benign epithelioid nerve sheath tumors display an infiltrative growth pattern in the lamina propria, composed of predominantly S-100-positive epithelioid cells with frequent nuclear pseudoinclusions. Variable CD34 staining can be seen in supporting cells.

Other Rare Mesenchymal Tumors

Inflammatory fibroid tumors are rare tumors affecting the proximal colon with histologic features identical to what is seen in their gastric counterpart. CD34 positivity is a useful marker for the diagnosis. Granular cell tumor is uncommon in the colon, and predominantly affects the proximal colon. Gastrointestinal stromal tumor (GIST) rarely affects the large bowel (5% of all GISTs). The epicenter of the tumor is the muscularis propria, and it rarely presents as polyp. Positivity of tumor cells for CD117 and DOG-1 confirms the diagnosis.

Miscellaneous Polyps

Cronkhite–Canada Syndrome

Cronkhite–Canada syndrome is a non-hereditary protein-losing enteropathy of unknown cause often classified with hamartomatous polyposis syndromes and most likely represents an immune dysregulation disorder. Patients with Cronkhite–Canada syndrome develop polyps in the gastrointestinal tract, including the large bowel, that resemble juvenile polyps with expanded and inflamed lamina propria and a broad base. The clinical context is necessary to establish the diagnosis.

Lymphoid Polyps

Benign lymphoid hyperplasia is common and a normal finding in the colon that sometimes can be biopsied; it usually is easily distinguished from lymphoma. Mantle cell lymphoma classically presents as a polyposis in the colon. Follicular lymphoma and large B-cell lymphoma can also present as polyps. Ancillary studies are necessary to classify the lymphoid proliferation.

Elastofibromatous Polyp

Accumulation of elastic fibers in the lamina propria and the submucosa, possibly secondary to an insult of the mucosa, can result in a polyp resembling an adenoma (Figure 11.20). Congo red and elastin stains may be necessary to exclude amyloidosis and identify elastic fibers.

Endometriosis

Endometriosis can sometimes present as a colonic polyp and be a challenging diagnosis (Figure 11.21). The presence of non-intestinal glands with surrounding stroma and hemosiderin should prompt the diagnosis.

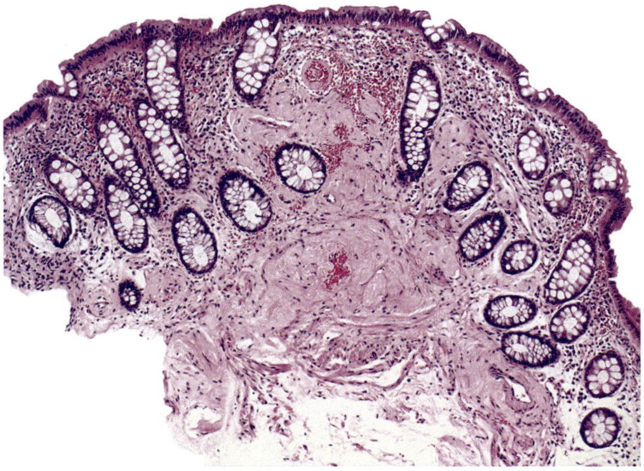

Figure 11.20 Colonic polyp with collagen bundles and thick eosinophilic elastic fibers located in lamina propria and submucosa.

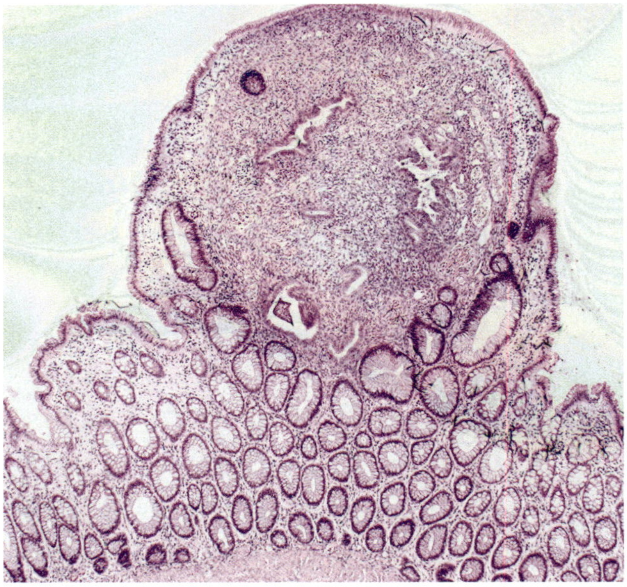

Figure 11.21 Colonic polypoid endometriosis with its typical glands being surrounded by dense spindly endometrioid stroma.

Further Reading

Alizart, M.M., Rosty, C., and Brown, I.S. (2011). Colonic mucosubmucosal elongated polyp: a Clinicopathologic study of 13 cases and review of the literature. *Am. J. Surg. Pathol.* 35: 1818–1822.

Anderson, J.C., Rangasamy, P., Rustagi, T. et al. (2011). Risk factors for sessile serrated adenomas. *J. Clin. Gastroenterol.* 45: 694–699.

Appelman, H.D. (2008). Con: high-grade dysplasia and villous features should not be part of the routine diagnosis of colorectal adenomas. *Am. J. Gastroenterol.* 103: 1329–1331.

Bauer, V.P. and Papaconstantinou, H.T. (2008) Management of serrated adenomas and hyperplastic polyps. *Clin Colon Rectal Surg.* 21(4):273-279. doi:10.1055/s-0028-1089942

Bettington, M., Brown, I.S., Kumarasinghe, M.P. et al. (2014). The challenging diagnosis of Cronkhite–Canada syndrome in the upper gastrointestinal tract: a series of 7 cases with clinical follow-up. *Am. J. Surg. Pathol.* 38: 215–223.

Bettington, M., Walker, N., Rosty, C. et al. (2014). Critical appraisal of the diagnosis of the sessile serrated adenoma. *Am. J. Surg. Pathol.* 38: 158–166.

Bettington, M.L., Walker, N.I., Rosty, C. et al. (2014). A clinicopathological and molecular analysis of 200 traditional serrated adenomas. *Mod. Pathol.* 28: 414–427.

Burgess, N.G., Tutticci, N.J., Pellise, M. et al. (2014). Sessile serrated adenomas/polyps with cytologic dysplasia: a triple threat for interval cancer. *Gastrointest. Endosc.* 80: 307–310.

Burkart, A.L., Sheridan, T., Lewin, M. et al. (2007). Do sporadic Peutz–Jeghers polyps exist? Experience of a large teaching hospital. *Am. J. Surg. Pathol.* 31: 1209–1214.

Burke, A.P. and Sobin, L.H. (1989). The pathology of Cronkhite–Canada polyps. A comparison to juvenile polyposis. *Am. J. Surg. Pathol.* 13: 940–946.

Chetty, R., Bateman, A.C., Torlakovic, E. et al. (2014). A pathologist's survey on the reporting of sessile serrated adenomas/polyps. *J. Clin. Pathol.* 67: 426–430.

Costantini, M., Sciallero, S., Giannini, A. et al. (2003). Interobserver agreement in the histologic diagnosis of colorectal polyps. The experience of the multicenter adenoma colorectal study (SMAC). *J. Clin. Epidemiol.* 56: 209–214.

Denis, B., Peters, C., Chapelain, C. et al. (2009). Diagnostic accuracy of community pathologists in the interpretation of colorectal polyps. *Eur. J. Gastroenterol. Hepatol.* 21: 1153–1160.

Ensari, A., Bilezikci, B., Carneiro, F. et al. (2012). Serrated polyps of the colon: how reproducible is their classification? *Virchows Arch.* 461: 495–504.

Farris, A.B., Misdraji, J., Srivastava, A. et al. (2008). Sessile serrated adenoma: challenging discrimination from other serrated colonic polyps. *Am. J. Surg. Pathol.* 32: 30–35.

Forsberg, A.M., Kjellstrom, L., Agreus, L. et al. (2012). Prevalence of colonic neoplasia and advanced lesions in the normal population: a prospective population-based colonoscopy study. *Scand. J. Gastroenterol.* 47: 184–190.

Gibson, J.A. and Hornick, J.L. (2009). Mucosal Schwann cell "hamartoma": clinicopathologic study of 26 neural colorectal polyps distinct from neurofibromas and mucosal neuromas. *Am. J. Surg. Pathol.* 33: 781–787.

Gill, P., Wang, L.M., Bailey, A. et al. (2013). Reporting trends of right-sided hyperplastic and sessile serrated polyps in a large teaching hospital over a 4-year period (2009–2012). *J. Clin. Pathol.* 66: 655–658.

Hamilton, S.R., Bosman, F.T., Boffetta, P. et al. (2010). Carcinoma of the colon and rectum. In: *World Health Organization Classification of Tumours of the Digestive System*, 4e (eds. F.T. Bosman, F. Carneiro, R.H. Hruban and N.D. Theise), 134–146. Lyon: International Agency for Research on Cancer (IARC).

Hancock, B.J. and Vajcner, A. (1988). Lipomas of the colon: a clinicopathologic review. *Can. J. Surg.* 31: 178–181.

Imperiale, T.F., Ransohoff, D.F., Itzkowitz, S.H. et al. (2004). Fecal DNA versus fecal occult blood for colorectal-cancer screening in an average-risk population. *N. Engl. J. Med.* 351: 2704–2714.

Imperiale, T.F., Wagner, D.R., Lin, C.Y. et al. (2000). Risk of advanced proximal neoplasms in asymptomatic adults according to the distal colorectal findings. *N. Engl. J. Med.* 343: 169–174.

Kelly, J.K. (1991). Polypoid prolapsing mucosal folds in diverticular disease. *Am. J. Surg. Pathol.* 15: 871–878.

Kim, M.J., Lee, E.J., Suh, J.P. et al. (2013). Traditional serrated adenoma of the colorectum: clinicopathologic implications and endoscopic findings of the precursor lesions. *Am. J. Clin. Pathol.* 140: 898–911.

Lee, B.G., Shin, S.H., Lee, Y.A. et al. (2012). Juvenile polyp and colonoscopic polypectomy in childhood. *Pediatr. Gastroenterol. Hepatol. Nutr.* 15: 250–255.

Lewin, M.R., Dilworth, H.P., Abu Alfa, A.K. et al. (2005). Mucosal benign epithelioid nerve sheath tumors. *Am. J. Surg. Pathol.* 29: 1310–1315.

Lin, O.S., Kozarek, R.A., Schembre, D.B. et al. (2006). Screening colonoscopy in very elderly patients: prevalence of neoplasia and estimated impact on life expectancy. *JAMA* 295: 2357–2365.

Lobert, P.F. and Appelman, H.D. (1981). Inflammatory cloacogenic polyp. A unique inflammatory lesion of the anal transitional zone. *Am. J. Surg. Pathol.* 5: 761–766.

Mahajan, D., Downs-Kelly, E., Liu, X. et al. (2013). Reproducibility of the villous component and high-grade dysplasia in colorectal adenomas <1 cm: implications for endoscopic surveillance. *Am. J. Surg. Pathol.* 37: 427–433.

Miettinen, M., Sarlomo-Rikala, M., and Sobin, L.H. (2001). Mesenchymal tumors of muscularis mucosae of colon and rectum are benign leiomyomas that should be separated from gastrointestinal stromal tumors – a clinicopathologic and immunohistochemical study of eighty-eight cases. *Mod. Pathol.* 14: 950–956.

Nakamura, S., Kino, I., and Akagi, T. (1992). Inflammatory myoglandular polyps of the colon and rectum. A clinicopathological study of 32 pedunculated polyps, distinct from other types of polyps. *Am. J. Surg. Pathol.* 16: 772–779.

Nielsen, J.A., Lager, D.J., Lewin, M. et al. (2013). Incidence of diagnostic change in colorectal polyp specimens after deeper sectioning at 2 different laboratories staffed by the same pathologists. *Am. J. Clin. Pathol.* 140: 231–237.

Pai, R.K., Hart, J., and Noffsinger, A.E. (2010). Sessile serrated adenomas strongly predispose to synchronous serrated polyps in non-syndromic patients. *Histopathology* 56: 581–588.

Pai, R.K., Mackinnon, A.C., Joseph, L. et al. (2010). Identification of histologically distinct conventional adenomas that arise predominately in patients with sessile serrated adenomas. *Am. J. Surg. Pathol.* 34: 355–363.

Regula, J., Rupinski, M., Kraszewska, E. et al. (2006). Colonoscopy in colorectal-cancer screening for detection of advanced neoplasia. *N. Engl. J. Med.* 355: 1863–1872.

Rex, D.K., Ahnen, D.J., Baron, J.A. et al. (2012). Serrated lesions of the colorectum: review and recommendations from an expert panel. *Am. J. Gastroenterol.* 107: 1315–1329.

Rosty, C. and Bettington, M. (2014). Serrated colorectal polyps and polyposis. *Diagn. Histopathol.* 20: 30–37.

Samowitz, W.S., Albertsen, H., Sweeney, C. et al. (2006). Association of smoking, CpG island methylator phenotype, and V600E BRAF mutations in colon cancer. *J. Natl. Cancer Inst.* 98: 1731–1738.

Schoenfeld, P., Cash, B., Flood, A. et al. (2005). Colonoscopic screening of average-risk women for colorectal neoplasia. *N. Engl. J. Med.* 352: 2061–2068.

Shekitka, K.M. and Sobin, L.H. (1994). Ganglioneuromas of the gastrointestinal tract. Relation to Von Recklinghausen disease and other multiple tumor syndromes. *Am. J. Surg. Pathol.* 18: 250–257.

Snover, D.C., Ahnen, D.J., Burt, R.W. et al. (2010). Serrated polyps of the colon and rectum and serrated polyposis. In: *WHO Classification of Tumours of the Digestive System* (eds. F.T. Bosman, F. Carneiro, R.H. Hruban and N.D. Theise), 160–165. Lyon: IARC Press.

Spring, K.J., Zhao, Z.Z., Karamatic, R. et al. (2006). High prevalence of sessile serrated adenomas with BRAF mutations: a prospective study of patients undergoing colonoscopy. *Gastroenterology* 131: 1400–1407.

Strul, H., Kariv, R., Leshno, M. et al. (2006). The prevalence rate and anatomic location of colorectal adenoma and cancer detected by colonoscopy in average-risk individuals aged 40–80 years. *Am. J. Gastroenterol.* 101: 255–262.

Terry, M.B., Neugut, A.I., Bostick, R.M. et al. (2002). Reliability in the classification of advanced colorectal adenomas. *Cancer Epidemiol. Biomarkers Prev.* 11: 660–663.

Toon, C.W., Walsh, M.D., Chou, A. et al. (2013). BRAFV600E immunohistochemistry facilitates universal screening of colorectal cancers for lynch syndrome. *Am. J. Surg. Pathol.* 37: 1592–1602.

Torlakovic, E.E., Gomez, J.D., Driman, D.K. et al. (2008). Sessile serrated adenoma (SSA) vs. traditional serrated adenoma (TSA). *Am. J. Surg. Pathol.* 32: 21–29.

Tsai JH, Liau JY, Lin YL, et al. Traditional serrated adenoma has two pathways of neoplastic progression that are distinct from the sessile serrated pathway of colorectal carcinogenesis. *Mod. Pathol.* 2014, 27:1375-85.

Van Putten, P.G., Hol, L., van Dekken, H. et al. (2011). Interobserver variation in the histological diagnosis of polyps in colorectal cancer screening. *Histopathology* 58: 974–981.

Vasen, H.F., Watson, P., Mecklin, J.P. et al. (1999). New clinical criteria for hereditary nonpolyposis colorectal cancer (HNPCC, lynch syndrome) proposed by the international collaborative group on HNPCC. *Gastroenterology* 116: 1453–1456.

Walker, R.G., Landmann, J.K., Hewett, D.G. et al. (2010). Hyperplastic polyposis syndrome is associated with cigarette smoking, which may be a modifiable risk factor. *Am. J. Gastroenterol.* 105: 1642–1647.

Walsh, M.D., Buchanan, D.D., Pearson, S.A. et al. (2012). Immunohistochemical testing of conventional adenomas for loss of expression of mismatch repair proteins in lynch syndrome mutation carriers: a case series from the Australasian site of the colon cancer family registry. *Mod. Pathol.* 25: 722–730.

WHO Classification of Tumors Editorial Board. Digestive System Tumors. Lyon (France): International Agency for Research on Cancer; 2019 (WHO classification of tumors series; 5th ed.; vol 1)

Wiland, H.O., Shadrach, B., Allende, D. et al. (2014). Morphologic and molecular characterization of traditional serrated adenomas of the distal colon and rectum. *Am. J. Surg. Pathol.* 38: 1290–1297.

Williams, G.T., Bussey, H.J.R., and Morson, B.C. (1985). Inflammatory cap polyps of the large intestine. *Br. J. Surg.* 72 (Suppl): 133.

Wong, N.A., Hunt, L.P., Novelli, M.R. et al. (2009). Observer agreement in the diagnosis of serrated polyps of the large bowel. *Histopathology* 55: 63–66.

12

Epithelial Neoplasms of the Large Bowel

Christophe Rosty[1], *Michael B. Wallace*[2] *and Till S. Clauditz*[3]

[1]*Envoi Specialist Pathologists, Brisbane, QLD, Australia*
[2]*Mayo Clinic, Jacksonville, Florida, USA*
[3]*Department of Pathology, University-Medical-Center Hamburg-Eppendorf, Hamburg, Germany*

The previous chapter covered the benign epithelial and non-epithelial neoplasms of the large bowel presenting as polyps. Conventional adenomas and serrated polyps are the most common neoplasms and, for some of them, may progress to carcinomas through different morphologic and molecular pathways. In this chapter, we will emphasize on the genetic predisposition to colorectal carcinoma, the molecular pathogenesis and clinical management. A specific section on malignant polyps is also included. A large variety of non-epithelial neoplasms of the large bowel has been considered in the previous chapter; here we will cover more in detail neuroendocrine neoplasms and lymphomas.

Colorectal Carcinoma

Definition, General Features, and Predisposing Factors

Colorectal carcinomas are malignant epithelial neoplasms of the large bowel that usually develop from a precursor polyp progressing through a sequence of cumulative molecular alterations. There is a marked variation in the incidence of colorectal carcinoma worldwide with the highest incidence in North America, Europe, and Australasia. The mortality rates from colorectal carcinoma have declined in many developed countries, with higher mortality in some countries with low incidence and poorer resources. In most Westernized countries including the United States, colorectal carcinoma is the second leading cause of cancer death after lung cancer. Environmental factors are likely to account for a large proportion of different incidences worldwide (Table 12.1).

A family history of colorectal carcinoma is found in up to 30% of affected individuals, indicative of a genetic predisposition to the disease and possibly shared environmental factors. Moreover, having a first degree relative with colorectal carcinoma increases the risk of the disease approximately twofold. However, genetically defined syndromes predisposing mutation carriers to an increased risk of colorectal are found in only 5% of all incident cases. Lynch syndrome is the most common of these conditions found in 3–4% of all incident colorectal carcinomas and is defined by the identification of a germline defect in DNA mismatch repair (MMR) genes *MLH1*, *MSH2*, *MSH6,* or *PMS2* or in *EPCAM*. Neoplasms in Lynch syndrome patients demonstrate high levels of microsatellite instability (MSI). The Amsterdam I criteria were developed in 1991 to define hereditary nonpolyposis colorectal cancer (HNPCC), a term coined to separate familial predisposition to colorectal carcinoma from the known polyposis syndromes (familial adenomatous polyposis (FAP) and hamartomatous polyposis syndromes). However, not all HNPCC individuals have Lynch syndrome and not all Lynch syndrome individuals fulfill the clinical criteria for HNPCC. Up to 50% of HNPCC individuals do not have Lynch syndrome. The other half comprises patients with a colorectal carcinoma showing MSI but no identified mutations in an MMR gene (Lynch-like or suspected Lynch syndrome) and patients with colorectal carcinoma with no MSI, referred to as familial colorectal cancer type 2 (FCCTX). Other known genetic conditions associated with a high risk of colorectal carcinoma are listed in Table 12.2, including FAP, *MUTYH*-associated polyposis, and hamartomatous polyposis syndromes.

FAP is an autosomal dominant syndrome characterized by the development of hundreds to thousands of

Gastrointestinal Pathology: Correlative Endoscopic and Histologic Assessment, First Edition. Edited by Gregory Y. Lauwers and Michael B. Wallace.

Table 12.1 Environmental factors affecting the risk of colorectal carcinoma.

Predisposing factors
Dietary habits
Animal fat
Grilled and processed beef meat
Some dietary fibers
Lifestyle
Alcohol, in particular beer consumption for rectal cancer
Cigarette smoking
Low physical activity
Protective factors
Dietary habits
Cruciferous vegetables (spinach, cabbage)
Whole grains
Calcium and vitamin D
Lifestyle
Physical exercise
Drugs
Estrogen replacement therapy
Long-term nonsteroidal anti-inflammatory drugs

conventional adenomas throughout the large bowel and the inevitable transformation to colorectal carcinoma, justifying total coloproctectomy early in adulthood. Neoplasms in the stomach and the small intestine also commonly occur. Caused by a mutation in *APC*, FAP can be diagnosed in 30–50% of patients with no familial history of colorectal carcinoma or polyps, usually secondary to a de novo mutation. The location of the mutation in the *APC* gene correlates with the phenotype, including attenuated forms of polyposis (<100 polyps) and variants of FAP. Gardner syndrome includes fibromatosis (desmoid tumor), epidermoid cysts, and osteoma; Turcot syndrome includes brain tumors (medulloblastoma).

Serrated polyposis, previously named hyperplastic polyposis, is a polyposis syndrome of unknown genetic basis, characterized by the development of multiple serrated polyps and an increased risk of colorectal carcinoma in affected individuals and their first degree relatives. Prospective studies with long-term follow-up of serrated polyposis patients are lacking; so the exact risk of colorectal carcinoma compared with the risk in the general population is currently not known.

Other predisposing conditions to colorectal carcinoma are ulcerative colitis and Crohn's disease as well as prior radiation therapy, in particular for distal colorectal carcinoma in patients who received high-dose irradiation for cancer of the uterine cervix, bladder, and prostate.

Clinical Features and Endoscopic Characteristics

Colorectal neoplasia is typically asymptomatic until it becomes invasive. It may then present with symptoms based on the location. Distal colon and rectal cancers typically present bleeding (bright red blood per stool), anemia, or narrowing of bowel caliber. Proximal colon cancers are more likely to present as anemia or obstruction. Endoscopically, invasive cancers are usually easily detected as mass forming, ulcerated, friable lesions. A detailed discussion of national and international screening guidelines is beyond the scope of this book but can be found in the recent guidelines of the US Multi-society Task Force On Colorectal Cancer.

In brief, clinicians should offer those at average risk of CRC, screening beginning at age 50. Regarding specific methods of screening, multiple options are reasonable including colonoscopy, fecal immunochemical testing (FIT), multi-targeted stool DNA (MT-DNA), although only colonoscopy has the potential to detect and treat colorectal polyps in a single test.

Whichever test is used, colonscopy if required is a non-colonoscopy test is positive. At colonoscopy, all detected lesions should be assessed with regard to neoplastic potential using common classifications systems such as the shape (Paris classification) and surface features (Narrow Band Imaging International Classification for Endoscopy, NICE or Japan NBI Expert Team, JNET classification). Detailed guidelines on polyp management are reported by the US Multisociety Task Force. It is key for pathologist to recognize that endoscopists, with high-definition, high-magnification endoscopes, can now accurately distinguish non-neoplastic (particularly rectosigmoid hyperplastic) polyps that do not require resection, noninvasive neoplasms for routine polypectomy, and superficially invasive neoplasms for advanced reaction (endoscopic mucosal resection and submucosal dissection). The latter cases are considered definitive for a subset of cancers (differentiated, superficial submucosal invasion, negative margins, no lymphovascular invasion) and thus pathology should include reports of those features as would be done for a surgical tumor case.

Microscopic Features

The histologic diagnosis of colorectal carcinoma is usually straightforward. By definition, a carcinoma invades through the lamina muscularis mucosae into the submucosa and the deeper portion of the bowel wall. An epithelial neoplasm that is confined to the large bowel mucosa has no potential to metastasize and is usually reported as

Table 12.2 Genetic conditions associated with a risk of colorectal carcinoma.

	Gene	Inheritance	Risk of CRC	Other cancers	Large bowel lesion
Lynch syndrome	*MLH1, MSH2, MSH6, PMS2, EPCAM*	Autosomal dominant	20–60%	Endometrium, hepatopancreatobiliary tract, stomach, small intestine, urinary tract, brain, ovary, sebaceous glands	Low number of conventional adenomas
Familial adenomatous polyposis	*APC*	Autosomal dominant	100%	Small intestine, stomach, fibromatosis, hepatoblastoma, some brain and thyroid tumors, osteoma	Multiple (>100) conventional adenomas
MUTYH-associated polyposis	*MUTYH*	Autosomal recessive	70%	Duodenum	Multiple (>10) up to >100 conventional adenomas
Peutz–Jeghers syndrome	*STK11 (LKB1)*	Autosomal dominant	Mild increase	Small intestine, stomach, pancreas, esophagus, ovary, lung, uterus, breast	Hamartomatous polyps with arborizing muscle
Juvenile polyposis	*SMAD4, BMPR1A*	Autosomal dominant	Mild increase	Small intestine, stomach	Hamartomatous polyps with inflamed lamina propria with cystic crypts
PTEN hamartoma syndrome (Cowden syndrome)	*PTEN*	Autosomal dominant	Mild increase	Thyroid, breast, endometrium	Juvenile-type hamartomatous polyps, lipoma, ganglioneuroma, lymphoid hyperplasia
Hereditary mixed polyposis syndrome	*GREM1*	Autosomal dominant	Not finally distinguished	Not finally distinguished	Conventional adenomas, serrated polyps and hamartomatous polyps

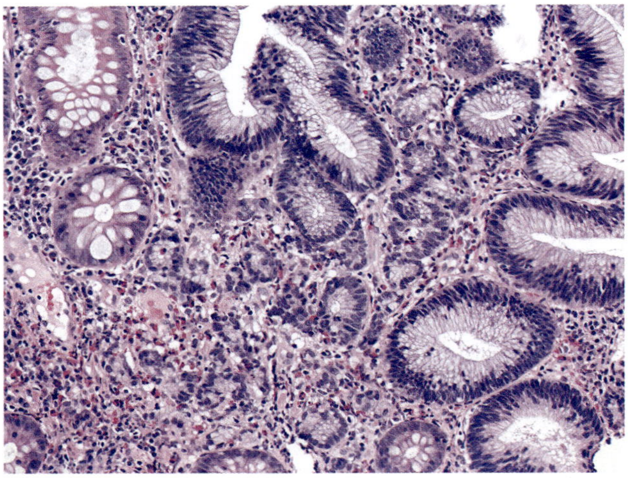

Figure 12.1 Cecal polyp showing invasion of the lamina propria by small atypical glands in a tubulovillous adenoma. No submucosa is present in the biopsy specimen. This case may be reported as intramucosal adenocarcinoma or high-grade adenoma suspicious for adenocarcinoma. The subsequent surgical specimen showed a small adenocarcinoma invading into the submucosa.

high-grade adenoma. Invasion in the lamina propria is reported by some pathologists, in particular in Japan, as intramucosal/in situ carcinoma. This terminology can sometimes be used for unusual intramucosal neoplasms with poor differentiation and suspicious for true invasion into the submucosa that cannot be unequivocally identified in a biopsy specimen (Figure 12.1).

Grossly, tumors may present as a large fungating mass with primarily intraluminal growth, more frequently found in the cecum, or as an infiltrative and ulcerating lesion with primarily intramural growth. Other gross presentation of colorectal carcinomas include a plaque-like or annular appearance (Figure 12.2). Rectal carcinoma after neoadjuvant therapy may regress and present as a small eroded scar.

Histologic typing and grading of colorectal carcinoma may be problematic in biopsy specimens due to sampling issues. At this stage, the importance is to make a diagnosis of carcinoma and to exclude other types of malignancy (i.e. lymphoma, melanoma); other histologic parameters such as grading are unlikely to affect patient management. Microscopically, 80–90% of colorectal carcinoma are adenocarcinomas of usual type composed of glandular structures with intestinal differentiation showing variability in size and configuration, containing mucus and cellular debris in the lumen. Adenocarcinomas are graded into well, moderately or poorly differentiated tumors depending on the proportion of gland formation in the least differentiated component of the tumor away from the invasive edge. The World Health Organization (WHO) recommends a two-tiered histologic grading system. Low-grade adenocarcinomas comprise well- and moderately differentiated tumor displaying 50–100% gland formation while high-grade adenocarcinomas consists of poorly differentiated tumor with <50% gland formation. The significance of poor differentiation may be different depending on the MSI status of the adenocarcinoma. Poorly differentiated colorectal adenocarcinomas with MSI behave as low-grade tumors. Other histologic types of colorectal carcinoma are not graded; some of them carry their own prognostic significance. Mucinous carcinomas and signet ring cell carcinomas are associated with poor prognosis, expect for tumors with MSI. Medullary carcinomas are rare tumors, almost invariably MSI, and of good prognosis (Figure 12.3). Serrated adenocarcinoma, micropapillary carcinoma, and cribriform comedo-type adenocarcinoma have been recently introduced in the WHO classification (Table 12.3) and are associated with other adverse histologic features and poor prognosis. Unusual histologic subtypes of colorectal carcinoma that may cause diagnostic problems are adenosquamous carcinoma combining a squamous cell carcinoma component and an adenocarcinoma component, spindle cell carcinoma showing a sarcomatoid component, and undifferentiated carcinoma.

Immunohistochemical Studies and Molecular Features

Immunohistochemical studies are rarely needed for the diagnosis of colorectal carcinoma in biopsy sample (see Section "Differential Diagnosis").

The DNA MMR status of newly diagnosed colorectal carcinoma is being increasingly tested in pathology departments as universal screening for Lynch syndrome. Upfront immunohistochemistry for the four DNA MMR proteins (MLH1, PMS2, MSH2, and MSH6) is a highly sensitive and specific test to analyze the tumor for MMR deficiency. Alternatively, PMS2 and MSH6 only can be tested first, complemented by the testing of the corresponding dimer if one marker is lost: MLH1 for PMS2 loss, MSH2 for MSH6 loss. Approximately 15% of colorectal carcinomas demonstrate MMR deficiency, most commonly caused by somatic hypermethylation of the promoter of the *MLH1* gene, resulting in loss of expression of MLH1 (Figure 12.4) and PMS2 by immunohistochemistry. Colorectal carcinoma in Lynch syndrome patients due to germline mutation in *MLH1* will exhibit a similar immunophenotype. To help separating both conditions, $BRAF^{V600E}$ mutation testing in the tumor can be performed. The presence of a $BRAF^{V600E}$ mutation will almost exclude Lynch syndrome. The absence of $BRAF^{V600E}$ mutation makes Lynch syndrome likely and usually results in *MLH1* germline mutation testing from patient's blood DNA. Testing the tumor for *MLH1*

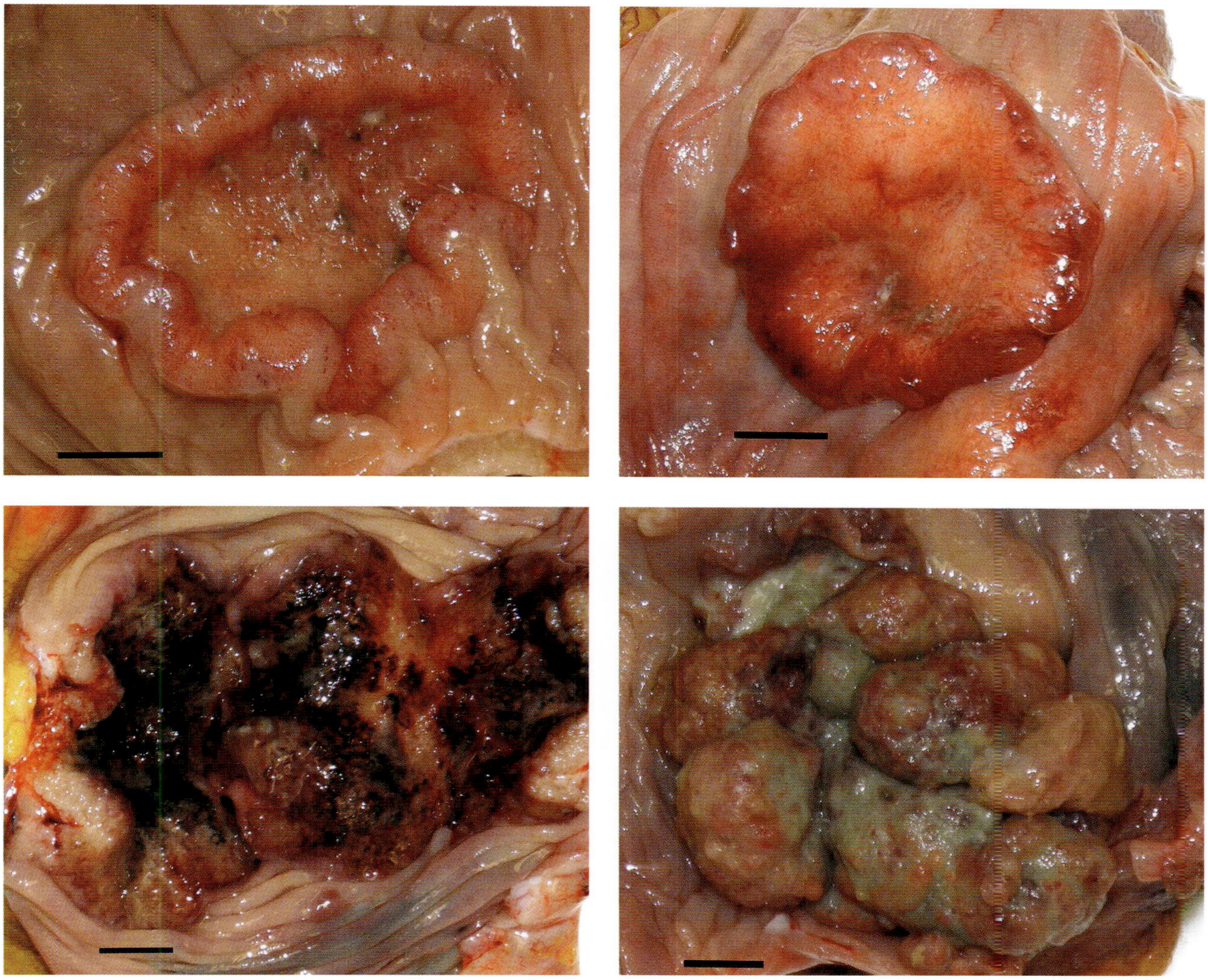

Figure 12.2 Various macroscopic appearances of colorectal carcinoma presenting as an annular tumor with elevated border and central erosion (upper left), as a plaque-like lesion with sharp demarcation (upper right), as a large circumferential ulcerated tumor (lower left), or as a bulky fungating mass (lower right). Scale bar is 10 mm.

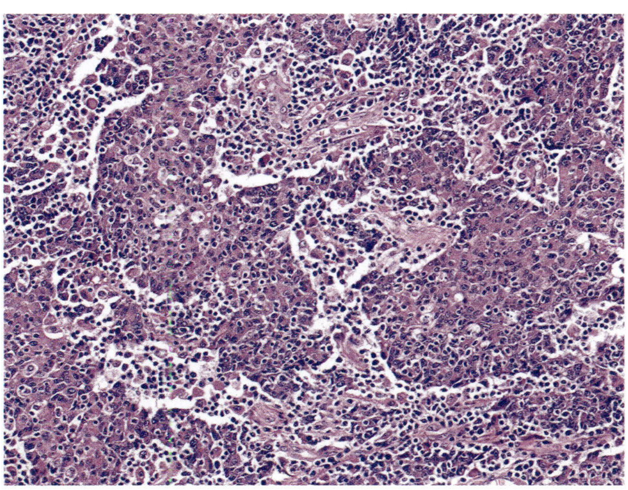

Figure 12.3 Medullary carcinoma of the proximal colon consisting of sheets of large carcinoma cells with eosinophilic cytoplasm and vesicular nuclei, associated with a prominent infiltration of lymphocytes.

Table 12.3 Histological classification of colorectal carcinoma according to the WHO classification.

1) Adenocarcinoma NOS
2) Serrated adenocarcinoma
3) Micropapillary adenocarcinoma
4) Mucinous adenocarcinoma
5) Poorly cohesive carcinoma
6) Signet-ring cell carcinoma
7) Medullary adenocarcinoma
8) Adenosquamous carcinoma
9) Carcinoma, undifferenciated, NOS
10) Carcinoma with sarcomatoid component

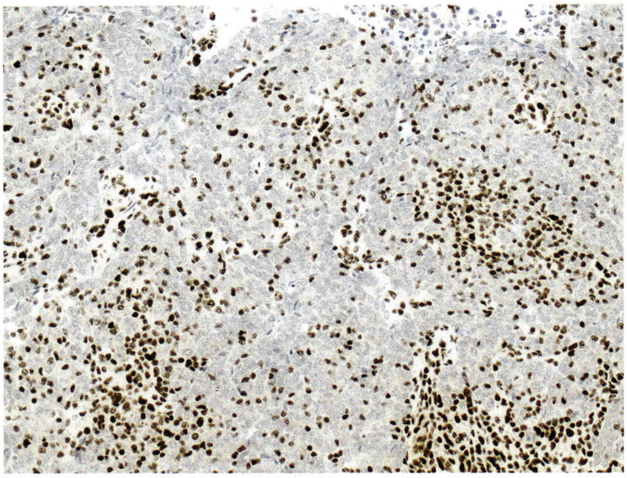

Figure 12.4 Loss of immunohistochemical expression of MLH1 in a medullary carcinoma. Note the conspicuous tumor infiltrating lymphocytes showing a preserved nuclear staining of MLH1.

methylation is another approach to separate sporadic from inherited cause; if *MLH1* methylation is present, Lynch syndrome is almost excluded.

Other Abnormal Immunohistochemical Results in Tumors, Suggestive of Lynch Syndrome

These include the loss of

1) MSH2 and MSH6, suggestive of a mutation in *MSH2*.
2) PMS2 only, suggestive of a mutation in *PMS2* or *MLH1* if *PMS2* is normal.
3) MSH6 only, suggestive of a mutation in *MSH6* or *MSH2* if *MSH6* is normal.

Caveats in the Interpretation of the Results

1) Loss of MSH6 expression caused by secondary somatic mutation in *MSH6* (containing a microsatellite sequence in a coding region) in an MSI tumor caused by an alteration in another DNA MMR gene (usually *MLH1*).
2) Patchy and partial of MSH6, secondary to the effect of chemoradiation therapy in rectal carcinoma.
3) Partial and/or focal loss of expression in any MMR protein from an MSI tumor with a gene mutation causing loss of function but preserved immunoreaction with the antibody used for immunohistochemistry. MSI testing by molecular method is warranted in these situations or if the clinical presentation is highly suggestive of Lynch syndrome and the tumor shows normal immunohistochemical expression of all MMR proteins.

The molecular pathogenesis of colorectal carcinoma is among the best known in human tumors. For the purpose of molecular classification with prognostic implication, the different classifiers are usually used: first, chromosomal instability (CIN), characterized by abnormal numbers and structures of chromosomes leading to aneuploidy, frequent deletions, and duplications of chromosomal segments. This pathway drives the progression of the majority (70–80%) of colorectal carcinoma and is associated with DNA hypomethylation, *APC* mutation, and *TP53* mutation. Another one is MSI, defined by variation in lengths of repeat nucleotide sequences (microsatellites) due to altered function of DNA MMR enzymes that do not correct errors during DNA replication. DNA MMR genes include *MLH1*, *MSH2*, *PMS2*, and *MSH6*. Germline or somatic alterations in any of these genes result in MMR deficiency and MSI, present in 15% of all colorectal carcinomas. Tumors with functional DNA MMR are called MMR proficient or microsatellite stable (MSS). The majority of colorectal carcinoma with MSI are caused by somatic hypermethylation of the promoter region of *MLH1*, usually part of a global hypermethylation of the tumor DNA, referred to as CpG island methylator phenotype (CIMP). CIMP-positive tumors are virtually never associated with CIN and these two molecular alterations are mutually exclusive. Germline mutations in any of the four DNA MMR genes are a less common cause of MMR deficiency and defines Lynch syndrome. At least mutation in genes of the MAP kinase signaling pathway as *BRAF* and *KRAS* are two key oncogenes from this pathway. They are mutated in approximately 15 and 35% of all colorectal carcinomas, respectively. *BRAF* mutation is strongly associated with CIMP and the subset of MSI carcinomas caused of somatic hypermethylation of *MLH1*. The presence of a mutation in the *KRAS* gene is a negative predictive marker of response to anti-EGFR therapy for advanced-stage colorectal carcinoma patients. Mutations in *KRAS* and *BRAF* are mutually exclusive. The mutation status of these two genes also bears some prognostic significance in subsets of colorectal carcinoma: poor prognosis of *BRAF* mutation in MSS tumors; poor prognosis of *KRAS* mutation in CIMP-negative tumors (CIN tumors).

Using these molecular classifiers, colorectal carcinomas can be divided into subtypes of tumors with phenotypic correlation and prognostic significance (Table 12.4).

Differential Diagnosis

The leading differential diagnosis on colon biopsy is the distinction between invasive adenocarcinoma and high-grade adenoma. Deeper sections from the tissue block may be helpful to prove invasive growth (e.g. angio- and/or perineural invasion, presence of thick bundles of muscle and/or large vessels). If invasive growth cannot be proven, a comment mentioning suspicion for an invasive component not sampled in the biopsy may be necessary. However, the diagnosis of high-grade dysplasia from a biopsy of a mass lesion may

Table 12.4 Classification of colorectal carcinomas according to molecular characteristics with clinical and pathologic correlates and prognosis.

Groups	Proportion (%)	Precursor lesion	Molecular hallmarks	Clinicopathologic correlates	Prognosis
1.	10	Sessile serrated lesion	MSI, CIMP+, *BRAF*-mutated	Older patients, female predominance, proximal colon, poor differentiation, mucinous differentiation, pushing margin, tumor infiltrating lymphocytes	Good
2.	5	Subset of serrated polyps	MSS, CIMP+, *BRAF*-mutated	Older patients, female predominance, proximal colon, poor differentiation, cribriform carcinoma, adverse histologic features	Very poor
3.	30	Subset of serrated polyps (traditional serrated adenoma, TSA) and conventional adenoma (tubulovillous adenoma, TVA)	MSS, CIMP−, *KRAS*-mutated	Distal colorectum, adverse histologic features, serrated adenocarcinoma	Poor
4.	50	Conventional adenoma	MSS, CIMP−, *BRAF*- and *KRAS*-wildtype	Distal colorectum, adenocarcinoma of usual type	Reference
5.	3	Conventional adenoma	MSI, CIMP−, *BRAF*-wildtype	Lynch syndrome, proximal colon, poor differentiation, mucinous differentiation, pushing margin, tumor infiltrating lymphocytes	Good

lead to refer the patient to surgery, depending on clinical appearance and radiologic findings. The distinction between deeply invasive carcinoma and noninvasive or superficially invasive has become critical as endoscopic mucosal resection (for noninvasive) and endoscopic submucosal dissection (for superficially T1sm1) invasive cancers is now considered curative, and preferred over surgery according to the US Multisociety Task Force guidelines. To estimate depth of invasion, several criteria have been developed including shape (depressed more likely to be malignant), and surface patterns (highly irregular/loss of pattern indicative of invasion).

To confirm the diagnosis of carcinoma for tumors showing an undifferentiated pattern and excluding other malignancy (i.e. lymphoma, melanoma) a small immunohistochemical panel such as pan-cytokeratin marker (AE1/AE3), CD45, CD20, and S100 (Figure 12.5) may be helpful. Furthermore, solid tumor masses might be identified as neuroendocrine carcinomas (NECs) as well. These tumor typically show suggestive morphology in H&E (e.g. nuclear features: "salt and pepper" chromatin) and can be verified using immunohistochemical stains like chromogranin and synaptophysin.

However, secondary carcinomas infiltrating the large bowel may have to be excluded. For example, pelvic carcinomas could extend into the rectal wall (e.g. prostate adenocarcinoma, carcinoma from the bladder, uterus or kidney) and can be excluded histomorphologically and/or immunohistochemically. Furthermore, metastatic disease,

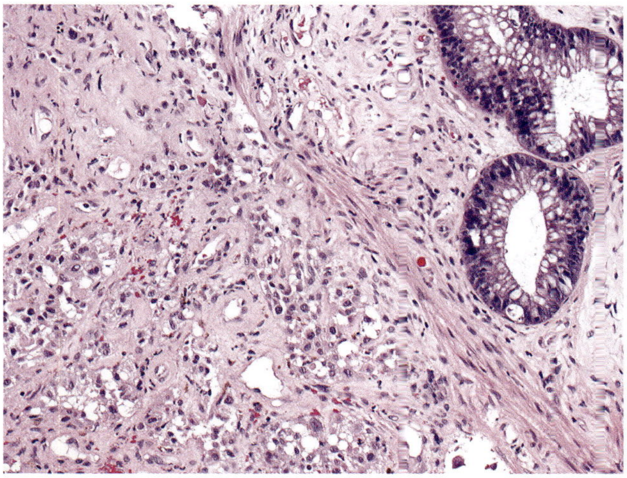

Figure 12.5 Metastatic melanoma in the sigmoid colon infiltration of the colonic mucosa by large epitheloid cells with clear or eosinophilic cytoplasm and melanin pigment.

such as lobular carcinoma of the breast, intestinal carcinoma from other parts of the gastrointestinal (GI) tract (e.g. gastric adenocarcinoma), or pancreatobiliary carcinoma, may involve the large bowel.

Rarely benign lesions like endometriosis may mimic well-differentiated primary colorectal carcinoma (Figures 12.6 and 12.7). This differential can be excluded by immunohistochemistry showing estrogen-positive benign glands surrounded by CD10-positive stroma cells.

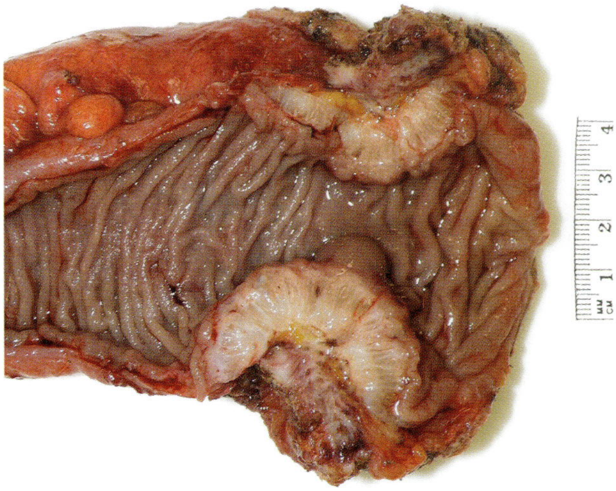

Figure 12.6 Endometriosis presenting as a large mass in the upper rectum, mimicking a primary rectal tumor.

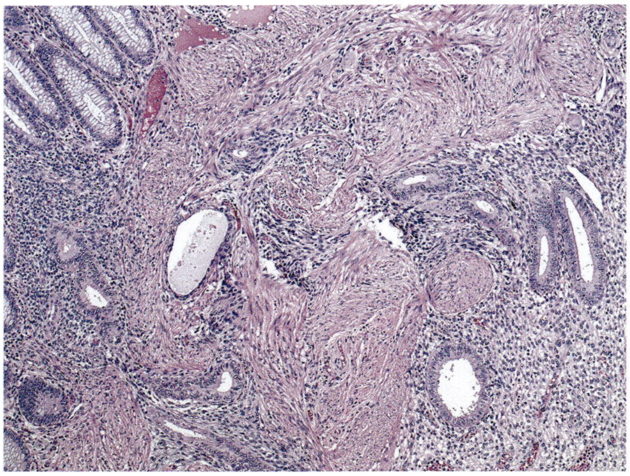

Figure 12.7 Endometriosis in the rectal mucosa: Endometrial glands surrounded by stroma, infiltrating the rectal mucosa and the submucosa, mimicking an adenocarcinoma.

Poorly differentiated and undifferentiated colorectal carcinomas, frequently found in the proximal colon, are less likely to demonstrate the usual immunophenotype of colonic carcinoma: positivity for cytokeratin 20 and for CDX2; therefore, negativity for these markers does not exclude a colonic origin.

Treatment/Prognosis/Evolution Most noninvasive polyps are removed at the time of routine screening colonoscopy; however larger polyps, and especially laterally spreading large polyps, require specialized endoscopic resection techniques. Traditionally, these were sent for surgery, and many still are, but these can be effectively and safely removed by endoscopic mucosal or submucosal resection methods with lower morbidity, mortality, and cost than surgery.

Malignant Colorectal Polyp

Definition, General Features, and Predisposing Factors

Endoscopically removed polyps that contain carcinoma at microscopic examination are defined as malignant colorectal polyps (MCPs). Up to 6% of all colorectal polyps are MCPs and are usually found in the distal colon. MCPs can present as invasive carcinoma arising from a pre-existing adenoma or, less frequently, polypoid carcinoma with no evident precursor lesion. The role of the pathologist is to provide the gastroenterologist and surgeon with a risk assessment analysis for the presence of residual disease based on a set of histologic features. Polypectomy may be an adequate curative treatment for patients if no adverse histologic features are present.

The predisposing factors to MCPs are the same as for any colorectal carcinoma described above.

Clinical Features and Endoscopic Characteristics (with Guidelines)

MCP can present as a sessile polyp or a pedunculated polyp (Figure 12.8).

Microscopic Features

Besides the conventional histomorphological appearance of polyps (as described in this chapter) MCPs are characterized by an invasive component infiltrating the submucosa and sometimes lymphatic and/or blood vessels. MCPs are mainly adenocarcinomas composed of at least a tubular component and sometimes with additional tumor cell clusters or solid sheets. Mucinous carcinomas can sometimes be found and is often considered as an adverse feature. Adverse histological features with high risk of residual disease include qualitative parameters and quantitative parameters (Table 12.5). These adverse factors are cumulative to predict the risk of residual disease in the surgical resection specimen. Histologic parameters most consistently found to be associated with residual disease are the presence of a poorly differentiated component and large size of the invasive component, which is most reproducibly measured in mm. Lymphovascular invasion and tumor budding have also been associated with residual disease by some but not all studies.

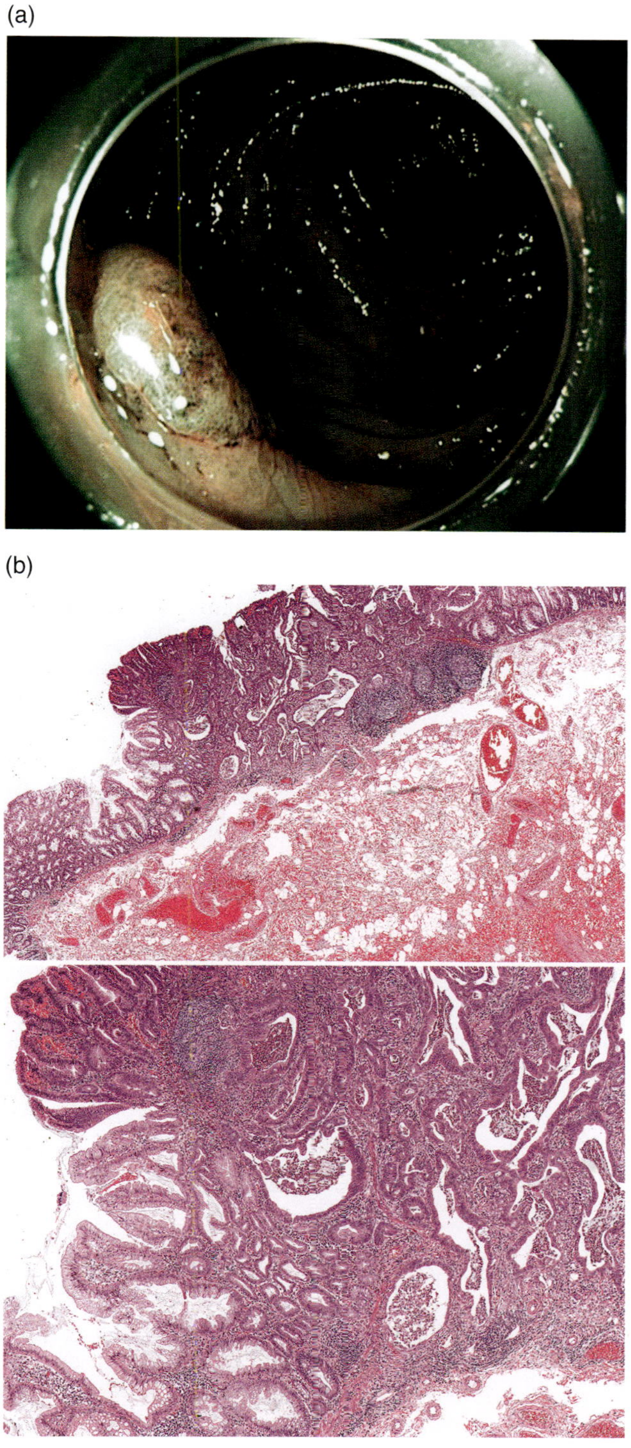

Figure 12.8 (a) Endoscopical appearance of malignant sessile colon polyp with typical features of a highly irregular surface, plaque-like appearance, and puckering of the adjacent folds. (b) Malignant colorectal polyp: moderately differentiated adenocarcinoma arising from a sessile serrated lesion with dysplasia (SSLD) (top) and infiltrating the submucosa (bottom).

Table 12.5 Adverse histologic parameters in malignant colorectal polyps resected by endoscopy and associated with high risk of residual disease.

Qualitative parameters
Poor differentiation (high grade)
Lymphatic and venous space invasion
Tumor budding (buds of <5 tumor cells at the leading edge of the invasive component)
Quantitative parameters
Size of invasive tumor: Haggitt level 4 for pedunculated polyps, Kikuchi levels Sm2 and Sm3 for sessile polyps, depth of invasion >2 mm, width of invasion >4 mm
Positive polypectomy margin (tumor reaching the cauterized margin or <1 mm)

Immunohistochemical Studies and Molecular Features

Special stains and immunohistochemical studies in MCPs may be necessary in the following contexts:

1) Lymphatic invasion, using an endothelial marker for lymphatic vessels (D2–40).
2) Venous invasion, using an elastic stain.
3) Neuroendocrine differentiation, using chromogranin and synaptophysin.
4) MMR proteins MLH1, MSH2, PMS2, and MSH6 to screen for Lynch syndrome and to identify MLH1 deficiency in carcinoma arising from an advanced sessile serrated lesion.

Differential Diagnosis

A particular diagnostic issue specific of MCP is the distinction between adenocarcinoma arising from a precursor polyp and pseudoinvasion. Pseudoinvasion refers to the misplacement of adenomatous glands or non-neoplastic epithelium in the submucosa, mimicking invasive adenocarcinoma (Figure 12.9). It is also almost exclusively seen in large pedunculated polyps of the sigmoid colon and the descending colon, which are often removed in patients who undergo screening colonoscopy after positive fecal blood test as these polyps are often ulcerated and bleed. This issue often represents a major histological diagnostic conundrum with low level of interobserver agreement even for groups of expert pathologists.

Favoring invasive carcinoma is an infiltrative pattern of the glandular structures, in particular in the deepest part of the lesion showing irregularly shaped glands infiltrating into the submucosa. A desmoplastic reaction would favor carcinoma but it may be difficult to

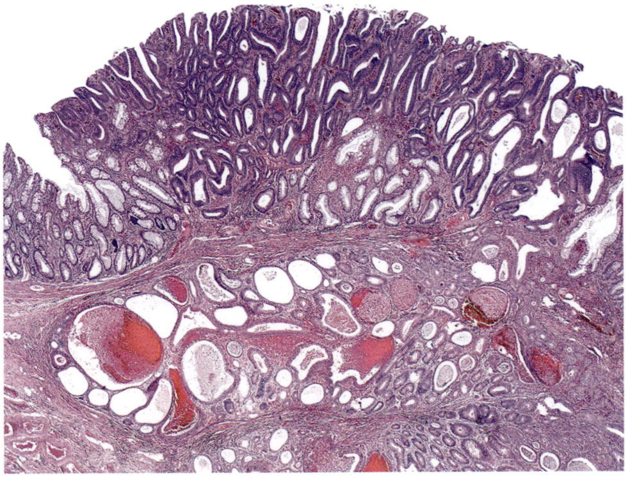

Figure 12.9 Pseudoinvasion in the stalk of a large pedunculated tubular adenoma of the sigmoid colon. Misplaced adenomatous glands with regular border are present in the submucosa, surrounded by lamina propria and associated with hemorrhage and hemosiderin pigment.

distinguish desmoplasia from the lamina propria surrounding misplaced glands or from a fibroblastic reaction secondary to reparative changes. A cellular mucin pools and hemosiderin are usually found in the surrounding of misplaced glands. However, these features associated with trauma and torsion of a polyp can also be seen in true MCPs or in polyps showing both misplaced glands and invasive carcinoma. Special stains are not helpful for the most problematic cases; deeper sections in the tissue block are more informative and should be performed. For very difficult cases, the most important parameter is the completeness of excision as these problematic polyps, if truly malignant, are well-differentiated, do not show any adverse histologic features and are therefore curatively treated by endoscopy if the base of the polyp is identified and clear.

Treatment/Prognosis/Evolution

The management of intramucosal and superficial, low-risk submucosal cancers is discussed above with regard to endoscopic management. Deeply (more than sm1) invasive cancers and those with other high risk (poorly differentiated, lymphovascular invasion) should be resected surgically with standard bowel and lymph node removal. To exclude synchronous lesions, pre-operative a full colonoscopy should be performed. In the case of an obstructing cancer, when the proximal colon cannot be assessed, patients should undergo surveillance colonoscopy as soon as possible after surgery.

Neuroendocrine Neoplasms

Definition, General Features, and Predisposing Factors

Neuroendocrine neoplasms represent <0.5% of all neoplasms of the large bowel and comprise neuroendocrine tumors (NET), (NEC; large cell and small cell), and mixed adenoneuroendocrine carcinoma (MANEC), according to the 2010 WHO classification. Although obsolete, carcinoid is a terminology still often used to describe grade 1 neuroendocrine tumor. No definite and specific predisposing factor is known for colorectal neuroendocrine neoplasms. The most common site is the rectum, followed by the cecum and the sigmoid colon.

Clinical Features and Endoscopic Characteristics (with Guidelines)

Colorectal NETs are usually small, submucosal tumors, not often found in the rectum. These are often detected unexpectedly when a pathology same from a polypectomy notes NET.

Microscopic Features

Neuroendocrine neoplasms of the rectum are almost always well-differentiated tumors with low proliferation rate, found incidentally during colonoscopy as a small (<10 mm) polyp. The usual microscopic growth pattern consists of rosettes, anastomosing ribbons, nodules, trabecules, or short cords of uniform cells (Figure 12.10). Cytomorphologically, NETs consist of uniform, round cells with a round to ovoid nucleus with disperse granular (salt

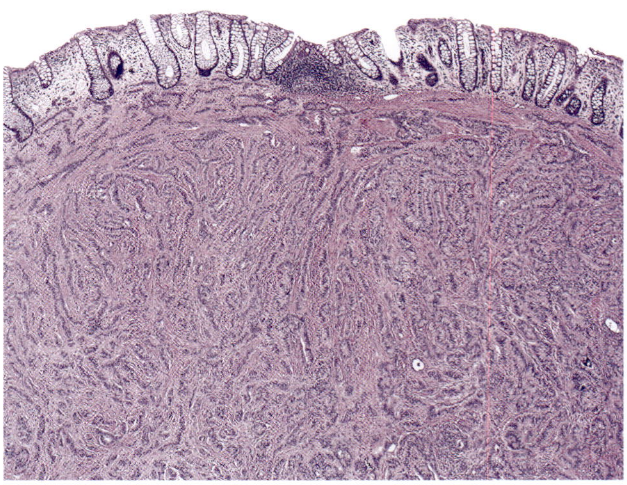

Figure 12.10 NET of the rectum showing an anastomosing ribbon pattern infiltrating the submucosa, with overlying normal mucosa.

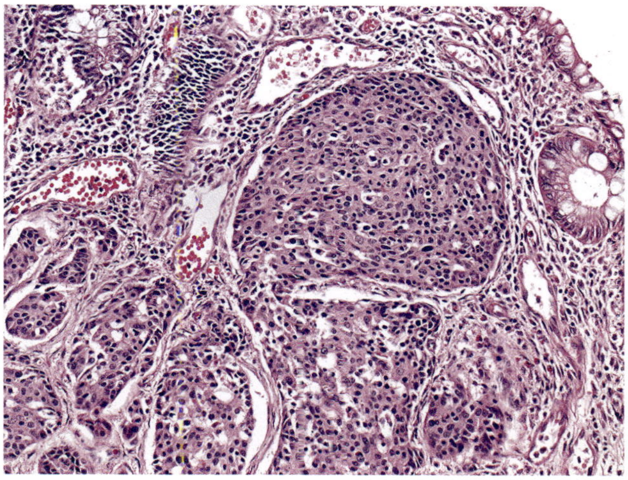

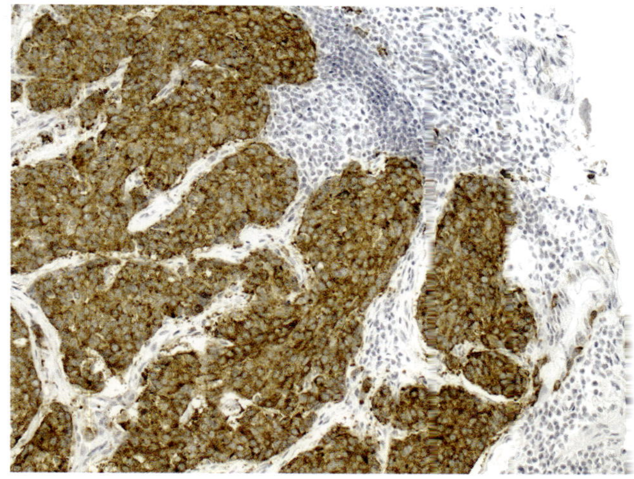

Figures 12.11 and 12.12 Large cell neuroendocrine carcinoma of the rectum showing an undifferentiated appearance in hematoxylin-and-eosin stained sections and positive expression of synaptophysin by immunohistochemistry.

Table 12.6 Grading of neuroendocrine tumors/carcinomas of the colon according to the recent WHO classification.

Grade	Mitotic count	Ki67 index (%)
G1	<2 per 10 HPF	<3
G2	2–20 per 10 HPF	3–20
G3	>20 per 10 HPF	>20

and pepper like) chromatin structure and few mitotic figures. Different morphologic appearances for NETs have been described, i. e. lipid-rich, rhabdoid, and oncocytic variants, which might be challenging to diagnose.

NECs resemble their counterparts in the lung. The majority are large cell type (Figures 12.11 and 12.12), while small cell NECs are more frequent in the anus. An overlying adenoma or conventional adenocarcinoma can be found in some NECs.

NETs are graded by mitotic activity and/or immunohistochemically evaluated proliferative activity with the Ki67 (MIB-1) stain (Table 12.6). The mitotic activity should be evaluated after counting at least 50 HPF, whereas the Ki67 labeling index is recommended to be calculated in the so-called "hot spot" evaluating between 500 and 2000 tumor cells. If different results are found (mitotic count vs. Ki67%), the higher grade should be assumed.

Recently, a group of pancreatic NETs showing histomorphological low-grade appearance with mitotic activity akin to G2 and G3 Ki67-index defined (i.e. NEC according to the WHO criteria) has been reported. Whether similar cases also exist in the colon and are missed since immunohistochemistry for Ki67 was not performed.

Immunohistochemical Studies and Molecular Features

The most important for all neuroendocrine neoplasms immunohistochemical stain is Ki-67 since it is prognostically relevant.

Morphologically challenging cases need to be stained with specific markers such as chromogranin and synaptophysin to verify the neuroendocrine differentiation. It is important to mention that rectal NET may be negative for chromogranin. A less specific marker of neuroendocrine differentiation such as CD56 may be helpful if the previous markers are negative.

Recent studies of pancreatic NET found the inactivating mutations in *DAXX* and *ATRX* and mutations in *MEN1* were exclusively found in well-differentiated neoplasms. Also contrary to pancreatic NEC, well-differentiated tumors do not show an inactivation of *TP53* and *Rb/p16* pathways. These findings may also play a role in neuroendocrine neoplasias of the large bowl. A recent study reported of *BRAF V600E* mutation in colorectal neuroendocrine neoplasia.

Differential Diagnosis Sequentially Presented on (i) Clinical Presentation; (ii) Microscopic Appearance; and (iii) Results of Ancillary Studies (When Performed)

- Undifferentiated carcinoma: absence of chromogranin and synaptophysin expression.
- Prostate adenocarcinoma for rectal carcinoid: both are positive for prostatic acid phosphatase but only prostate adenocarcinoma is positive for PSA.

(a) (b)

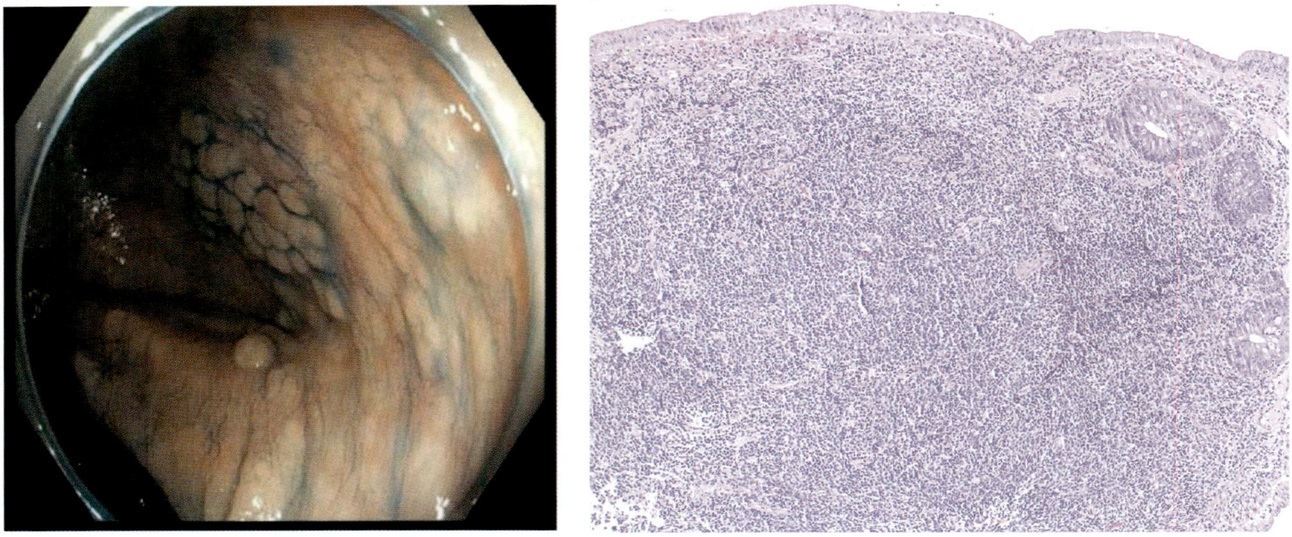

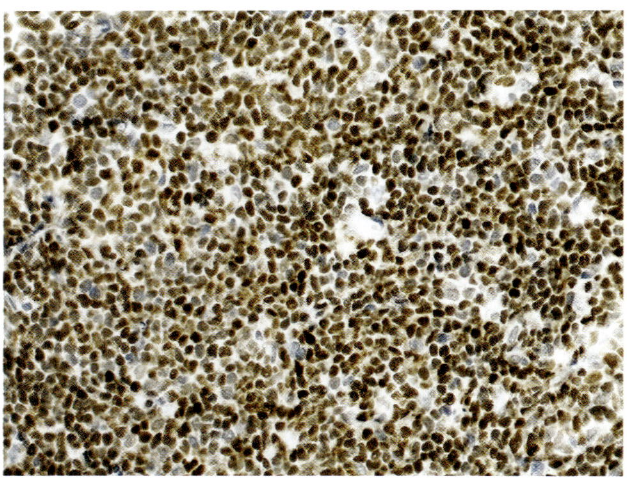

Figures 12.13 and 12.14 Endoscopic appearance of mucosal-associated lymphoid tissue (MALT) lymphoma of the proximal colon (12.13a). The patient was treated with rituximab for cure. Biopsy from a lymphomatous polyposis of the colon showing infiltration of the mucosa by monotonous lymphoid cells of small to medium size (12.13b) with immunohistochemical expression of cyclin D1 (12.14), diagnostic of a mantle cell lymphoma.

Treatment/Prognosis/Evolution

- In endoscopically resected cases, it is imperative to assess if the lesion was completely excised (negative margins) and the risk of occult metastases. Often they are not fully removed and require subsequent definitive resection, either by endoscopic mucosal or submucosal resection, or more recently by endoscopic full-thickness resection using specialized, dedicated full-thickness resection devices. For completely resected lesions, the main issue is the risk of occult metastases, and the need for further staging and surgery. Current consensus guidelines suggest that local (endoscopic or local surgical) resection is adequate for small lesions, <10 mm although even these have a 3–4% risk of metastases, so further staging, such as whole-body Gallium-68 Dotatate scanning is warranted.

Lymphomas of the Large Bowel

Definition, General Features, and Predisposing Factors

Primary lymphoma of the large bowel is uncommon (<1%) and most frequently encountered in the cecum and the rectum. The morphologic and molecular characteristics of colorectal lymphomas are comparable to those from their nodal counterparts. Immunodeficiency is the major predisposing

Table 12.7 Most common lymphomas of the colon.

	DLBCL-NOS	MALT lymphoma	Mantle cell lymphoma	Follicular lymphoma
Histomorphology	More common in older adults	Centrocytes like or monocytoid lymphoid cells ± plasma cell differentiation	Monotonous small/medium size cells	Centrocytes and centroblasts (grade 1–2, or 3)
Growth pattern	Diffuse growth Large cells: centroblasts and/or immunoblasts and/or anaplastic cells	Lymphoepithelial lesions, reactive and colonialized follicles. Abundant T-cells	Mantle, nodular, or diffuse pattern of growth. Follicles usually absent	Neoplastic follicles
Immunophenotype	CD20+, CD79a+, CD10−/+, BCL6+/−, MUM1+/−, BCL2+/−, MYC−/+, Ki67 < 90%	CD5−/+, CD10−, CD43−/+, BCL6−, IRTA1+. Monotypic plasma cells (30%)	CD5+, cyclin D1+, SOX11+, CD23−, CD43+, BCL2+, BCL6−, CD10−	CD5−, BCL2+, BCL6+, CD10+
Genetics	*BCL6, MYC* (or *BCL2*) rearrangement in a subset of cases (no double hit)	t(11;18)(q21;q21)/*API2-MALT1* t(1;14)(p22;q32)/*BCL10-IGH*	t(11;14)(q13;q32)/*CCND1-IGH*	(14;18)(q32;q21)/*IGH-BCL2*
Clinical features	Rare cases EBV+ (EBV+ DLBCL NOS)	Indolent, responding to antibiotic therapy	Usually aggressive	Indolent

EBV: Epstein Barr virus; NOS: not otherwise specified.

factor for lymphoma. The most common subtype is the diffuse large B-cell lymphoma (50%), followed by marginal zone B-cell lymphoma (MALT lymphoma; approximately 25%), follicular lymphoma, and mantle cell lymphoma. Lymphomatous polyposis is an endoscopic presentation of mantle cell lymphoma (Figure 12.13a).

Clinical Features and Endoscopic Characteristics (with Guidelines)

Primary colorectal lymphomas are rare, but may present with nodular mucosal, sometimes resembling a granular, lateral spreading polyp (Figures 12.13a, b and 12.14).

Microscopic Features, Immunohistochemical Studies and Molecular Features

Lymphomas consist of blue, small to medium large cells on the one end to medium to large blastoid cells on the other end. Lymphomas of the small cell type include MALT-, follicular-, and mantel cell lymphomas. In contrast, diffuse large B-cell lymphomas (DLBCL) show aggregates of large atypical lymphoid cells resembling centor- and/or immunoblasts.

The histomorphologic findings of lymphomas of the large bowl do not differ from gastric lymphomas described in Chapter 6. The diagnostic features of the most common lesions of the large bowl are summarized in Table 12.7.

Differential Diagnosis

Benign lymphoid aggregates and focal lymphoid hyperplasia (including "rectal tonsils") may appear like a high-grade lymphoma.

Another differential is the enteropathy-associated T-cell lymphoma (EATL), which is classified into type 1 and type 2. EATL type 1 is commonly associated to celiac disease, whereas type 2 arises sporadically. In general EATL is more common in the small bowl but is can arise in the colon as well.

DLBCL may have to be distinguished from Burkitt–Lymphoma, which would have a major effect on outcome and therapy.

Treatment/Prognosis/Evolution

GI lymphomas management is beyond the scope of this article; however, key issues related to endoscopy and pathology are detailed in the national comprehensive cancer center guidelines (http://nccn.org) for non-gastric lymphomas.

Further Reading

Basturk, O., Yang, Z., Tang, L.H. et al. (2015). The high-grade (WHO G3) pancreatic neuroendocrine tumor category is morphologically and biologically heterogenous and includes both well differentiated and poorly differentiated neoplasms. *Am. J. Surg. Pathol.* 39 (5): 683–690.

WHO Classification of Tumors Editorial Board. Digestive System Tumors. Lyon (France): International Agency for Research on Cancer; 2019 (WHO classification of tumors series; 5th ed.; vol 1)

Botteri, E., Iodice, S., Bagnardi, V. et al. (2008). Smoking and colorectal cancer: a meta-analysis. *JAMA* 300: 2765–2778.

Center, M.M., Jemal, A., Smith, R.A. et al. (2009). Worldwide variations in colorectal cancer. *CA Cancer J. Clin.* 59: 366–378.

Cho, E., Smith-Warner, S.A., Spiegelman, D. et al. (2004). Dairy foods, calcium, and colorectal cancer: a pooled analysis of 10 cohort studies. *J. Natl. Cancer Inst.* 96: 1015–1022.

Cicek, M.S., Lindor, N.M., Gallinger, S. et al. (2011). Quality assessment and correlation of microsatellite instability and immunohistochemical markers among population- and clinic-based colorectal tumors results from the Colon Cancer Family Registry. *J. Mol. Diagn.* 13: 271–281.

Cooper, H.S., Deppisch, L.M., Kahn, E.I. et al. (1998). Pathology of the malignant colorectal polyp. *Hum. Pathol.* 29: 15–26.

Rex, D.K., Boland, C.R., Dominitz, J.A. et al. (2017). Colorectal cancer screening: recommendations for physicians and patients from the U.S. Multi-Society Task Force on Colorectal Cancer Rex. *Gastrointest. Endosc.* 86 (1): 18–33.

Foukas, P.G. and de Leval, L. (2015). Recent advances in intestinal lymphomas. *Histopathology* 66 (1): 112–136.

Galiatsatos, P. and Foulkes, W.D. (2006). Familial adenomatous polyposis. *Am. J. Gastroenterol.* 101: 385–398.

Hamilton, S.R., Bosman, F.T., Boffetta, P. et al. (2010). Carcinoma of the colon and rectum. In: *World Health Organization Classification of Tumours of the Digestive System*, 4e (eds. F.T. Bosman, F. Carneiro, R.H. Hruban and N.D. Theise), 134–146. Lyon: International Agency for Research on Cancer (IARC).

Hampel, H., Frankel, W.L., Martin, E. et al. (2005). Screening for the Lynch syndrome (hereditary nonpolyposis colorectal cancer). *N. Engl. J. Med.* 352: 1851–1860.

Hassan, C., Zullo, A., Risio, M. et al. (2005). Histologic risk factors and clinical outcome in colorectal malignant polyp: a pooled-data analysis. *Dis Colon Rectum* 48: 1588–1596.

Heald, B., Plesec, T., Liu, X. et al. (2013). Implementation of universal microsatellite instability and immunohistochemistry screening for diagnosing lynch syndrome in a large academic medical center. *J. Clin. Oncol.* 31: 1336–1340.

Hoang, M.P., Hruban, R.H., and Albores-Saavedra, J. (2001). Clear cell endocrine pancreatic tumor mimicking renal cell carcinoma: a distinctive neoplasm of von Hippel–Lindau disease. *Am. J. Surg. Pathol.* 25: 602–609.

Hong, Y.S., Woo, Y.S., Park, G. et al. (2016). Endoscopic findings of enteropathy-associated T-cell lymphoma type II: a case series. *Gut Liver* 10 (1): 147–151.

Jass, J.R. (2007). Classification of colorectal cancer based on correlation of clinical, morphological and molecular features. *Histopathology* 50: 113–130.

Kim, J.Y. and Hong, S.M. (2016). Recent updates on neuroendocrine tumors from the gastrointestinal and pancreatobiliary tracts. *Arch. Pathol. Lab. Med.* 140 (5): 437–448.

Larsson, S.C., Rutegard, J., Bergkvist, L. et al. (2006). Physical activity, obesity, and risk of colon and rectal cancer in a cohort of Swedish men. *Eur. J. Cancer* 42: 2590–2597.

Lindor, N.M. (2009). Familial colorectal cancer type X: the other half of hereditary nonpolyposis colon cancer syndrome. *Surg. Oncol. Clin. N. Am.* 18: 637–645.

Lynch, H.T. and de la Chapelle, A. (2003). Hereditary colorectal cancer. *N. Engl. J. Med.* 348: 919–932.

Mandair, D. and Caplin, M.E. (2012). Colonic and rectal NET's. *Best Pract. Res. Clin. Gastroenterol.* 26 (6): 775–789.

Meier, B., Albrecht, H., Wiedbrauck, T. et al. (2020). Full-thickness resection of neuroendocrine tumors in the rectum. *Endoscopy* 52 (01): 68–72.

Nelson, H.D., Humphrey, L.L., Nygren, P. et al. (2002). Postmenopausal hormone replacement therapy: scientific review. *JAMA* 288: 872–881.

Park, C., Ha, S.Y., Kim, S.T. et al. (2016). Identification of the BRAF V600E mutation in gastroenteropancreatic neuroendocrine tumors. *Oncotarget* 7 (4): 4024–4035.

Phipps, A.I., Limburg, P.J., Baron, J.A. et al. (2015). Association between molecular subtypes of colorectal cancer and patient survival. *Gastroenterology* 148: 77–87.e2.

Ramage, J.K., De Herder, W.W., Delle Fave, G. et al. (2016). ENETS consensus guidelines update for colorectal neuroendocrine neoplasms. *Neuroendocrinology* 103 (2): 139–143.

Rindi, G., Arnold, R., Bosman, F.T. et al. (2010). Nomenclature and classification of neuroendocrine neoplasms of the digestive system. In: *World Health Organization Classification of Tumours of the Digestive System* (eds. F.T. Bosman, F. Carneiro, R.H. Hruban and N.D. Theise), 13–14. Lyon: International Agency for Research on Cancer (IARC).

Rosty, C., Parry, S., and Young, J.P. (2011). Serrated polyposis: an enigmatic model of colorectal cancer predisposition. *Pathol. Res. Int.* 2011: 157073.

Rosty, C., Williamson, E.J., Clendenning, M. et al. (2014). Should the grading of colorectal adenocarcinoma include microsatellite instability status? *Hum. Pathol.* 45: 2077–2084.

Sano, Y., Hirata, D., and Saito, Y. (2018). Japan NBI expert team classification: narrow-band imaging magnifying endoscopic classification of colorectal tumors. *Dig. Endosc.* 30 (4): 543–545. https://doi.org/10.1111/den 13072.

Sekiguchi, M., Matsuda, T., and Saito, Y. (2016). Surveillance after endoscopic and surgical resection of colorectal cancer. *Best Pract. Res. Clin. Gastroenterol.* 30 (6): 959–970.

Shia, J., Erlandson, R.A., and Klimstra, D.S. (2004). Whorls of intermediate filaments with entrapped neurosecretory granules correspond to the "rhabdoid" inclusions seen in pancreatic endocrine neoplasms. *Am. J. Surg. Pathol.* 28: 271–273.

Shia, J., Holck, S., Depetris, G. et al. (2013). Lynch syndrome-associated neoplasms: a discussion on histopathology and immunohistochemistry. *Familial Cancer* 12: 241–260.

Siegel, R., Desantis, C., and Jemal, A. (2014). Colorectal cancer statistics, 2014. *CA Cancer J. Clin.* 64: 104–117.

Singh, R., Basturk, O., Klimstra, D.S. et al. (2006). Lipid-rich variant of pancreatic endocrine neoplasms. *Am. J. Surg. Pathol.* 30 (2): 194–200.

Swerdlow, S.H. (ed.) (2017). *WHO Classification of Tumours of Haematopoietic and Lymphoid Tissues*, 4e. Lyon: International Agency for Research on Cancer.

Taylor, D.P., Burt, R.W., Williams, M.S. et al. (2010). Population-based family history-specific risks for colorectal cancer: a constellation approach. *Gastroenterology* 138: 877–885.

Tonya, K., Anderson, J.C., Burke, C.A. et al. (2020). Endoscopic removal of colorectal lesions – recommendations by the US Multi-Society Task Force on Colorectal Cancer. *Gastrointest. Endosc.* 91 (3): 486–519.

Toon, C.W., Walsh, M.D., Chou, A. et al. (2013). BRAFV600E immunohistochemistry facilitates universal screening of colorectal cancers for lynch syndrome. *Am J. Surg. Pathol.* 37: 1592–1602.

Trock, B., Lanza, E., and Greenwald, P. (1990). Dietary fiber, vegetables, and colon cancer: critical review and meta-analyses of the epidemiologic evidence. *J. Natl. Cancer Inst.* 82: 650–661.

Ueno, H., Mochizuki, H., Hashiguchi, Y. et al. (2004). Risk factors for an adverse outcome in early invasive colorectal carcinoma. *Gastroenterology* 127: 385–394.

Vasen, H.F. (2000). Clinical diagnosis and management of hereditary colorectal cancer syndromes. *J. Clin. Oncol.* 18: 81S–92S.

Vasen, H.F., Mecklin, J.P., Khan, P.M. et al. (1991). The International Collaborative Group on Hereditary Non-Polyposis Colorectal Cancer (ICG-HNPCC). *Dis. Colon Rectum* 34: 424–425.

de Wilde, R.F., Heaphy, C.M., Maitra, A. et al. (2012). Loss of ATRX or DAXX expression and concomitant acquisition of the alternative lengthening of telomeres phenotype are late events in a small subset of MEN-1 syndrome pancreatic neuroendocrine tumors. *Mod. Pathol.* 25 (7): 1033–1039.

Williams, J.G., Pullan, R.D., Hill, J. et al. (2013). Management of the malignant colorectal polyp: ACPGBI position statement. *Color. Dis.* 15 (Suppl 2): 1–38.

Yachida, S., Vakiani, E., White, C.M. et al. (2012). Small cell and large cell neuroendocrine carcinomas of the pancreas are genetically similar and distinct from well-differentiated pancreatic neuroendocrine tumors. *Am. J. Surg. Pathol.* 36 (2): 173–184.

Zhang, J.C., Wang, Y., Wang, X.K. et al. (2016). Type I enteropathy-associated T-cell lymphoma in the colon of a 29-year-old patient and a brief literature review. *Oncol. Targets. Ther.* 9: 863–868.

13

Inflammatory Conditions of the Anus

Thomas Arnason[1] and Michael B. Wallace[2]

[1]*Department of Pathology, Dalhousie University, Halifax, Canada*
[2]*Mayo Clinic, Jacksonville, Florida, USA*

The anal canal, for which the anorectal ring and anal verge represent the proximal and distal boundaries, respectively, is divided at the halfway point by the dentate line and has three types of mucosa, including colorectal mucosa proximally, transitional mucosa immediately proximal to the dentate line, and nonkeratinizing squamous mucosa distally. This chapter discusses inflammatory and infectious diseases that involve the anal canal and perianal skin (located within 5 cm of the anal verge).

Anal Fissure

Definition, General Features, and Predisposing Factors

Anal fissures are linear tears developing in the distal anal canal mucosa below the dentate line. Their development is usually related to increased internal anal sphincter tone or spasm, with local ischemia. These are increasingly diagnosed in postpartum women, and in patients with a low fiber diet and constipation. Inflammatory bowel disease (IBD) and infections such as human immunodeficiency virus and syphilis are also known risk factors.

Clinical Features and Endoscopic Characteristics

Patients commonly present with pain and bleeding. The majority of anal fissures will heal within six weeks of onset. Others are of longer duration and are referred to as chronic.

Microscopic Features

The microscopic findings are nonspecific, with mucosal ulceration and inflammation, usually with granulation tissue, representing the diagnostic features. The surrounding squamous mucosa can be hypertrophic and can display reactive changes. In its extreme form, a polypoid projection at the dentate line known as a sentinel tag or a hypertrophied anal papilla can be observed. In chronic lesions, extensive fibrosis can develop, at times involving the anal sphincter muscle (Figure 13.1).

Differential Diagnosis

In chronic anal fissures, secondary causes such as IBD should be considered.

Treatment/Prognosis/Evolution

Treatment of chronic anal fissures typically starts with medical therapy including fiber supplementation to loosen stools, warm sitz baths to relax the anal sphincter, and topical vasodilators/smooth muscle relaxants such as nifedipine or nitroglycerin. If these measures fail, surgical therapy is typically more effective. Surgery is primarily based on releasing the sphincter muscle with a lateral internal sphincterotomy. This heals fissures in approximately 95% of individuals. The major risk of surgery is fecal incontinence, which occurs in approximately 14%, although only about 1% have major fecal soilage.

Hemorrhoids

Definition, General Features, and Predisposing Factors

Hemorrhoids are polypoid protrusions composed of dilated and commonly prolapsed submucosal blood vessels that may arise proximal to the dentate line (internal hemorrhoid)

Gastrointestinal Pathology: Correlative Endoscopic and Histologic Assessment, First Edition. Edited by Gregory Y. Lauwers and Michael B. Wallace.

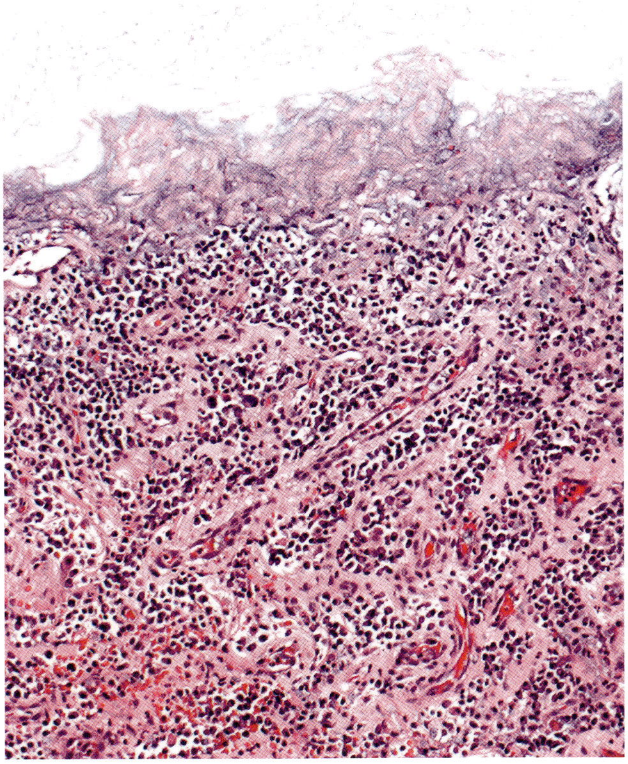

Figure 13.1 Example of anal fissure lined by inflamed granulation tissue and with ulceration of the mucosa.

or distal to it (external hemorrhoids). Causes leading to increased abdominal pressure such as constipation, pregnancy, ascites, and large intra-abdominal masses are risk factors. Increased anal sphincter tone and straining at defecation are also predisposing conditions.

Clinical Features and Endoscopic Characteristics

Hemorrhoids may be asymptomatic or present with bleeding, discomfort, or acute pain. They can be visualized with either direct examination, anoscopy, or during colonoscopy with retroflexion of the endoscope in the rectum (Figure 13.2a). There is a continuum of severity from prominent anal vein to large thrombosed hemorrhoids.

Microscopic Features

Hemorrhoids appear as dilated, thick-walled submucosal blood vessels. Thrombi and hemorrhage are frequently observed. Colorectal or transitional type mucosa lines internal hemorrhoids, while squamous epithelium lines external hemorrhoids (Figure 13.2b, c).

Treatment/Prognosis/Evolution

Treatment is typically topical corticosteroids or astringent agents (witch hazel) although in severe cases, especially with internal hemorrhoids, various devices are available to induce thrombosis and eradication such as rubber band ligation.

Anal (Rectal) Tonsil

Definition, General Features, and Predisposing Factors

Anal (rectal) tonsil is a discrete polypoid lesion formed by hyperplastic mucosal-associated lymphoid tissue. In most patients, no distinct etiology is recognized. The role of infection has been suggested in part because of the role of chlamydial infection in one report.

Clinical Features and Endoscopic Characteristics

Anal tonsil presents as small nodules, usually measuring about 1 cm in size just proximal to the dentate line. Patients may present with rectal bleeding or constipation. The lesion may also be an incidental finding on digital rectal exam or endoscopy.

Microscopic Features

The diagnostic features are the expansion of the mucosa and submucosal tissue by benign lymphoid tissue with occasional germinal centers. Cryptitis and increased intraepithelial lymphocytes can be observed in the overlying mucosa.

Histochemical, Immunohistochemical, and Molecular Features

An immunohistochemical panel may be helpful to rule out lymphoma if there is any doubt, particularly if the follicular architecture is distorted by crush artifact. In a benign tonsil, the lymphoid follicles are characterized by a preserved CD21 or CD23-positive dendritic cell network, while CD20-positive B cells are confined to the follicles, and CD3-positive T cells are limited to the interfollicular zone. Intraepithelial lymphocytes in a benign process are typically CD3-positive. Lymphomas may need to be ruled out, including extranodal marginal zone lymphoma, mantle cell lymphoma, and follicular lymphoma. In marginal zone lymphoma, the B-cell infiltrate extends beyond the follicles and into the crypts. B cells may demonstrate aberrant CD43 expression and monotypic kappa or lambda light chain

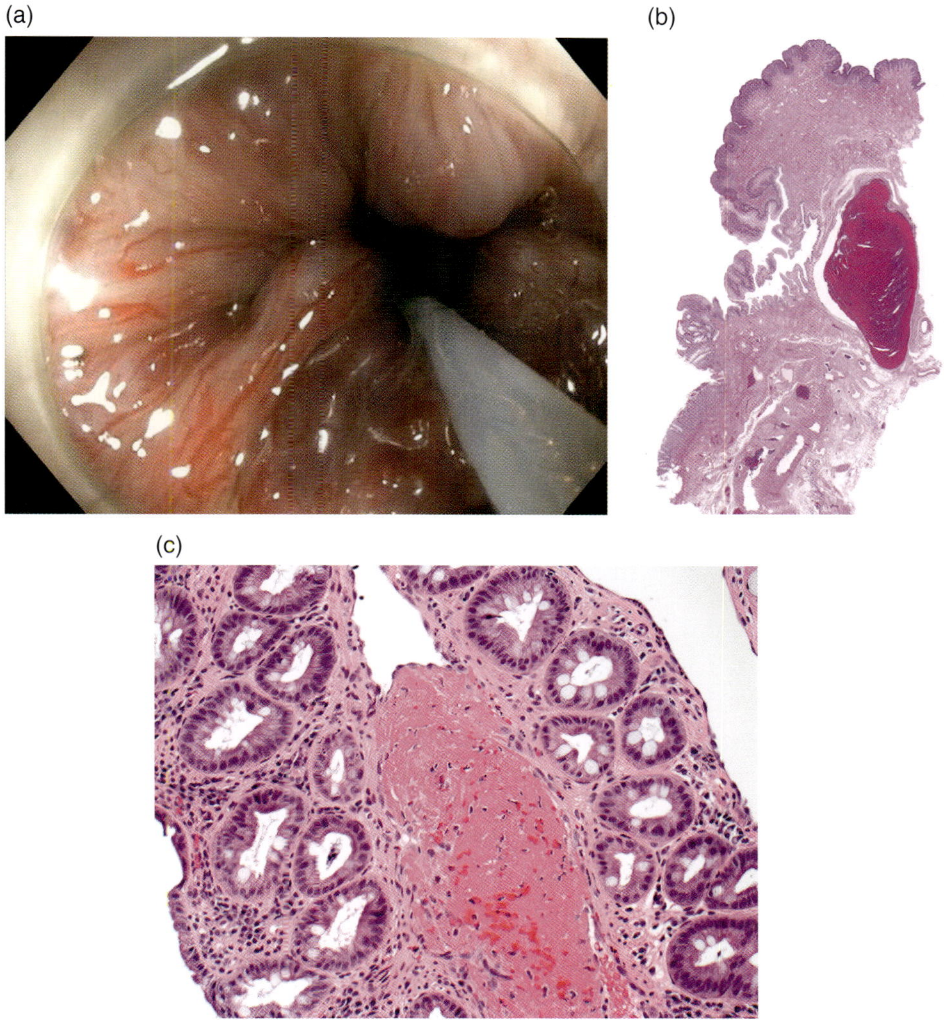

Figure 13.2 (a) Large external hemorrhoid seen via anoscopy. A snare device is used to demonstrate the lumen. (b) Characteristic appearance of hemorrhoid with markedly dilated blood vessel underlying the squamocolumnar junctional mucosa of the anal canal. (c) Fibrin thrombus present in a smaller branch of a hemorrhoid blood vessel.

expression. In mantle cell lymphoma, immunopositivity for CD5 and cyclinD1 in the neoplastic B cells is a distinctive feature. Finally, in follicular lymphoma, the follicles typically co-express CD20, CD10, BCL-2, and BCL-6.

Differential Diagnosis

Endoscopically, the differential includes small polyps, i.e. rectal adenomas, hyperplastic polyp, an anal canal hemorrhoid, or a fibroepithelial polyp. Histologically, it is most critical not to confuse this entity with a lymphoproliferative disorder. A panel of immunohistochemical stains, as described above, can help resolve this differential. Lymphoid follicular proctitis is another condition with similar histologic features to anal tonsil, but with a much different endoscopic picture, since it tends to diffusely involve the rectum and distal sigmoid.

Treatment/Prognosis/Evolution

Anal tonsil lesions are typically found incidentally as an atypical polyp or nodule and may be diagnosed by endoscopic polypectomy or biopsy. Once diagnosed and other more sinister (lymphoma) diagnoses are excluded, no specific therapy is needed. Most lesions resolve spontaneously.

Hidradenitis Suppurativa

Definition, General Features, and Predisposing Factors

Hidradenitis suppurativa is a chronic inflammatory disease involving the skin and subcutaneous tissue at sites with apocrine glands. Obesity and smoking have been identified as risk factors.

Clinical Features and Endoscopic Characteristics

Young adults are most commonly affected. Common symptomatology includes pruritus and burning sensation, and pain or tenderness. Abscesses superficial fistulas, and sinuses can develop as well.

Microscopic Features

The histologic features of hidradenitis suppurativa are not entirely specific. Early findings include occlusion of hair follicles by keratin plugs and perifolliculitis. There is a mixed lymphoplasmacytic infiltrate extending into the submucosa. If the disease progresses, ulcers, abscesses, and sinus tracts develop. Scattered giant cells are often identified, but well-formed granulomas are usually not present. Late in the course of the disease, fibrous scarring occurs.

Differential Diagnosis

Fistulas secondary to Crohn's disease (CD) and fistulas arising from anal gland abscesses need to be excluded. Patients with Crohn's often have known intestinal disease. The fistula tracts of Crohn's tend to be located the most deeply, often tracking deep to both internal and external sphincter muscles, and arise more proximally in the low rectal mucosa. Well-formed granulomas may be present in Crohn's. The fistulas secondary to anal gland abscesses often involve the intersphincteric space. In contrast, the sinuses and fistulas of hidradenitis suppurativa tend to be superficial to the sphincter muscle and arise only in the distal anal canal and perianal skin, which contains the inciting hair follicles and adnexal structures.

Treatment/Prognosis/Evolution

Malignant transformation is a rare but well-described complication of long-standing hidradenitis suppurativa. High-risk HPV (specifically HPV-16) has been identified in a majority of squamous cell carcinomas arising in this setting. Hydradenitis is classified by severity using the Hurley scale from mild to severe. Treatment is usually supportive and multifactorial including avoidance of skin trauma, anorectal hygiene, wound dressing, smoking cessation, and diet (avoidance of sugary, high glycemic index foods). Other specific therapies include topical antibiotics, surgical unroofing, and in severe cases, monoclonal antibody therapy with anti-TNF agents similar to CD.

Anal Abscess and Fistula

Definition, General Features, and Predisposing Factors

Anal abscesses are thought to arise from infection in the anal glands, perhaps due to stasis or obstruction of the duct or gland orifice. They arise in a perianal, submucosal, intersphincteric, ischiorectal, or supralevator location.

Fistulas arise when an anal gland abscess develops a drainage tract to the anal mucosa or the perianal skin. Anal fistulas also arise secondary to CD, which is discussed in the next section. Some anal "fistulas" are actually sinuses, because they have only one epithelial surface opening. Anal fistulas have been classified as low, originating below the dentate line, or high, originating above the dentate line. The Parks classification system is more anatomically precise, and categorizes fistulas as superficial, intersphincteric, transsphincteric, suprasphincteric, and extrasphincteric.

Anal abscesses and fistulas are two to three times more common in males than females, and are more common in the third and fourth decades of life. They occur more commonly in patients with hematologic disease, including leukemia. Cigarette smoking as a risk factor has been recently identified.

Clinical Features and Endoscopic Characteristics

Anal abscesses tend to present with pain, often worse with defecation, or an erythematous, tender mass. Patients may develop a fever. Fistulas may have drainage.

Microscopic Features

Anal abscesses and fistulas display the features of an acute suppurative inflammatory process, with abundant neutrophilic inflammation and a border lined by granulation tissue. Foreign body-type giant cells may be present as a response to fecal matter, and should not be construed as evidence of CD. Fat necrosis, local vasculitis, and skeletal muscle degeneration are often appreciated in the surrounding area.

Differential Diagnosis

It is important to distinguish anal abscesses and fistulas secondary to idiopathic gland obstruction from anal CD, but this may not be possible based on histologic examination of a fistula tract biopsy in isolation. Correlation with the clinical picture and biopsies from other sites is essential. Fistulas associated with Crohn's tend to be more deeply located, and concurrent to intestinal CD. Rarely, perianal tuberculosis also may cause an anal abscess or fistula, but these also are associated with caseating granulomas. Examples of the parasites *Enterobius vermicularis* and *Trichuris trichiura* causing anal abscesses have been reported.

Treatment/Prognosis/Evolution

Treatment is surgical drainage with antibiotics usually reserved for immunosuppressed patients or those at risk for endocarditis.

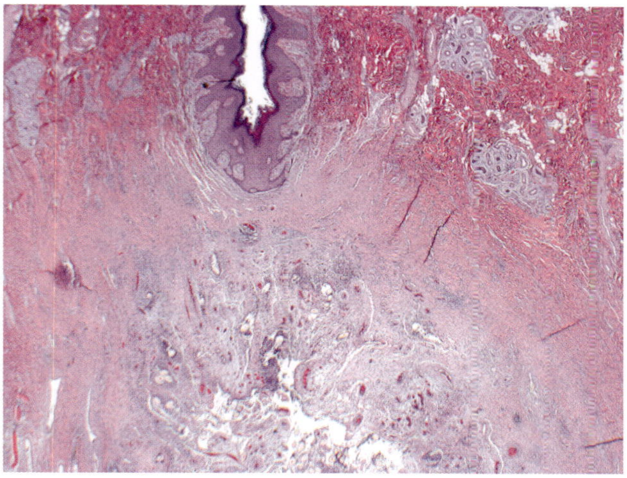

Figure 13.3 Anal involvement by Crohn's disease with granulomatous inflammation underlying the squamous mucosa with inflammatory changes in a patient with an established diagnosis.

Inflammatory Bowel Disease

Definition, General Features, and Predisposing Factors

CD and ulcerative colitis (UC) have characteristic anal and perianal skin manifestations.

Clinical Features and Endoscopic Characteristics

CD is characteristically associated with anal fistulas, which usually have a path located deep to the sphincter muscles. Perianal abscesses, anal strictures, and fissures can also develop. The perianal skin may show ulceration and fibroepithelial polyps (skin tags). While patients with UC tend to have fewer manifestations, they do have increased hemorrhoidal disease, perianal abscesses, and anal fissures when compared to the general population.

Microscopic Features

Abscesses, ulcers, fissures, and fistula tracts have nonspecific features of an inflammatory process, including granulation tissue, mixed inflammation, and healing with fibrosis. Granulomas may be present in Crohn's (Figure 13.3).

Histochemical, Immunohistochemical, and Molecular Features

Histochemical stains may be helpful to rule out infectious mimics, including Ziehl–Neelsen for acid-fast bacilli, Grocott–Gomori's Methenamine Silver (GMS) or periodic acid–Schiff (PAS) for fungi, and Warthin–Starry or Steiner stains for spirochetes. Immunohistochemical stains can be used to identify herpes virus infection. Polymerase chain reaction (PCR) and serology tests are available for a number of infectious diseases that can involve this area, including syphilis, lymphogranuloma venereum, granuloma inguinale, chancroid, and tuberculosis.

Differential Diagnosis

Endoscopic findings diagnostic and biopsies of CD or UC from other sites in the gastrointestinal tract are essential to establish the diagnosis. If the inflammatory changes are confined to the anus and low rectum, there should be a high degree of suspicion for infectious diseases, particularly if there are risk factors for sexually transmitted infections, immunosuppression, or tuberculosis.

Treatment/Prognosis/Evolution

In addition to the symptoms of inflammatory anal disease in CD and UC, patients with IBD have an increased risk of anal carcinomas. Patients with anal CD are at increased risk of both squamous cell carcinoma and adenocarcinoma, although the latter type is more common. The adenocarcinomas include both the usual colorectal type and the rare anal mucinous adenocarcinoma arising from a perianal fistula. There is an increased risk for anal canal adenocarcinoma in patients with UC, which persists following colectomy. At least 15 cases of adenocarcinoma in the anal cuff have been reported in post-colectomy UC patients.

Anorectal Tuberculosis

Definition, General Features, and Predisposing Factors

Anorectal tuberculosis is uncommon but represents an important mimicker of perianal CD, particularly in patients from countries where tuberculosis is endemic. A large proportion of patients have coexisting active pulmonary tuberculosis. The risk is also increased in HIV patients.

Clinical Features and Endoscopic Characteristics

Presenting symptoms include perianal pain and anal discharge. Findings on examination include anal abscess and fistula.

Microscopic Features

The characteristic feature is chronic inflammation including caseating granulomas. Some biopsies reveal only noncaseating granulomas or nonspecific chronic inflammatory changes, raising the differential diagnosis of CD.

Histochemical, Immunohistochemical, and Molecular Features

A Ziehl–Neelsen stain should be performed to identify acid-fast bacilli, but the sensitivity of the stain is notoriously relatively poor. PCR of tissue obtained at biopsy for *Mycobacterium tuberculosis* improves the sensitivity to 64–75%, with 100% specificity. Culture of fresh tissue, fluid, or pus can also be performed.

Differential Diagnosis

The main differentials are anal CD and anal gland abscess or fistula, but the finding of caseating granulomas strongly suggests tuberculosis. When the characteristic granulomas are not present, a high index of suspicion should be considered in higher risk populations.

Treatment

Treatment of any active tuberculosis involves multidrug anti-tuberculin antibiotics. Careful assessment of pulmonary Tb is essential given the public health risk of disease dissemination.

Syphilis

Definition, General Features, and Predisposing Factors

Syphilis, caused by the spirochete *Treponema pallidum,* is divided into primary, secondary, and tertiary stages, of which the first two may involve the anorectum. The incidence of syphilis declined through much of the twentieth century, but has increased since the year 2000 in the United States. Syphilis can be acquired through anoreceptive intercourse. There is an increased risk of anorectal syphilis in men who have sex with men.

Clinical Features and Endoscopic Characteristics

Primary syphilis presents with a chancre (ulcer) at the site of infection within two to six weeks. Secondary syphilis has onset a few weeks later and typically presents with a maculopapular skin eruption, often affecting the palms and soles. The condyloma lata of secondary syphilis are warty lesions that can involve the anus.

Microscopic Features

The histologic features of syphilis proctitis include mucosal ulceration, a plasma cell-rich inflammatory infiltrate of the lamina propria, and ill-formed granulomas. Features of active proctitis including cryptitis and crypt abscesses can be present. Condyloma lata involving the anal squamous mucosa is characterized by acanthosis and papillomatosis, with wide and elongated rete pegs. Edema and neutrophilic inflammation are present in the superficial squamous mucosa, and a dense plasma cell rich infiltrate is present in the lamina propria (Figure 13.4a, b).

Histochemical, Immunohistochemical, and Molecular Features

Silver stains (i.e. Warthin–Starry and Steiner) can be used to identify spirochetes. An immunohistochemical stain is also available. PCR of biopsy tissue for syphilis is possible. Serological tests such as Venereal Disease Research Laboratory (VDRL) or rapid plasma reagin (RPR) and the more specific anti-treponemal tests such as the fluorescent treponemal antibody absorption test can be used to make the diagnosis.

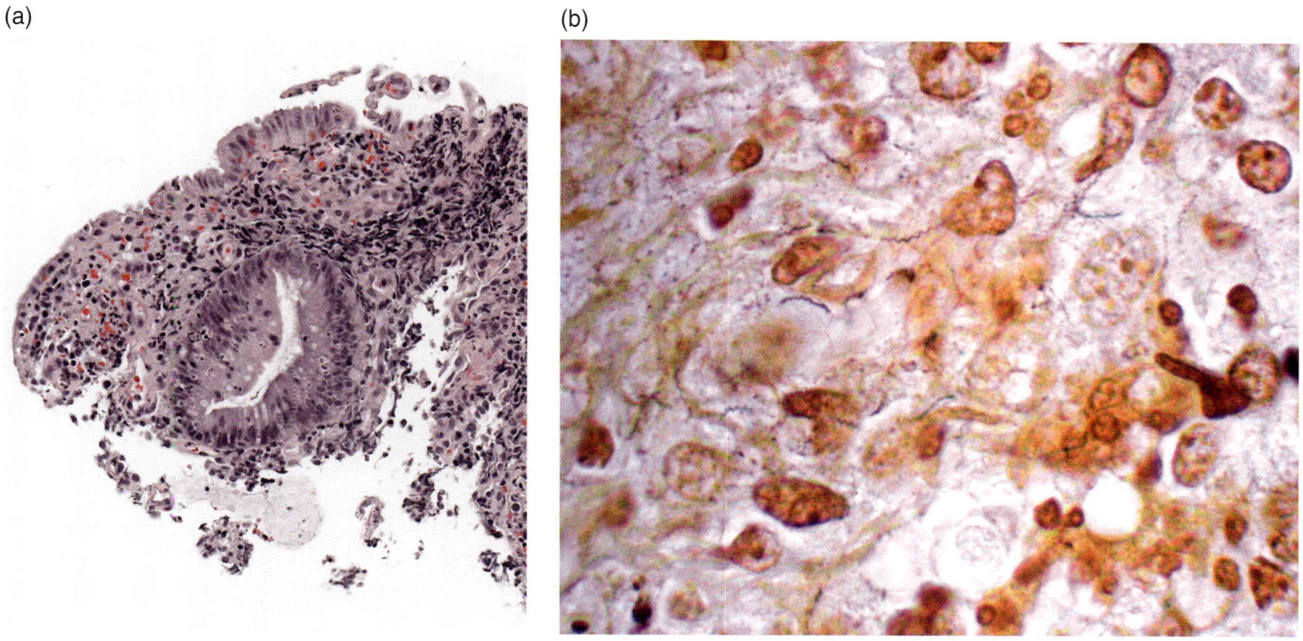

Figure 13.4 (a) Syphilis proctitis: Cryptitis and expanded lamina propria inflammatory infiltrate, typically rich in plasma cells, are present. The histology can mimic inflammatory bowel disease. *Source:* Photo courtesy Dr. Erica Schollenberg. (b) A Steiner stain highlights the spirochetes (*Treponema pallidum*) in a case of syphilis proctitis. *Source:* Photo courtesy Dr. Erica Schollenberg.

Differential Diagnosis

Crohn's disease is the main differential diagnosis, with significant clinical and histologic overlap. Other infectious diseases such as tuberculosis and lymphogranuloma venereum should be entertained.

Treatment/Prognosis/Evolution

Syphilis is usually responsive to penicillin (2.4 million units intramuscular (IM) weekly) for three weeks. Alternatives include doxycycline or ceftriaxone.

Lymphogranuloma Venereum

Definition, General Features, and Predisposing Factors

Lymphogranuloma venereum is a sexually transmitted infection caused by the Gram-negative bacterium *Chlamydia trachomatis*. Men who have sex with men are at the greatest risk of infection, particularly those who are HIV-positive. Anoreceptive intercourse is a risk factor for lymphogranuloma proctitis.

Clinical Features and Endoscopic Characteristics

The presentation and features depend on the site of infection, which occurs at a site of direct mucocutaneous contact, and the time interval since inoculation. The infection tends to spread to the inguinal and femoral lymph nodes with genital infection and to the perirectal or pelvic nodes with inguinal infection. There are three chronologic stages. The first, occurring within a month, is a painless papule at the site of infection that evolves into an ulcer. In the second stage, usually a few weeks later, tender lymphadenopathy (i.e. "buboes") can develop, which may form fistula tracts to the skin. The proctitis occurs in the third stage, and includes symptoms of bloody diarrhea and tenesmus, often with onset months to years after infection. The proctitis is characterized by granular, erythematous mucosa with exudative erosions and ulceration, localized to the distal rectum and increasing in severity distally.

Microscopic Features

The nonspecific features of active proctocolitis include cryptitis, crypt abscesses, and ulceration, with an increased chronic inflammatory cell infiltrate in the lamina propria.

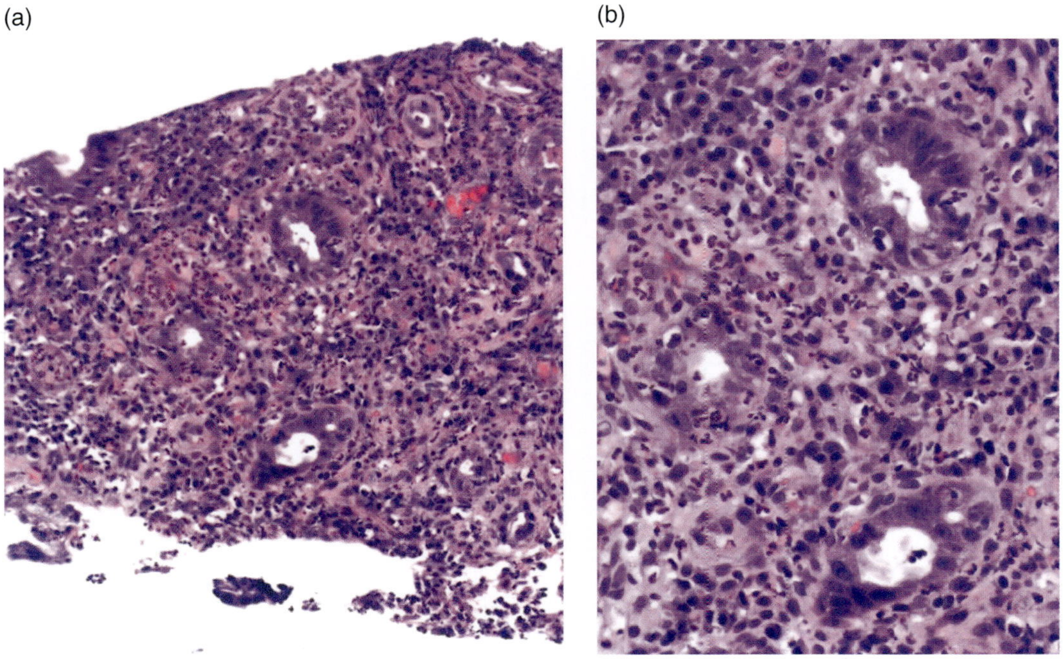

Figure 13.5 (a) Columnar mucosa with expanded lamina propria inflammatory infiltrate, cryptitis, and surface erosion in a biopsy from a case of confirmed lymphogranuloma venereum. (b) Lymphogranuloma venereum: a higher magnification view highlights the plasma cell rich lamina propria inflammatory infiltrate and cryptitis.

Granulomas, some with central stellate abscesses typical of lymph node infection, are occasionally identified. Features of chronicity, i.e. crypt architectural distortion and basal lymphoplasmacytic inflammation, can be present, but usually to a lesser degree than seen in IBD (Figure 13.5a, b).

Histochemical, Immunohistochemical, and Molecular Features

The organisms are not easily identified on light microscopy, but can be detected using histochemical stains such as Brown–Hopps and Warthin–Starry. However, nucleic acid amplification tests for *C. trachomatis* using PCR are more sensitive and specific.

Differential Diagnosis

The major differential diagnosis is IBD. Clinical suspicion should arise from a history of risk factors and limitation of the disease to the distal rectum and anus. Crypt architectural distortion and basal lymphoplasmacytic inflammation are uncommon in lymphogranuloma venereum, but cannot be relied upon to definitively differentiate lymphogranuloma venereum from IBD. Rarely, lymphogranuloma venereum can be complicated by transmural inflammation, and such cases are essentially histologically indistinguishable from Crohn's. Other infections may have a similar histologic appearance, but viral infections (e.g. cytomegalovirus (CMV) and herpes) can be confirmed with immunohistochemical stains. Tuberculosis and syphilis tend to have more granulomatous inflammation, and the organisms can be identified by special stains or ancillary molecular or serologic tests.

Treatment, Prognosis, Evolution

Antibiotic treatment is recommended with standard doxycycline 100 mg twice daily for 21 days with erythromycin 500 mg daily as second line therapy. Sexual partners should also be tested and treated. Late-stage disease is characterized by fibrosis and strictures as well as elephantiasis and fistulae, which may not resolve with antibiotics.

Granuloma Inguinale

Definition and General Features

Granuloma inguinale, also known as donovanosis, is a sexually transmitted infection caused by the Gram-negative bacterium *Klebsiella (Calymmatobacterium) granulomatis*. It is relatively more common in tropical and subtropical countries than in North America.

Clinical Features and Endoscopic Characteristics

The disease is most common in young adult males. The infection causes a non-painful anal ulcer.

Microscopic Features

Mucosal ulceration is the cardinal feature, associated with a mixed acute and chronic inflammatory infiltrate. Numerous large histiocytes can be seen (25–90 µm in diameter) containing the diagnostic Donovan bodies, which are bacterial organisms measuring 0.5–0.7 wide by 1–1.5 µm long. Adjacent pseudoepitheliomatous hyperplasia of the squamous mucosa should not be mistaken for a squamous cell carcinoma.

Histochemical, Immunohistochemical, and Molecular Features

Giemsa stain is helpful in highlighting the chromatin at each end of the bacterium in blue, in a pattern resembling a safety pin. Warthin–Starry stain also highlights the organisms. Ancillary tests including serology, viral culture, and viral PCR are also available.

Differential Diagnosis

The differential diagnosis of anal ulceration includes IBD and other infectious diseases of the anorectum.

Treatment/Prognosis/Evolution

Antibiotics are effective against granuloma inguinale including doxycycline 100 mg twice daily, azithromycin 1 g weekly, or ciprofloxacin 750 mg twice a day (BID) among others, all for 21 days.

Chancroid

Definition and General Features

Chancroid is a sexually transmitted infection caused by the Gram-negative bacterium *Haemophilus ducreyi*. Chancroid is more common in developing countries than in the West. HIV infection increases the susceptibility to infection.

Clinical Features and Endoscopic Characteristics

Patients present with painful ulcers several days after sexual contact. While involvement of the genitalia is more common, patients may present with perianal ulcers and tender, enlarged regional lymph nodes.

Microscopic Features

The ulcers may display three distinct zones. The narrow superficial layer is composed of fibrinopurulent debris. The middle layer is composed of inflamed and edematous stroma with dilated thin-walled blood vessels that are associated with neutrophilic inflammation and degenerate at the junction with the superficial zone. The deep zone contains a dense predominantly plasmacytic infiltrate, with a smaller contingent of lymphocytes.

Histochemical, Immunohistochemical, and Molecular Features

A Gram stain may identify Gram-negative coccobacilli in the superficial fibrinopurulent exudate of the ulcer. Serology, culture, and PCR amplification are more specific.

Differential Diagnosis

Other sexually transmitted infections causing perianal ulceration including herpes simplex virus, syphilis, and lymphogranuloma venereum should be considered.

Treatment/Prognosis/Evolution

Recommended treatments include azithromycin 1 g PO ("per os" meaning "taken by mouth") daily or ceftriaxone 250 mg IM both as a single dose. Prognosis is good with treatment response in two to three days in most individuals. Infected individuals should refrain from sexual contact until all lesions are healed. Sexual partners should be treated regardless of whether they are symptomatic.

Herpes Simplex Virus

Definition, General Features, and Predisposing Factors

Anal herpes infections are usually sexually transmitted and historically secondary to HSV-2 DNA virus infection. However, the proportion of anogenital infection associated with HSV-1 has increased.

Herpes infection is commonly spread by anoreceptive intercourse or oral-anal contact. The infection can also spread to the anus from genital infection.

Clinical Features and Endoscopic Characteristics

The main presenting symptoms are anal pain, pruritus, or discharge. The lesions are fluid filled vesicles that ulcerate.

Microscopic Features

The squamous mucosa is usually ulcerated, while a neutrophilic infiltrate and crypt abscesses may be seen in the rectal mucosa. The squamous cells at the lip of the ulcer are the best site to identify the characteristic viral cytopathic effects, i.e. multinucleation, margination of chromatin, nuclear molding, and increased nuclear size. Intranuclear inclusions (Cowdry A inclusions) may be present.

Histochemical, Immunohistochemical, and Molecular Features

Immunohistochemical stains for HSV-1 and HSV-2, as well as viral culture, viral DNA detection by PCR, and serology can be performed to support and/or confirm the diagnosis in difficult cases.

Differential Diagnosis

CMV infections are rare in the anus and occur mainly in immunocompromised individuals, including AIDS patients.

TTreatment/Prognosis/Evolution

Anal HSV is treated similarly to other genital HSV infections, with oral antiviral agents. Preferred agents include acyclovir, famciclovir, and valacyclovir, typically for five days. Complete response rates range from 54 to 59%. Recurrent cases are treated with chronic suppressive antiviral agents.

Further Reading

Anderson, M.J. Jr. and Dockerty, M.B. (1958). Perianal hidradenitis suppurativa; a clinical and pathologic study. *Dis. Colon Rectum* 1 (1): 23–31.

Bodsworth, N.J., Crooks, R.J., Borelli, S. et al. (1997). Valaciclovir versus aciclovir in patient initiated treatment of recurrent genital herpes: a randomised, double blind clinical trial. International Valaciclovir HSV Study Group. *Genitourin. Med.* 73 (2): 110.

Boer, J. and Weltevreden, E.F. (1996). Hidradenitis suppurativa or acne inversa. A clinicopathological study of early lesions. *Br. J. Dermatol.* 135 (5): 721–725.

Bouguen, G., Siproudhis, L., Bretagne, J.F. et al. (2010). Nonfistulizing perianal Crohn's disease: clinical features, epidemiology, and treatment. *Inflamm. Bowel Dis.* 16 (8): 1431–1442.

Brown, A.C., Sumfest, J.M., and Rozwadowski, J.V. (1989). Histopathology of the internal anal sphincter in chronic anal fissure. *Dis. Colon Rectum* 32 (8): 680–683.

Carter, J.S., Bowden, F.J., Bastian, I. et al. (1999). Phylogenetic evidence for reclassification of Calymmatobacterium granulomatis as Klebsiella granulomatis comb. *Int. J. Syst. Bacteriol.* 49 (Pt 4): 1695–1700.

Chambers, W.M. and Mc, C.M.N.J. (2007). Should ileal pouch-anal anastomosis include mucosectomy? *Color. Dis.* 9 (5): 384–392.

Cramer, S.F., Romansky, S., Hulbert, B. et al. (2009). The rectal tonsil: a reaction to chlamydial infection? *Am. J. Surg. Pathol.* 33 (3): 483.

Culp, C.E. (1983). Chronic hidradenitis suppurativa of the anal canal. A surgical skin disease. *Dis. Colon Rectum* 26 (10): 669–676.

Cunningham, S.E., Johnson, M.D., and Laczek, J.T. (2012). Lymphogranuloma venereum proctitis. *Gastrointest. Endosc.* 75 (6): 1269–1270.

Davis, B.T., Thiim, M., and Zukerberg, L.R. (2006). Case records of the Massachusetts General Hospital. Case 2-2006. A 31-year-old, HIV-positive man with rectal pain. *N. Engl. J. Med.* 354 (3): 284–289.

Devaraj, B., Khabassi, S., and Cosman, B.C. (2011). Recent smoking is a risk factor for anal abscess and fistula. *Dis. Colon Rectum* 54 (6): 681–685.

Devon, K.M., Brown, C.J., Burnstein, M., and McLeod, R.S. (2009). Cancer of the anus complicating perianal Crohn's disease. *Dis. Colon Rectum* 52 (2): 211–216.

Farris, A.B., Lauwers, G.Y., Ferry, J.A., and Zukerberg, L.R. (2008). The rectal tonsil: a reactive lymphoid proliferation that may mimic lymphoma. *Am. J. Surg. Pathol.* 32 (7): 1075–1079.

Feigen, G.M. (1987). Suppurative anal cryptitis associated with Trichuris trichiura. Report of a case. *Dis. Colon Rectum* 30 (8): 620–622.

Freinkel, A.L. (1987). Histological aspects of sexually transmitted genital lesions. *Histopathology* 11 (8): 819–831.

Furman, D.L., Patel, S.K., and Arluk, G.M. (2008). Endoscopic and histologic appearance of rectal syphilis. *Gastrointest. Endosc.* 67 (1): 161. commentary-2.

Gallegos, M., Bradly, D., Jakate, S., and Keshavarzian, A. (2012). Lymphogranuloma venereum proctosigmoiditis is a mimicker of inflammatory bowel disease. *World J. Gastroenterol.* 18 (25): 3317–3321.

Garg, P., Garg, M., and Menon, G.R. (2013). Long-term continence disturbance after lateral internal

sphincterotomy for chronic anal fissure: a systematic review and meta-analysis. *Color. Dis.* 15 (3): e104–e117.
Haddow, L.J., Dave, B., Mindel, A. et al. (2006). Increase in rates of herpes simplex virus type 1 as a cause of anogenital herpes in western Sydney, Australia, between 1979 and 2003. *Sex. Transm. Infect.* 82 (3): 255–259.
Hadfield, T.L., Lamy, Y., and Wear, D.J. (1995). Demonstration of Chlamydia trachomatis in inguinal lymphadenitis of lymphogranuloma venereum: a light microscopy, electron microscopy and polymerase chain reaction study. *Mod. Pathol.* 8 (9): 924–929.
Hamzaoglu, I. and Hodin, R.A. (2005). Perianal problems in patients with ulcerative colitis. *Inflamm. Bowel Dis.* 11 (9): 856–859.
Hart, C.A. and Rao, S.K. (1999). Donovanosis. *J. Med. Microbiol.* 48 (8): 707–709.
Hoentjen, F. and Rubin, D.T. (2012). Infectious proctitis: when to suspect it is not inflammatory bowel disease. *Dig. Dis. Sci.* 57 (2): 269–273.
Hulme-Moir, M. and Bartolo, D.C. (2001). Hemorrhoids. *Gastroenterol. Clin. N. Am.* 30 (1): 183–197.
Jacobs, E. (1976). Anal infections caused by herpes simplex virus. *Dis. Colon Rectum* 19 (2): 151–157.
Jonas, M. and Scholefield, J.H. (2001). Anal Fissure. *Gastroenterol. Clin. N. Am.* 30 (1): 167–181.
King, R., Gough, J., Ronald, A. et al. (1996). An immunohistochemical analysis of naturally occurring chancroid. *J. Infect. Dis.* 174 (2): 427–430.
Lagergard, T., Bolin, I., and Lindholm, L. (2011). On the evolution of the sexually transmitted bacteria Haemophilus ducreyi and Klebsiella granulomatis. *Ann. N. Y. Acad. Sci.* 1230: E1–E10.
Lavogiez, C., Delaporte, E., Darras-Vercambre, S. et al. (2010). Clinicopathological study of 13 cases of squamous cell carcinoma complicating hidradenitis suppurativa. *Dermatology* 220 (2): 147–153
Maitra, R.K., Bowling, T., Venkatesan, P., and Maxwell-Armstrong, C. (2012). Crohn's disease or TB – the perennial question and diagnostic pitfalls. *BMJ Case Rep.* 2012.
Mansour, M. and Weston, L A. (2010). Perianal infections: a primer for nonsurgeons. *Curr. Gastroenterol. Rep.* 12 (4): 270–279.
Martin, I.M., Alexander, S.A., Ison, C.A. et al. (2006). Diagnosis of lymphogranuloma venereum from biopsy samples. *Gut* 55 (10): 1522–1523.
McCallion, K. and Gardiner, K.R. (2001). Progress in the understanding and treatment of chronic anal fissure. *Postgrad. Med. J.* 77 (914): 753–758.
Mortensen, N.J. and Thomson, J.P. (1984). Perianal abscess due to Enterobius vermicularis. Report of a case. *Dis. Colon Rectum* 27 (10): 677–678.
Nagot, N., Ouedraogo, A., Ouangre, A. et al. (2005). Is sexually transmitted infection management among sex workers still able to mitigate the spread of HIV infection in West Africa? *J. Acquir. Immune Defic. Syndr.* 39 (4): 454–458.
O'Farrell, N. (2002). Donovanosis. *Sex. Transm. Infect.* 78 (6): 452–457.
Papagrigoriadis, S. and Rennie, J.A. (1998). Lymphogranuloma venereum as a cause of rectal strictures. *Postgrad. Med. J.* 74 (869): 168–169.
Parks, A.G. (1961). Pathogenesis and treatment of fistuila-in-ano. *Br. Med. J.* 1 (5224): 463–469.
Parks, A.G., Gordon, P.H., and Hardcastle, J.D. (1976). A classification of fistula-in-ano. *Br. J. Surg.* 63 (1): 1–12.
Puy-Montbrun, T., Ganansia, R., Lemarchand, N. et al. (1990). Anal ulcerations due to cytomegalovirus in patients with AIDS. Report of six cases. *Dis. Colon Rectum* 33 (12): 1041–1043.
Sheer, T.A. and Coyle, W.J. (2003). Gastrointestinal tuberculosis. *Curr. Gastroenterol. Rep.* 5 (4): 273–278.
Shelat, V.G., Ng, S.R., and Sim, R. (2011). Perianal abscess secondary to enterobius vermicularis infestation. *Ann. Acad. Med. Singap.* 40 (3): 149.
Su, J.R., Beltrami, J.F., Zaidi, A.A., and Weinstock, H.S. (2011). Primary and secondary syphilis among black and Hispanic men who have sex with men: case report data from 27 states. *Ann. Intern. Med.* 155 (3): 145–151.
Tai, W.C., Hu, T.H., Lee, C.H. et al. (2010). Ano-perianal tuberculosis: 15 years of clinical experiences in Southern Taiwan. *Color. Dis.* 12 (7Online): e114–e120.
Vanhueverzwyn, R., Delannoy, A., Michaux, J.L., and Dive, C. (1980). Anal lesions in hematologic diseases. *Dis. Colon Rectum* 23 (5): 310–312.
Wollina, U., Tilp, M., Meseg, A. et al. (2012). Management of severe anogenital acne inversa (hidradenitis suppurativa). *Dermatol. Surg.* 38 (1): 110–117.
Workowski, K.A. and Bolan, G.A. (2015). Centers for Disease Control and Prevention. Sexually transmitted diseases treatment guidelines, 2015. *MMWR Recomm. Rep.* 64: 1.
Yilmaz, M., Memisoglu, R., Aydin, S. et al. (2011). Anorectal syphilis mimicking Crohn's disease. *J. Infect. Chemother.* 17 (5): 713–715.

14

Polyps and Neoplastic Lesions of the Anus

Thomas Arnason[1], Michael B. Wallace[2] and Till S. Clauditz[3]

[1]Department of Pathology, Dalhousie University, Halifax, Canada
[2]Mayo Clinic, Jacksonville, Florida, USA
[3]Department of Pathology, University-Medical-Center Hamburg-Eppendorf, Hamburg, Germany

This chapter addresses neoplastic and non-neoplastic polyps of the anal canal and perianal skin. There is detailed discussion of the more common neoplasms of the anus including anal intraepithelial neoplasia (AIN), squamous cell carcinoma, adenocarcinoma, melanoma, and Paget's disease. Several uncommon neoplasms are discussed briefly.

Inflammatory Cloacogenic Polyp

Definition, General Features, and Predisposing Factors

This benign mucosal polyp represents a prolapse of the anal transitional zone. These polyps have features similar to mucosal prolapse polyps at other locations, including solitary rectal ulcer syndrome, inflammatory fibrin cap polyps, inflammatory myoglandular polyps, and prolapsing folds of diverticular disease. Whether straining at defecation has a role in the development of inflammatory cloacogenic polyps is not well established.

Clinical Features and Endoscopic Characteristics

Rectal bleeding, anal pruritus, and anal tenderness associated with defecation are among the common complaints. In some patients the polyp can be observed protruding from the anal verge. Anoscopy reveals a polyp with a stalk originating in the anal transitional zone.

Microscopic Features

The frequently eroded and inflamed surface of inflammatory cloacogenic polyp is usually composed of a combination of reactive colonic, squamous, and transitional type mucosa. A common finding is proctitis cystica profunda, formed of colonic crypts misplaced in the submucosa, along with splaying of the muscularis mucosa into the lamina propria. Acellular mucin pools, if present, should not be misconstrued as evidence of neoplasia (Figure 14.1a, b).

Immunohistochemistry

In some cases, special stains might be useful to obviate cancers or dysplasia. Ki67, p16, and p53 have been reported to be helpful to rule out squamous and columnar dysplasia.

Differential Diagnosis

Clinically, the differential diagnosis includes other causes of anal polyps such as hemorrhoids, fibroepithelial polyps, and low-lying rectal adenomas.

Treatment/Prognosis/Evolution

Cloacogenic polyps are benign and generally do not require resection unless causing bleeding, or become large enough to cause fecal seepage. Conservative treatment includes avoidance of straining with stool softeners and fiber supplementation, and topical emollients and corticosteroids. In severe cases, minor surgical resection is required similar to hemorrhoidectomy or suture ligation.

Gastrointestinal Pathology: Correlative Endoscopic and Histologic Assessment, First Edition. Edited by Gregory Y. Lauwers and Michael B. Wallace.

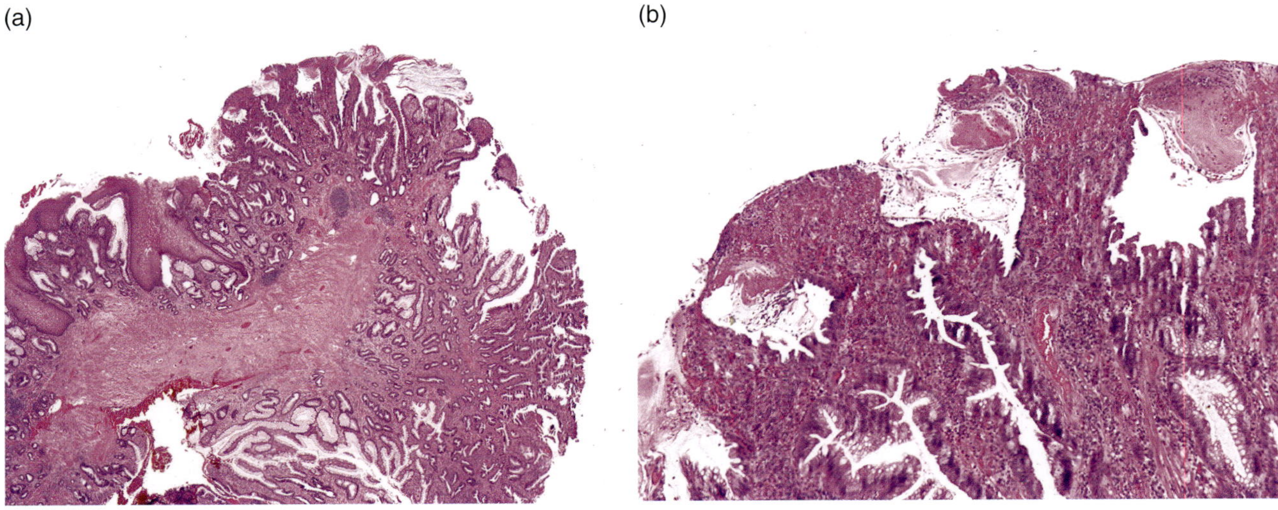

Figure 14.1 (a) Inflammatory cloacogenic polyp: The polyp is composed of elongated, slightly serrated crypts with splaying of the muscularis mucosa between the crypts. (b) Inflammatory cloacogenic polyp: The surface of the polyp is eroded with associated reactive changes in the epithelium, including nuclear enlargement and mucin depletion.

Fibroepithelial Polyp

Definition, General Features, and Predisposing Factors

This common benign lesion is sometimes reported as anal tag or hypertrophied anal papilla. Fibroepithelial polyps are likely reactive in nature, perhaps secondary to local irritation or infection, and are thought to arise from enlargement of the anal papillae.

Clinical Features and Endoscopic Characteristics

Fibroepithelial polyps arise from papillae at the level of the dentate line, and resemble hemorrhoids. They are usually small, but rare examples of giant fibroepithelial polyp causing bowel obstruction have been observed.

Microscopic Features

The bulk of the polyp is composed of expanded connective tissue with various areas of fibroblasts and myofibroblasts with occasional smooth muscle within a variably collagenous or myxoid stroma. Mast cells are typically observed. Scattered bizarre multinucleated fibroblasts or myofibroblasts, which are large and stellate, may be seen occasionally. The overlying benign squamous mucosa is often hyperplastic and may show hyperkeratosis, parakeratosis, or ulceration. The superficial keratinocytes often contain large cytoplasmic vacuoles containing homogenous eosinophilic material (Figure 14.2).

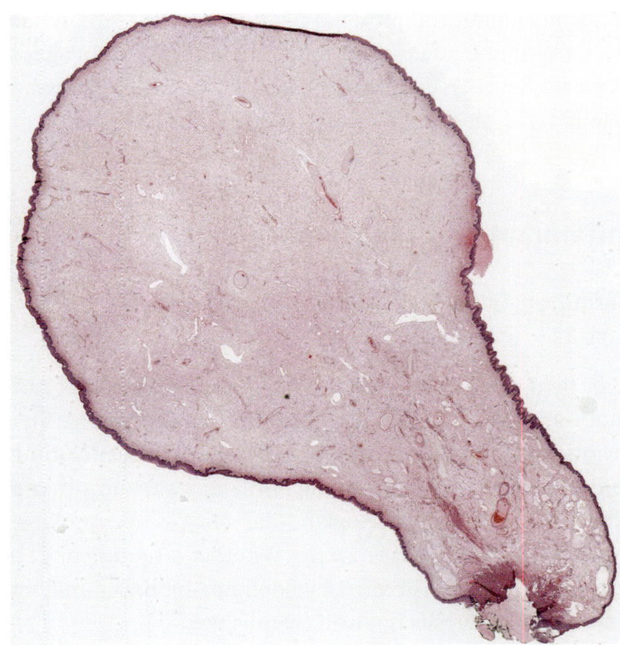

Figure 14.2 Fibroepithelial polyp: The polyp has a core containing variably collagenous or more myxoid stroma. The surface is benign squamous mucosa.

Immunohistochemistry

Increased CD34 immunopositivity has been identified in the stromal cells, but special studies are otherwise not helpful.

Differential Diagnosis

Hemorrhoids have a similar clinical appearance.

Treatment/Prognosis/Evolution

Fibroepithelial polyps are often associated with anal fissures. The polypoid components are managed in the same way as cloacogenic polyps. Management of anal fissure is discussed elsewhere.

Hidradenoma Papilliferum

Definition and General Features

This rare benign skin adnexal tumor is believed to be derived from apocrine glands. Notably, most cases have been reported in women.

Clinical Features and Endoscopic Characteristics

Most lesions are small (<1.0 cm) and mobile, and can be painful.

Microscopic Features

The lesion forms a well-circumscribed nodule in the superficial submucosa, and is composed of papillary and/or glandular structures lined by two cell layers. The surface layer is composed of columnar and eosinophilic cells with apical cytoplasmic blebs, while the inner layer is formed of cuboidal cells with eosinophilic cytoplasm (Figure 14.3a, b).

Histochemistry

Characteristically, the columnar lining cell layer often contains periodic acid-Schiff stain (PAS)-positive, diastase-resistant material.

Differential Diagnosis

Clinically, these lesions are often suspected to be other benign polypoid lesions, but the distinctive histology should confirm the diagnosis.

Treatment/Prognosis/Evolution

Hidradenoma papilliferum typically occurs in females in the anogenital region and may be associated with Bartholin's cysts and abscesses. If symptomatic, they are managed with incision and drainage. Most lesions are benign but rare progression to adenocarcinoma has been reported.

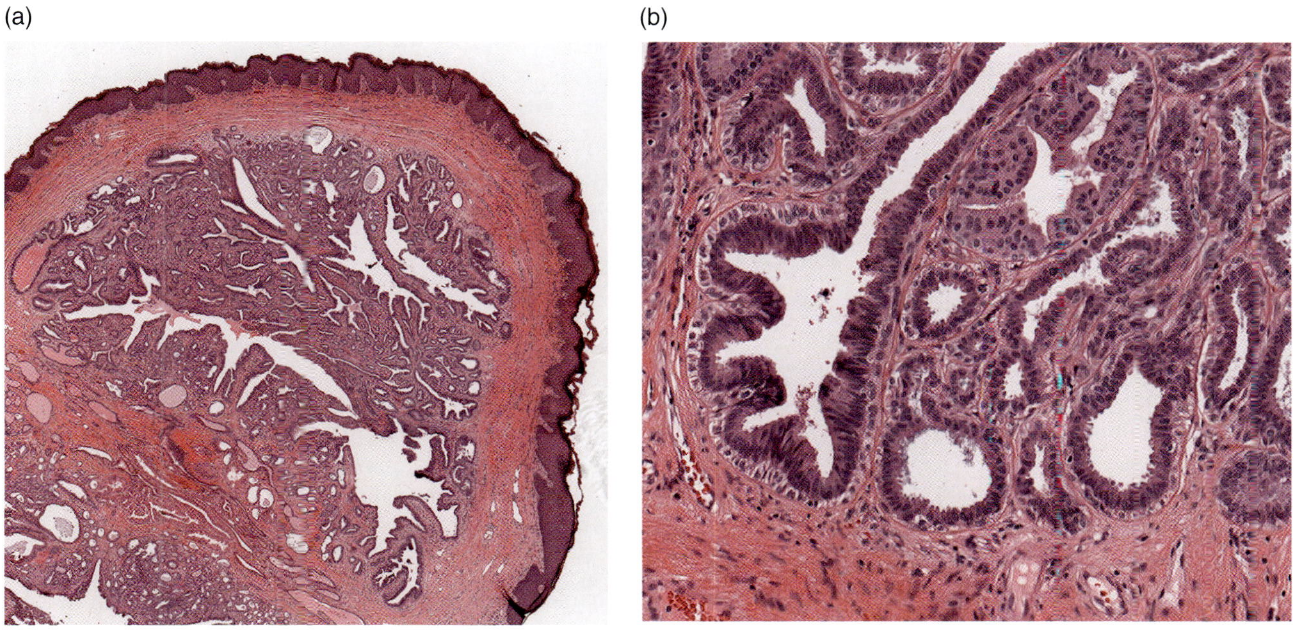

Figure 14.3 (a) Hidradenoma papilliferum: A submucosal proliferation of papillary and glandular structures with two cell layers (photo courtesy Dr. Rosalynn Nazarian). (b) Hidradenoma papilliferum: The surface layer has columnar cells with abundant eosinophilic cytoplasm and apical blebs. The outer layer is composed of cuboidal cells. *Source:* Photo courtesy Dr. Rosalynn Nazarian.

Squamous Hyperplasia and "Leukoplakia"

Definition, General Features, and Predisposing Factors

Leukoplakia is a clinical term referring to the observation of a white plaque covering the squamous mucosa that corresponds to a wide range of histopathologic conditions, including AIN, lichen planus, and lichen sclerosus et atrophicus. Squamous hyperplasia is a descriptive term referring to the changes observed in many of the lesions biopsied for the finding of "leukoplakia" that do not fall into one of the more specific diagnostic categories previously mentioned.

The cause of squamous hyperplasia is not entirely clear. It may be secondary to local irritation, or it may be due to metaplasia on the surface of a prolapsing hemorrhoid. Squamous hyperplasia can also be identified in the mucosa adjacent to squamous cell carcinoma. Lichen planus and lichen sclerosus et atrophicus are chronic inflammatory skin conditions that also lack clear etiologies, although an immune-mediated mechanism is thought to be involved.

Clinical Features and Endoscopic Characteristics

Leukoplakia is a white plaque in the squamous mucosa, often with a hard granular surface.

Microscopic Features

Squamous hyperplasia refers to a spectrum of changes including acanthosis, parakeratosis, and hyperkeratosis. A mild chronic inflammatory infiltrate of the lamina propria may be observed in association (Figure 14.4).

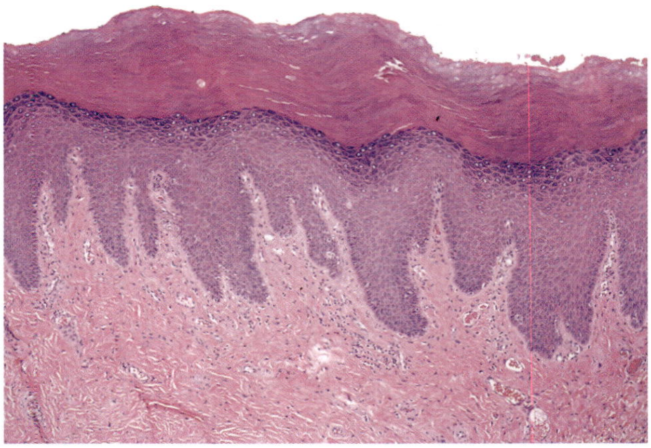

Figure 14.4 Squamous hyperplasia: The squamous mucosa has acanthosis (thickening) with an overlying dense layer of hyperkeratosis.

Immunohistochemistry

Squamous hyperplasia lacks the strong, diffuse, nuclear, and cytoplasmic immunopositivity for p16 associated with high-grade squamous intraepithelial lesions (HSILs).

Differential Diagnosis

The clinical differential diagnosis for leukoplakia has been previously described. Histologically, squamous hyperplasia should be differentiated from lichen sclerosus et atrophicus, lichen planus, and AIN. Lichen sclerosus et atrophicus classically shows atrophy of the squamous epithelium and homogenization of the collagen in the superficial lamina propria, with an underlying lymphoid infiltrate. Lichen planus shows band-like interface lymphocytic inflammation with acanthosis and pointed rete ridges, imparting a "sawtooth"-like appearance to the epithelium. Hypergranulosis and Civatte bodies (eosinophilic colloid bodies) may be seen in the squamous epithelium in lichen planus. In squamous hyperplasia, the cellular crowding and cytologic atypia of AIN are notably absent.

Treatment/Prognosis/Evolution

Anal leukoplakia is poorly understood. Case reports suggest it is associated with chronic anal irritation such as pruritis ani, or chronic use of hemorrhoidal creams. Although it is considered benign, given the differential diagnosis, biopsy should be considered to exclude other neoplastic lesions.

Condyloma Acuminatum

Definition, General Features, and Predisposing Factors

This is terminology for an anogenital viral wart associated with human papillomaviruses (HPV), most commonly low-risk HPV type 6 and HPV type 11. Condyloma is part of the spectrum of low-grade squamous intraepithelial lesions (LSILs), which is discussed in detail under AIN/ASIL (anal squamous intraepithelial lesion). HPV is transmitted by mucocutaneous contact. Risk factors for anal condyloma acuminata include HIV infection, immunocompromised status, and anoreceptive intercourse.

Clinical Features and Endoscopic Characteristics

Condyloma acuminata are soft, polypoid lesions with an irregular cauliflower-like appearance. They are usually small, measuring less than 1 cm in diameter, and can present several pigmentations (skin colored, erythematous, hypopigmented, or hyperpigmented).

Microscopic Features

The squamous mucosa shows acanthosis and papillomatosis with surface parakeratosis and hyperkeratosis. The keratinocytes often have a prominent perinuclear clear halo and membrane irregularity (koilocytosis). Binucleation can be observed. Occasional mitoses can be seen above the basal cell layer; however, there is orderly maturation of squamous cells (Figure 14.5a, b).

Immunohistochemistry

Ki67 is useful in differentiating condyloma acuminatum from non-HPV associated lesions, such as perianal skin with inflammation and reactive changes or a fibroepithelial polyp. Nuclear Ki67 expression is generally limited to the basal two or three layers of keratinocytes in the latter non-HPV associated lesions, but is increased in condyloma acuminatum, staining at least a few keratinocytes in the upper 2/3 of the squamous epithelium. A p16 stain is helpful in the differential of condyloma acuminatum (which is considered part of the spectrum of LSIL) from high-grade squamous intraepithelial lesion (HSIL). Condyloma acuminatum should show negative, very weak, or patchy/discontinuous cytoplasmic and nuclear staining for p16, while HSILs will have diffuse, moderate to strong intensity nuclear staining in at least the lower third of the squamous epithelium. HPV can be detected by in situ hybridization, but this is less widely available. Polymerase chain reaction (PCR) can be applied to identify HPV infection.

Differential Diagnosis

Clinically, the differential diagnosis includes hemorrhoids and fibroepithelial polyp. Microscopically, condyloma with marked koilocytosis can be difficult to differentiate from HSIL, with more differentiation toward the epithelial surface in condyloma. Condyloma also lack the high nuclear density and crowding associated with high-grade dysplasia. In difficult cases, p16 and Ki67 can be useful, as described above.

Treatment/Prognosis/Evolution

Most condyloma acuminata are benign. However, a small proportion of warts harbor infection with high-risk HPV (types 16 and 18), which raises the theoretical possibility of higher risk for progression to squamous cell carcinoma. Some of these cases are revealed when an area of HSIL is identified within a condyloma. However, morphologic changes diagnostic of HSIL are not always present in condyloma infected with high-risk HPV. Thus, histologic examination of warts lacks 100% sensitivity for HPV infection with oncogenic potential. Occult squamous cell carcinomas are identified in a small proportion (3% in one series) of surgically excised warts submitted for histologic examination.

(a) (b)

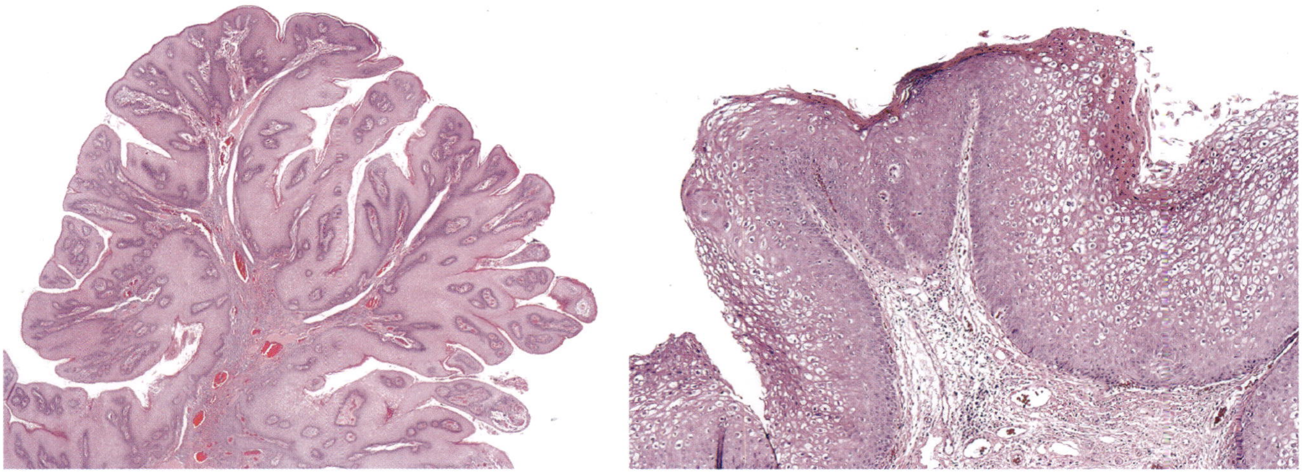

Figure 14.5 (a) Condyloma acuminatum: There is acanthosis of the squamous mucosa and the lesion has a papillary architecture. (b) Condyloma acuminatum: Many superficial keratinocytes have irregular nuclear contours and a clear perinuclear halo, referred to as koilocytosis.

Anal Intraepithelial Neoplasia (AIN)/Anal Squamous Intraepithelial Lesion (ASIL)

Definition, General Features, and Predisposing Factors

AIN (or its equivalent, ASIL) refers to dysplastic changes of the anal mucosa, usually caused by infection with HPV. Perianal dysplasia, including perianal intraepithelial neoplasia (PAIN) and Bowen's disease, occurs outside of the anal opening, and is discussed separately. There are two commonly used grading systems. Currently, the two-tiered grading system of LSIL or HSIL is favored by most authorities including the College of American Pathologists and the World Health Organization, although the latter organization uses the terms AIN-L (low grade) and AIN-H (high grade) for the equivalent lesions. The three-tiered system of AIN-1 (low grade dysplasia), AIN-2 (moderate grade dysplasia), and AIN-3 (severe dysplasia) is less favored due to interobserver variability in distinguishing the two high-grade lesions (AIN-2 vs. AIN-3) and an improved understanding of the biology of HPV-related lesions. LSILs are thought to represent transient HPV infections, which for the most part resolve spontaneously. In contrast, HSILs (including both AIN-2 and AIN-3) are thought to represent true precursors to squamous cell carcinoma. In 2012, working groups from the College of American Pathologists and the American Society for Colposcopy and Cervical Pathology recommended use of the two-tiered grading system for pathology reporting, with an option to further subclassifying lesions based on the three-tiered system.

The most important predisposing factor for AIN is HPV infection, which is detected in approximately 90% of cases. High risk-HPV (most commonly types 16, 18, 31, and 33) is identified in at least 70% of HSIL cases and in a minority of LSIL cases. Low-risk HPV types (including types 6, 11, and 70) are commonly identified in LSIL and are present in a small proportion of HSIL cases. The risk of dysplasia increases with persistent high-risk HPV infection and when multiple HPV types are present. Additional risk factors for AIN include HPV-related dysplasia at other sites in the genital tract, receptive anal intercourse, HIV infection (particularly with low CD4 count), immunosuppression from other causes, cigarette smoking, and radiation.

Clinical Features and Endoscopic Characteristics

The zone of transitional mucosa in the region of the dentate line is the most common area affected.

Microscopic Features

Dysplasia is characterized by the extension of cells with a high nuclear-to-cytoplasmic ratio from the usual basal location toward the mucosal surface. It is accompanied by increased nuclear size, nuclear pleomorphism, nuclear membrane irregularity, and increased mitotic figures above the basal layer. Grading depends on the degree of maturation (see Table 14.1.). In AIN-1, the immature basaloid cells and mitoses are confined to the lower third of the epithelium. In AIN-2, there is a lack of maturation in the lower 2/3, and in AIN-3 more than 2/3 of the mucosa show immaturity and often demonstrate mitoses. AIN-3 includes dysplasia involving the full thickness of the mucosa, which has also been termed "carcinoma in situ." Koilocytes, which have a low nuclear-to-cytoplasmic ratio with prominent perinuclear haloes, nuclear membrane irregularity, and occasional binucleate forms, are a sign of HPV viral cytopathic effect that may be seen in any grade of dysplasia, but are most prominent in low-grade lesions (Figures 14.6 and 14.7).

Using ASIL terminology, the general principle is that AIN-1 lesions and condyloma acuminatum are grouped under the category of LSIL, while AIN-2 and AIN-3 are grouped under the HSIL category, although recent consensus definitions refine these principles slightly. LSIL is

Table 14.1 Comparison of the two-tiered (squamous intraepithelial lesion) and three-tiered (intraepithelial neoplasia) grading systems for squamous dysplasia of the anal canal.

2-Tier	3-Tier	Description
LSIL	Condyloma acuminatum	A viral wart with acanthosis and papillomatosis
	AIN-1	Low-grade dysplasia where immature basaloid cells and mitoses are confined to the lower third of the squamous mucosa
HSIL	AIN-2	Lack of maturation in the lower 2/3 of the squamous mucosa
	AIN-3	Immaturity (and often mitoses) extend into the upper third of the squamous mucosa

LSIL, low-grade squamous intraepithelial lesion; HSIL, high-grade squamous intraepithelial lesion; AIN, anal intraepithelial neoplasia.

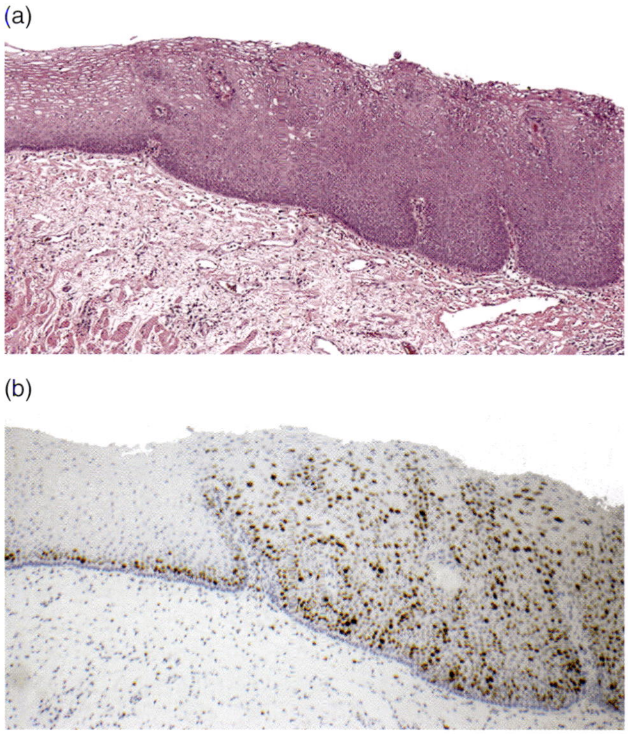

Figure 14.6 Anal intraepithelial neoplasia grade 1/low-grade squamous intraepithelial lesion: Panel A shows immature basaloid cells in the lower third of the mucosa with overlying koilocytes. At left, there is a junction with normal mucosa for comparison. panel B shows Ki67 immunohistochemistry, which is increased in the lesion compared to normal mucosa.

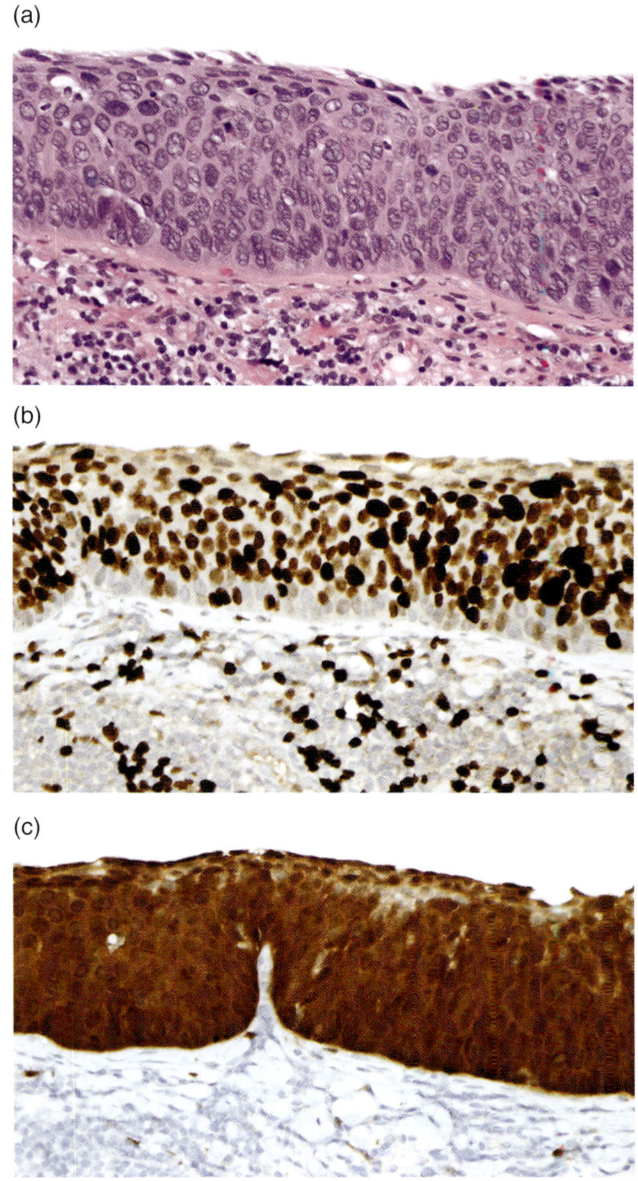

Figure 14.7 Anal intraepithelial neoplasia grade 3/high-grade squamous intraepithelial lesion: Panel A shows immature basaloid cells with nuclear atypia and mitoses reach the upper third of the mucosa. Panel B shows increased staining for Ki67 throughout the full thickness of the mucosa. Panel C shows strong nuclear and cytoplasmic "block" positivity for p16 by immunohistochemistry.

defined as having little maturation in the basal third, with maturation "beginning" in the middle third and normal in the upper third, and mitoses limited to the lower third. HSIL is defined as having little or no cytoplasmic differentiation in the middle to upper third and mitoses are typically present above the basal third. Lesions with abnormal mitotic figures and marked nuclear pleomorphism are graded as HSIL even if they show differentiation satisfying LSIL criteria. The WHO's AIN-L and AIN-H grading system has similar criteria.

Immunohistochemical and Molecular Features

While much of the data on p16 immunohistochemistry in HPV-related squamous dysplasia comes from studies in the uterine cervix, there are increasing data supporting similar diagnostic utility for p16 in ASIL. For example, p16 is helpful in differentiating HSIL from a non-HPV related lesion such as reactive transitional zone mucosa or immature squamous metaplasia. In HSIL, there will be strong diffuse nuclear and cytoplasmic staining in at least the lower third of the mucosa, but often extending into the middle and upper third. In non-HPV related histologic mimics of HSIL, p16 staining will be negative, highlight scattered single cells, or appear weak and patchy. The other situation where a p16 stain is useful is in cases that have a moderate degree of dysplasia, where there is uncertainty about whether to categorize the lesion as LSIL or HSIL. LSIL usually does not have the strong diffuse p16 positivity of HSIL. However, p16 should not entirely replace morphologic assessment, because a small proportion of morphologically unequivocal

LSIL cases do have diffuse p16 staining. Ki67 can be helpful, but is less specific than p16 for high-grade lesions. Ki67 immunopositivity is normally confined to the basal two or three layers of the mucosa, and its expression is progressively increased with increasing grades of dysplasia, often involving the upper third in high-grade lesions. While Ki67 may help separating HPV-related lesions from non-HPV related lesions, it is less helpful in differentiating low- and high-grade lesions. Immunohistochemistry and in situ hybridization for HPV are available, but they have little diagnostic significance for grading lesions. PCR for HPV is the best test to identify high-risk and low-risk HPV types.

Differential Diagnosis

The most important differential diagnosis is non-HPV related histologic mimics of HSIL, such as reactive or inflammatory changes in the transitional mucosa and immature squamous metaplasia. Histologically, there is a greater degree of nuclear crowding, overlap, pleomorphism, atypia, and suprabasal mitoses in HSIL than in reactive lesions. As described above, p16 may be useful in difficult cases.

Treatment/Prognosis/Evolution

ASIL lesion are premalignant and require close monitoring and therapy when the risk of progression is high. Risk factors include HIV-associated immunosuppression and low CD-4 counts, HPV infection, particularly high-risk HPV subtypes. Prevention with HPV vaccine should be considered in high-risk individuals. Treatment for patients with HSIL is recommended including ablation of small localized lesions, or topical trichloroacetic acid for more diffuse lesions.

Perianal Intraepithelial Neoplasia (PAIN), Bowen's Disease, and Bowenoid Papulosis

Definition, General Features, and Predisposing Factors

PAIN is the presence of dysplasia in the skin arising within 5 cm of the anal opening. Bowen's disease refers to squamous cell carcinoma in situ, and is equivalent to PAIN-3 or HSIL using current terminology. Bowenoid papulosis is histologically indistinguishable from PAIN or Bowen's, but has a distinct clinical picture characterized by the presence of transient papules with spontaneous regression. The risk factors and association with HPV for PAIN are similar to those described for AIN. High-risk HPV types (16, 18, 31, 33) are identified in most Bowenoid papulosis lesions.

Clinical Features and Endoscopic Characteristics

While PAIN tends to have onset in middle age, Bowenoid papulosis tends to affect younger adults, often in their 20s and 30s PAIN tends to present as a scaling, erythematous, or white plaque with sharp borders, ranging in size from a few millimeters to a few centimeters. Bowenoid papulosis presents as multiple small papules in the anogenital region, some of which have a verrucous appearance.

Microscopic Features

The histologic appearance of PAIN and Bowenoid papulosis is essentially the same as for AIN. There is more parakeratosis, hyperkeratosis, and dyskeratosis than in the anal canal, attributable to the cutaneous rather than mucosal location. The lesions can be graded as LSIL/HSIL or as PAIN-1/2/3 (Figure 14.8a–c).

Immunohistochemistry

Immunohistochemistry for p16 may be used in similar fashion to anal canal lesions.

Differential Diagnosis

These lesions need to be distinguished clinically from inflammatory skin diseases such as psoriasis, dermatitis (eczema), lichen planus, and lichen sclerosus et atrophicus. Biopsy resolves this differential. PAIN and Bowenoid papulosis are histologically indistinguishable, and must be differentiated by clinical parameters.

Treatment/Prognosis/Evolution

While most cases of Bowenoid papulosis resolve following treatment or regress spontaneously, rare cases have been identified concurrently with anal squamous cell carcinoma.

Extramammary Paget's Disease

Definition, General Features, and Predisposing Factors

Extramammary Paget's disease is a rare intraepidermal neoplastic condition that can involve the perianal skin. While mammary Paget's is almost always associated with

(a) (b) (c)

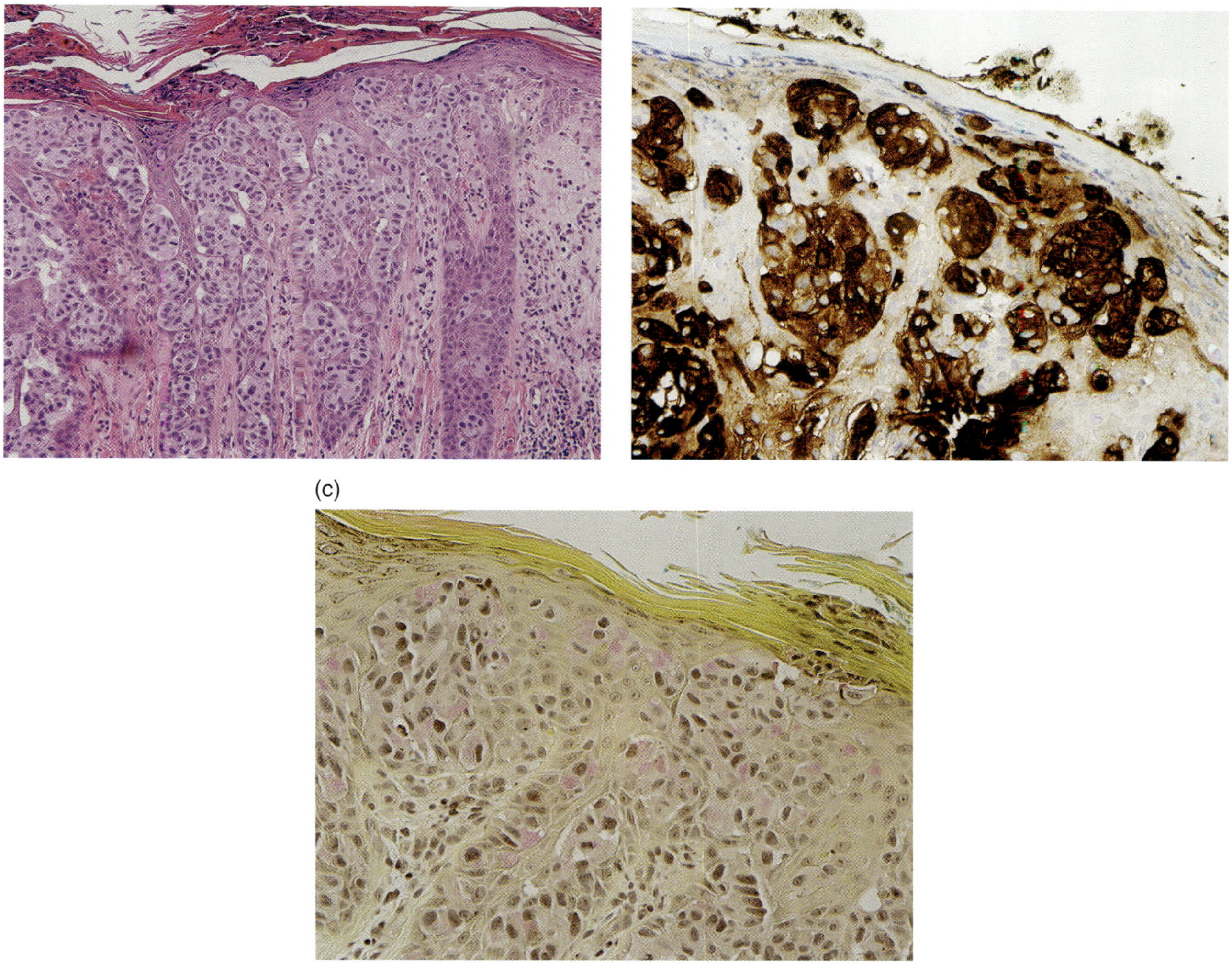

Figure 14.8 (a) Perianal Paget's disease: Paget's cells are scattered throughout the epidermis. (b) Perianal Paget's disease: CEA (carcinoembryonic antigen) immunohistochemistry highlights the Paget's cells within the epidermis. (c) Perianal Paget's disease: Mucicarmine highlights intracytoplasmic mucin in Paget's cells.

an underlying breast ductal carcinoma (often ductal carcinoma in situ), extramammary Paget's disease is associated with underlying malignancy in only approximately 40% of cases. It is generally accepted that cases not associated with an underlying internal malignancy arise from skin adnexal structures.

Most cases are sporadic, although a few familial examples have been reported. A review of 193 cases revealed that 31% of the cases were associated with a synchronous neoplasm, and 10% had neoplasms diagnosed prior to or following the diagnosis. Twenty-one percent had synchronous rectal adenocarcinoma and 9% had metachronous rectal adenocarcinoma. Rare cases were associated with rectal adenomatous polyps, skin adnexal carcinomas, or distant adenocarcinomas in the colon, prostate, or lung.

Clinical Features and Endoscopic Characteristics

Perianal Paget's presents as a patch or plaque of varying size, which may be erythematous or white. The lesions may show ulceration, weeping, and scaling. Symptoms frequently include pruritus and occasionally pain.

Microscopic Features

The diagnostic Paget's cells, which tend to be large with abundant pale to clear cytoplasm, are scattered individually or as small clusters throughout the epidermis. They present with a vesicular nucleus that may be central, or peripherally located with a signet ring cell-like appearance.

Histochemical and Immunohistochemical Features

Special stains can be used to discriminate Paget's disease from other neoplasms, particularly melanoma in situ or HSIL with a pagetoid pattern of atypical keratinocytes (the latter is sometimes called "pagetoid Bowen's disease"). Intracytoplasmic mucin can be highlighted with a PAS diastase, mucicarmine, or Alcian Blue stain. An immunohistochemical stain for CEA (carcinoembryonic antigen) or epithelial membrane antigen (EMA) also highlights the diagnostic cells. Melanocytic markers such as S100, Melan-A, and MITF (microphthalmia-associated transcription factor) are positive in melanoma in situ and not in Paget's cells. A high molecular weight keratin stain such as CK5/6 will be positive in the atypical cells in HSIL (pagetoid Bowen's), but not in Paget's disease. Immunohistochemical stains also may be helpful in distinguishing Paget's disease secondary to rectal adenocarcinoma from primary the cases that are suspected to arise from skin appendages. Those associated rectal adenocarcinomas are typically CK20 positive and GCDFP-15 (gross cystic disease fluid protein-15) negative, while primary Paget's cells are CK20 negative and GCDFP positive. CK7 is not particularly discriminatory, since primary Paget's is usually CK7 positive, and rectal adenocarcinoma shows variable CK7 reactivity.

Differential Diagnosis

From a clinical point of view, Paget's disease must be differentiated from inflammatory skin disease such as eczema, psoriasis, and lichen sclerosus et atrophicus. This differential can be resolved with tissue biopsy. Histologically, the differential diagnosis includes melanoma in situ and HSIL (see discussion above). In differentiating primary from secondary Paget's associated to underlying malignancy, the stains described above may be helpful, in addition to endoscopic examination.

Treatment/Prognosis/Evolution

Perianal Paget's disease has a high rate of local recurrence (33–60%), even following wide local excision with margins greater than 1 cm.

Squamous Cell Carcinoma

Definition, General Features, and Predisposing Factors

Squamous cell carcinoma is the most common malignancy of the anal canal, and is commonly associated with HPV infection. Perianal squamous cell carcinoma shares similar risk factors and morphology to anal canal tumors, and differs mainly based on location in the skin within 5 cm of the anal opening rather than in the canal. Perianal squamous cell carcinomas do have a slightly better prognosis than tumors of the anal canal.

The main risk factor is infection with high-risk HPV, isolated in the West from nearly 90% of invasive lesions. About 70% of cases are associated with HPV type 16. Anoreceptive intercourse, an increased lifetime number of sexual partners, and other sexually transmitted infections are noted risk factors. Men who have sex with men are also at higher risk. HIV/AIDS and other causes of immunosuppression such as solid organ transplantation have been associated with increased risk of anal squamous cell carcinoma. Smoking and Crohn's disease also increase the risk.

Clinical Features and Endoscopic Characteristics

Patients often present with rectal bleeding, a palpable mass, or anal pain. In some cases, involvement of the anal sphincter muscles may cause incontinence (Figure 14.9).

Microscopic Features

Most tumors display more than one pattern of differentiation and arise in a background mucosa showing HSIL/AIN2–3 changes. The presence of tumor cells with abundant eosinophilic cytoplasm, individual cell keratinization, formation of keratin pearls, and intercellular bridges are characteristic of the keratinizing pattern. Non-keratinizing tumors lack the distinctive keratinization but may retain

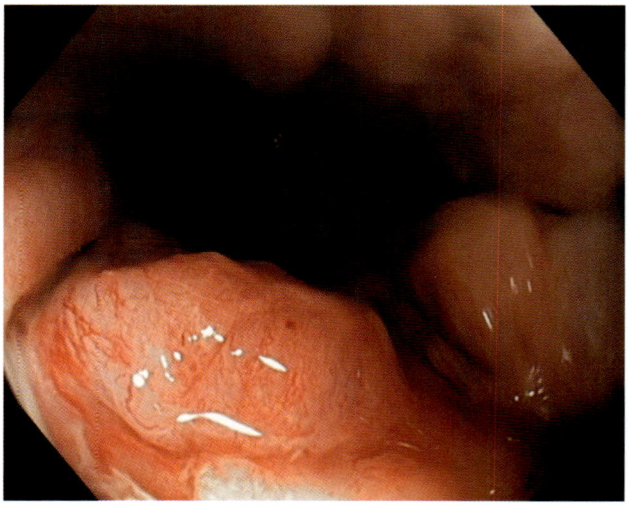

Figure 14.9 Endoscopic view of anal squamous cell carcinoma at the 6 o'clock position. Note the dilated vessels and irregular mucosal surface.

(a)

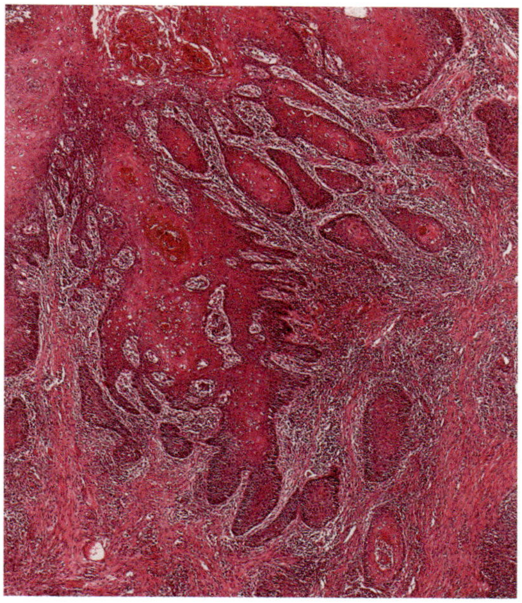

(b)

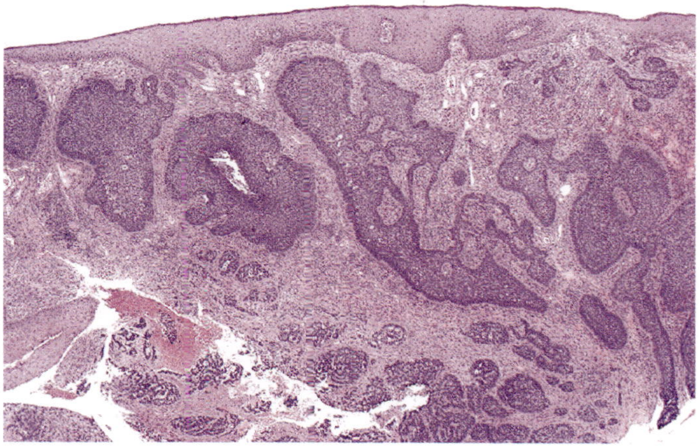

(c)

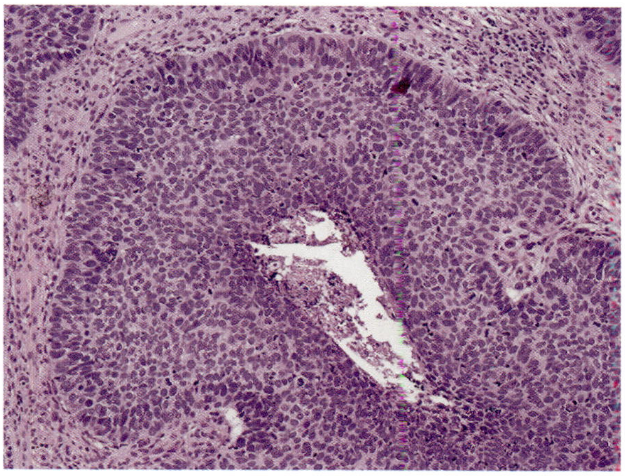

Figure 14.10 (a) Invasive squamous cell carcinoma, keratinizing, with infiltrative architecture. Some of the invasive nests of tumor form keratin pearls. (b) Invasive basaloid: squamous cell carcinomas with basaloid differentiation show higher nuclear: cytoplasmic ratio, peripheral palisading, and areas of central necrosis within islands of tumor. (c) Invasive squamous cell carcinoma, basaloid: higher magnification highlights the peripheral palisading and central necrosis.

visible intercellular bridges. Basaloid differentiation (also known historically as cloacogenic carcinoma) includes nests or infiltrative sheets of cells with a high nuclear-to-cytoplasmic ratio and scant basophilic cytoplasm. Peripheral palisading is common, and central necrosis may be observed. Ductal differentiation can be seen in about 25% of the cases, the majority of which contain mucin that can be demonstrated with a PAS–diastase stain. This has also been described as formation of mucinous microcysts. A few cases of basaloid squamous cell carcinoma have been described as having an adenoid cystic pattern. These cases show prominent basement membrane-like material within and surrounding the tumor nests, and have occasional mucinous microcysts (Figure 14.10a, b).

Immunohistochemical and Molecular Features

Immunohistochemical stains can be helpful in distinguishing poorly differentiated squamous cell carcinoma from other poorly differentiated malignancies, including poorly differentiated adenocarcinoma, neuroendocrine tumors (both large cell and small cell), and melanoma. In this differential, p63 and p40 are the most specific markers for squamous cell carcinoma, with specificity over 95%. While squamous cell carcinomas are typically CK5/6 positive, this is a less specific marker, as approximately 20% of adenocarcinomas and neuroendocrine tumors are immunoreactive as well. Adenocarcinomas of the colorectal type are typically CK20 positive, CDX-2 positive, and CEA positive, with variable CK7 expression. Neuroendocrine tumors are typically CD56 and synaptophysin positive, with variable chromogranin expression. Melanoma markers including HMB45, Melan-A, and S100 can be helpful at times. PCR-based methods can be used to identify high-risk HPV. Furthermore, p16 and HPV testing are reccomended for anal squamous dysplasia in the current WHO classification.

Differential Diagnosis

Clinically, the differential diagnosis for squamous cell carcinoma includes other malignant tumors arising in the anal canal, such as adenocarcinoma and melanoma. While the differential can usually be resolved easily by histologic examination, certain scenarios are challenging, particularly with small biopsies. Poorly differentiated malignancies (squamous cell carcinoma, melanoma, adenocarcinoma, and neuroendocrine tumors) can show overlapping features. Most squamous cell carcinomas will demonstrate characteristic squamous differentiation, such as individual cell keratinization and intercellular bridges, at least focally. Immunohistochemical stains, as described above, can also help to resolve this differential. Squamous cell carcinoma is distinguished from verrucous carcinoma (giant condyloma of Buschke and Löwenstein) by the presence of infiltrative growth, and in the former, usually more cytologic atypia. The differential diagnosis of squamous cell carcinoma with basaloid differentiation from perianal basal cell carcinoma can be challenging.

Basal cell carcinoma tends not to originate in the anal canal, but to spread from the perianal skin and should be differentiated from basaloid squamous cell carcinomas. Histologically, basaloid squamous cell carcinomas are also composed of basaloid cells, but tend to have less peripheral palisading, less retraction artifact, a more infiltrative growth pattern, more squamous differentiation, occasional keratin pearl formation, more nuclear pleomorphism, and more atypical mitoses. One study of 10 cases found that Ber-EP4 is positive in basal cell carcinoma, but negative in basaloid squamous cell carcinoma. It also showed that basaloid squamous cell carcinomas were immunopositive for CEA and EMA, while basal cell carcinomas were negative. The distinction is critical, since there is a stark contrast in the behavior of these two tumors. Basaloid squamous cell carcinoma of the anal canal can metastasize and has a significant five-year mortality, while the prognosis of basal cell carcinoma is excellent after complete excision. Metastases and direct spread of malignancy originating in the female genital tract should also be considered in the differential diagnosis of anal squamous cell carcinoma.

Treatment/Prognosis/Evolution

Anal squamous cell carcinomas spread more often via lymphatics than hematogenously, and the pattern of regional lymph node involvement depends on the location of the tumor. The anorectal, perirectal, and paravertebral nodes are involved more often if the tumor is located above the dentate line, while the superficial inguinal nodes are more often involved if the tumor arises below the dentate line. Distant metastases occur in 10–17% of patients, and most often are to the liver or lungs.

The American Joint Committee on Cancer (AJCC) 8th edition tumor nodes metastasis (TNM) staging system for tumors of the anal canal is summarized in Table 14.2. The AJCC TNM system does not subdivide T1 tumors (<2 cm), but other organizations, including the College of American Pathologists, recommend reporting microinvasive squamous cell carcinoma using the criteria of invasion ≤3 mm from the basement membrane or point of origin and

Table 14.2 American Joint Committee on Cancer (AJCC), 8th edition TNM staging for tumors of the anal canal.

Primary tumor (T)	
TX	Primary tumor cannot be assessed
T0	No evidence of primary tumor
Tis	Carcinoma in situ (Bowen's disease," high-grade squamous intraepithelial lesion [HSIL], anal intraepithelial neoplasia 2–3 [AIN2–3]
T1	Tumor 2 cm or less in greatest dimension
T2	Tumor more than 2 cm but not more than 5 cm in greatest dimension
T3	Tumor more than 5 cm in greatest dimension
T4	Tumor of any size invades adjacent organ(s), e.g. vagina, urethra, bladder
Regional lymph nodes (N)	
NX	Regional lymph nodes cannot be assessed
N0	No regional lymph node metastasis
N1a	Metastasis in inguinal, mesorectal, or internal iliac lymph
N1b	Metastasis in external iliac lymph nodes
N1c	Metastasis in external iliac with any N1a nodes
Distant metastasis (M)	
M0	No distant metastasis
M1	Distant metastasis

Source: Based on Edge, S.B., Byrdm, D.R., Compton, C.C. et al. (2010). *AJCC Cancer Staging Manual Seventh Edition*. New York: Springer.

≤7 mm in lateral extent. Microinvasive squamous cell carcinomas are thought to have a better prognosis, and may be amenable to conservative, sphincter sparing local excision. Until the 1970s, larger tumors were also treated surgically, often with abdominoperineal resection. However, several studies starting in the 1970s showed that combined chemoradiation resulted in much improved outcomes. Consequently, chemoradiation has been recommended as the primary treatment modality for anal squamous cell carcinoma, with resection reserved for recurrent disease. A recent retrospective study of 6696 patients with stage I–III squamous cell carcinoma showed improved five-year survival in patients who received chemoradiation therapy according to guidelines (64.2%, 95% CI: 63.3–65.1%) compared to those who did not receive chemoradiation (58.1%, 95% CI: 56.6–59.6%).

Verrucous Carcinoma (Giant Condyloma of Buschke and Löwenstein)

Definition, General Features, and Predisposing Factors

Verrucous carcinomas (or giant condyloma of Buschke and Löwenstein) are very large warty lesions involving the anogenital region.

Immunosuppression is the main risk factor, with a recent review specifically identifying HIV/AIDS, solid organ transplantation, hematologic malignancy, long-term corticosteroid use, diabetes, pregnancy, and alcohol abuse as predisposing factors. In many cases, HPV types 6 and 11 have also been isolated from the tumors.

Clinical Features and Endoscopic Characteristics

These tumors are often large, with many reported cases measuring over 10 cm in diameter. The tumor surface is warty and is often described as "cauliflower-like." Common symptoms include pelvic pain, pelvic discharge, rectal bleeding, altered bowel habit, and weight loss.

Microscopic Features

The tumors have features that resemble condyloma acuminatum, including marked acanthosis, papillomatosis, parakeratosis, hyperkeratosis, and increased mitoses above the basal layer. Koilocytes are often present. There is a broad, "pushing" border of invasion, without the typical infiltrative growth pattern of conventional squamous cell carcinomas. The squamous cells show minimal cytologic atypia. In many cases, HSIL and a classic infiltrative squamous cell carcinoma have been reported to occur in a background of verrucous carcinoma.

Differential Diagnosis

The large size and broad "pushing" border of invasion distinguishes these tumors from condyloma acuminata. The lack of cytologic atypia and infiltrative growth differentiates verrucous carcinoma from typical squamous cell carcinoma.

Treatment/Prognosis/Evolution

Verrucous carcinoma is generally thought to be a locally aggressive tumor with limited metastatic potential, unless the tumor transforms to a more classical invasive squamous cell carcinoma. However, transformation to invasive squamous cell carcinoma is reported to be relatively common, occurring in up to 56% of cases. The main treatment for these tumors is surgical resection, usually by wide local excision initially. There is a high rate of local recurrence, reported to be approximately 50%. Some patients have multiple recurrences, which can be treated with a more radical re-excision (often abdominoperineal resection), or by chemoradiation. There is a high degree of morbidity due to difficulty in wound healing following excision and re-excision.

Adenocarcinoma

Definition, General Features, and Predisposing Factors

The vast majority of adenocarcinomas of the anal canal are of colorectal type. These tumors arise from the colorectal type mucosa in the proximal anal canal, above the dentate line. In contrast, adenocarcinoma of the anal ducts or glands is thought to arise from submucosal structures rather than the surface mucosa. Adenocarcinoma arising in fistula tracts and abscesses, which are typically mucinous adenocarcinomas, are also rare, and can be related to Crohn's disease.

There are no well-described predisposing factors for anal duct adenocarcinomas. A single case of synchronous anal duct adenocarcinoma and squamous cell carcinoma in situ with weak in situ hybridization for HPV types 16 and 18 raises the possibility of association with HPV, but this has not been confirmed. The fistula associated tumors are associated with long-standing anal fistulas or abscesses with or without Crohn's disease. Chronic inflammation along fistulous tracts, immunosuppression related to Crohn's treatment, and smoking are believed to be contributory.

Clinical Features and Endoscopic Characteristics

The most common presenting symptoms are bleeding, a palpable mass (sometimes mistaken initially for hemorrhoids), or pain.

Microscopic Features

Various patterns can be observed, and the grading for anal adenocarcinomas is the same as for colorectal adenocarcinomas. The most common colorectal type adenocarcinomas have morphology similar to their counterparts in the colorectum.

Anal duct adenocarcinomas are typically centered in the submucosa underlying an uninvolved benign squamous mucosa. They are typically composed of small glands, which resemble the normal anal ducts. The cells lining the glands are often cuboidal with a high nuclear-to-cytoplasmic ratio, and produce little mucin. There are a few cases where the neoplasm is in direct continuity with the anal glands or with cytologic atypia in the adjacent anal glands, raising the possibility of a preinvasive dysplastic change in the anal glands. Mucinous differentiation and pagetoid spread of tumor cells in the overlying squamous mucosa have been reported as well.

Mucinous adenocarcinomas associated with anal fistulas or abscesses often are deeply situated within the muscularis propria. The morphology resembles colorectal mucinous adenocarcinoma, and the glands are usually well differentiated. The associated fistula tracts are often lined by colorectal type mucosa, which may show adenomatous dysplastic changes. There may be mucin pools and granulomatous inflammation adjacent to the tumor.

Immunohistochemistry

Normal anal glands have a two-cell-thick lining in their most distal portions that thickens to three cell layers and to a thicker transitional type mucosa at the interface with the anal canal squamous mucosa. The ductal luminal cells are positive for CK7 and negative for CK20 and CDX-2, while the basal and intermediate cells are p63 and CK5/6 positive. Anal duct adenocarcinomas show a similar pattern of immunopositivity for CK7 and immunonegativity for CK20 and CDX-2. The p63 and CK5/6-positive basal/intermediate cells are lost in anal duct adenocarcinomas, confirming the invasive nature of the process. This staining pattern contrasts with colorectal type adenocarcinomas, which are often CK7 negative (only a minority are positive), and are almost always positive for CK20 and CDX-2. Mucinous adenocarcinomas are reported to have an immunophenotype more closely resembling colorectal adenocarcinomas.

Differential Diagnosis

Anal duct adenocarcinoma must be differentiated from colorectal type adenocarcinoma. Morphological clues include an intact overlying squamous mucosa, the small gland architecture with scant mucin, and rarely contiguity with anal ducts or glands. The CK7/CK20/CDX-2 immunohistochemical profile described above is also helpful in directing the diagnosis.

Mucinous adenocarcinomas associated with fistula tracts are often well differentiated and must not be confused with a benign process such as mucin extravasation or misplaced benign glandular epithelium from fistula tracts or associated with prolapse, analogous to colitis cystic profunda.

Treatment/Prognosis/Evolution

Treatment for patients with anal canal adenocarcinoma is usually surgical with local excision or abdominoperineal resection. Survival outcomes are much poorer than observed in anal squamous cell carcinoma. Five-year survival was less than 20% in five series with long-term follow-up.

Malignant Melanoma

Definition, General Features, and Predisposing Factors

The anal squamous mucosa and transitional zone mucosa are normally populated by melanocytes, from which these tumors are thought to arise. Although uncommon, melanoma of the anal canal is the most common site of mucosal melanoma, and it is the third most common type of malignant tumor in the anal canal.

Anal canal melanomas most commonly affect older adults, with a mean age at presentation of 66–68 years old. Females are affected almost twice as often as males. There is some evidence suggesting HIV/AIDS is a predisposing factor. The rate of anal melanoma in males aged 25–44 tripled in the San Francisco area during the decade between 1982 and 1992, coinciding with the HIV/AIDS epidemic.

Clinical Features and Endoscopic Characteristics

Patients typically present with rectal bleeding or anal discomfort, often initially mistaken for hemorrhoids. Perhaps due to their location, anal melanomas are typically much larger in size at presentation than their counterparts in the skin. The tumors can present due to symptoms from metastases in lymph nodes or distant organs.

Microscopic Features

There is wide variation in the histologic appearance. The tumor cells are most commonly epithelioid or spindled, but lymphoma-like and pleomorphic cell types also have been described. Frequent mitoses are usually present. In a series of 17 cases, pigmentation was identified in 35% of the cases. A junctional component was present in 60% of cases with a mucosal surface that could be assessed (Figure 14.11).

Histochemical, Immunohistochemical, and Molecular Features

The immunohistochemical staining profile of anal canal melanomas is similar to the cutaneous tumors. In the same series of 17 cases, S100 immunopositivity was present in 100% of cases, HMB-45 in 16 of 17, Melan A in 14 of 15, and tyrosinase in 12 of 14 cases. All cases were negative for a pan-keratin stain. CD117 (c-kit) expression is detected by immunohistochemistry in half of cases. In a series of 40

(a) (b) (c) (d)

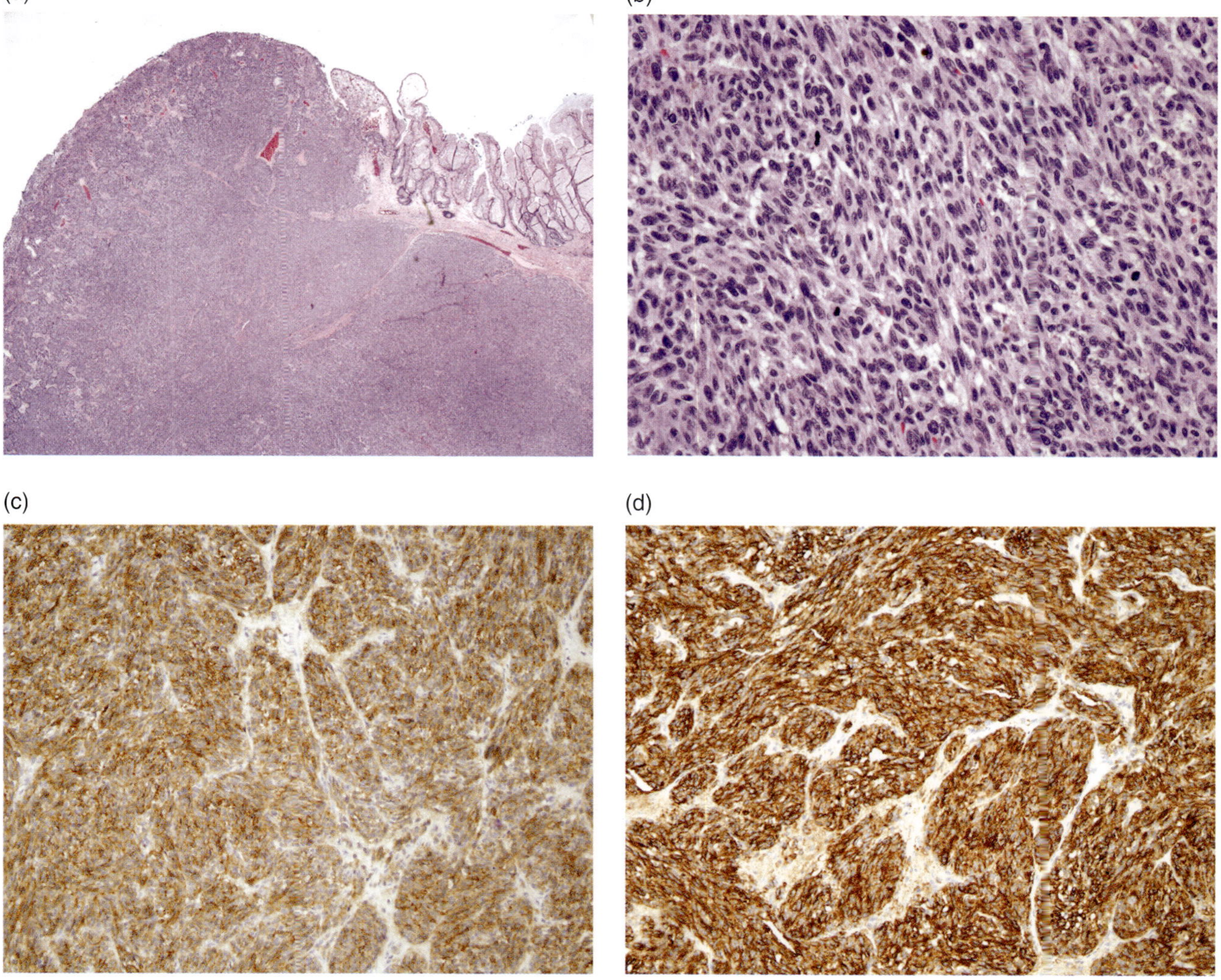

Figure 14.11 Malignant melanoma: Panel A shows a densely cellular lesion adjacent the columnar mucosa. Higher power (panel B) reveals malignant spindle cells with frequent mitoses. Immunohistochemistry for S100 (panel C) and HMB-45 (panel D) confirm melanocytic differentiation in the tumor cells.

cases, c-kit mutations were identified in seven tumors, and BRAF mutations were present in two tumors.

Differential Diagnosis

Due to its variable morphology, the histologic differential diagnosis is broad. Melanomas composed of epithelioid cells must be distinguished from poorly differentiated squamous cell carcinoma and adenocarcinoma, which are cytokeratin immunopositive. Melanomas with spindle cell morphology can resemble spindle cell squamous cell carcinoma, sarcomas, and gastrointestinal stromal tumor (GIST). The latter is a particular pitfall in the diagnosis of anal canal melanoma, as both GIST and melanoma are often CD117 positive by immunohistochemistry. Consequently, there should be a low threshold for performing melanoma markers in poorly differentiated and spindle cell neoplasms arising in the anus.

Treatment/Prognosis/Evolution

Treatment for anal canal melanoma is surgical, with transanal excision or abdominoperineal resection. A recent study of 183 patients has shown no difference in outcomes for anal melanoma for the two surgical techniques, despite similar baseline characteristics. Anal melanoma has a very poor prognosis, with a five-year survival rate of less than 25% and a mean survival of 15 months. Outcomes are dismal in patients presenting with lymph node or distant metastases, which respectively have five-year survival rates of 9.8 and 0% and median survival of 17 months and 8 months.

Miscellaneous and Rare Tumors

Rare neoplasms can involve the anal canal. These include small cell carcinomas that should be considered in the differential diagnosis of poorly differentiated malignancies, and can be identified with immunohistochemical markers such as CD56, synaptophysin, and chromogranin, although staining may be focal in some biopsies. Anorectal lymphomas are also rare and are mostly of B-cell lineage, often diffuse large B-cell lymphoma (DLBCL). Notably, there is an increased risk of Epstein–Barr virus-related anorectal B-cell lymphoma in patients with HIV/AIDS. Both benign and malignant soft tissue tumors can occur in the anal canal. They include lipomas and leiomyomas. Sarcomas are rare, but a few cases of leiomyosarcoma, rhabdomyosarcoma, and liposarcoma have been reported. Kaposi's sarcoma has been diagnosed in the perianal skin in a few patients with HIV.

Further Reading

Alvarez-Canas, M.C., Fernandez, F.A., Rodilla, I.G., and Val-Bernal, J.F. (1996). Perianal basal cell carcinoma: a comparative histologic, immunohistochemical, and flow cytometric study with basaloid carcinoma of the anus. *Am. J. Dermatopathol.* 18 (4): 371–379.

Anthony, T., Simmang, C., Lee, E.L., and Turnage, R.H. (1997). Perianal mucinous adenocarcinoma. *J. Surg. Oncol.* 64 (3): 218–221.

Balachandra, B., Marcus, V., and Jass, J.R. (2007). Poorly differentiated tumours of the anal canal: a diagnostic strategy for the surgical pathologist. *Histopathology* 50 (1): 163–174.

Barrett, W.L., Callahan, T.D., and Orkin, B.A. (1998). Perianal manifestations of human immunodeficiency virus infection: experience with 260 patients. *Dis. Colon Rectum* 41 (5): 606–611; discussion 11-2.

Bean, S.M., Eltoum, I., Horton, D.K. et al. (2007). Immunohistochemical expression of p16 and Ki-67 correlates with degree of anal intraepithelial neoplasia. *Am. J. Surg. Pathol.* 31 (4): 555–561.

Bean, S.M., Meara, R.S., Vollmer, R.T. et al. (2009). p16 improves interobserver agreement in diagnosis of anal intraepithelial neoplasia. *J. Low. Genit. Tract Dis.* 13 (3): 145–153.

Beer, T.W. and Carr, N.J. (1999). Fibroepithelial polyps of the anus with epithelial vacuolation. *Am. J. Surg. Pathol.* 23 (4): 488–489.

Bender, M.D. and Lechago, J. (1976). Leukoplakia of the anal canal. *Am J Dig Dis* 21 (10): 867–872.

Benson, A.B. 3rd, Arnoletti, J.P., Bekaii-Saab, T. et al. (2012). Anal carcinoma, version 2.2012: featured updates to the NCCN guidelines. *J. Natl. Compr. Cancer Netw.* 10 (4): 449–454.

Bilimoria, K.Y., Bentrem, D.J., Ko, C.Y. et al. (2008). Squamous cell carcinoma of the anal canal: utilization and outcomes of recommended treatment in the United States. *Ann. Surg. Oncol.* 15 (7): 1948–1958.

Cagir, B., Whiteford, M.H., Topham, A. et al. (1999). Changing epidemiology of anorectal melanoma. *Dis. Colon Rectum* 42 (9): 1203–1208.

Carpenter-Kling, J.T. and Jacyk, W.K. (1994). Anogenital flat papules. Bowenoid papulosis of the genitalia. *Arch. Dermatol.* 130 (10): 1311–1314.

Caruso, M.L. and Valentini, A.M. (1999). Different human papillomavirus genotypes in ano-genital lesions. *Anticancer Res.* 19 (4B): 3049–3053.

Chang, G.J., Gonzalez, R.J., Skibber, J.M. et al. (2009). A twenty-year experience with adenocarcinoma of the anal canal. *Dis. Colon Rectum* 52 (8): 1375–1380.

Chetty, R., Bhathal, P.S., and Slavin, J.L. (1993). Prolapse-induced inflammatory polyps of the colorectum and anal transitional zone. *Histopathology* 23 (1): 63–67.

Chetty, R., Serra, S., and Hsieh, E. (2005). Basaloid squamous carcinoma of the anal canal with an adenoid cystic pattern: histologic and immunohistochemical reappraisal of an unusual variant. *Am. J. Surg. Pathol.* 29 (12): 1668–1672.

Chu, Q.D., Vezeridis, M.P., Libbey, N.P., and Wanebo, H.J. (1994). Giant condyloma acuminatum (Buschke-Lowenstein tumor) of the anorectal and perianal regions. Analysis of 42 cases. *Dis. Colon Rectum* 37 (9): 950–957.

Chute, D.J., Cousar, J.B., and Mills, S.E. (2006). Anorectal malignant melanoma: morphologic and immunohistochemical features. *Am. J. Clin. Pathol.* 126 (1): 93–100.

Clark, M.A., Hartley, A., and Geh, J.I. (2004). Cancer of the anal canal. *Lancet Oncol.* 5 (3): 149–157.

Clemmensen, O.J. and Fenger, C. (1991). Melanocytes in the anal canal epithelium. *Histopathology* 18 (3): 237–241.

Daling, J.R., Madeleine, M.M., Johnson, L.G. et al. (2004). Human papillomavirus, smoking, and sexual practices in the etiology of anal cancer. *Cancer* 101 (2): 270–280.

Darragh, T.M., Colgan, T.J., Cox, J.T. et al. (2012). The lower anogenital squamous terminology standardization project for HPV-associated lesions: background and consensus recommendations from the College of American Pathologists and the American Society for Colposcopy and Cervical Pathology. *J. Low. Genit. Tract Dis.* 16 (3): 205–242.

Demitsu, T., Gonda, K., Tanita, M. et al. (1999). Extramammary Paget's disease in two siblings. *Br. J. Dermatol.* 141 (5): 951–953.

Devon, K.M., Brown, C.J., Burnstein, M., and McLeod, R.S. (2009). Cancer of the anus complicating perianal Crohn's disease. *Dis. Colon Rectum* 52 (2): 211–216.

Donaldson, D.R., Jass, J.R., and Mann, C.V. (1987). Anal leukoplakia. *Gut* 28: A1368.

Amin, M.B., Edge, S., Greene, F. et al. (2017). *AJCC Cancer Staging Manual*, 8e. New York: Springer.

Engstrom, P.F., Benson, A.B. 3rd, Chen, Y.J. et al. (2005). Anal canal cancer clinical practice guidelines in oncology. *J. Natl. Compr. Cancer Netw.* 3 (4): 510–515.

Fenger, C. and Morson, B.C. (1989). Anal duct carcinoma. *Dis. Colon Rectum* 32 (4): 355–357.

Galanis, I., Dragoumis, D., Tsolakis, M. et al. (2009). Obstructive ileus due to a giant fibroepithelial polyp of the anus. *World J. Gastroenterol.* 15 (29): 3687–3690.

Gholam, P., Enk, A., and Hartschuh, W. (2009). Successful surgical management of giant condyloma acuminatum (Buschke–Lowenstein tumor) in the genitoanal region: a case report and evaluation of current therapies. *Dermatology* 218 (1): 56–59.

Gormley, R.H. and Kovarik, C.L. (2012). Human papillomavirus-related genital disease in the immunocompromised host: part I. *J. Am. Acad. Dermatol.* 66 (6): 867.e1–867.e14; quiz 81-2.

Gormley, R.H. and Kovarik, C.L. (2012). Human papillomavirus-related genital disease in the immunocompromised host: part II. *J. Am. Acad. Dermatol.* 66 (6): 883.e1–883.e17. quiz 99-900.

Grodsky, L. (1960). Extramammary Paget's disease of the perianal region. *Dis. Colon Rectum* 3: 502–510.

Groisman, G.M. and Polak-Charcon, S. (1998). Fibroepithelial polyps of the anus: a histologic, immunohistochemical, and ultrastructural study, including comparison with the normal anal subepithelial layer. *Am. J. Surg. Pathol.* 22 (1): 70–76.

Helwig, E.B. and Graham, J.H. (1963). Anogenital (extramammary) Paget's disease. A clinicopathological study. *Cancer* 16: 387–403.

Hobbs, C.M., Lowry, M.A., Owen, D., and Sobin, L.H. (2001). Anal gland carcinoma. *Cancer* 92 (8): 2045–2049.

Hoots, B.E., Palefsky, J.M., Pimenta, J.M., and Smith, J.S. (2009). Human papillomavirus type distribution in anal cancer and anal intraepithelial lesions. *Int. J. Cancer* 124 (10): 2375–2383.

Iddings, D.M., Fleisig, A.J., Chen, S.L. et al. (2010). Practice patterns and outcomes for anorectal melanoma in the USA, reviewing three decades of treatment: is more extensive surgical resection beneficial in all patients? *Ann. Surg. Oncol.* 17 (1): 40–44.

Ioachim, H.L., Antonescu, C., Giancotti, F. et al. (1997). EBV-associated anorectal lymphomas in patients with acquired immune deficiency syndrome. *Am. J. Surg. Pathol.* 21 (9): 997–1006.

Jaworski, R.C., Biankin, S.A., and Baird, P.J. (2001). Squamous cell carcinoma in situ arising in inflammatory cloacogenic polyps: report of two cases with PCR analysis for HPV DNA. *Pathology* 33 (3): 312–314.

Kessler, K.J., Kerlakian, G.M., and Welling, R.E. (1996). Perineal and perirectal sarcomas: report of two cases. *Dis. Colon Rectum* 39 (4): 468–472.

Leonard, D., Beddy, D., and Dozois, E.J. (2011). Neoplasms of anal canal and perianal skin. *Clin. Colon Rectal Surg.* 24 (1): 54–63.

Lisovsky, M., Patel, K., Cymes, K. et al. (2007). Immunophenotypic characterization of anal gland carcinoma: loss of p63 and cytokeratin 5/6. *Arch. Pathol. Lab. Med.* 131 (8): 1304–1311.

Longacre, T.A., Kong, C.S., and Welton, M.L. (2008). Diagnostic problems in anal pathology. *Adv. Anat. Pathol.* 15 (5): 263–278.

Marchesa, P., Fazio, V.W., Oliart, S. et al. (1997). Long-term outcome of patients with perianal Paget's disease. *Ann. Surg. Oncol.* 4 (6): 475–480.

Mazoujian, G., Pinkus, G.S., and Haagensen, D.E. Jr. (1984). Extramammary Paget's disease – evidence for an apocrine origin. An immunoperoxidase study of gross cystic disease fluid protein-15, carcinoembryonic antigen, and keratin proteins. *Am. J. Surg. Pathol.* 8 (1): 43–50.

Meeker, J.H., Neubecker, R.D., and Helwig, E.B. (1962). Hidradenoma papilliferum. *Am. J. Clin. Pathol.* 37: 182–195.

Melbye, M., Cote, T.R., Kessler, L. et al. (1994). High incidence of anal cancer among AIDS patients. The AIDS/ Cancer Working Group. *Lancet* 343 (8898): 636–639.

Meriden, Z. and Montgomery, E.A. (2012). Anal duct carcinoma: a report of 5 cases. *Hum. Pathol.* 43 (2): 216–220.

Minicozzi, A., Borzellino, G., Momo, R. et al. (2010). Perianal Paget's disease: presentation of six cases and literature review. *Int. J. Color. Dis.* 25 (1): 1–7.

Murphy, R. (2010). Lichen sclerosus. *Dermatol. Clin.* 28 (4): 707–715.

Ni, S., Huang, D., Chen, X. et al. (2012). c-kit gene mutation and CD117 expression in human anorectal melanomas. *Hum. Pathol.* 43 (6): 801–807.

UK Co-ordinating Committee on Cancer Research (1996). Epidermoid anal cancer: results from the UKCCCR randomised trial of radiotherapy alone versus radiotherapy, 5-fluorouracil, and mitomycin. UKCCCR Anal Cancer Trial Working Party. UK Co-ordinating Committee on Cancer Research. *Lancet* 348 (9034): 1049–1054.

Nowak, M.A., Guerriere-Kovach, P., Pathan, A. et al. (1998). Perianal Paget's disease: distinguishing primary and secondary lesions using immunohistochemical studies including gross cystic disease fluid protein-15 and cytokeratin 20 expression. *Arch. Pathol. Lab. Med.* 122 (12): 1077–1081.

Ordonez, N.G., Awalt, H., and Mackay, B. (1987). Mammary and extramammary Paget's disease. An immunocytochemical and ultrastructural study. *Cancer* 59 (6): 1173–1183.

Owens, S.R. and Greenson, J.K. (2007). Immunohistochemical staining for p63 is useful in the diagnosis of anal squamous cell carcinomas. *Am. J. Surg. Pathol.* 31 (2): 285–290.

Papaconstantinou, H.T., Lee, A.J., Simmang, C.L. et al. (2005). Screening methods for high-grade dysplasia in patients with anal condyloma. *J. Surg. Res.* 127 (1): 8–13.

Parfitt, J.R. and Shepherd, N.A. (2008). Polypoid mucosal prolapse complicating low rectal adenomas: beware the inflammatory cloacogenic polyp! *Histopathology* 53 (1): 91–96.

Paterson, C.A., Young-Fadok, T.M., and Dozois, R.R. (1999). Basal cell carcinoma of the perianal region: 20-year experience. *Dis. Colon Rectum* 42 (9): 1200–1202.

Pelle, M.T., Parc, Y., and Mourra, N. (2009). C-kit expression in spindle cell melanoma – a diagnostic pitfall in anorectal biopsy. *Arch. Pathol. Lab. Med.* 133 (8): 1189–1191.

Penn, I. (1986). Cancers of the anogenital region in renal transplant recipients. Analysis of 65 cases. *Cancer* 58 (3): 611–616.

Pirog, E.C., Quint, K.D., and Yantiss, R.K. (2010). P16/ CDKN2A and Ki-67 enhance the detection of anal intraepithelial neoplasia and condyloma and correlate with human papillomavirus detection by polymerase chain reaction. *Am. J. Surg. Pathol.* 34 (10): 1449–1455.

Ramalingam, P., Middleton, L.P., Tamboli, P. et al. (2003). Invasive micropapillary carcinoma of the breast metastatic to the urinary bladder and endometrium: diagnostic pitfalls and review of the literature of tumors with micropapillary features. *Ann. Diagn. Pathol.* 7 (2): 112–119.

Regauer, S. (2006). Extramammary Paget's disease – a proliferation of adnexal origin? *Histopathology* 48 (6): 723–729.

Rock, B., Shah, K.V., and Farmer, E.R. (1992). A morphologic, pathologic, and virologic study of anogenital warts in men. *Arch. Dermatol.* 128 (4): 495–500.

Rudlinger, R. and Buchmann, P. (1989). HPV 16-positive bowenoid papulosis and squamous-cell carcinoma of the anus in an HIV-positive man. *Dis. Colon Rectum* 32 (12): 1042–1045.

Sakai, Y. and Matsukuma, S. (2002). CD34+ stromal cells and hyalinized vascular changes in the anal fibroepithelial polyps. *Histopathology* 41 (3): 230–235.

Schlecht, H.P., Fugelso, D.K., Murphy, R.K. et al. (2010). Frequency of occult high-grade squamous intraepithelial neoplasia and invasive cancer within anal condylomata in men who have sex with men. *Clin. Infect. Dis.* 51 (1): 107–110.

Shia, J. (2010). An update on tumors of the anal canal. *Arch. Pathol. Lab. Med.* 134 (11): 1601–1611.

Shia, J., Tang, L.H., Weiser, M.R. et al. (2008). Is nonsmall cell type high-grade neuroendocrine carcinoma of the tubular gastrointestinal tract a distinct disease entity? *Am. J. Surg. Pathol.* 32 (5): 719–731.

Tseng, H.F., Morgenstern, H., Mack, T.M., and Peters, R.K. (2003). Risk factors for anal cancer: results of a population-based case – control study. *Cancer Causes Control* 14 (9): 837–846.

Valenzuela, N., Barnadas, M.A., Matias-Guiu, X. et al. (2004). Lethal perianal Buschke–Lowenstein tumor in a female patient with AIDS. *Dermatology* 208 (4): 349–350.

Walts, A.E., Lechago, J., and Bose, S. (2006). P16 and Ki67 immunostaining is a useful adjunct in the assessment of biopsies for HPV-associated anal intraepithelial neoplasia. *Am. J. Surg. Pathol.* 30 (7): 795–801.

Welton, M.L., Lambert, R., and Bosman, F.T. (2010). Tumours of the anal canal. In: *WHO Classification of Tumors of the Digestive System*, 4e (eds. F.T. Bosman, F. Carneiro, R.H. Hruban and N.D. Theise), 183–193. Lyon: International Agency for Research on Cancer (IARF).

Welton, M.L., Lambert, R., and Bosman, F.T. (2010). Tumours of the anal canal. In: *WHO Classification of Tumors of the Digestive System*, 4e (eds. F.T. Bosman, F. Carneiro, R.H. Hruban and N.D. Theise), 183–193. Lyon: International Agency for Research on Cancer (IARF).

Welton, M.L., Lambert, R., and Bosman, F.T. (2010). Tumours of the anal canal. In: *WHO Classification of Tumors of the Digestive System*, 4e (eds. F.T. Bosman, F. Carneiro, R.H. Hruban and N.D. Theise), 183–193. Lyon: International Agency for Research on Cancer (IARF).

Welton, M.L., Lambert, R., and Bosman, F.T. (2010). Tumours of the anal canal. In: *WHO Classification of Tumors of the Digestive System*, 4e (eds. F.T. Bosman, F. Carneiro, R.H. Hruban and N.D. Theise), 183–193. Lyon: International Agency for Research on Cancer (IARF).

Welton, M.L., Sharkey, F.E., and Kahlenberg, M.S. (2004). The etiology and epidemiology of anal cancer. *Surg. Oncol. Clin. N. Am.* 13 (2): 263–275.

Welton, M.L., Sharkey, F.E., and Kahlenberg, M.S. (2004). The etiology and epidemiology of anal cancer. *Surg. Oncol. Clin. N. Am.* 13 (2): 263–275.

WHO Classification of Tumors Editorial Board. Digestive System Tumors. Lyon (France): International Agency for Research on Cancer; 2019 (WHO classification of tumors series; 5th ed.; vol 1).

Wong, A.K., Chan, R.C., Aggarwal, N. et al. (2010). Human papillomavirus genotypes in anal intraepithelial neoplasia and anal carcinoma as detected in tissue biopsies. *Mod. Pathol.* 23 (1): 144–150.

Wong, A.Y., Rahilly, M.A., Adams, W., and Lee, C.S. (1998). Mucinous anal gland carcinoma with perianal Pagetoid spread. *Pathology* 30 (1): 1–3.

Yeong, M.L., Wood, K.P., Scott, B., and Yun, K. (1992). Synchronous squamous and glandular neoplasia of the anal canal. *J. Clin. Pathol.* 45 (3): 261–263.

Index

Gastrointestinal Pathology: Correlative Endoscopic and Histologic Assessment, First Edition. Edited by Gregory Y. Lauwers and Michael B. Wallace.